A Comprehensive Review for the Certification and Recertification Examinations for PAs

A Comprehensive Review for the Certification and Recertification Examinations for PAs

Seventh Edition

Co-Editor

Claire Babcock O'Connell, DrPH, PA-C

Associate Professor
Physician Assistant Program
School of Health Professions
Rutgers Biomedical and Health Sciences
Piscataway, New Jersey

Co-Editor

Thea Cogan-Drew, DScPAS, PA-C

Lecturer
Physician Assistant Program
School of Health Professions
Rutgers Biomedical and Health Sciences
Piscataway, New Jersey

Published in Collaboration with AAPA and PAEA

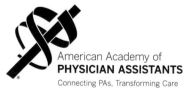

American Academy of
PHYSICIAN ASSISTANTS
Connecting PAs, Transforming Care

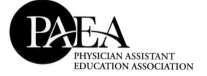

PHYSICIAN ASSISTANT
EDUCATION ASSOCIATION

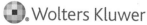 Wolters Kluwer

Philadelphia · Baltimore · New York · London
Buenos Aires · Hong Kong · Sydney · Tokyo

Acquisitions Editor: Matt Hauber
Development Editor: Andrea Vosburgh
Editorial Coordinator: Priyanka Alagar
Marketing Manager: Phyllis Hitner
Production Project Manager: Catherine Ott
Design Coordinator: Steve Druding
Manufacturing Coordinator: Margie Orzech
Prepress Vendor: S4Carlisle Publishing Services

Seventh Edition

10 9 8 7 6 5 4 3 2

Printed in Mexico

Library of Congress Cataloging-in-Publication Data
ISBN-13: 978-1-975158-20-0
Cataloging-in-Publication data available on request from the Publisher.

shop.lww.com

QUADM0423

In memory of my parents, Thomas G. Babcock, Jr. and Claire Smith Babcock, RN, MEd.
—*Claire Babcock O'Connell*

With loving thanks to my family: Daniel, Leo, and Thomas Cogan-Drew.
—*Thea Cogan-Drew*

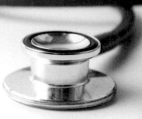

Acknowledgments

The assistance, support, and encouragement from excellent colleagues have guided the efforts needed to continue to produce this high-quality text and review book. We are indebted to the colleagues and administration at the Rutgers Department of Physician Assistant Studies and Practice. Their confidence in us provides encouragement and support in our growth as PAs and educators. We are also grateful to the contributing authors, item writers, and reviewers; the personnel at Wolters Kluwer; and the leadership of the Physician Assistant Education Association and American Academy of Physician Assistants. Finally, we wish to thank our family and friends (and our dogs) for their endless patience and constant support and love.

—*Claire Babcock O'Connell and*
Thea Cogan-Drew

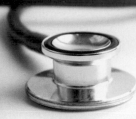

Preface

Taking certification and recertification examinations is a fact of life for practicing physician assistants (PAs). The certification examination is taken upon graduation from an accredited PA program, and the recertification examination is taken every 10 years thereafter. The National Commission on Certification of Physician Assistants (NCCPA), using test data from the National Board of Medical Examiners (NBME) as well as the experience and aptitude of test item writers, develops the two examinations and refines them on an annual basis to keep current with clinical practice and medical advances.

Traditionally, test preparation books have consisted of practice questions, answers, and explanations. This format provided the opportunity for both new and experienced PAs to improve their test-taking skills by becoming more accustomed to the test experience, and by reading the answers and explanations provided with each question, the candidate could learn from his or her successes and mistakes.

This edition continues to include content outline and review test items. Each chapter contains a set of test items and explanations to review major concepts contained in the chapter. All of these test items plus several hundred more are available online to simulate the computer format of the certification and recertification examinations. All test items have been written by experienced, NBME-trained PA educators and compiled using the proportions per subject area and skill areas as delineated in the NCCPA guidelines. Each test question is also written according to the NCCPA structure for multiple-choice format, an especially important feature of the last several editions. For further information and explanation of the NCCPA subject and skill areas, see http://www.nccpa.net.

In addition to the practice questions and answers, this book provides, in a condensed outline format, all the necessary information not only to take and successfully complete the tests but also to refer to in clinical practice. Each chapter has been completely reviewed and rewritten to reflect changes in clinical practice. In other words, this book is a practical, "real-time" educational tool for busy practitioners—a handy resource to be used on the front line of patient care.

The chapters are carefully formatted to give general characteristics of diseases (e.g., incidence, pathophysiology, prognosis), clinical signs and symptoms, diagnostic and laboratory evaluation, and treatment. These chapters, as well as the accompanying questions and their explanations, closely mirror the body of knowledge that is tested on the certification examinations and is needed for the reality of clinical practice. Regardless of their practice setting, PAs can use this book to review and test themselves on the material most likely to be included in their examination.

The American Academy of Physician Assistants (AAPA) and the Physician Assistant Education Association (PAEA) have continued their close collaboration in the development of this book. This partnership serves to enhance the value and credibility of the book and to ensure that it meets certification and continuing medical education needs of the PA constituency.

We believe that you will find this book helpful in preparing to take either of the NCCPA examinations. Equally important, however, we hope that you use this book as a quick and valuable reference in clinical practice. We encourage you to make the book a permanent addition to your library not only upon graduation and every 10 years thereafter but also on a daily basis for the most important use of all—providing quality care to your patients.

Contributors

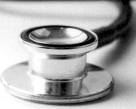

Frank Acevedo, MS, PA-C
Assistant Professor
New York Institute of Technology
Old Westbury, New York
Surgical Intensive Care Physician Assistant
Winthrop-University Hospital
Mineola, New York

Michael Cirone, MS, PA-C
Lead Physician Assistant
Skylands Urgent Care
Franklin, New Jersey

Thea Cogan-Drew, DScPAS, PA-C
Lecturer
Physician Assistant Program
School of Health Professions
Rutgers Biomedical and Health Sciences
Piscataway, New Jersey

Sheryl L. Geisler, MS, PA-C
Associate Professor
Physician Assistant Program
School of Health Professions
Rutgers Biomedical and Health Sciences
Piscataway, New Jersey

Frank R. Giannelli, PhD, PA-C
Lecturer
School of Health Professions
Rutgers Biomedical and Health Sciences
Piscataway, New Jersey

Jessica R. M. Gomes, MS, PA-C
Lecturer
School of Health Professions
Rutgers Biomedical and Health Sciences
Piscataway, New Jersey

Michael A. Johnson, DHSc, PA-C
Physician Assistant
Good Samaritan Clinic
Gulf Breeze, Florida

Jennifer Joseph, DHSc, PA-C
Assistant Professor
Physician Assistant Program
School of Health Professions
Rutgers Biomedical and Health Sciences
Piscataway, New Jersey

Kathy Kemle, MS, PA-C, DFAAPA
Assistant Professor
Department of Family Medicine
The Medical Center/Navicent Health
Macon, Georgia

Susan LeLacheur, DrPH, PA-C
Associate Professor
Department of Physician Assistant Studies
School of Medicine & Health Sciences
George Washington University
Washington, District of Columbia

Nkechi E. Mbadugha, MS, PA-C
Lecturer
Physician Assistant Program
School of Health Professions
Rutgers Biomedical and Health Sciences
Piscataway, New Jersey

Claire Babcock O'Connell, DrPH, MPH, PA-C
Associate Professor
Physician Assistant Program
School of Health Professions
Rutgers Biomedical and Health Sciences
Piscataway, New Jersey

Lori Parlin Palfreyman, DHSc, PA-C
Assistant Professor
Program Director Physician Assistant Program
School of Health Professions
Rutgers Biomedical and Health Sciences
Piscataway, New Jersey

Allan Platt, PA-C, MMSc, DFAAPA
Assistant Professor
Director of Admissions
Physician Assistant Program
Emory University School of Medicine
Atlanta, Georgia

Erich Vidal, MS, PA-C
Assistant Professor
Physician Assistant Program
School of Health Professions
Rutgers Biomedical and Health Sciences
Piscataway, New Jersey

Matthew Wright, MS, PA-C
Lecturer
Physician Assistant Program
School of Health Professions
Rutgers Biomedical and Health Sciences
Piscataway, New Jersey

Andrew M. Zolp, MSM, PA-C
Assistant Professor
Department of Physician Assistant
Western Michigan University
Kalamazoo, Michigan

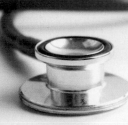

Reviewers

Raquel C. Barreto, MPAS, PA-C
Adjunct Faculty
School of Health Professions
Rutgers Biomedical and Health Sciences
Piscataway, New Jersey
Department of Surgery
Memorial Sloan Kettering Cancer Center
New York, New York

Mirela Bruza-Augatis, MS, PA-C
Assistant Professor
Physician Assistant Program
School of Health and Medical Science
Seton Hall University
Nutley, New Jersey

Alyssa Carbajal, MS, PA-C
Lecturer
Physician Assistant Program
School of Health Professions
Rutgers Biomedical and Health Sciences
Piscataway, New Jersey

Christine Fernandez, MD
Medical Director
Physician Assistant Program
School of Health and Medical Science
Seton Hall University
Nutley, New Jersey

Michelle McWeeney, PhD, PA-C
Assistant Professor
Physician Assistant Program
School of Health and Medical Science
Seton Hall University
Nutley, New Jersey

Abby Saunders, PhD, MS, PA-C
Assistant Professor
Physician Assistant Program
School of Health and Medical Science
Seton Hall University
Nutley, New Jersey

Dipali Yeh, MS, PA-C
Assistant Professor
Physician Assistant Program
School of Health Professions
Rutgers Biomedical and Health Sciences
Piscataway, New Jersey

Contents

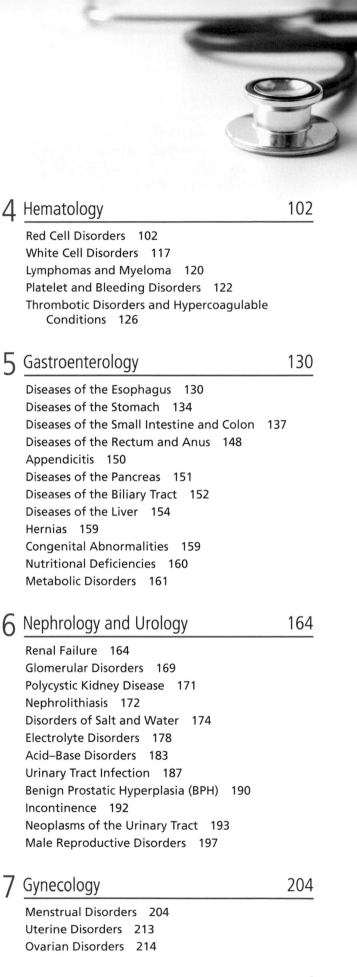

Ophthalmology and Otolaryngology | 1

Erich Vidal and Claire Babcock O'Connell

Disorders of the Eyes

A. Disorders of the globe

1. **Trauma**

   a. General characteristics

   (1) Traumatic disorders affecting the globe include blunt or penetrating trauma, foreign bodies, and chemical burns.

   (2) All management steps should be taken as soon as possible, especially with penetrating trauma and foreign bodies. Document when and how the accident, trauma, or burn occurred.

   (3) Consult an ophthalmologist for any sight-threatening injury (open globe injuries, protruding foreign body, or vitreous extrusion). Avoid further manipulation or topical medication.

   b. Physical examination

   (1) Observe: inspect, noticing any abnormalities; keep the head elevated to 45 degrees.

   (a) Orbit: for edema, hematoma, or ecchymosis

   (b) Lids: for laceration, hematoma, edema, or foreign bodies

   (c) Pupils: for irregularity, which may be benign or an indication of neurologic pathology; teardrop pupil indicates rupture of the globe with iris prolapse.

   (d) Extraocular muscles: for unequal, limited, or decreased movement, which may indicate laceration or entrapment of eye muscles

   (e) Anterior chamber: for hyphema, which indicates intraocular trauma

   (f) Interior of eye with funduscope: for ruptured retinal vessels, which may indicate physical abuse, such as shaken baby syndrome or retinal detachment

   (2) Palpate orbital rim: for irregularity, which may indicate a fracture. If rupture of the globe is suspected, do not palpate.

   c. Measurements

   (1) Visual acuity is tested using the Snellen chart. This is important to establish a baseline; any new or acute loss of vision indicates serious trauma.

   (2) Pupillary reactions should be checked. Unequal reactions might indicate severe trauma to the globe, head trauma, or nerve palsies.

   (3) Check for intraocular pressure (IOP). After appropriate topical anesthesia, carefully measure using the Schiötz tonometer.

   (4) The cornea is inspected for lesions or abrasions using fluorescein dye and a blue-light filter.

> Ophthalmic Danger Signs: open globe, protruding foreign body, vitreous extrusion.

d. Treatment

(1) Penetrating trauma

  (a) The object should not be removed. Do not apply pressure. Shield the eye but avoid manipulation.

  (b) The patient should be transported to the emergency department for consult with an ophthalmologist.

  (c) Pain can be alleviated with systemic analgesia or sedatives. Avoid eye drops. Parenteral antibiotics are recommended prophylactically.

(2) Foreign body

  (a) Patients will complain of pain, irritation, and a sensation of foreign body in the eye.

  (b) The eyelids should be carefully everted, stained with fluorescein, and observed with a blue light (Wood's lamp) (Fig. 1-1).

  (c) Gently attempt to remove the foreign body using a moistened, cotton-tipped swab. Embedded objects may need removal via blunt edge or needle tip after anesthetics are applied.

  (d) Patching may be beneficial if a large corneal abrasion occurs. Patching should be limited to 24 hours. Reexamine the next day.

  (e) A rust ring on the cornea indicates metallic foreign bodies. These may be removed with a rotating burr, or the patient may be referred to an ophthalmologist.

(3) Chemical burns (acid or alkali)

  (a) The eye should be irrigated with water or normal saline for at least 30 minutes. Use sterile solution if available. A chemical burn can continue to cause damage even after flushing.

  (b) An eye shield should be placed on the eye.

  (c) Because an acid or alkali burn is severe, transport the patient to the emergency department and refer to an ophthalmologist.

2. Blow-out fracture

a. General characteristics

  (1) The orbital floor is composed of maxillary, palatine, and zygomatic bones. These bones are very thin and fragile.

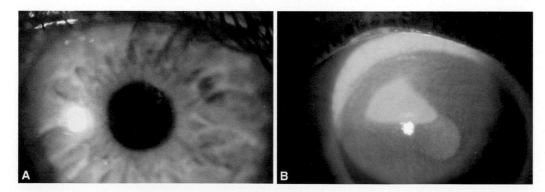

Figure 1-1 ▶ A: Remaining corneal epithelial defect (1 o'clock pupil edge) immediately post-foreign body removal. Trace fluorescein dye pooling is seen in the defect. **B:** A triangular corneal abrasion is evident superiorly with the cobalt blue light after fluorescein stain. There is some punctate epithelial staining surrounding the abrasion. (**A:** Reprinted with permission from Rosenfield M, Lee EM, Goodwin D. *Clinical Cases in Eye Care.* Wolters Kluwer; 2019, Fig. 33-2. **B:** Reprinted with permission from Rapuano CJ. *Wills Eye Hospital Color Atlas & Synopsis of Clinical Ophthalmology: Cornea.* 3rd ed. Wolters Kluwer; 2019, Fig. 11-4B.)

(2) Blunt trauma, such as that from a fist or a ball, causes the floor to fracture, trapping the orbital structures inferiorly.

b. Clinical features

(1) Patients present with swelling and misalignment of the eyes. Movement of the globe is restricted, specifically an inability to look up because of entrapment of the infraorbital nerve and the musculature.

(2) Double vision is common.

(3) Subcutaneous emphysema and exophthalmos are commonly present.

(4) Computed tomography (CT) scan is recommended to delineate extent of the damage.

c. Treatment

(1) Prompt referral to an ophthalmologist is essential.

(2) Patients should be kept calm and avoid sneezing or anything that would increase pressure.

(3) Nasal decongestants, ice packs or cold compresses, and antibiotics are started during transport.

> Fracture of orbital floor ("blowout") results in the inability to look up.

3. Corneal abrasion (corneal epithelial defect)

a. General characteristics: It is usually caused by minor trauma, such as that from a fingernail, contact lens, eyelash, or small foreign body.

b. Clinical features

(1) Pain and sensation of a foreign body can be accompanied by photophobia, tearing, injection, and blepharospasm.

(2) Record visual acuity before examining or treating. Patients may complain of blurred vision.

(3) A slit-lamp examination or fluorescein staining will reveal an epithelial defect but a clear cornea. A search for foreign bodies is required.

c. Treatment

(1) Topical anesthetic will provide immediate relief; however, it should be used only to assist in confirming the diagnosis and should not be prescribed because it may retard healing.

(2) Saline irrigation will loosen debris. Antibiotic ointment, such as gentamicin or sulfacetamide, should be applied. Acetaminophen is given for analgesia.

(3) Patching for no longer than 24 hours is recommended only for large abrasions (>5 to 10 mm) to promote healing. Patching for longer than 24 hours may retard healing and cause vision problems.

(4) Daily follow-up of all abrasions is essential. Failure to heal should prompt referral to an ophthalmologist.

> For corneal abrasion, treat with topical antibiotics and short-term patching *only* for large abrasions.

4. Corneal ulcer

a. General characteristics

(1) Corneal ulcers may result from inflammation or infection.

(2) Risk factors include trauma, contact lens use, or poor lid apposition.

b. Clinical features

(1) Patients will present with pain, photophobia, and tearing.

(2) Examination will reveal circumcorneal injection and watery to purulent discharge.

(3) Fluorescein staining will reveal a dense corneal infiltrate with overlying epithelial defect. A dendritic lesion indicates herpes keratitis.

c. Treatment

(1) All corneal ulcers should be referred to an ophthalmologist.

         (2) Lesions should be stained and cultured to identify cause and guide treatment options.

         (3) Avoid topical steroids because they will cause further tissue loss and increase risk of perforation.

         (4) Patching should be avoided.

    5. Retinal disorders

       a. Retinal detachment

         (1) General characteristics

           (a) The underlying pathogenesis is a separation of the retina from the pigmented epithelial layer, causing the detached tissue to appear as flapping in the vitreous humor.

> The most common retinal detachment involves the superior temporal segment.

           (b) The tear most commonly begins at the superior temporal retinal area.

           (c) The tear can happen spontaneously or be secondary to trauma; extreme myopia; or inflammatory changes in the vitreous, retina, or choroid.

         (2) Clinical features

           (a) The patient may report acute onset of painless blurred or blackened vision that occurs over several minutes to hours and progresses to complete or partial monocular blindness. Bilateral detachment occurs in 10% of cases.

           (b) It is classically described as a curtain being drawn over the eye from top to bottom.

           (c) The patient may sense floaters or flashing lights at the initiation of symptoms. IOP is normal or reduced.

           (d) There will be a relative afferent pupillary defect. Funduscopic examination may reveal the ridges (rugae) of the displaced retina flapping in the vitreous humor.

         (3) Treatment

           (a) An emergency consult with an ophthalmologist regarding possible laser surgery or cryosurgery is needed.

           (b) Patients with retinal detachment should remain supine, with the head turned to the side of the retinal detachment.

           (c) Prognosis is good: 80% will recover without recurrence, 15% will require retreatment, and 5% will never reattach.

       b. Macular degeneration

         (1) This disorder may be age related or secondary to the toxic effects of drugs such as chloroquine or phenothiazine. It is the leading cause of irreversible central visual loss.

> Prevalence of age-related macular degeneration (ARMD) increases after age 50 years.

         (2) Drusen deposits accumulate in Bruch membrane, leading to degenerative changes, loss of nutritional supply, and atrophy (dry macular degeneration), and, later in the disease, neovascular degeneration, which causes hemorrhage and fibrosis (wet macular degeneration).

         (3) ARMD usually has an insidious onset, and its chief clinical feature is gradual loss of central vision. Metamorphopsia is the phenomenon of wavy or distorted vision and can be measured with an Amsler grid. Visual loss deteriorates quickly with the onset of neovascular degeneration (wet ARMD).

         (4) Mottling, serous leaks, and hemorrhages may be seen on the retina. Scarring of the macula develops in end-stage disease.

         (5) There is no effective treatment. If detected early, laser therapy or intravitreal injections of vascular endothelial growth factor (VEGF) inhibitors may slow the progression of wet macular degeneration.

(6) Age-Related Eye Diseases Study (AREDS) compound is a combination of vitamin C, vitamin E, lutein, zeaxanthin, zinc, and copper; there is evidence of its role in slowing the progression of ARMD.

c. Retinal artery occlusion

   (1) General characteristics

   (a) Central retinal artery occlusion is considered to be an ophthalmic emergency; prognosis is poor, even with immediate treatment.

   (b) Common causes are emboli, thrombotic phenomenon, and vasculitides.

   (c) It must be differentiated from giant-cell arteritis (fever, headache, scalp tenderness, jaw claudication, visual loss).

> Retinal vascular occlusion causes a *painless* loss of vision.

   (2) Clinical features

   (a) Central retinal arterial occlusion is characterized by sudden, painless, and marked unilateral loss of vision.

   (b) Funduscopy reveals pallor of the retina, arteriolar narrowing, separation of arterial flow (box-carring), retinal edema, and perifoveal atrophy (cherry red spot). Ganglionic death leads to optic atrophy and a pale retina (blindness).

   (c) Peripheral arterial occlusions are less severe and cause focal visual loss.

   (3) Treatment

   (a) Emergency referral to an ophthalmologist is necessary. Recumbent position and gentle ocular massage may help reduce the extent of damage. Vessel dilation and paracentesis are attempted to save the eye.

   (b) Workup and management of atherosclerotic disease or arrhythmias are warranted to reduce the risk of recurrence.

d. Retinal vein occlusion

   (1) This usually occurs secondary to a thrombotic event. Risks include diabetes, hyperlipidemia, glaucoma, and hyperviscosity states (e.g., polycythemia, leukemia).

   (2) Patients present with sudden, unilateral, painless blurred vision or complete visual loss. Peripheral occlusion will be less severe in presentation.

   (3) Examination reveals an afferent pupillary defect, optic disc swelling, and a "blood and thunder" retina (dilated veins, hemorrhages, edema, and exudates).

   (4) Vision typically is resolved with time, at least partially. A workup for further thrombosis is warranted.

   (5) Neovascularization can be treated with intravitreal injection of VEGF inhibitors.

e. Retinopathy

   (1) Hypertensive retinopathy

   (a) States of acute or accelerated hypertension, such as preeclampsia/eclampsia, pheochromocytoma, or sudden discontinuation of antihypertensive medication, confer the greatest risk.

   (b) Signs include diffuse arteriolar narrowing, copper or silver wiring, and arteriovenous nicking (atherosclerosis).

   (c) The key to treatment and prevention is control of hypertension.

   (2) Diabetic retinopathy

   (a) This is the leading cause of blindness in adults in the United States. Patients with diabetes should have yearly dilated ophthalmoscopic examinations.

> Diabetes is the leading cause of blindness in the United States.

   (b) Nonproliferative: venous dilation, microaneurysms, retinal hemorrhages, retinal edema, hard exudates

   (c) Proliferative: neovascularization, vitreous hemorrhage

(3) Treatment includes optimized glucose control, regulation of blood pressure, laser photocoagulation, and vitrectomy. Severe disease is permanent.

6. **Cataract**

   a. General characteristics

   (1) A cataract is any opacity of the natural lens of the eye caused by progressive increase in the proportion of insoluble protein. It may involve a small part of the lens or the entire lens.

   (2) Cataracts may develop secondary to the natural aging process (senile cataract, most common type) or because of trauma, congenital causes, systemic disease (e.g., diabetes), or medication use (e.g., corticosteroids, statins).

   (3) Excess sun exposure predisposes to cataract development.

   b. **Clinical features**

   (1) A gradual diminution of vision is characteristic. Patients also may complain of double vision, excess glare, fixed spots, or reduced color perception. The insidious onset of decreased vision is the main clinical feature; it is typically bilateral, although often asymmetrical.

   (2) On examination, there is a translucent, yellow discoloration in the lens. On funduscopic examination, the cataract appears dark against a red background. Once mature, the retina is no longer visible.

   c. **Treatment**

   (1) Treatment is warranted to improve activities of daily living, prevent secondary glaucoma, and permit visualization of the fundus.

   (2) Treatment involves intracapsular or extracapsular extractions of the cataract with lens replacement.

   (3) Prognosis is excellent; postoperative bleeding occurs in less than 0.1%.

> In cataracts, patients present with painless gradual loss of vision; surgical lens replacement offers an excellent prognosis.

7. **Glaucoma**

   a. General characteristics

   (1) This condition is defined as increased IOP with optic nerve damage. Any impediment to the flow of aqueous humor through the trabecular meshwork and canal of Schlemm will increase pressure in the anterior chamber which exerts pressure onto the back of the eye.

   (2) Glaucoma may be acute (angle-closure glaucoma) or chronic (open-angle glaucoma).

   (3) Open-angle glaucoma is more common. It generally affects people older than 40 years and is more common in African Americans and patients with a family history of glaucoma or diabetes.

   b. **Clinical features**

   (1) Angle-closure glaucoma is an ophthalmic emergency resulting from complete closure of the angle and thus complete destruction of the aqueous humor.

   (a) Painful eye and loss of vision are important clinical features.

   (b) Nausea, vomiting, and diaphoresis are common.

   (c) Physical examination reveals circumlimbal injection, steamy cornea, fixed mid-dilated pupil, decreased visual acuity, and tearing.

   (d) The anterior chamber is narrowed; IOP is acutely elevated.

   (2) Open-angle glaucoma

   (a) This is a chronic, asymptomatic, and potentially blinding disease that affects 2% of the population.

   (b) It manifests as increased IOP, defects in the peripheral visual field, and increased cup-to-disc ratios.

    (c) Patients are typically asymptomatic until late in disease. Loss of peripheral vision is the main symptom.

    (d) Elevated IOP without optic disc damage is known as ocular hypertension. Close monitoring is warranted.

    (e) Optic nerve damage without increased IOP is also seen. Subsequent monitoring typically reveals increasing IOP.

c. Treatment

  (1) Angle-closure glaucoma

    (a) These patients must be referred immediately to an ophthalmologist. Start intravenous (IV) carbonic anhydrase inhibitor (i.e., acetazolamide), topical β-blocker, and an osmotic diuretic (i.e., mannitol).

    (b) Mydriatics should not be administered to these patients.

    (c) Optimal treatment is via laser or surgical iridotomy.

  (2) Open-angle glaucoma

    (a) Patients should be referred to an ophthalmologist for close monitoring and chronic treatment.

    (b) Treatment consists of topical and/or systemic medications to decrease the IOP by decreasing aqueous production (β-blockers, carbonic anhydrase inhibitors) and/or increasing outflow (prostaglandin-like medications, cholinergic agents, epinephrine components). α-Agonists (brimonidine) provide both mechanisms.

> Angle-closure glaucoma is painful; open-angle glaucoma is often asymptomatic.

8. Orbital cellulitis

a. General characteristics

  (1) Orbital cellulitis is more common in children than in adults. Median age is 7 to 12 years.

  (2) Orbital cellulitis is primarily associated with sinusitis. Other underlying causes include dental infections, facial infections, infection of the globe or eyelids, and infections of the lacrimal system. Less often, it results from trauma.

  (3) Common causative agents include *Streptococcus pneumoniae*, *Staphylococcus aureus*, *Haemophilus influenzae*, and Gram-negative bacteria. An increase in methicillin-resistant *S. aureus* (MRSA) has been noted.

b. Clinical features

  (1) Orbital cellulitis presents with ptosis, eyelid edema, exophthalmos, purulent discharge, and conjunctivitis.

  (2) Examination will reveal fever, restricted range of motion in the eye muscles, edema and erythema of the lids and surrounding skin, and a sluggish pupillary response.

> When considering or differentiating orbital cellulitis, consider the surrounding edema and erythema, sluggish pupils, restriction in extraocular eye movements, and the systemic symptom of fever.

c. Diagnostic studies

  (1) Cellulitis is a systemic disorder. Workup includes complete blood count (CBC), blood cultures, and cultures of any drainage. White blood cell (WBC) count will be elevated.

  (2) CT is recommended to determine the extent of disease. CT will show broad infiltration of the orbital soft tissue.

d. Treatment

  (1) Orbital cellulitis constitutes a medical emergency requiring hospitalization, IV antibiotics, and surgical drainage if recalcitrant or recurrent. Inadequate treatment can lead to meningeal or cerebral infection.

  (2) Antibiotics should be broad spectrum until the causative agent is identified. Continue IV administration until fever subsides, then complete 2 to 3 weeks of oral antibiotics.

(3) Recommended regimens include nafcillin and metronidazole or clindamycin; second- or third-generation cephalosporin; and fluoroquinolones. If MRSA is suspected, treat with vancomycin.

B. Disorders of the adnexa

    1. Disorders of the lacrimal system

> Obstructed lacrimal duct in infants typically resolves by 9 months of age.

        a. Dacryostenosis is common in the newborn and occurs when the duct does not open.

            (1) The obstruction usually resolves by 9 months of age.

            (2) Treatment includes warm compresses and massage; if no resolution, surgical probe is indicated.

        b. Dacryocystitis is an inflammation of the lacrimal sac caused by obstruction. Common pathogens include *S. aureus*, β-hemolytic streptococci, *Staphylococcus epidermidis*, and, rarely, *Candida* sp.

            (1) Pain, swelling, tenderness, redness, and tearing and/or purulent discharge are characteristic.

            (2) Treatment consists of warm compresses and systemic antibiotics.

            (3) If an abscess forms, incision and drainage (I&D) may be required. Surgical interventions may help if the condition is recalcitrant (dacryocystorhinostomy or dacryocystectomy).

    2. Eyelids

        a. **Blepharitis** is chronic inflammation of the lid margins.

            (1) Causes include seborrhea, staphylococcal or streptococcal infection, and dysfunction of the meibomian glands.

            (2) Anterior blepharitis involves the eyelid skin, eyelashes, and associated glands. It may be ulcerative (*S. aureus*) or seborrheic.

            (3) Posterior blepharitis is inflammation of the meibomian glands. It may be infectious (*S. aureus*) or caused by glandular dysfunction.

            (4) **Clinical features**

                (a) Anterior blepharitis presents with red rims, scales, and adherent eyelashes.

                (b) Posterior blepharitis presents with hyperemic lid margins and telangiectasias with prominent meibomian gland opening.

                (c) Dandruff-like deposits (scurf) and fibrous scales (collarettes) may be seen.

                (d) The conjunctiva is clear or slightly erythematous.

                (e) Thick, cloudy discharge will be visible if the meibomian glands are obstructed.

                (f) Complications include recurrent disease, hordeola, chalazia, trichiasis, entropion, and corneal disease.

> Thorough lid hygiene and avoidance of makeup are key to clearing blepharitis.

            (5) **Treatment**

                (a) Lid scrubs using warm compresses and diluted baby shampoo on cotton-tipped swabs are helpful. Massage to express meibomian glands.

                (b) Topical antibiotics can be used if infection is suspected. Systemic antibiotics are reserved for recalcitrant cases.

        b. **Hordeolum (sty)**

            (1) General characteristics

                (a) A hordeolum is an acute development of a small, mildly painful nodule or pustule within a gland in the upper or lower eyelid.

                (b) Types

                    i. Internal hordeola are caused by the inflammation and infection of a meibomian gland, with pustular formation in that gland. They are situated deep from the palpebral margin.

ii. External hordeola are caused by the inflammation and infection of the glands of Moll or Zeis, with pustular formation in those glands. They are situated immediately adjacent to the edge of the palpebral margin.

(c) Causal pathogen is typically *S. aureus*.

(d) Hordeolum is not contagious.

(2) Clinical features

(a) Hordeolum is characterized by acute onset of pain and edema of the involved eyelid.

(b) There is a palpable, indurated area in the involved eyelid, which has a central area of purulence with surrounding erythema.

(3) Treatment

(a) Warm compresses should be applied several times per day for 48 hours.

(b) Topical antibiotics can be used if secondary infection develops.

(c) I&D may be indicated if it does not resolve within 48 hours.

> The majority of hordeola and chalazia resolve with local treatment only, warm compresses.

c. **Chalazion**

(1) General characteristics

(a) This is a relatively painless, indurated granulomatous lesion deep from the palpebral margin.

(b) It is often secondary to a chronic inflammation of an internal hordeolum of the meibomian gland.

(2) Clinical features

(a) The chalazion is characterized by insidious onset with minimal irritation. The lesion may appear white to grayish.

(b) It can become pruritic and cause erythema of the involved lid and adjacent conjunctiva.

(3) Treatment involves warm compresses and, if no resolution, a referral to an ophthalmologist for an elective excision or steroid injection.

d. **Entropion and ectropion**

(1) Entropion: The lid and lashes are turned in secondary to scar tissue or a spasm of the orbicularis oculi muscles.

(2) Ectropion: The edge of the eyelid everts secondary to advanced age, trauma, infection, or palsy of the facial nerve.

(3) Treatment involves surgical repair if the condition causes trauma (trichiasis), excessive tearing, exposure keratitis, or cosmetic distress.

> Trichiasis is corneal irritation secondary to inverted lashes.

C. Disorders of the conjunctiva

1. **Viral conjunctivitis**

a. General characteristics

(1) Viral infection in the conjunctiva usually is caused by adenovirus type 3, 8, or 19.

(2) Viral conjunctivitis is highly contagious. Transmission is by direct contact, usually via the fingers, with the contralateral eye or with other persons.

(3) Viral conjunctivitis can be transmitted in swimming pools (epidemic keratoconjunctivitis), and it is most common in midsummer to early fall.

b. **Clinical features**: Viral conjunctivitis is characterized by the acute onset of unilateral or bilateral erythema of the conjunctiva, copious watery discharge, and ipsilateral tender preauricular lymphadenopathy.

c. **Treatment**

(1) Therapy includes eye lavage with normal saline twice a day for 7 to 14 days; vasoconstrictor–antihistamine drops also may have beneficial effects.

> In bacterial cases of conjunctivitis, discharge is usually purulent; in viral cases, preauricular lymphadenopathy is common.

(2) Warm to cool compresses reduce discomfort.

(3) Ophthalmic sulfonamide drops may prevent secondary bacterial infection in patients at increased risk but are not routinely required.

2. **Bacterial conjunctivitis**

  a. General characteristics: Bacterial infection in the conjunctiva may occur with common or rare pathogens.

    (1) Common pathogens include *S. pneumoniae*, *S. aureus*, *H. aegyptius*, and *Moraxella* sp.

      (a) Transmission is via direct contact or fomites. Autoinoculation, from one eye to the other, usually via the fingers, is typical.

      (b) The natural history of an infection caused by these common pathogens usually is self-limiting, but a secondary keratitis can develop.

    (2) Rare pathogens include *Chlamydia trachomatis* and *Neisseria gonorrhoeae*.

      (a) Transmission is by direct contact or fomites, including nonchlorinated swimming sources. It also can be transmitted via sexual contact or to a neonate via vaginal delivery.

      (b) The natural history of an infection caused by these rare pathogens is severe conjunctivitis and keratitis with development of permanent visual impairment.

  b. **Clinical features**

    (1) Bacterial conjunctivitis is characterized by the acute onset of purulent discharge from both eyes.

    (2) Patients may have a mild decrease in visual acuity and mild discomfort. The eyes may be "glued" shut on awakening.

    (3) *Neisseria* causes copious purulent discharge. It is commonly unilateral.

    (4) *Chlamydia* causes a mucopurulent discharge with a marked follicular response on the inner lids. Nontender preauricular adenopathy is common.

  c. Diagnostic studies

    (1) Common pathogens: Gram stain should show the presence of polymorphonuclear cells (PMNs) and a predominant organism although this is not routinely done.

    (2) If rare pathogens are suspected, Gram stain and Giemsa stain should be done. PMNs will predominate.

      (a) *C. trachomatis*: No organisms will be seen.

      (b) *N. gonorrhoeae*: Intracellular Gram-negative diplococci will be present.

> In Neisseria conjunctivitis, discharge is copious and usually remains unilateral.

  d. **Treatment**

    (1) Attention to hygiene, including handwashing and avoidance of contamination, should be stressed.

    (2) Specific therapy includes application of topical antibiotics. Sulfonamides, fluoroquinolones, and aminoglycosides are commonly prescribed. Drops are more effective than ointment.

    (3) For the rare pathogens, treatment also may require concurrent systemic antibiotics.

3. **Pinguecula**

  a. General characteristics: It may be the result of chronic actinic exposure, repeated trauma, or dry and windy conditions.

  b. **Clinical features**

    (1) Elevated, yellowish, fleshy conjunctival mass found on the sclera adjacent to the cornea, typically on the nasal side

(2) Painless inflammation may occur (pingueculitis).

c. Treatment

(1) No treatment is necessary.

(2) If it is cosmetically undesirable or chronically inflamed, it can be resected.

4. Pterygium

a. General characteristics

(1) Slowly growing thickening of the bulbar conjunctiva

(2) It can be unilateral or bilateral.

b. Clinical features

(1) A highly vascular, triangular mass grows from the nasal side toward the cornea.

(2) It eventually encroaches on the cornea and interferes with vision.

c. Treatment

(1) Excision is warranted if it interferes with vision.

(2) Recurrence is common and may be more aggressive.

> Pinguecula are of cosmetic concern only; Pterygia should be excised when the lesion overlies the cornea.

D. Optic nerve and visual pathways

1. Papilledema

a. This condition is defined as an increase in intracranial pressure.

b. Causes are numerous but may include malignant hypertension, hemorrhagic strokes, acute subdural hematoma, and pseudotumor cerebri.

c. The disc appears swollen, and the margins are blurred, with an obliteration of the vessels.

d. The patient may be asymptomatic or may complain of transient visual alterations that last for seconds.

e. Treatment consists of therapy for the underlying cause.

2. Blurred vision and decreased visual acuity

a. The location of the lesion determines the effect on vision (Fig. 1-2).

(1) Lesions anterior to the optic chiasm will affect only one eye.

(2) Lesions at the optic chiasm will affect both eyes partially.

(3) Lesions posterior to the chiasm will yield corresponding defects in both visual fields.

b. The quality of visual loss helps to determine the diagnosis.

(1) Transient visual loss may be secondary to a transient ischemic attack (TIA), an embolus (amaurosis fugax), or a giant-cell (temporal) arteritis.

(a) Giant-cell arteritis is characterized by a tender temporal artery, fever, malaise, and a strikingly increased erythrocyte sedimentation rate (ESR).

(b) Prompt treatment with systemic corticosteroids is necessary to prevent permanent blindness.

(2) Sudden visual loss may be secondary to central retinal vein or branch vein occlusion, optic neuropathy, papillitis, and retrobulbar neuritis.

(3) Gradual visual loss may be secondary to macular degeneration, tumors, cataracts, or glaucoma.

3. Strabismus

a. Strabismus is a condition in which binocular fixation is not present.

b. Strabismus may occur in one eye or both. A corneal light reflex test will reveal misalignment (manifest or heterotropia strabismus). A cover–uncover test may reveal latent (heterophoria) strabismus, which may not be readily apparent otherwise.

c. Inward misalignment is termed *esotropia*; outward misalignment is termed *exotropia*.

> The most common cause of amblyopia is strabismus.

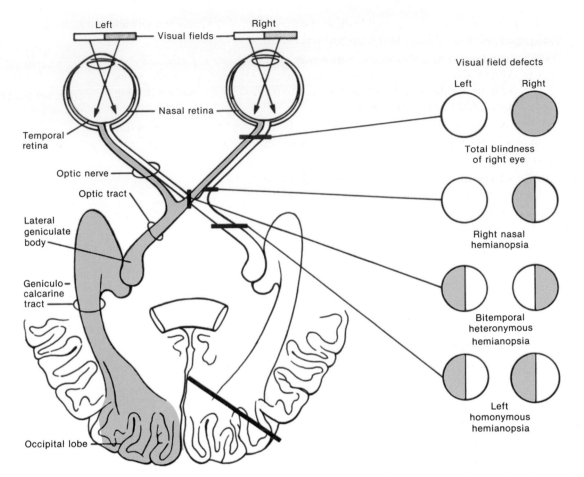

Figure 1-2 ▶ Optic pathways. (Reprinted with permission from Harwood-Nuss A, Wolfson AB, Linden CH, et al. *The Clinical Practice of Emergency Medicine.* 3rd ed. Lippincott Williams & Wilkins; 2001, Fig. 9.2.)

    d. Strabismus may be corrected with eye exercises (patch therapy) or, in severe cases, with surgery. If left untreated after the age of 2 years, amblyopia will result.

  4. Amblyopia

    a. Amblyopia is reduced visual acuity not correctable by refractive means.

    b. It may be caused by strabismus (most commonly); uremia; or toxins such as alcohol, tobacco, lead, and other toxic substances.

  5. Icterus or jaundice, which is a yellowing of the sclera, is caused by the retention of bilirubin.

  6. Blue or cyanotic sclera may be normal in newborns; persistence is seen in infants with osteogenesis imperfecta.

Disorders of the Ears

A. Hearing loss

  1. General characteristics

    a. The etiology may be conductive or sensorineural.

    b. The most common causes of hearing impairment/loss are cerumen impaction, eustachian tube dysfunction (secondary to upper respiratory tract infection [URI]), and increasing age (presbycusis).

    c. Using a 512-Hz tuning fork, the Weber test (tuning fork held to middle of forehead) and the Rinne test (tuning fork held to mastoid process until cessation of sound, then moved to near external auditory meatus [EAM]) can help with distinguishing between conductive and sensorineural hearing loss (Fig. 1-3).

> **(1)** With conductive loss, the Weber test results in lateralization to the affected ear. With mild or greater conductive hearing loss, the Rinne test may also show greater bone conduction (tuning fork on mastoid) than air conduction (tuning fork near EAM) on the affected side.

> **(2)** With sensorineural loss, the Weber test results in lateralization to the better or unaffected side. The Rinne test will show greater air conduction than bone conduction.

d. Patients with hearing loss should have audiologic testing unless there is an obvious treatable cause (e.g., cerumen buildup or an ear infection).

2. Conductive hearing loss is caused by impaired sound transmission to the inner ear. There are several common causes:

a. Blockage/obstruction caused by cerumen impaction or exudate from otitis externa

b. Cerumen can be mechanically removed (ear curette/loop). Other methods include detergent drops, suction, and irrigation.

c. Otitis media with effusion

d. Otosclerosis (abnormal bony growth of the middle ear)

e. Ossicular chain disruption (e.g., ear trauma/injury, infection)

3. Sensorineural hearing loss occurs with damage/impairment of the inner ear (cochlea) or neural pathways.

a. **Presbycusis**

> **(1)** Presbycusis is the most common etiology of sensorineural hearing loss.

> **(2)** It is a gradual impairment typically of higher sound frequencies that occurs with increasing age.

> The most common causes of hearing loss are correctable: cerumen impaction and eustachian tube dysfunction.

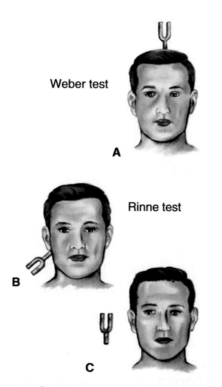

Weber test

A

Rinne test

B

C

Figure 1-3 ▶ A–C: Weber/Rinne hearing test. (Reprinted with permission from Hickey JV. *The Clinical Practice of Neurological and Neurosurgical Nursing.* 8th ed. Wolters Kluwer; 2020, Fig. 6.11.)

b. Ménière disease

(1) General characteristics

(a) Also known as endolymphatic hydrops, Ménière disease has an unknown etiology.

(b) Symptoms appear to be related to distension of the inner ear's endolymphatic compartment.

(2) Clinical features

(a) The typical syndrome involves recurrent vertigo (episodes lasting minutes to hours), with lower range hearing loss, tinnitus, and one-sided aural pressure.

(b) With caloric testing, nystagmus is lost on the impaired side.

(3) Treatment

(a) Initial treatment consists of a low-sodium diet and diuretics (i.e., acetazolamide).

(b) Meclizine or diazepam can help with acute symptoms.

(c) Unresponsive cases may be treated with more invasive procedures (i.e., intratympanic corticosteroid therapy, surgery).

> Patients with Meniere's disease will complain of low range hearing loss along with tinnitus, aural pressure, and episodic vertigo.

c. Acoustic trauma

(1) It is another common cause of sensory hearing loss.

(2) Sounds at 85 dB or louder can cause cochlear damage. There is an increased risk with chronic exposure.

d. Acoustic neuroma (vestibular schwannoma)

(1) This is an intracranial benign tumor affecting the eighth cranial nerve.

(2) It is usually unilateral and may present with progressive one-sided hearing loss with impaired speech discrimination. The hearing loss may also present more acutely. Other symptoms include tinnitus and vertigo, which is usually continuous rather than episodic.

(3) Diagnosis is by magnetic resonance imaging (MRI).

(4) Treatment takes into account patient age, health status, and tumor size and can involve surgery or focused radiation.

4. Drug-induced hearing loss

a. Some common examples of ototoxic agents include aminoglycosides, loop diuretics, and platinum-based anticancer drugs (e.g., cisplatin).

b. Permanent damage can occur despite correct dosing.

c. Monitoring of hearing acuity and drug levels can help reduce the risk.

5. Infancy and childhood hearing loss

a. Congenital causes include hereditary factors, anoxia, erythroblastosis, and intrauterine infections (e.g., rubella).

b. Acquired causes include otitis media, measles, mumps, meningitis, influenza, and head injury.

> The most common cause of congenital hearing loss is maternal rubella infection.

c. Clinical features include inattentiveness to human voices or lack of reaction to noise.

d. Treatment involves correction of underlying causes.

B. Acute otitis media (AOM)

1. General characteristics

a. The typical scenario involves a viral URI that leads to eustachian tube dysfunction or blockage. A bacterial infection occurs with the subsequent buildup of fluid and mucus. Less common causes include anatomic deformities or chronic edema.

b. It is most common in infants and children, but any age group can be affected. The most common offending agents are *S. pneumoniae*, *H. influenzae*, *Moraxella catarrhalis*, and *S. pyogenes*.

> The common symptoms and findings for AOM are ear pain, fever, hearing impairment, with an erythematous or bulging tympanic membrane.

2. Clinical features

  a. Symptoms can include fever, ear pain (otalgia), ear pressure, and hearing impairment.

  b. Otoscopic examination may reveal tympanic membrane erythema and limited mobility with pneumotoscopy.

  c. Bulging and eventual rupture of the tympanic membrane may occur with significant empyema, leading to otorrhea and abruptly decreased pain.

3. Treatment

  a. Watchful waiting may be adequate for older children without severe pain or fever, but adults are typically treated.

  b. First line antibiotic therapy is amoxicillin. In resistant cases, amoxicillin–clavulanate, cefuroxime, or cefpodoxime may be helpful. Other options with known significant penicillin allergy include doxycycline, azithromycin, or clarithromycin.

  c. With recalcitrant or recurring cases, more invasive procedures such as tympanostomy, tympanocentesis, and myringotomy (with severe pain/complications) can be considered.

  d. Recurrent cases may also be treated with prophylactic antibiotics (e.g., daily sulfamethoxazole or amoxicillin) for several months.

  e. Mastoiditis can occur with inadequate treatment of otitis media. Signs and symptoms are spiking fever and postauricular pain, erythema, and fluctuant painful mass. CT can help with diagnosis (i.e., mastoid air cell coalescence). Treatment is initially IV antibiotics (e.g., cefazolin) and myringotomy (for culture as well as drainage) followed by a full course of oral antibiotics. If such measures are ineffective, surgery (mastoidectomy) is indicated.

> Untreated otitis media may progress to mastoiditis— fever, pain, and fluctuant painful mass.

C. Chronic otitis media

  1. General characteristics

    a. It can occur from repeated episodes of AOM or trauma (persistent tympanic membrane perforation).

    b. Compared with AOM, different causative organisms are involved (e.g., *Pseudomonas aeruginosa*, *S. aureus*, *Proteus*, anaerobes).

  2. Clinical features

    a. The main findings are a perforated tympanic membrane and chronic ear discharge with or without pain.

    b. Tympanic membrane and/or ossicular damage can result in conductive hearing loss.

  3. Treatment

    a. Medical treatment is usually successful and includes ear hygiene, avoidance of aural water exposure, and topical antibiotic drops (e.g., ofloxacin, ciprofloxacin with dexamethasone). Systemic antibiotics may be used for targeted penetration to the affected area.

    b. Definitive treatment may include surgery (tympanic membrane repair/reconstruction) but only if medical therapy fails.

D. Otitis externa

  1. General characteristics

    a. Also known as "swimmer's ear," otitis externa is commonly associated with water exposure, trauma (i.e., ear scratching/cleaning), or exfoliative skin conditions (e.g., psoriasis, eczema).

    b. Etiology most commonly includes *P. aeruginosa*, *S. epidermidis,* and *S. aureus.*

2. Clinical features

a. Patients complain of ear pain (especially with movement of the tragus/auricle).

b. Signs include redness and swelling of the ear canal. Purulent exudate is also common.

3. Treatment

a. Treatment involves topical antibiotic otic drops (aminoglycoside or fluoroquinolone ± corticosteroids) and avoiding further moisture or ear injury.

b. In diabetic or immunocompromised patients, malignant otitis externa may develop, which is a necrotizing infection extending to the blood vessels, bone, and cartilage; this may require parenteral antibiotics transitioning to oral with clinical improvement.

E.   Vertigo (Table 1-1)

1. General characteristics

a. Vertigo is the sensation of movement (spinning, tumbling, or falling) in the absence of any actual movement or an overresponse to movement.

b. Peripheral causes of vestibular dysfunction include labyrinthitis, benign paroxysmal positioning vertigo (BPPV), endolymphatic hydrops (Ménière syndrome), vestibular neuronitis, and head injury.

c. Central causes of vertigo include brainstem vascular disease, arteriovenous malformations, tumors, multiple sclerosis, and vertebrobasilar migraine.

2. Clinical features

a. Duration and presence of hearing loss/nystagmus can help with diagnosis.

b. Peripheral vertigo is associated with sudden onset, nausea/vomiting, tinnitus, hearing loss, and nystagmus (typically horizontal with a rotatory component).

Table 1-1 | Differentiation Among Common Causes of Vertigo

Condition	Onset/Characteristic	Associated Neurologic Symptoms	Auditory Symptoms	Other Notes
BPPV	Recurrent, brief (seconds); associated with head movement	None	None	Dix–Hallpike test will induce symptoms
Labyrinthitis	Acute, severe, lasts several days to a week	None	Hearing loss	
Vestibular neuritis	Single episode, acute onset, lasts days; may be associated with viral illness	Falls toward the side of lesion	Usually none	Head thrust test usually abnormal
Ménière disease	Recurrent episodes, lasts minutes to several hours	None	Ear fullness or pain, unilateral hearing loss, tinnitus	Audiometry reveals unilateral low-frequency sensorineural hearing loss
Vestibular migraine	Recurrent episodes, lasting several minutes to hours	Migraine headache and/or other migrainous symptoms	Usually none	History of migraine headache
Vertebrobasilar TIA	Single or recurrent episodes lasting several minutes to hours	Usually other brainstem symptoms	Usually none	Typically, older patient with vascular risk factors
Brainstem infarction	Sudden onset, persists over days to weeks	Usually other brainstem symptoms, especially lateral medullary signs	Usually none unless anterior inferior cerebellar syndrome	Typically, older patient with vascular risk factors; MRI is indicated
Cerebellar infarction or hemorrhage	Sudden onset, persists over days to weeks	Gait impairment; headache; limb dysmetria	None	CT and/or MRI required to demonstrate lesion

MRI, magnetic resonance imaging; CT, computed tomography; TIA, transient ischemic attack; BPPV, benign paroxysmal positional vertigo.

   c. Central vertigo is associated with a more gradual onset and vertical nystagmus. Unlike peripheral vertigo, it does not present with auditory symptoms. Central vertigo is commonly associated with motor, sensory, or cerebellar deficits.

3. Diagnostic studies

   a. With BPPV, the Dix–Hallpike maneuver (i.e., quickly turning the patient's head 90 degrees while the patient is in the supine position) will produce a delayed fatigable nystagmus. If the nystagmus is nonfatigable, a central cause for the vertigo is more likely.

   b. Other testing, such as audiometry, caloric stimulation, electronystagmography (ENG), MRI, and evoked potentials, is indicated with persistent vertigo or with suspected central nervous system (CNS) involvement.

4. Treatment

   a. Therapy is based on the underlying etiology.

   b. Vestibular suppressants (e.g., diazepam, meclizine) may help with acute symptoms.

   c. BPPV may respond to physical therapy maneuvers (Epley maneuver).

   d. Some cases may require interventional/surgical therapies (e.g., to restore blood flow in brainstem vascular disease or surgical excision of tumors).

> BPPV is differentiated from other causes of vertigo by its lack of neurologic symptoms or hearing loss.

F. Labyrinthitis

1. General

   a. This is an inflammatory disorder of the inner ear that may manifest unilaterally or bilaterally.

   b. It is often secondary to local or systemic bacterial infection or an autoimmune disorder.

2. Clinical features

   a. It typically presents as an acute continuous severe vertigo, with hearing loss and vertigo of several days to a week.

   b. Patients may also experience tinnitus, nausea/vomiting, aural fullness or pain, or gait instability.

   c. The vertigo progressively improves over a few weeks, but the hearing loss may or may not resolve. Etiology is unknown.

3. Treatment

   a. Antimicrobials are indicated with associated fever or signs of bacterial infection.

   b. Vestibular suppressants (e.g., meclizine, diazepam) are helpful during the initial acute symptoms.

   c. Glucocorticoids in tapering doses have been shown effective if started early in the course of the illness.

   d. Symptomatic treatment may include antiemetics, antihistamines, or anticholinergics.

G. Barotrauma

1. General characteristics

   a. Barotrauma is the inability to equalize barometric pressure on the middle ear and is associated with eustachian tube dysfunction (from congenital narrowing or acquired mucosal edema).

   b. It can occur with flying (especially descent), rapid altitude changes, or diving underwater.

   c. Such pressure differences can cause rupture of the tympanic membrane.

2. Clinical features: Barotrauma presents with ear pain and hearing loss that persists past the inciting event.

3. Treatment

   a. Patient measures, such as swallowing, yawning, and autoinflation (with descent), as well as the use of systemic or topical nasal decongestants (prior to arrival), can be helpful to prevent or relieve initial symptoms.

   b. Persistent symptoms after landing can be treated with analgesics and repeated autoinflation.

   c. With severe or persistent pain/hearing loss, myringotomy should be considered.

 Barotrauma that does not resolve with auto-inflation methods may require myringotom.

H. Tympanic membrane perforation

   1. Rupture can occur from infection (AOM) or trauma (i.e., barotrauma, direct impact, or explosion).

   2. Most cases will resolve on their own; however, surgical repair of the tympanic membrane as well as the ossicular chain (with persistent hearing loss) may be necessary.

   3. Water/moisture to the ear should be avoided to prevent a secondary infection that can impede closure.

Disorders of the Nose, Sinus, and Throat

A. Acute sinusitis

   1. General characteristics

   a. Inflammation of the area near the osteomeatal complex is an important component differentiating sinusitis from allergic or viral rhinitis; hence, the alternate term "rhinosinusitis."

   b. Sinusitis often follows a URI and can be viral or bacterial in nature. Bacterial etiology is the same as that for otitis media (e.g., *S. pneumoniae*, *H. influenzae*, and, less often, *S. aureus* and *M. catarrhalis*).

   c. Risk factors include cigarette smoke or exposure to secondary smoke, history of trauma, chronic allergies or dental disease, and presence of a foreign body.

   2. Clinical features

   a. With acute bacterial sinusitis, symptoms and signs include purulent nasal discharge, facial pain and pressure, nasal obstruction or congestion, and fever.

   b. Physical examination may reveal tenderness to palpation over the affected sinus. Decreased light transmission with transillumination of the sinuses may be suggestive as well but is not always apparent.

   c. Possible complications include orbital cellulitis, osteomyelitis, or cavernous sinus thrombosis.

   3. Diagnostic studies

   a. Acute bacterial sinusitis is typically a clinical diagnosis.

   b. Routine sinus x-rays are not recommended, but they can be useful with an unclear clinical presentation, treatment failure, or indications of a more serious infection.

   c. CT is sensitive but lacks specificity and is not routinely performed. MRI is indicated if malignancy or intracranial spread of infection is suspected.

   4. Treatment

   a. Treatment includes nonsteroidal anti-inflammatory drugs (NSAIDs) (for pain), saline washes, steam, and oral and/or nasal decongestants. Intranasal corticosteroids can be helpful for moderate to severe disease.

   b. Many patients improve within 2 weeks without antimicrobial therapy.

   c. Antibiotics should be recommended in the presence of extended duration of symptoms (10 to 14 days) or more significant symptoms (fever, facial pain, or swelling).

   d. Amoxicillin–clavulanate is the first-line drug; course is usually 5 to 7 days (or longer with a higher dose in more severe cases). Doxycycline or clindamycin with a

 Treatment for acute sinusitis involves symptom management, and antibiotics are not required unless symptoms are prolonged or severe.

third-generation cephalosporin (e.g., cefixime, cefpodoxime) can be used if the patient is penicillin-allergic. Quinolones, such as levofloxacin or moxifloxacin, could also be used with penicillin allergy if no other alternatives.

B. Rhinitis

    1. General characteristics

        a. Rhinitis refers to any inflammation of the nasal mucosa.

        b. There are three basic types: allergic rhinitis, vasomotor rhinitis, and rhinitis medicamentosa.

            (1) Allergic rhinitis is an immunoglobulin E (IgE)–mediated reactivity to airborne antigens (e.g., pollen, molds, dander, dust). It commonly occurs in people who have other atopic diseases (e.g., asthma, eczema, atopic dermatitis) and those with a family history.

            (2) Vasomotor rhinitis is rhinorrhea caused by increased secretion of mucus from the nasal mucosa. It may be precipitated by changes in temperature or humidity, odors, or alcohol, or caused by vidian nerve sensitivity.

            (3) Rhinitis medicamentosa is caused by the overzealous use of decongestant drops or sprays containing oxymetazoline or phenylephrine. This causes a rebound congestion, which prompts increased use of the agent, creating a repetitive cycle.

    2. Clinical features

        a. Allergic rhinitis

            (1) Symptoms may be confused with those of a common cold except they are typically persistent and can vary by season.

            (2) Signs may include allergic shiners (bluish discoloration below the eyes); rhinorrhea; itchy or watery eyes; sneezing; nasal congestion; dry cough; and pale, boggy, or bluish mucosa. Children may develop a horizontal nasal crease (the allergic salute) from habitual rubbing of the nose.

            (3) The discharge usually is clear and watery.

        b. Vasomotor rhinitis

            (1) Vasomotor rhinitis consists of bogginess of the nasal mucosa associated with a complaint of stuffiness and rhinorrhea in response to nonspecific irritants as previously described.

            (2) Symptoms are labile and can clear quickly.

        c. Rhinitis medicamentosa

            (1) Patients experience rebound congestion with inflamed red nasal mucosa after decongestant withdrawal.

            (2) Discharge is typically minimal.

    3. Treatment

        a. Allergic rhinitis: Avoid any known allergens and use antihistamines, cromolyn sodium, intranasal corticosteroids (most effective), nasal saline drops or washes, and immunotherapy.

        b. Vasomotor rhinitis: Milder cases—irritant avoidance. For more significant symptoms, saline or antihistamine nasal sprays, intranasal corticosteroids, or decongestants may be helpful.

        c. Rhinitis medicamentosa: Discontinue the irritant. The use of topical corticosteroids is warranted through the withdrawal period to help with symptoms.

C. Acute pharyngitis

    1. General characteristics

        a. Sore throat, a common reason for outpatient visits, is associated with about half of outpatient antibiotic use.

> Vasomotor rhinitis is characterized by acute and labile symptoms in response to local environmental factors such as change in humidity or odors.

> Topical corticosteroids are often needed to break the cycle of rhinitis medicamentosa.

   b. Etiology is more commonly viral than bacterial. It is important to differentiate and treat cases that are caused by group A β-hemolytic streptococci (GABHS) to prevent complications as well as to limit unnecessary antibiotic use.

2. Clinical features

   a. GABHS-suggestive manifestations include fever (38°C or 100.4°F or greater), tender anterior cervical adenopathy, lack of cough, and pharyngotonsillar exudate.

   b. Presence of all four strongly suggests GABHS (per Centor criteria). Two to three indicates intermediate likelihood, but the patient may benefit from testing. With only one, GABHS is not likely.

3. Diagnostic studies

   a. Rapid streptococci screening for GABHS has 90% to 99% sensitivity.

   b. Throat culture also has 90% to 95% sensitivity with even greater specificity (95% to 99%).

4. Treatment

   a. Oral penicillin or cefuroxime can be used, and intramuscular (IM) penicillin can be used if patient compliance is in doubt. Erythromycin or another macrolide can be substituted in cases of penicillin allergy.

   b. Inadequate treatment can lead to complications, such as scarlet fever, glomerulonephritis, acute rheumatic fever, and abscess formation.

> 💡 Coryza, hoarseness, and cough do *not* support a diagnosis of streptococcal pharyngitis.

D. **Peritonsillar abscess/cellulitis (quinsy)**

   1. General characteristics: It results from penetration of infection through the tonsillar capsule and involvement of neighboring tissue.

   2. Clinical features

   a. It can present with a significant sore throat, pain with swallowing, trismus, deviation of the soft palate/uvula, and muffled "hot potato" voice.

   b. Deviation of the soft palate and asymmetric rise of the uvula are highly suggestive of abscess.

   3. Treatment

   a. Treatment involves aspiration, I&D, and/or antibiotics. Tonsillectomy may also be considered in about 10% of patients.

   b. Examples of recommended antimicrobial therapy include parenteral amoxicillin, amoxicillin–sulbactam, and clindamycin. In less severe cases, oral antibiotics can be used for 7 to 10 days (e.g., amoxicillin, amoxicillin–clavulanate, clindamycin).

   c. Patients are typically treated with IV antibiotics until symptoms abate and then continue oral antibiotics to complete the course.

> 💡 An asymmetric rise of the uvula indicates peritonsillar abscess.

E. **Laryngitis**

   1. General characteristics

   a. Etiology is usually viral and follows a URI.

   b. Bacterial causes, although rare, include *M. catarrhalis* and *H. influenzae.*

   2. Clinical features

   a. Hoarseness is the hallmark symptom, although cough can also be present.

   b. Pain is atypical.

   3. Treatment

   a. Supportive therapy is typically sufficient. Hydration, humidification and vocal rest, and avoidance of singing or shouting are recommended.

   b. Continued trauma to the vocal cord can cause vocal fold hemorrhage, polyp, or cyst formation.

    c. If bacterial, erythromycin can decrease hoarseness/cough, but there is no strong evidence to show effectiveness of antibiotic treatment.

    d. Oral or IM corticosteroids may also hasten recovery for performers but requires vocal fold evaluation before starting therapy.

F. **Aphthous ulcers (canker sores, ulcerative stomatitis)**

  1. General characteristics: Etiology is not clear, but they may be associated with human herpesvirus 6.

  2. **Clinical features**: They present as single or multiple painful, round ulcers with yellow-gray centers and red halos. They occur on nonkeratinized mucosa (i.e., buccal or labial mucosa) and are usually recurrent.

  3. **Treatment**

    a. Treatment is nonspecific, but topical therapies, such as corticosteroids, can provide symptomatic relief.

    b. Other topical therapies (e.g., diclofenac in hyaluronan, doxymycine–cyanoacrylate, enzyme-containing mouthwashes) can be effective.

    c. A 1-week oral prednisone taper can also be helpful for severe cases.

    d. Cimetidine can be used as maintenance therapy in recurrent cases.

G. **Oral candidiasis**

  1. General characteristics

    a. *Candida albicans* is a common yeast.

    b. Outside of the newborn period, infection is more likely in patients who wear dentures; those with diabetes or immunocompromised states; undergoing chemotherapy or radiation, or undergoing treatment with corticosteroids or broad-spectrum antibiotics.

  2. **Clinical features**

    a. It can cause throat or mouth pain and appears as creamy white patches that can be scraped off to reveal underlying erythematous mucosa.

    b. The diagnosis is usually clinical, but wet prep or biopsy can be done.

  3. **Treatment** is with antifungals, which are available in several forms (i.e., ketoconazole or fluconazole orally, clotrimazole troches, nystatin liquid rinses).

> Oral candidiasis presents as nonadherent creamy white patches; treatable with antifungals.

H. **Leukoplakia**

  1. This is also a white oral lesion; however, unlike oral candidiasis, it is painless and cannot be rubbed or scraped off.

  2. Lesions are often linked with tobacco, alcohol, or denture use.

  3. Some are dysplastic or squamous cell carcinomas.

  4. If there is an associated erythematous appearance (erythroplakia), there is a higher risk of dysplasia or cancer (90%).

I. **Epiglottitis (supraglottitis)**

  1. General characteristics

    a. This is a potentially serious infection of the epiglottis and nearby tissues that can lead to airway compromise. Once, it was more common in children but can occur at any age. It is more common in adults since the onset of the vaccine against *H. influenzae*.

  2. **Clinical features**

    a. In adults, it is suspected with a history of a quickly developing sore throat or pain on swallowing with a relatively benign oral examination. Use caution when examining the oral cavity.

    b. Other classic findings include fever, drooling, and, in children, a tripod or sniffing posture to improve air exchange.

> The incidence of epiglottitis has significantly declined since the widespread distribution of the H flu vaccine.

3. Diagnostic studies

    a. Laryngoscopy reveals a swollen, erythematous epiglottis. The procedure can cause airway spasm and should be done in a controlled environment.

    b. Lateral soft-tissue neck x-rays may also show an enlarged epiglottis ("thumb sign").

4. **Treatment**

    a. Treatment involves IV antibiotics (e.g., ceftizoxime or cefuroxime) and IV corticosteroids (i.e., dexamethasone). As the patient improves, antibiotic therapy can be switched to oral forms to complete a 10-day course, and steroids can be tapered.

    b. If there is dyspnea or such a rapid course that airway compromise is likely to occur before the medications take effect, intubation is indicated (about 10% of adults). Even without intubation, patients should be closely monitored (i.e., pulse oximetry, intensive care unit [ICU]).

> Most nosebleeds are anterior and can be treated with pressure alone.

J. **Epistaxis**

1. General characteristics/clinical features

    a. Nosebleeds most commonly occur anteriorly from the Kiesselbach plexus.

    b. Risk factors include nasal trauma (i.e., nose picking), dry nasal mucosa, hypertension, nasal cocaine, or alcohol use.

    c. Typical presentation is unilateral anterior bleeding.

    d. Posterior bleeding is much less frequent (5%, Woodruff plexus) and is associated with hypertension and atherosclerosis.

2. **Treatment** (anterior)

    a. Most anterior epistaxis cases can be treated with direct pressure to the area. The patient is placed in a sitting position while leaning forward slightly (to lessen swallowing of blood). The nares are compressed for about 15 minutes.

    b. If the bleeding continues, the site of bleeding should be identified.

    c. Topical decongestants (i.e., oxymetazoline) and topical anesthetics (i.e., lidocaine) can be used as an anesthetic and vasoconstrictor. Topical cocaine can be used as well.

    d. With a visible bleeding source, cautery (i.e., silver nitrate, electrocautery) can be used. If unsuccessful, anterior packing can also be considered.

3. **Treatment** (posterior)

    a. Posterior packing is more difficult and carries a high risk for complications; therefore, specialist evaluation and inpatient monitoring are recommended.

    b. With life-threatening cases of continued bleeding, surgery is indicated (i.e., nasal arterial supply ligation).

K. **Nasal polyps**

1. General characteristics/clinical features

    a. Nasal polyps appear as pale, boggy masses on the nasal mucosa.

    b. Patients commonly also have allergic rhinitis. With a history of nasal polyps and asthma, aspirin is contraindicated because of the possibility of causing severe bronchospasm, also known as triad asthma (Samter triad).

    c. Patients may complain of chronic congestion and a decreased sense of smell.

2. **Treatment**

    a. A several (1 to 3) month course of topical nasal corticosteroid is the initial treatment choice. This is effective for small polyps and can reduce the need for surgical intervention. Oral steroids (6-day taper) can also help reduce size.

    b. Surgical removal may be necessary if therapy is unsuccessful or if polyps are large.

Practice Questions

Directions: *Each of the numbered items or incomplete statements in this section is followed by a list of answers or completions of the statement. Select the ONE lettered answer or completion that is BEST in each case.*

1. A 9-year-old is brought to the clinic with severe, worsening earache. The pain started a week ago. His mother gave him a few doses of antibiotics she had left over from a urinary tract infection (UTI). Today, the child has a fever and pain, erythema, and swelling behind the left ear. What is the best treatment option?
   A. IV antibiotics and myringotomy
   B. Local I&D with cultures
   C. Mastoidectomy
   D. Skull series to map out lesions prior to definitive treatment
   E. Check sodium, plan management per results

2. A 19-year-old female presents with copious purulent discharge from the right eye. Gram staining shows PMNs and Gram-negative diplococci. What is the recommended treatment?
   A. IVIG and high-dose antivirals
   B. Laser photocoagulation
   C. IM penicillin once
   D. Systemic and topical antibiotics
   E. Urgent iridectomy

3. Exposure to which of the following most strongly increases the risk of developing cataracts?
   A. Contact lens
   B. Particulate ambient matter
   C. Secondary smoke
   D. Sun
   E. Vitaminosis

4. A 73-year-old describes sudden unilateral painless blurred vision of the left eye. Vision has slowly resolved in the 2 days since the event. Fundus is with swollen disc, dilated veins, hemorrhages, and exudates. What else is most likely to be found on physical examination?
   A. Afferent pupillary defect
   B. Box-carring of vasculature
   C. Hyphema and ciliary injection
   D. Increased ocular pressure
   E. Perifoveal atrophy

5. A 62-year-old presents for follow-up of chronic central visual loss. He describes a phenomenon of wavy or distorted vision that has deteriorated rather quickly. Presence of what finding on examination would indicate a poor prognosis?
   A. Drusen deposits
   B. Fibrotic plaques
   C. Mottling
   D. Neovascularization
   E. Serous leaks

6. A patient with severe myopia presents with flashers and floaters followed by loss of vision in one-half of one eye. Examination reveals an afferent pupillary defect and the presence of rugae in the vitreous. What is the immediate treatment?
   A. Acetazolamide, mannitol, and topical β-blocker
   B. Decrease IOP by reducing aqueous production
   C. Intravitreal injection of VEGF
   D. Remain supine, turn head to the side of vision loss
   E. Remain supine, turn head away from the side of vision loss

7. A 13-year-old was hit in the right eye with a billiard ball. The area is ecchymotic and swollen. He complains of pain, rated 6 out of 10. Which of the following examination findings is most supportive of the likely diagnosis?
   A. Double vision
   B. Loss of accommodation
   C. Proptosis
   D. Restricted range of motion (ROM)
   E. Subcutaneous emphysema

8. A 18-year-old presents day 4 of a high fever and sore throat. He is febrile and wan with tender cervical and occipital lymph nodes. Tonsils are asymmetrically enlarged and touching; the uvula is displaced. What is the most likely etiologic agent?
   A. *Candida albicans*
   B. Cytomegalovirus
   C. Epstein–Barr virus
   D. Herpesvirus
   E. GABHS

9. A 30-year-old describes episodes of vertigo that come on suddenly with movement; they are not associated with tinnitus or hearing loss. Which of the following will most likely be found on physical examination?
   A. Claudication pain with resisted temporomandibular joint (TMJ) movement
   B. Delayed fatigable nystagmus on Dix–Hallpike maneuver
   C. Photophobia and facial twitching with strobe light
   D. Tenderness and bogginess of the mastoid area
   E. Vertical nystagmus at rest

10. An elderly person complains of acute hearing loss. Examination reveals a canal occluded with cerumen. Irrigation is successful and hearing was restored. What was likely found on physical examination?
    A. Air/fluid behind thickened tympanic membrane
    B. Bulging tympanic membrane with dilated vessels
    C. Loss of extreme degrees of sounds
    D. Weber lateralized to affected ear
    E. Rinne air conduction < bone conduction

11. A 20-year-old contact lens wearer complains of pain and photophobia. Eyes are injected with cloudy discharge unilaterally. A dense corneal infiltrate is visible with fluorescein staining. What is the best next step?
    A. Culture the discharge and begin topical antibiotics
    B. Irrigate the eye until the pH falls below 5.0
    C. Laser photocoagulation is needed.
    D. Systemic antiviral medications
    E. Topical corticosteroid

12. A 6-year-old is brought to the nurse's office because of a nosebleed. This is the third event in the past 2 weeks. What is the most likely underlying cause?
    A. Acute leukemia
    B. Allergic rhinitis
    C. Local trauma
    D. Immune thrombocytopenia (ITP)
    E. von Willebrand disease

Practice Answers

1. A. *EENT; Clinical Intervention; Mastoiditis*

Mastoiditis most commonly arises from inadequately treated otitis media. Localized abscess presentation includes swelling, redness, and tenderness. The child should be started on broad-spectrum IV antibiotics and undergo drainage via myringotomy. Keep the area well drained, and switch to oral antibiotics once responding. A mastoidectomy is an option if the child does not improve with medical care.

2. D. *EENT; Pharmacology; Conjunctivitis, Neisseria*

Neisseria gonorrhoeae conjunctivitis presents as copious unilateral discharge. Patients should be treated with antibiotics both topically and systemically. Severe viral illness, herpes virus, presents with dendritic lesion. Iridectomy is for acute glaucoma. Photocoagulation is for proliferative diseases.

3. D. *EENT; History and Physical Examination (PE); Cataracts*

Excessive unprotected sun exposure is the strongest modifiable risk factor for the development of cataracts. Risk is increased in aging; trauma; congenital defects; systemic disease such as diabetes; and medications such as steroids or statins.

4. A. *EENT; History and PE; Central Venous Occlusion*

The patient is describing the resolving phase of an acute venous occlusion. The "blood and thunder" retina is likely caused by thrombotic disease and associated with an afferent pupillary defect. An acute arterial occlusion is likely embolic and may cause box-carring in the vasculature, cherry red spot (perifoveal atrophy), and hyphema or increased pressure.

5. D. *EENT; History and PE; Age-Related Macular Degeneration*

The presence of neovascularization heralds "wet" ARMD. The pathology typically *begins* with Drusen deposits compromising Bruch's membrane, blocking nutrient arrival. The disease progresses and affects central vision. ARMD is the leading cause of irreversible central visual loss. There is no effective treatment. Wet ARMD can be slowed by up to 25% with AREDS supplement, which is vitamin C, vitamin E, β-carotene (vitamin A), zinc oxide, and copper as cupric oxide.

6. D. *EENT; Clinical Intervention; Retinal Detachment*

This patient describes the development of a retinal detachment. Severe myopia is a strong risk factor. Turn the patient's head toward the side of the vision loss to use gravity to prevent further detachment. The sooner the intervention by ophthalmology, the better the outcome. Acute glaucoma is treated with acetazolamide, mannitol, and a β-blocker. VEGF is indicated in wet ARMD.

7. D. *EENT; History and PE; Blow-Out Fracture*

A blow-out fracture is strongly suspect in the presence of trauma and restricted movement, especially upward gaze.

Subcutaneous emphysema is common but a less specific finding. The eye is usually sunken. Visual complaints are variable.

8. E. *EENT; Basic Science; Peritonsillar Abscess*

Asymmetrically enlarged tonsils with a displaced uvula indicate peritonsillar abscess (quinsy throat). The organism is most commonly Group A Streptococci. *Candida* causes thrush—adherent cheesy white exudate. Cytomegalovirus is associated with small scattered ulcers on the mucosa. Epstein–Barr virus causes mononucleosis; in this case, the tonsils would be symmetric if indeed enlarged. Herpesvirus presents as grouped vesicles.

9. B. *EENT; History and PE; Vertigo*

BPPV is the most common peripheral vertigo. Dix–Hallpike maneuvers result in delayed onset of nystagmus that quickly fatigues. Patients may have nausea but rarely vomit. Central vertigo will show nystagmus at rest, usually vertical, not fatigued. Tenderness and bogginess at mastoid indicates mastoiditis. Claudication pain supports a diagnosis of giant-cell (temporal) arteritis. Photophobia and movement with strobe light supports a diagnosis of seizure.

10. D. *EENT; History and PE; Hearing Loss*

Cerumen impaction causes an obstructive hearing loss: Weber lateralizes to the affected ear; Rinne result is bone conduction < air conduction. Bulging indicates otitis media; air/fluid levels are a sequela. Presbycusis is loss of extreme spectrum of hearing.

11. A. *EENT; Pharmacology; Corneal Ulcer*

This patient has developed a corneal ulcer. The discharge should be cultured for definitive organism and sensitivities. Meanwhile, treat with a broad-spectrum antibiotic topically. The eye does not need to be irrigated. Antivirals would be warranted in the face of a dendritic lesion, herpesvirus. Topical corticosteroids are contraindicated because they may cause further tissue loss and risk of perforation.

12. C. *EENT; Diagnosis; Nosebleed*

Local trauma, i.e., picking, is by far the most common cause of recurrent nosebleeds in children. Local care with pressure and petroleum jelly is all that is needed. If an underlying disorder is suspected, a screening cell count and smear would reveal any rare pathology; but screening blood work is not recommended until further investigation regarding local trauma is complete.

Pulmonology | 2

Jessica R. M. Gomes

Infectious Disorders

A. Pneumonia

  1. Pneumonia denotes inflammation in the alveoli or interstitium of the lung caused by microorganisms that infect the lower respiratory tract.

  2. Pneumonia is one of the leading causes of morbidity and mortality worldwide.

  3. Risk factors: alcohol use, asthma, tobacco use, and chronic obstructive pulmonary disease (COPD)

B. Classic community-acquired pneumonia (CAP)

  1. General characteristics

    a. It is acquired in the home or nonhospital environment.

    b. In most cases of CAP, the causative agent is not identified. However, in those cases where an agent is identified, bacterial etiology is more common.

    c. Common causative agents (Table 2-1) include *Streptococcus pneumoniae*, *Haemophilus influenzae*, *Moraxella catarrhalis*, *Staphylococcus aureus*, *Klebsiella pneumoniae*, and other Gram-negative bacilli. Atypical agents include *Legionella*, *Mycoplasma*, and *Chlamydia*. Viral causes include influenza virus, respiratory syncytial virus (RSV), adenovirus, and parainfluenza virus.

  2. Clinical features

    a. Typical presentation is a 1- to 10-day history of increasing cough, purulent sputum, shortness of breath, tachycardia, tachypnea, dyspnea, pleuritic chest pain, fever or hypothermia, sweats, and rigors.

    b. Physical examination may reveal altered breath sounds and inspiratory crackles, dullness to percussion if an effusion is present, and bronchial breath sounds over an area of consolidation. *Note*: The chest examination alone is not sufficient to confirm or exclude the diagnosis.

    c. Table 2-2 provides classic descriptions of pneumonias caused by specific organisms. Although these characteristics may help in attempting to identify specific pathogens, exceptions and less typical presentations are common.

    d. Table 2-3 lists the pathogens more likely to occur in certain patient groups. *S. pneumoniae* remains the most common cause of bacterial pneumonia in all groups.

  3. Diagnostic studies

    a. Organisms may be detected with conventional sputum Gram stain or sputum culture, although typically this is not done before initiating treatment. The most common bacterial pathogen identified is *S. pneumoniae*.

    b. Chest radiography (CXR) may show lobar or segmental infiltrates, air bronchograms, and pleural effusions. There is no pathognomonic radiographic presentation.

    c. White blood cell (WBC) count is typically elevated. Procalcitonin levels rise in response to a proinflammatory stimulus, especially bacterial infection. Elevated levels support a bacterial versus viral origin.

> **Bacterial CAP:**
> Patient will have cough, sputum, dyspnea, and fever, with possible altered breath sounds on examination and elevated WBC and procalcitonin.

Table 2-1 | Common Etiologies of Pneumonia

Common	*Streptococcus pneumoniae* (pneumococcus) (*most common*) *Haemophilus influenzae* *Moraxella catarrhalis* *Staphylococcus aureus* *Klebsiella pneumoniae*
Atypical	*Legionella* *Mycoplasma* *Chlamydia*
Viral	Influenza virus Respiratory syncytial virus Adenovirus Parainfluenza virus

Table 2-2 | Typical Manifestations of Pneumonia per Pathogen

Organism	Typical Manifestations
Mycoplasma pneumoniae	Low-grade fever Cough Bullous myringitis Cold agglutinins Hemolytic anemia
Pneumocystis jiroveci (nee *carinii*)	Slower onset, immunosuppression Increased lactate dehydrogenase More hypoxemic than appears on chest radiography Interstitial infiltrates Pneumothorax
Legionella pneumoniae	Chronic cardiac or respiratory disease Hyponatremia Diarrhea, other systemic symptoms
Chlamydia pneumoniae	Longer prodrome Sore throat, hoarseness
Streptococcus pneumoniae	Single rigor Rust-colored sputum
Klebsiella pneumoniae	Currant jelly sputum Chronic illness, including alcohol abuse

Table 2-3 | Pathogens More Likely to Cause Pneumonia in Certain Patient Groups

Patient Characteristics	Pathogen More Likely Seen in This Group
Alcohol abuse	*Klebsiella pneumonia*
COPD	*Haemophilus pneumoniae*
Cystic fibrosis	*Pseudomonas* sp.
Young adults, college settings	*Mycoplasma pneumoniae* *Chlamydia pneumoniae*
Air conditioning/aerosolized water	*Legionella pneumoniae*
Postsplenectomy	Encapsulated organisms *Streptococcus pneumoniae* *Haemophilus pneumoniae*
Leukemia, lymphoma	Fungus
Children, <1 year	Respiratory syncytial virus
Children, <2 year	Parainfluenza virus

COPD, chronic obstructive pulmonary disease.

4. **Management**

  a. The patient who is otherwise healthy and free of respiratory distress or complications may be treated as an outpatient with oral antibiotics and appropriate supportive care (fluids, antipyretics, analgesics, relative rest).

  b. A macrolide (clarithromycin, azithromycin) or doxycycline is the appropriate choice for outpatient treatment if the patient is otherwise healthy and without risk factors for drug-resistant organisms. A fluoroquinolone (levofloxacin, moxifloxacin) or a macrolide plus a β-lactam is the top choice for patients with underlying chronic disease, prior antibiotic use in the last 3 months, >65 years old, or immunosuppression.

  c. Neutropenia, involvement of more than one lobe, or poor host resistance indicates a need for hospitalization. Also consider hospitalization for patients older than 50 years of age with comorbidities, altered mental status, or hemodynamic instability.

  d. If inpatient treatment is necessary, consider coverage of *S. pneumoniae* and *Legionella* sp. with a fluoroquinolone or a combination of β-lactam (i.e., ceftriaxone or cefotaxime) plus a macrolide (i.e., azithromycin).

  e. Treat with antibiotics for a minimum of 5 days or until clinically stable and afebrile for at least 48 to 72 hours.

5. Prevention

  a. There are two pneumococcal vaccines currently available: the 13-valent pneumococcal conjugate vaccine (PCV13, Prevnar) and the 23-valent pneumococcal polysaccharide vaccine (PPSV23, Pneumovax).

  b. The Advisory Committee on Immunization Practice (ACIP) recommendations call for a dose of PCV13 followed 1 year later with a dose of PPSV23 for all adults >65 years old (unless they have received a previous vaccine), immunocompromised, and children >2 years old with underlying medical conditions putting them at risk of pneumococcal disease.

  c. Dosage and timing recommendations for the two vaccines varies according to age and risk group. Further information should be sought at www.cdc.gov.

C. **Atypical CAP**

  1. General characteristics

  a. As the term *atypical* implies, this form of pneumonia has a clinical presentation different from that of classic CAP.

  b. *Mycoplasma pneumoniae* is the most common cause of atypical pneumonias. Other causes include viruses (influenza types A and B and adenoviruses), *Chlamydia pneumoniae*, *Legionella* sp., and *Moraxella* sp.

  2. **Clinical features**

  a. The typical presentation of atypical pneumonia is a low-grade fever with relatively mild pulmonary symptoms, which are self-limited, occurring in young, otherwise healthy adults. A nonproductive chronic cough, myalgia, and fatigue are common.

  b. *Mycoplasma* may cause reddened tympanic membranes or bullous myringitis—a rare but unique feature.

  c. *Legionella* infection is associated with exposure to contaminated water droplets from cooling and ventilation systems. Acute development of high fever, dry cough, dyspnea, and systemic symptoms is common.

  d. Viral pneumonias are variable in presentation but are often associated with epidemics and upper respiratory symptoms (for COVID, see Chapter 14).

  e. Complications: empyema, cavitations, endocarditis

> Empiric treatment of CAP must cover Pneumococcus, atypical bacteria.

> Atypical pneumonia and unique characteristics: Mycoplasma, bullous myringitis; Leigonella, contaminated water droplets; viral, endemic to some areas.

3. Diagnostic studies

    a. Organisms are usually not detected with conventional stain or culture of sputum.

    b. The WBC count is normal or only slightly elevated.

    c. Radiography may show segmental unilateral lower lung zone infiltrates or diffuse infiltrates.

4. Management

    a. Antibiotic treatment is started empirically based on the clinical features. Regimens include erythromycin or doxycycline (for suspected *M. pneumoniae* and *Legionella* infection) and tetracycline (for suspected *Chlamydia* infection).

    b. Viral pneumonias are treated with supportive measures (analgesics, fluids, cough suppressants) unless influenza is suspected. Amantadine and rimantadine are no longer recommended in the treatment of influenza because of increasing resistance. Neuraminidase inhibitors (inhaled zanamivir or oral oseltamivir) may be used if antiviral therapy is indicated.

> 💡 HAP is defined as having symptoms develop 48 hours or more after admission.

D. **Hospital-acquired (nosocomial) pneumonia**

  1. General characteristics

    a. Hospital-acquired pneumonia is caused by organisms that colonize ill patients, staff, and equipment, producing clinical infection >48 hours after admission to the hospital. Those at highest risk are intensive care unit (ICU) patients on mechanical ventilation.

    b. Pneumonia is the second most common cause of hospital-acquired infection after urinary tract infection (UTI).

    c. The causative organisms are unique, and the mortality rate is 10% but can vary greatly among subgroups.

      (1) The usual organisms are *S. aureus* and Gram-negative bacilli, which are easy to recover from respiratory secretions.

      (2) *Pseudomonas aeruginosa* is the most likely pathogen in ICUs and carries the worst prognosis. Others include *S. aureus*, *Klebsiella* sp., *Escherichia coli*, and *Enterobacter* sp.

  2. Clinical features are similar to those with CAP. Signs/symptoms include a new or progressive lung infiltrate and ≥2 of the following compatible findings: fever, leukocytosis/leukopenia, purulent secretions.

  3. Diagnostic studies: Diagnosis is clinical and supported with Gram stain and culture of sputum and blood. The CXR may help to support the diagnosis.

  4. Management includes use of appropriate empiric antibiotics.

    a. There is no consensus on the best regimen. If the patient is at low risk for multiple drug resistance, consider use of a single antibiotic such as ceftriaxone, a respiratory fluoroquinolone, imipenem, or piperacillin–tazobactam.

    b. If patient is at high risk for multiple drug-resistant pathogens, cover with two agents as long as they are from separate classes. Once an organism is isolated, therapy should be narrowed based on the culture and sensitivity results. Patients may need aggressive supportive measures, including mechanical ventilation as appropriate. Treat with antibiotics for at least 7 days.

> 💡 Although Pneumocystis pneumonia develops most commonly in patients with HIV disease, the most common cause of pneumonia in patients with HIV is Strep pneumococcal.

E. **Pneumonia: human immunodeficiency virus (HIV) related**

  1. General characteristics

    a. *Streptococcus* is the most common cause of bacterial pneumonia in patients with HIV infection.

    b. *Pneumocystis jiroveci* (formerly *Pneumocystis carinii*) is one of the most common opportunistic infections in patients with HIV disease, typically with CD4 counts of <200 cells per μL. *Pneumocystis* infection also occurs in patients with cancer, malnourished states, and immunosuppression.

   c. Other pathogens common in patients with HIV and pneumonia include *Haemophilus*, *Pseudomonas*, and *Mycobacterium* sp.

2. Clinical features

   a. Pneumocystis pneumonia typically presents with fever, tachypnea, dyspnea, and nonproductive cough which ranges in severity.

   b. Nonpneumocystis pneumonia typically follows a more fulminant course in patients with HIV than in non–HIV-infected persons.

3. Diagnostic studies

   a. CXR aids in diagnosis, typically showing diffuse or bilateral perihilar infiltrates; no effusions are seen.

   b. Lymphopenia and a low CD4 count are typical.

   c. Sputum staining, via either induced sputum or bronchoalveolar lavage, with Wright Giemsa stain or direct fluorescence antibody (DFA), establishes the definitive diagnosis in >90% of patients.

4. Management

   a. Trimethoprim–sulfamethoxazole (Bactrim) is the treatment of choice in Pneumocystis.

   b. There is an extremely high mortality rate (near 100%) if not treated.

   c. Prophylaxis is recommended in all patients with a CD4 count of <200 cells per μL or with a history of *Pneumocystis* infection. Trimethoprim–sulfamethoxazole is the antibiotic of choice.

> TMP-SMX is both therapeutic and preventive against Pneumocystis.

F. **Tuberculosis (TB)**

1. General characteristics

   a. *Mycobacterium tuberculosis* infection is acquired by inhaling organisms within aerosol droplets expelled during coughing by an individual with active disease.

   b. Most exposed people mount an immune response sufficient to prevent progression from initial infection to clinical illness. T cells and macrophages surround the organism in forming a granuloma. Overall, 10% of persons infected with TB will develop the disease. This is primary TB.

   c. Approximately 5% of exposed people fail to contain the primary infection and progress to active TB; this is known as progressive primary TB.

   d. Approximately 90% of infected persons will contain the bacterium without becoming symptomatic. This is known as latent TB infection (LTBI). These patients are not considered to be infectious nor can they spread the disease. They are asymptomatic and have inactive TB in their body, most commonly in the apices of the lungs. Reactivation TB illness develops from LTBI in the setting of immune compromise, gastrectomy, silicosis, diabetes, and HIV.

   e. Outbreaks since the mid-1990s have seen an emergence of organisms resistant to multiple antituberculous drugs.

   f. Risk factors include household exposure to patients with active disease, incarceration, drug use, and travel to endemic areas.

2. Clinical features

   a. Cough is the most common symptom. It begins as a dry cough and progresses to productive cough, with or without hemoptysis, typically over 3 weeks or longer.

   b. The classic symptom complex includes fever, drenching night sweats, anorexia, fatigue, and weight loss. Other common pulmonary symptoms include pleuritic chest pain, dyspnea, and hemoptysis. Post-tussive rales are classic.

   c. On examination, the patient may appear chronically ill and malnourished.

3. Diagnostic studies

   a. Radiography: chest x-ray

> For TB, the classic symptoms are dry cough, fever, drenching night sweats, anorexia, fatigue, and weight loss.

(1) Primary TB: homogeneous infiltrates, hilar/paratracheal lymph node enlargement, segmental atelectasis, cavitations with progressive disease

(2) Reactivation TB: fibrocavitary apical disease, nodules, infiltrates, posterior and apical segments of the right upper lobe, apical–posterior segments of the left upper lobe, superior segments of the lower lobes

(3) HIV patients may display lower lung zone diffuse or miliary infiltrates and pleural effusions.

(4) Ghon's complexes (calcified primary focus) and Ranke complexes (calcified primary focus and calcified hilar lymph node) represent healed primary infection.

> The BCG vaccine against tuberculosis is not recommended in the United States.

b. The tuberculin skin test (TST) identifies individuals who have been infected, but it does not differentiate between active and latent infection. Tuberculin skin testing (such as the purified protein derivative [PPD; Mantoux test]) is reported according to the diameter of induration not erythema (Table 2-4).

c. Definitive diagnosis requires the identification of *M. tuberculosis* from cultures (6 to 8 weeks to grow) or by DNA or RNA amplification techniques (1 to 2 days). Demonstration of acid-fast bacilli on sputum supports, but does not confirm, a diagnosis of TB.

d. Biopsy revealing caseating granulomas (also known as necrotizing granulomas) is the histologic hallmark.

4. **Management**

a. Any confirmed or suspected cases should be reported to public health agencies who will investigate contacts. Patients with active disease should be isolated until a minimum of 2 weeks of treatment is completed.

b. Antituberculous drugs, including isoniazid (INH), rifampin (RIF), pyrazinamide (PZA), and ethambutol (EMB), are the cornerstone of therapy. Diligent compliance is essential to reduce the risk of emerging drug-resistant TB. Directly observed therapy (DOT) may be recommended to improve compliance.

> Treat for LTBI only after active TB is ruled out because active TB is treated with a multidrug regimen.

c. The Centers for Disease Control and Prevention (CDC) recommends multiple drug regimens such as the following (Table 2-5):

(1) LTBI: INH for 9 months *or* RIF for 4 months *or* RIF and PZA for 2 months (only if in contact with TB-resistant persons)

(2) Active TB: INH/RIF/PZA/EMB for 2 months, followed by 4 months of additional multidrug treatment based on culture and sensitivity results

Table 2-4 | Classification of Positive Tuberculin Skin Test Reactions

Reaction Size (mm)	Group
≥5	HIV-positive persons Recent contacts of those with active tuberculosis Persons with evidence of tuberculosis on chest radiography Immunosuppressed patients on steroids TNF-α antagonist or organ transplant
≥10	Recent immigrants from countries with high rate of tuberculosis HIV-negative injection drug users Mycobacteriology laboratory personnel Residents/employees of high-risk congregate settings: prisons, jails, health care facilities, mycobacteriology labs, and homeless shelters Persons with certain medical conditions: diabetes mellitus, silicosis, chronic renal failure, etc. Malignancy Children younger than 4 years of age Infants, children, and adolescents exposed to adults at high risk
≥15	Persons with no risk factors for tuberculosis

HIV, human immunodeficiency virus; TNF-α, tumor necrosis factor-α.

Table 2-5 | Antituberculosis Regimens

	Regimen	Notes
LTBI	INH 9 months RIF 4 months INH + RIF × 3 months RIF + PZA for 2 months (if INH resistant)	Treat for LTBI only after active TB is ruled out INH × 1 year if HIV+
Active TB	INH/RIF/PZA/EMB for 2 months, followed by additional, based on culture and sensitivities Requires 4 months of treatment	Isolation precautions during initial 2–4 weeks of treatment
Drug-resistant TB	Seek expert advice, www.cdc.gov	

LTBI, latent TB infection; INH, isoniazid; RIF, rifampin; PZA, pyrazinamide; EMB, ethambutol; TB, tuberculosis; HIV, human immunodeficiency virus

    (3) Drug-resistant TB: Other regimens are recommended for patients who are drug resistant. Expert advice should be sought if the clinician is unfamiliar with drug-resistant TB.

    (4) For more information and alternative treatment regimens, see www.cdc.gov

  d. Antituberculous class-specific side effects (Table 2-6)

    (1) INH: hepatitis, peripheral neuropathy (coadminister vitamin B_6 [pyridoxine] to reduce the risk), central nervous system (CNS) effects

    (2) RIF: hepatitis, flu syndrome, orange body fluid (e.g., orange urine)

    (3) EMB: optic neuritis (red–green vision loss)

    (4) PZA: hyperuricemia and hepatotoxicity (need to assess uric acid level)

  e. Patients with active disease require combination chemotherapy for 6 to 9 months; patients infected with HIV require therapy for at least 1 year.

  f. INH for 6 to 12 months is indicated for prophylaxis in patients who have tested negative in the past but are now positive with known or unknown exposure (recent converters).

  g. Persons exposed to active TB should be screened with TST. Indurations >5 mm should be treated aggressively if indicated.

  h. The Bacille Calmette–Guérin (BCG) vaccine can be administered to a tuberculin-negative person in settings with a high risk for intense, prolonged exposure to untreated or ineffectively treated cases of infectious TB. This practice is not recommended in the United States, but it is common in areas with endemic TB.

  i. Children, adolescents, and the immunocompromised who have been in close contact with a person with active TB should be offered treatment until a TST is negative 12 weeks after exposure. Treatment of other cases should be dictated by TST status.

Table 2-6 | Common Side Effects of Antituberculin Medications

Medication	Side Effect
INH	Hepatitis Peripheral neuropathy (Vitamin B_6 [pyridoxine] to reduce risk) Rash CNS effects
RIF	Hepatitis Flu syndromes Orange body fluid (urine, sweat)
EMB	Optic neuritis (red–green vision) (reversible)
PZA	Hyperuricemia Hepatotoxicity

CNS, central nervous system; INH, isoniazid; RIF, rifampin; EMB, ethambutol; PZA, pyrazinamide.

G. **Acute bronchitis**

1. General characteristics

a. More than 90% of cases are caused by viruses, including rhinovirus, coronavirus, and RSV.

b. Bronchitis is defined as inflammation of the airways (trachea, bronchi, bronchioles) characterized by cough.

c. In patients with chronic lung disease, causes also include *H. influenzae*, *S. pneumoniae*, and *M. catarrhalis*.

2. **Clinical features**

a. Signs and symptoms include cough (with or without sputum), dyspnea, fever, sore throat, headache, myalgias, substernal discomfort, and expiratory rhonchi or wheezes.

b. Bronchitis can be difficult to distinguish from pneumonia, so the examination should be conducted to identify comorbid conditions that may influence the treatment.

3. Diagnostic studies

a. Generally, no laboratory evaluation is required unless there is a strong need to differentiate bronchitis from pneumonia.

b. The CXR will be negative in acute bronchitis.

4. **Management**

a. Supportive measures include hydration, expectorants, analgesics, β_2-agonists, and antitussives such as dextromethorphan, guaifenesin, dexbrompheniramine/pseudoephedrine, and bromhexine. Do not use nonprescription cough and cold products in children under 2 years of age.

b. For acute exacerbations of chronic bronchitis, in which bacterial causes are more likely, empiric first-line treatment is a second-generation cephalosporin; second-line treatment is a second-generation macrolide or trimethoprim–sulfamethoxazole.

c. Antibiotics are indicated for the following: elderly patients, those with underlying cardiopulmonary diseases and a cough for more than 7 to 10 days, and any patient who is immunocompromised.

d. For acute exacerbations in otherwise healthy adults, no empiric antibiotic treatment is needed.

H. **Acute bronchiolitis**

1. General characteristics

a. Bronchiolitis refers to inflammation of the bronchioles (airways <2 mm in diameter). It is primarily an illness of infants and young children <2 years.

b. RSV is the most common cause; other agents include parainfluenza virus, adenovirus, and rhinovirus. Most infections occur during wintertime epidemics.

2. **Clinical features**

a. Signs and symptoms include rhinorrhea, sneezing, wheezing, and low-grade fever.

b. Bronchiolitis typically begins with upper respiratory tract infection (URI) prodrome which progresses with signs of lower respiratory distress, including nasal flaring, tachypnea, and retractions. Severe disease may lead to apnea.

3. Diagnostic studies

a. Diagnosis should be made on history and physical examination without the need for laboratory and radiologic studies.

b. Pulse oximetry may be helpful if hospital admission being considered.

c. Viral Antigen Identification from nasal swab aids in diagnosis.

In bronchitis, sputum color is not predictive of bacterial involvement. Signs of pneumonia such as tachypnea and tachycardia should be absent.

RSV is the most common cause of bronchiolitis; treatment is supportive; add ribavirin for preemies or those with underlying chronic disease.

4. Management

    a. Supportive care with primary goals of ensuring oxygenation and hydration

    b. If RSV is present, consider hospitalization and administration of aerosolized rib-avirin especially of high-risk patients such as infants born premature, those with underlying chronic conditions, or those who are severely ill.

    c. Supportive measures, such as nebulized albuterol, intravenous (IV) fluids, antipyretics, chest physiotherapy, and humidified oxygen, are important.

I. **Acute epiglottitis**

    1. General characteristics

        a. This is a severe, life-threatening infection of the epiglottis.

        b. It may be of viral or bacterial origin.

        c. It may occur at any age; in children, it is most common between ages 2 and 7 years. In adults, most cases occur in the 45- to 65-year-old age group, and more commonly in patients with diabetes.

        d. The widespread administration of the *H. influenzae* type B (Hib) vaccine has decreased the incidence of epiglottitis in children. Many older adults, however, have not been immunized; therefore, the incidence of Hib-induced epiglottitis has increased in this population. The other common etiologies in adults include group A *Streptococcus*, *S. pneumoniae*, *H. parainfluenzae*, and *S. aureus*.

    2. Clinical findings

        a. Sudden onset of high fever, rapidly developing into a sore throat, odynophagia, respiratory distress, severe dysphagia, drooling, and muffled voice are characteristics.

        b. Examination may reveal mild stridor with little or no coughing; patients usually sit upright with their necks extended.

    3. Diagnostic studies

        a. Direct visualization with indirect laryngoscopy of the epiglottis is diagnostic in adults. Manipulation should be done under very controlled circumstances in children as it may initiate sudden, fatal airway obstruction.

        b. Once the airway is secured, obtain a complete blood count (CBC) and blood and epiglottic cultures.

        c. A lateral neck radiograph shows a swollen epiglottis (thumbprint sign) (Fig. 2-1).

    4. Management

        a. Secure airway: In pediatric patients, do not move or upset the child unless prepared to manage the airway.

        b. Administer broad-spectrum second- or third-generation cephalosporin such as cefotaxime or ceftriaxone for 7 to 10 days. Dexamethasone may also be indicated to reduce inflammation.

        c. Protect airway if needed with intubation.

J. **Croup**

    1. General characteristics

        a. Also known as acute viral laryngotracheobronchitis, which more commonly affects children aged 6 months to 5 years

        b. Most common cause is the parainfluenza virus types 1 and 2; RSV, adenovirus, influenza, and rhinovirus are also implicated.

    2. Clinical findings

        a. Harsh, barking, seal-like cough is characteristic; other symptoms include inspiratory stridor, hoarseness, aphonia, low-grade fever, and rhinorrhea.

> Lateral neck films: epiglottitis=thumbprint; croup=steeple sign.

> Croup is usually diagnosed clinically with the characteristic seal-like, barking cough; inspiratory stridor; low fever; and rhinorrhea.

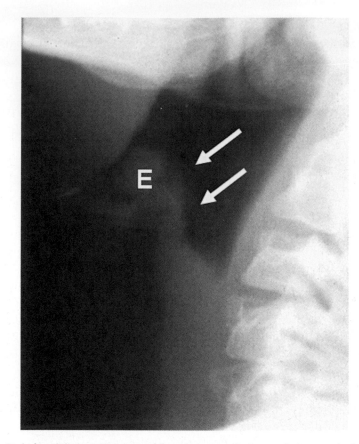

Figure 2-1 ▶ Epiglottitis in a 3-year-old girl. Lateral view of the neck shows thickening of the epiglottis (*E*) and aryepiglottic folds (*arrows*). (Reprinted with permission from Siegel MJ, Coley B. *Core Curriculum: Pediatric Imaging*. Lippincott Williams & Wilkins; 2005, Fig. 1.26.)

3. Diagnostic studies

   a. Diagnosis is usually made clinically with characteristic findings on history and physical examination.

   b. Posteroanterior (PA) neck film may show subglottic narrowing (steeple sign). The lateral neck film will differentiate croup from epiglottitis (thumbprint) (Fig. 2-2).

4. **Management**

   a. Mild croup does not usually require treatment as it is self-limited. Patients should stay well hydrated.

   b. Corticosteroids, humidified air or oxygen, and nebulized epinephrine may also be recommended in moderate to severe disease.

   c. Hospitalization may be required for patients with severe symptoms.

Neoplastic Diseases

A. **Bronchogenic carcinoma**

   1. General characteristics

      a. Bronchogenic carcinoma is the leading cause of cancer deaths in men and women. There are more deaths from lung cancer than from colon, breast, and prostate combined.

      b. The overall 5-year survival rate is 15%.

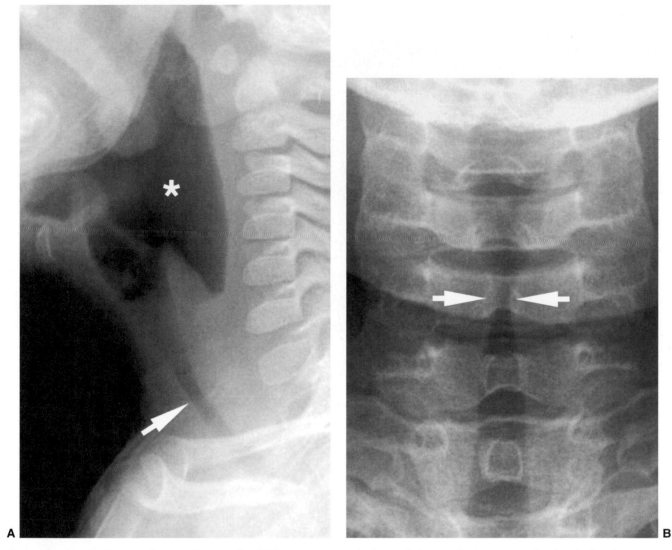

Figure 2-2 ▶ Viral croup in an 18-month-old boy. **A:** Lateral view of the neck shows marked subglottic tracheal narrowing (*arrow*) and distension of the hypopharynx (*asterisk*). **B:** Frontal view in another patient shows narrowing of the subglottic trachea (*arrows*). (Reprinted with permission from Siegel MJ, Coley B. *Core Curriculum: Pediatric Imaging*. Lippincott Williams & Wilkins; 2005, Fig. 1.27.)

   c. Smoking is the number one risk factor causing 85% to 95% of cases.

   d. Other risk factors: exposure to environmental tobacco smoke, radon, asbestos, diesel exhaust, ionizing radiation, metals (arsenic, chromium, nickel, iron oxide), and industrial carcinogens

   e. Bronchogenic carcinoma is divided into two major categories based on staging and treatment options: small-cell lung cancer (SCLC) and non-SCLC (NSCLC).

      (1) SCLC (oat cell)

         (a) Accounts for 13% of cases

         (b) Divided into two categories

            i. Limited (30%): Tumor is limited to the unilateral hemithorax.

            ii. Extensive disease (70%): Tumor extends beyond the hemithorax.

         (c) More likely to spread early and is rarely amenable to surgery (mean survival is 6 to 18 weeks if untreated).

Bronchogenic (lung) cancer is the cause of more deaths than colon, breast, and prostate cancers combined, with adenocarcinoma being the leading type.

(d) Tends to originate in the central bronchi and metastasize to regional lymph nodes.

(e) It is prone to early metastasis and an aggressive clinical course; assume micrometastases at presentation.

(2) NSCLC

(a) Grows more slowly and is more amenable to surgery. NSCLC includes squamous cell carcinoma, adenocarcinoma, and large cell carcinoma.

(b) Squamous cell carcinoma represents 23% of cases; is bronchial in origin and a centrally located mass; is more likely to present with hemoptysis and therefore more likely to be diagnosed via sputum cytology.

(c) Adenocarcinoma, the most common type of bronchogenic carcinoma, accounts for 47% of cases and is typically metastatic to distant organs. This tumor arises from mucous glands, usually appears in the periphery of the lung, and is not amenable to early detection through sputum examination.

  i. Bronchoalveolar cell carcinoma, a subtype of adenocarcinoma, is a low-grade carcinoma.

(d) Large cell carcinoma is a heterogeneous group of undifferentiated types that do not fit elsewhere; cytology typically shows large cells; doubling time is rapid; and metastasis is early; there may be central or peripheral masses.

2. **Clinical features**

  a. Symptoms include a new or changing cough, hemoptysis, pain, anorexia, weight loss, or asthenia.

  b. Patients may also exhibit lymphadenopathy, hepatomegaly, and clubbing of the fingers.

  c. Paraneoplastic syndromes occur in 10% to 20% of patients with lung cancer (Table 2-7).

3. Diagnostic studies

  a. CXR and computed tomography (CT) scans usually demonstrate abnormalities.

  b. Cytologic examination of sputum, if adequate cells are obtained, permits definitive diagnosis of a specific cell type in many cases.

  c. Bronchoscopy, examination of pleural fluid, and biopsy are used to establish a diagnosis by looking at specific cell types through direct visualization.

Table 2-7 | Paraneoplastic Syndromes

Lung Cancer Histologic Type	Classification	Syndrome
Small cell Squamous cell Large cell	Endocrine/metabolic	Cushing syndrome
		SIADH
		Hypercalcemia
		Gynecomastia
Small cell	Neuromuscular	Peripheral neuropathy
		Myasthenia (Eaton–Lambert)
		Cerebellar degeneration
Adenocarcinoma	Cardiovascular	Thrombophlebitis
All	Hematologic	Anemia
		DIC
		Eosinophilia
		Thrombocytosis
All	Cutaneous	Acanthosis nigricans

SIADH, syndrome of inappropriate antidiuretic hormone secretion; DIC, disseminated intravascular coagulation.

d. Positron emission tomography (PET) scans may also aid in diagnosis and avoid unnecessary surgery.

e. Tumor tissue analysis for epidermal growth factor receptor (EGFR) and K-RAS mutations which can guide chemotherapy selection

4. Management: All patients should be counseled to stop smoking.

   a. For NSCLC, surgery remains the treatment of choice if patient can tolerate the procedure and complete resection is possible. Cure is unlikely without resection. Adjuvant or neoadjuvant chemotherapy may be considered to improve survival.

   b. For SCLC, combination chemotherapy is the treatment of choice and results in improved median survival, although patients rarely live for >5 years after the diagnosis is established.

   c. Complications common to all types of bronchogenic carcinoma are listed in Table 2-8.

5. Screening

   a. The U.S. Preventive Services Task Force (USPSTF) recommends yearly screening with low-dose CT for lung cancer in those aged 50 to 80 years with a 20 pack-year smoking history who currently smoke or have quit in the past 15 years.

   b. Discontinue screening if a patient has not smoked for >15 years, has a medical condition that limits life expectancy, the ability or willingness to undergo lung surgery.

B. **Solitary pulmonary nodule**

   1. General characteristics (Table 2-9)

   a. Pulmonary nodules are also known as coin lesions. If the lesion measures >3 cm, it is referred to as a mass. They are completely surrounded by aerated lung and have no associated atelectasis, hilar enlargement, or pleural effusions.

> In SCLC, surgery is NOT recommended. In all other cancer types, surgery is an option along with chemotherapy.

Table 2-8 | SPHERE of Lung Cancer Complications

SVC syndrome	Compression of **S**VC: plethora, headache, mental status changes
Pancoast tumor	Tumor of the lung apex Causes Horner's syndrome and shoulder pain Affects brachial plexus and cervical sympathetic nerve
Horner's syndrome	Unilateral facial anhidrosis, ptosis, miosis
Endocrine	Carcinoid syndrome: flushing, diarrhea, telangiectasias
Recurrent laryngeal nerve	Hoarseness
Effusions	Exudative

SVC, superior vena cava.

Table 2-9 | Solitary Pulmonary Nodules

	Benign	**Malignant**
Characteristics	<30 years old Round, oval Sharply circumscribed margins Up to 3 cm Surrounded by normal tissue May be calcified	Older ages Round, oval, uneven Indistinct margins Usually >2 cm Rapidly progressive
Management	Low risk: CT every 3 months for a year Intermediate risk: hospitalize, biopsy, high-resolution CT or PET scan	If high probability: resect

CT, computed tomography; PET, positron emission tomography.

b. Solitary nodules are more often infectious granulomas from old or active TB, fungal infection, or foreign body reaction. Approximately 40% are malignant and represent carcinoma, hamartoma, or metastasis (but these are usually multiple) as well as bronchial adenoma (the majority of which are carcinoid tumors).

c. Malignant lesions have ill-defined margins, lobular in appearance, sparse calcifications that are typically stripped or eccentric.

d. Benign lesions are smooth with well-defined margins and dense calcifications in a central or laminated pattern.

e. Malignancy is rare in patients younger than 30 years of age. Smokers have an increased risk of malignancy; this increased risk rises with the number of pack-years.

2. Clinical features

a. Most pulmonary nodules are found unexpectedly at radiography and are asymptomatic.

b. Risk stratification guides clinical approach.

3. Diagnostic studies

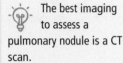

The best imaging to assess a pulmonary nodule is a CT scan.

a. CT provides accurate assessment of physical features of the nodule. Definitive diagnosis requires biopsy, but this is not always required. A solitary pulmonary nodule is a round or oval, sharply circumscribed pulmonary lesion/mass (up to 3 cm in diameter) surrounded by normal lung tissue.

b. Central cavitation, calcification, or surrounding (satellite) lesions may occur.

c. A lesion that has not enlarged in >2 years suggests a benign cause. Most are infectious granulomas.

d. Malignant lesions are occasionally symptomatic, tend to occur in patients older than 45 years of age, are usually >2 cm in diameter, often have indistinct margins, exhibit rapid progression in size, and are rarely calcified.

4. Management

a. Lesions with a low probability of malignancy can be watched. Patients should undergo CT every 3 months for a year; if stable, frequency of CT can be reduced to every 6 months for the next 2 years.

b. Lesions with a high probability of malignancy should be resected as soon as possible. An interim biopsy of a solitary nodule is not recommended.

c. Lesions with intermediate probability of malignancy should be biopsied; use transthoracic needle biopsy or bronchoscopy if the lesion is peripheral. False-positive rates can be as high as 25%. High-resolution CT or PET may aid in establishing the diagnosis. High-resolution CT is best to delineate the mass and detect adenopathy or the presence of multiple nodules.

C. Carcinoid tumors

1. General characteristics

a. Also known as carcinoid adenomas or bronchial gland tumors, these are well-differentiated neuroendocrine tumors that affect men and women equally. Patients are usually younger than 60 years of age.

Carcinoid syndrome develops in about 10% of those with carcinoid tumor.

b. Carcinoid tumors are rare, low-grade malignant neoplasms. They grow slowly and rarely metastasize and are more commonly found in the gastrointestinal (GI) tract.

2. Clinical features

a. Usually asymptomatic but hemoptysis, cough, focal wheezing, and recurrent pneumonia can occur.

b. Carcinoid syndrome (flushing, diarrhea, wheezing, hypotension) is rare, occurring in 10% of patients.

3. Diagnostic studies

    a. Bronchoscopy reveals a pink or purple central lesion that is well vascularized. The lesion can be pedunculated or sessile.

    b. CT and octreotide scintigraphy localize the disease. CT will localize the lesion as well as monitor for growth.

4. Management: Surgical excision carries a good prognosis. The lesions are resistant to radiation therapy and chemotherapy. Octreotide, a somatostatin analog that blocks hormone secretion, can be used to treat symptoms.

Obstructive Pulmonary Diseases

A. Asthma

    1. General characteristics

        a. Asthma is characterized by three components: obstruction of airflow, bronchial hyperreactivity, and inflammation of the airway. It is a disease of chronic inflammation leading to airway narrowing and increased mucus production.

        b. Asthma affects 8% to 10% of the population. Prevalence, hospitalization, and mortality have risen during the past 20 years.

        c. Many asthma syndromes have been identified: extrinsic allergic, allergic intrinsic asthma, extrinsic nonallergic, aspirin sensitivity, exercise induced, and asthma associated with COPD.

        d. The strongest predisposing factor to asthma is atopy. The atopic triad consists of wheeze, eczema, and seasonal rhinitis.

        e. Table 2-10 lists common asthma triggers that may precipitate exacerbation of symptoms. Exacerbations are often correlated with common precipitants.

> Asthma triad: obstruction of airflow, bronchial hyperactivity, inflammation
> Atopy triad: wheeze, eczema, seasonal rhinitis.

Table 2-10 | Common Precipitants of Acute Asthma Exacerbations

Precipitant	Example
Allergens	Dust, dust mites Dander Cockroaches Pollen
Exercise	Moderate or vigorous
Respiratory tract infections	Viral upper respiratory tract infection Rhinorrhea Sinusitis Postnasal drip
Gastrointestinal disorder	GERD Gastritis Spicy foods, intolerance
Drugs	β-Blockers ACEi Aspirin, NSAIDs Tobacco Cocaine Methamphetamines
Stress	Emotional stress Cold air Change in the weather Environmental irritants Air pollution

GERD, gastroesophageal reflux disease; ACEi, angiotensin-converting enzymes inhibitors; NSAIDs, nonsteroidal anti-inflammatory drugs.

2. **Clinical features**

a. Patients have an intermittent occurrence of cough, chest tightness, breathlessness, and wheezing. One-third of children with asthma have no wheeze.

b. Pulsus paradoxus and retractions are often present in severe episodes.

c. Patients undergo asymptomatic periods between these attacks.

d. Asthma is classified according to the frequency of symptoms and pulmonary function testing. In children, especially those younger than 5 years, the classification of asthma severity is more aggressive (Table 2-11).

3. Diagnostic studies

a. Airflow obstruction is indicated by decreased ratio of forced expiratory volume in 1 second to forced vital capacity ($FEV_1/FVC < 75\%$). A $>12\%$ increase in FEV_1 after bronchodilator therapy is supportive of the diagnosis.

b. Arterial blood gas (ABG) measurements may be normal in mild cases, but in severe cases, they may reveal hypoxemia and hypercapnia, with a PaO_2 of <60 mm Hg and a $PaCO_2$ of >40 mm Hg. ABGs are rarely indicated or obtained unless the patient is severely ill or nonresponsive to treatment.

c. CXR may show hyperinflation. Radiography is only indicated if pneumonia is suspected, the asthma is complicated, or another disorder is suspected.

d. Handheld peak expiratory flow meters estimate variability and quantify the severity of attacks. Use of this objective device should be encouraged in patients with chronic disease. Self-monitoring of symptoms and status leads to better outcomes.

e. A histamine or methacholine challenge test (bronchial provocation test) may help to establish the diagnosis of asthma when spirometry is nondiagnostic. An FEV_1 decrease of $>20\%$ is diagnostic.

4. **Management**

a. The goals of treatment are to minimize chronic symptoms; prevent recurrent exacerbations and thus minimize the need for urgent care visits; and maintain near-normal pulmonary function. Adequate hydration and avoidance of triggers are essential.

> In diagnosing asthma: $FEV_1/FVC < 75\%$ and $>12\%$ increase in FEV_1 after bronchodilator, or FEV_1 decrease of $>20\%$ in bronchial provocation test.

Table 2-11 | Classification of Severity of Chronic Stable Asthma

Severity	Symptoms	Nighttime Symptoms	Use of Rescue Medication	Lung Function	Recommended Step for Initiating Treatment	
Intermittent	Symptoms ≤2 days/week	≤2 times/month	<2 days/week	FEV_1 >80% predicted	Step 1	
	No interference with daily activities			FEV_1/FVC normal		
Mild persistent	>2 days/week but not daily	3–4 times/month	>2 days/week but not daily and not more than once on any day	FEV_1 >80% predicted	Step 2	
	Minor limitation			FEV_1/FVC normal		
Moderate persistent	Daily symptoms	>1 time/week but not nightly	Daily	FEV_1 >60% but <80% predicted	Step 3	Consider using oral steroids
	Some limitation in daily activity			FEV_1/FVC reduced 5%		
Severe persistent	Continual symptoms throughout the day	Often 7 times/week	Several times/day	FEV_1 <60% predicted	Step 4	
	Extremely limited physical activities			FEV_1/FVC reduced >5%		

FEV_1, forced expiratory volume in 1 second; FVC, forced vital capacity.

From National Institutes of Health, U.S. Department of Health & Human Services. *National Asthma Education and Prevention Program Expert Panel report 3: Guidelines for the Diagnosis and Management of Asthma*. National Institutes of Health, U.S. Department of Health & Human Services; 2007. NIH publication 08-5846.

b. Asthma medications can be divided into long-term control (corticosteroids, cromolyn, nedocromil, long-acting bronchodilators, leukotriene modifiers, and theophylline) and quick-relief ("rescue") medications (short-acting inhaled β_2-agonists, ipratropium bromide, and systemic corticosteroids).

c. Treatment algorithms are based on both the severity of the patient's baseline asthma and the severity of asthma exacerbations. In children, especially those younger than 5 years, the stepwise approach to treatment is more aggressive (Fig. 2-3).

d. β-Adrenergic agonists (also known as short-acting β-agonists [SABAs]) should be available to induce bronchodilation during acute symptoms (rescue medication).

e. Inhaled corticosteroids are the most effective anti-inflammatory medications for the management of chronic asthma.

f. Patients should be educated about their disease and the use of peak flow monitoring. Daily evaluation of pulmonary function with a peak flow meter is an important component of optimal asthma management. This type of monitoring warns of changes in disease status and allows for adjustments on a daily basis if needed. Changes in peak flow will occur prior to clinical symptoms.

> A peak flow meter is an easy and inexpensive tool to help patient's gauge their asthma symptoms.

B. **Bronchiectasis**

1. General characteristics

a. Bronchiectasis is defined as an abnormal, permanent dilation of the bronchi and destruction of bronchial walls. It can be congenital (cystic fibrosis [CF]) or acquired from recurrent infections (TB, fungal infection, lung abscess) or obstruction (tumor).

b. Bronchiectasis results from bronchial injury subsequent to severe infection and/or inflammation.

c. Half of all cases occur in patients with CF.

2. **Clinical features**

a. Symptoms include chronic purulent sputum (often foul smelling), hemoptysis, chronic cough, and recurrent pneumonia. Dyspnea and wheezing occur in 75% of patients.

b. Physical examination may reveal localized chest crackles and clubbing of the fingers.

3. Diagnostic studies

a. High-resolution chest CT is the imaging diagnostic of choice; it reveals dilated, tortuous airways, tram tracks, and rings.

b. CXR in patients with clinically significant bronchiectasis is abnormal. The degree of abnormality depends on the extent and severity of the disease. Crowded bronchial markings and basal cystic spaces are characteristics. CXR may reveal tram-track lung markings, honeycombing, and atelectasis.

c. Bronchoscopy is warranted to evaluate hemoptysis, remove secretions, and rule out obstructing lesions.

(1) *H. influenzae* is the most common organism in non-CF patients.

(2) *P. aeruginosa* is the most common organism in CF patients.

> Bronchiectasis is most often seen in CF. Imaging in CF shows tortuous airways, tram track, honeycombing, and atelectasis.

4. **Management**

a. A productive cough should be managed with the appropriate antibiotic, bronchodilators, and chest physiotherapy.

b. Antibiotics are prescribed for 10 to 14 days for acute symptoms; suppressive therapy may be helpful in severe disease or in patients with rapid recurrence. Amoxicillin, amoxicillin–clavulanate, trimethoprim–sulfamethoxazole, and ciprofloxacin are effective choices.

c. Bronchodilators are helpful for maintenance and for treating acute exacerbations.

Treatment	Intermittent Asthma STEP 1	Management of Persistent Asthma				
		STEP 2	STEP 3	STEP 4	STEP 5	STEP 6■
Preferred	PRN SABA	Daily low-dose ICS and PRN SABA or PRN concomitant ICS and SABA⅄	Daily and PRN combination low-dose ICS-formoterol⅄	Daily and PRN combination medium-dose ICS-formoterol⅄	Daily medium- to high-dose ICS-LABA + LAMA and PRN SABA⅄	Daily high-dose ICS-LABA + oral systemic corticosteroids + PRN SABA
Alternative		Daily LTRA* and PRN SABA or Cromolyn,* Nedocromil,* Zileuton,* or Theophylline,* and PRN SABA	Daily medium-dose ICS and PRN SABA or Daily low-dose ICS-LABA, or daily low-dose ICS + LAMA, ⅄ or daily low-dose ICS + LTRA,* and PRN SABA or Daily low-dose ICS + Theophylline* or Zileuton,* and PRN SABA	Daily medium-dose ICS-LABA or daily medium-dose ICS + LAMA, and PRN SABA⅄ or Daily medium-dose ICS + LTRA,* or daily medium-dose ICS + Theophylline,* or daily medium-dose ICS + Zileuton,* and PRN SABA	Daily medium- to high-dose ICS-LABA or daily high-dose ICS + LTRA,* and PRN SABA	
		Steps 2–4: Conditionally recommend the use of subcutaneous immunotherapy as an adjunct treatment to standard pharmacotherapy in individuals ≥5 years of age whose asthma is controlled at the initiation, buildup, and maintenance phases of immunotherapy⅄			Consider adding Asthma Biologics (e.g., anti-IgE, anti-IL5, anti-IL5R, anti-IL4/IL13)**	

Assess Control

- First check adherence, inhaler technique, environmental factors, ⅄ and comorbid conditions.
- **Step up** if needed; reassess in 2–6 weeks
- **Step down** if possible (if asthma is well controlled for at least 3 consecutive months)

Consult with asthma specialist if Step 4 or higher is required. Consider consultation at Step 3.

Control assessment is a key element of asthma care. This involves both impairment and risk. Use of objective measures, self-reported control, and health care utilization are complementary and should be employed on an ongoing basis, depending on the individual's clinical situation.

Abbreviations: ICS, inhaled corticosteroid; LABA, long-acting beta$_2$-agonist; LAMA, long-acting muscarinic antagonist; LTRA, leukotriene receptor antagonist; SABA, inhaled short-acting beta$_2$-agonist

⅄ Updated based on the 2020 guidelines.

* Cromolyn, Nedocromil, LTRAs including Zileuton and montelukast, and Theophylline were not considered for this update, and/or have limited availability for use in the United States, and/or have an increased risk of adverse consequences and need for monitoring that make their use less desirable. The FDA issued a Boxed Warning for montelukast in March 2020.

** The AHRQ systematic reviews that informed this report did not include studies that examined the role of asthma biologics (e.g. anti-IgE, anti-IL5, anti-IL5R, anti-IL4/IL13). Thus, this report does not contain specific recommendations for the use of biologics in asthma in Steps 5 and 6.

■ Data on the use of LAMA therapy in individuals with severe persistent asthma (Step 6) were not included in the AHRQ systematic review and thus no recommendation is made.

Figure 2-3 ▶ Stepwise approach for managing asthma. (From National Institutes of Health, U.S. Department of Health & Human Services. *2020 Focused Updates to the Asthma Management Guidelines: Clinician's Guide.* National Institutes of Health, U.S. Department of Health & Human Services; 2020. NIH publication 20-HL-8141. Accessed October 2021. https://www.nhlbi.nih.gov/sites/default/files/publications/Asthma%20 Clinicians%20Guide%20508_02-03-21.pdf)

d. Patients with disabling symptoms or progressive bronchiectasis can be considered for lung transplant; however, surgical interventions have little long-term benefit.

C. COPD

1. General characteristics

a. COPD is a clinical and pathophysiologic syndrome of persistent respiratory symptoms and air flow restriction owing to airway and alveolar abnormalities caused by substantial exposure to toxic particles of gas. Most COPD has features of emphysema and chronic bronchitis.

b. These disorders have overlapping features, and because patients often have characteristics of more than one disorder, both are classified together as COPD (Table 2-12).

(1) Emphysema is a condition in which the air spaces are enlarged as a consequence of destruction of alveolar septa

(2) Chronic bronchitis is a disease characterized by a chronic cough that is productive of phlegm occurring daily for 3 months of the year for 2 or more consecutive years without an otherwise-defined acute cause.

c. Smoking is the strongest contributory factor of COPD. Other causes include environmental pollutants, occupational dust or chemicals, recurrent upper respiratory infections, eosinophilia, bronchial hyperresponsiveness, and α_1-antitrypsin deficiency.

d. Symptoms are commonly triggered by infection or environmental factors.

e. The disease is usually progressive with a long-term decline in lung function.

f. Moderate to severe disease typically presents in the fifth or sixth decade of life.

2. Clinical features

a. Patients present with a history of progressive shortness of breath, excessive cough, and sputum production. Patients with predominantly emphysematous COPD may have dry cough and weight loss.

b. The physical examination of a patient with advanced COPD may reveal asthenia, dyspnea, pursed-lip breathing, and grunting expirations.

c. Chest examination

(1) Signs of hyperinflation with an increase in the anteroposterior dimension are noted.

(2) Increased resonance to percussion

> Risk factors for COPD: smoking, pollutants, occupational dust, eosinophilia, bronchial hyperresponsiveness, alpha-1 antitrypsin deficiency.

Table 2-12 | Chronic Obstructive Pulmonary Disease Comparisons

	Emphysema Predominant	Bronchitis Predominant
"Classic" patient type	"Pink puffers"	"Blue bloaters"
Clinical findings	Exertional dyspnea Cough is rare Quiet lungs No peripheral edema Thin; recent weight loss Barrel chest Hyperventilation Pursed-lip breathing	Mild dyspnea Chronic productive cough Noisy lungs: rhonchi and wheeze Peripheral edema Overweight and cyanotic
Chest radiography	Decreased lung markings at apices Flattened diaphragms Hyperinflation Small, thin-appearing heart Parenchymal bullae and blebs	Increased interstitial markings at bases Diaphragms not flattened

(3) Auscultation reveals decreased breath sounds and early inspiratory crackles. The duration of expiration is prolonged.

(4) Wheezing may not be present at rest but can be evoked with forced expiration or exertion.

d. In patients with chronic bronchitis, rhonchi reflect secretions in the airways, and breathing is typically raspy and loud.

3. Diagnostic studies

a. CXR

(1) CXR may show hyperinflation of the lungs and flattened diaphragms; however, a CXR is not sensitive or specific enough to serve as a diagnostic or screening tool.

(2) If emphysema is the main clinical feature, parenchymal bullae or subpleural blebs are pathognomonic.

(3) In chronic bronchitis, nonspecific peribronchial and perivascular markings may be present.

> CXR in COPD may have the following characteristic findings: hyperinflation, flattened diaphragms, subpleural blebs, or nonspecific peribronchial markings.

b. Pulmonary function testing

(1) Airflow obstruction demonstrated on forced expiratory spirometry is suggestive.

(2) The FEV_1/FVC ratio is decreased.

c. The CBC may show polycythemia secondary to chronic hypoxemia.

d. Screening is recommended for α_1-antitrypsin deficiency in patients with possible COPD who are young, have a positive family history of COPD at a young age, or have emphysema.

4. **Management**

a. In symptomatic patients, the goal of treatment is to improve their functional state and relieve symptoms.

b. Smoking cessation is the single most important intervention.

c. Anticholinergic inhalers (ipratropium or tiotropium) are superior to β-adrenergic agonists in achieving bronchodilation in patients with COPD.

d. Short-acting bronchodilators should be prescribed for acute exacerbations of dyspnea.

e. These patients are at high risk for acute infections; therefore, oral antibiotics are frequently necessary.

> The most important component in the management of COPD is avoiding all contact with cigarette smoke.

f. Supplemental oxygen is the only therapy that may alter the course of COPD in patients with resting hypoxemia ($PaO_2 < 55$ mm Hg or $SaO_2 < 88\%$).

g. Graded aerobic physical exercise should be encouraged.

h. Steroids are effective but should be used with caution owing to systemic adverse effects.

i. Human α_1-antitrypsin replacement may be recommended for patients who are deficient.

j. Patients should receive the pneumococcal vaccine and yearly influenza vaccine.

D. **Cystic fibrosis**

1. General characteristics

a. CF is an autosomal recessive disorder that results in the abnormal production of mucus by almost all exocrine glands, causing obstruction of those glands and ducts.

b. Patients are at increased risk of malignancies of the GI tract, osteopenia, and arthropathies.

2. **Clinical features**

a. Most cases are identified in infancy or early childhood: meconium ileus 20%, respiratory symptoms 45%, failure to thrive 25%.

   b. The diagnosis should be suspected in any young patient who presents with a history of chronic lung disease (bronchiectasis), pancreatitis, or infertility.

   c. Symptoms include cough, excess sputum, decreased exercise tolerance, recurrent hemoptysis, sinus pain, purulent nasal discharge, steatorrhea, diarrhea, and abdominal pain.

   d. Signs include clubbing of the fingers, increased anteroposterior chest diameter, malnutrition, and apical crackles.

3. Diagnostic studies

   a. ABG studies reveal hypoxemia and, in advanced disease, a chronic, compensated respiratory acidosis.

   b. Pulmonary function tests reveal a mixed obstructive and restrictive pattern.

   c. CXR may reveal hyperinflation; peribronchial cuffing; mucous plugging; bronchiectasis; increased interstitial markings; small, round peripheral opacities; focal atelectasis; or pneumothorax.

   d. Thin-section CT may confirm the presence of bronchiectasis.

   e. An elevated quantitative pilocarpine iontophoresis sweat chloride test (>60 mEq/L) performed on two different days is diagnostic; however, a normal result does not exclude the diagnosis. If the diagnosis is strongly suspected, DNA testing (CFTR genotyping) can provide definitive evidence of cystic fibrosis.

4. Management

   a. Comprehensive multidisciplinary therapy improves the control of symptoms and the chances of survival. Median survival is 40 years.

   b. For patients ≤ 6 years of age, there is insufficient evidence to recommend the best treatment.

   c. Therapies focus on the following areas: clearance of airway secretions, reversal of bronchoconstriction, treatment of respiratory infections, replacement of pancreatic enzymes, and nutritional and psychosocial support.

   d. Lung transplant is the only definitive treatment.

   e. Screening family members and genetic counseling for those diagnosed with CF are recommended.

   f. Pneumococcal vaccine and yearly influenza are advised.

Pleural Diseases

A. **Pleural effusion** (Table 2-13)

   1. General characteristics

      a. Pleural effusion (the accumulation of significant volumes of pleural fluid) may result from inflammation of structures adjacent to the pleural space or lesions within the chest.

      b. Small effusions may not cause symptoms and may be first discovered on routine radiography.

      c. About 25% of effusions are associated with malignancy.

      d. There are four types of effusions:

        (1) Exudative effusions are associated with "leaky capillaries"; causes include infection, malignancy, and trauma.

        (2) Transudative effusions ("intact capillaries") are associated with increased hydrostatic or decreased oncotic pressure; examples include congestive heart failure, atelectasis, and renal or liver disease (cirrhosis).

        (3) An empyema is an infection within the pleural space.

CF includes pulmonary findings in 90% of patients and can also present with pancreatic insufficiency and multiple GI symptoms.

CF patients require aggressive supportive care, including preventive care and vaccines.

Table 2-13 Pleural Effusions

	Exudative	Transudative	Empyema	Hemothorax
Pathogenesis	Leaky capillaries	Increased hydrostatic or decreased oncotic pressure	Infection in pleural space	Bleeding into pleural space
Causes	Infection Malignancy Trauma	Congestive heart failure Atelectasis Renal disease Liver disease (cirrhosis)	Infection	Trauma
Pleural fluid findings	Protein to serum protein ratio >0.5 LDH to serum LDH ratio >0.6 LDH >2/3 the upper limit of normal for serum LDH	Protein to serum protein ratio <0.5 LDH to serum LDH ratio <0.6 LDH <2/3 the upper limit of normal for serum LDH	WBCs	Blood
Intervention	Drainage, pleurodesis	Treat underlying cause	Drainage and antibiotics	Drainage and further as needed

LDH, lactate dehydrogenase; WBC, white blood cell.

(4) A hemothorax indicates bleeding into the pleural space, commonly as a result of trauma or malignancy.

2. **Clinical features**

   a. With a small inflammatory effusion, patients are often asymptomatic.

   b. Large or bilateral pleural effusions may lead to dyspnea, but orthopnea is uncommon in the absence of congestive heart failure.

   c. A dull to flat percussion note over the area of fluid may be heard as well as reduced or absent breath sounds.

   d. The mediastinum is usually shifted away from the side of the large effusion.

3. Diagnostic studies

   a. Radiographic findings include blunting of the costophrenic angle, loss of sharp demarcation of the diaphragm and heart, and mediastinal shift to the uninvolved side.

   b. Lateral decubitus radiography can help to identify small effusions and differentiate free-flowing versus loculated fluid.

   c. CT may be useful if plain-film radiography cannot separate parenchymal and pleural densities.

   d. Thoracentesis is the gold standard; the fluid is sent for protein, lactate dehydrogenase (LDH), pH, total WBC and differential cell counts, glucose, cytology, and Gram stain with culture and sensitivity.

   e. Transudates versus exudates (Light's criteria): Fluid is considered to be an exudate if it meets any *one* of the following:

      (1) Pleural fluid protein to serum protein ratio of >0.5

      (2) Pleural fluid LDH to serum LDH ratio of >0.6

      (3) Pleural fluid LDH greater than two-thirds the upper limit of normal for serum LDH

4. **Management**

   a. Unless the cause has been clearly established and a viable plan initiated, the presence of fluid is an indication for thoracocentesis. Removal of fluid via thoracocentesis allows fluid examination, radiographic visualization of the lung parenchyma, and relief of symptoms.

   b. Transudate pleural effusions resolve when underlying causes are treated.

   c. Malignant effusions may require drainage and pleurodesis. The most commonly used irritants are doxycycline and talc.

   d. Empyema requires drainage and antibiotic therapy.

> Pleural effusion is associated with dullness or flat percussion on exam. Plain radiography is sufficient for confirmation.

B. Pneumothorax

1. General characteristics

a. Pneumothorax is the accumulation of air in the pleural space.

b. The cause may be spontaneous (primary or secondary pneumothorax), traumatic (penetrating or blunt), or iatrogenic (owing to a procedure).

(1) Primary pneumothorax occurs in the absence of lung disease.

(2) Secondary pneumothorax is a result of a complication of an underlying lung disease.

c. Tall, thin males between 10 and 30 years of age are at greatest risk of primary pneumothorax. Additional risk factors include smoking and family history.

d. Tension pneumothorax can be life-threatening and is secondary to a sucking chest wound or a pulmonary laceration that allows air to enter the chest with inspiration but does not allow it to leave on expiration (Fig. 2-4).

2. Clinical features

a. Pneumothorax is characterized by the acute onset of ipsilateral chest pain and dyspnea. Physical findings depend on the size of the pneumothorax and may include unilateral chest expansion, decreased tactile fremitus, hyperresonance, and diminished breath sounds.

b. Tension pneumothorax is associated with a mediastinal shift to the contralateral side and impaired ventilation, leading to cardiovascular compromise.

3. Diagnostic studies

a. Expiratory CXR reveals the presence of pleural air. The "deep sulcus" sign, an abnormal radiolucent costophrenic sulcus, is indirect evidence of pneumothorax. A visceral pleural line may be the only evidence of a small pneumothorax (Fig. 2-5).

b. ABG analysis, if done, reveals hypoxemia.

> 💡 Young, tall, thin males are at highest risk of developing pneumothorax.

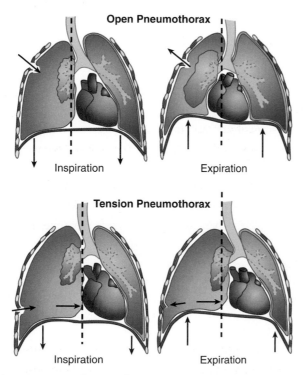

Figure 2-4 ▶ Tension pneumothorax. (Reprinted with permission from Hannon R. *Porth Pathophysiology.* 2nd ed. Wolters Kluwer Health; 2016, Fig. 29.4.)

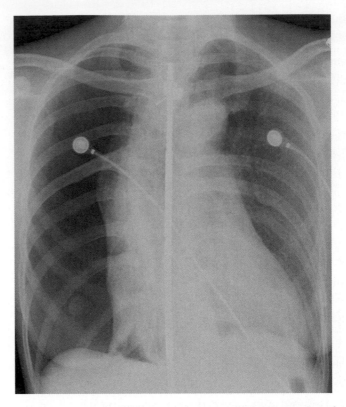

Figure 2-5 ▶ Primary spontaneous pneumothorax. Posteroanterior chest radiograph of a 46-year-old man with acute chest pain shows a right pneumothorax and collapse of the right lung. (Reprinted with permission from Collins J, Stern EJ. *Chest Radiology: The Essentials*. 3rd ed. Lippincott Williams & Wilkins/Wolters Kluwer; 2014, Fig. 9.31A.)

    4. Management depends on the severity.

        a. Small pneumothoraces (<15% of the diameter of the hemithorax) resolve spontaneously.

        b. For severely symptomatic or large pneumothoraces, chest tube placement is performed.

        c. Tension pneumothorax is a medical emergency. If it is suspected, a large-bore needle should be inserted through the chest wall (second or third intercostal space in the midclavicular line) to allow air to move out of the chest. Placement of a chest tube follows the decompression.

        d. Patients should be followed with serial CXR every 24 hours until resolved.

        e. Patients who smoke should be advised to discontinue owing to 50% recurrence if continued smoking.

Pulmonary Circulation

A. Pulmonary embolism (PE)

    1. General characteristics

        a. PE arises from thrombi in the systemic venous circulation or the right side of the heart, from tumors that have invaded the venous circulation, foreign body (IV drug users), septic emboli, parasitic eggs, and other sources.

        b. More than 90% of pulmonary emboli originate as clots in the deep veins of the lower extremities; others include air emboli from central lines, amniotic fluid from active labor, and fat from long bone (femur) fracture.

c. Risk factors revolve around Virchow's triad: hypercoagulable state (any exogenous hormones, Factor V Leiden, polycythemia vera), venous stasis (bedridden, obesity, cerebrovascular accident [CVA] patient, pregnancy), and vascular intimal inflammation or injury. Specific risks include surgical procedures (orthopedic, pelvic, abdominal), cancer, oral contraceptives, and pregnancy.

d. Approximately 50% to 60% of patients with deep vein thrombosis (DVT) will experience a PE; half of these will be asymptomatic; often the PE is found only on autopsy. Symptomatic PE is a serious and potentially fatal condition.

e. PE is the third leading cause of death in hospitalized patients.

2. **Clinical features**

a. Symptoms include sudden onset of pleuritic chest pain, dyspnea, apprehension, cough, hemoptysis, and diaphoresis.

b. Signs include tachycardia, tachypnea, crackles, accentuation of the pulmonary component of the second heart sound, and a low-grade fever. Homans' sign lacks sensitivity and specificity for DVT.

3. Diagnostic studies

> Diagnosing PE: a spiral CT is the initial imaging study of choice, instead of a ventilation–perfusion scan; CXR is not definitive; electrocardiography (ECG) may show a classic $S_1Q_3T_3$ pattern.

a. Spiral CT has now replaced ventilation–perfusion scans as the initial method of identifying pulmonary embolus.

b. ABG measurements can show acute respiratory alkalosis secondary to hyperventilation.

c. ECG is abnormal in 70% of PE patients; tachycardia and nonspecific ST–T wave changes are most common. The classic $S_1Q_3T_3$ pattern, indicating cor pulmonale, is seen in <20% of patients with symptomatic PE.

d. CXR may show nonspecific abnormalities such as basilar atelectasis. The main purpose of obtaining CXR is to rule out other abnormalities and aid in interpreting further imaging.

e. Venous ultrasound is done to assess the possibility of DVT. About 70% of PE patients will have a concurrent DVT. Although the majority of DVTs originate in the lower leg, the majority of those which embolize to the lungs originate in the thigh vessels.

f. A ventilation–perfusion lung scan may be indicated in patients unable to tolerate CT. It will show perfusion defects with normal ventilation. A normal scan rules out clinically significant thromboembolism. Nondiagnostic scans warrant further testing.

g. Measuring plasma dimerized plasmin fragment D (D-dimer) may be useful, especially to rule out PE if clinical suspicion is low and D-dimer is negative.

h. Pulmonary angiography remains the definitive test for diagnosis but is reserved for cases in which the diagnosis is uncertain after noninvasive testing.

4. **Management**

a. Anticoagulation therapy is initiated; heparin is the initial anticoagulant of choice. Low-molecular-weight heparin or warfarin is continued after the acute phase.

b. Newer agents such as factor Xa inhibitors (rivaroxaban, apixaban) and direct thrombin inhibitors are alternative options.

> Heparin is started in acute PE to prevent further propagation of clot.

c. Thrombolytic therapy (streptokinase, urokinase, recombinant tissue plasminogen activator [rt-PA]) may be appropriate for patients who are hemodynamically unstable despite heparin therapy.

d. Duration of therapy depends on the clinical situation. A minimum of 3 months is advised.

e. Vena cava interruption (filter) is helpful in patients at high risk of recurrence who are unable to tolerate anticoagulants or at high risk of bleeding and falls.

f. Prevention is the key. For high-risk patients, consider the following: early ambulation, intermittent pneumatic compression stockings, low-dose heparin and low-molecular-weight heparin, or a combination of mechanical and pharmacologic measures.

B. **Pulmonary hypertension (HTN)**

1. General characteristics

   a. Pulmonary HTN is present when the pulmonary arterial pressure rises to a level inappropriate for a given cardiac output. Once present, it is self-perpetuating.

   b. Hypoxia is the most important and potent stimulus of pulmonary arterial vasoconstriction. Other causes include acidosis and veno-occlusive conditions.

   c. The World Health Organization currently classifies pulmonary HTN by pathological mechanisms:

   (1) Group 1: Idiopathic pulmonary arterial HTN (formally primary), HIV infection, portal HTN, drug and toxins, heritable pulmonary arterial HTN, congenital heart disease

   (2) Group 2: Pulmonary venous HTN, left ventricular systolic or diastolic HTN, valvular heart disease

   (3) Group 3: Caused by advanced restrictive and obstructive lung disease, COPD, pulmonary fibrosis, interstitial lung disease, bronchiectasis

   (4) Group 4: Caused by thromboembolic occlusion of the proximal and distal pulmonary arteries

   (5) Group 5: Secondary to hematologic disorders such as chronic hemolytic anemia, myeloproliferative disorders, splenectomy, sarcoidosis, and vasculitis

   d. The clinical severity is classified by the New York Heart Association based on symptoms and functional status:

   (1) Class I: Without limitation of physical activity and asymptomatic

   (2) Class II: Slight limitation of physical activity. No symptoms at rest, though ordinary physical activity causes dyspnea, fatigue, chest pain, or near syncope.

   (3) Class III: Marked limitation of physical activity. No symptoms at rest, but less than ordinary physical activity causes dyspnea, fatigue, chest pain, or near syncope.

   (4) Class IV: Inability to perform any physical activity without symptoms. Evidence of right-sided heart failure with dyspnea and at rest and worsening with activity.

2. **Clinical features**

   a. Clinical manifestations may include dyspnea, angina-like retrosternal chest pain, weakness, fatigue, jugular venous distension, edema, ascites, cyanosis, and effort syncope.

   b. Signs may include narrow splitting and accentuation of the second heart sound and a systolic ejection click.

3. Diagnostic studies

   a. CXR and CT scans may show enlarged pulmonary arteries.

   b. Electrocardiography is usually normal, but advanced disease may show right ventricular hypertrophy, atrial hypertrophy, and right ventricular strain.

   c. Echocardiography may be useful in estimating pulmonary arterial pressure, but right heart catheterization offers more precise hemodynamic monitoring and assesses vasodilator response. Mean pulmonary arterial pressure ≥25 mm Hg is diagnostic.

   d. Pulmonary angiography is currently the standard for definitive diagnosis.

4. **Management**

   a. Treatment of primary pulmonary HTN may include chronic oral anticoagulants, calcium channel blockers to lower systemic arterial pressure, and prostacyclin (a potent pulmonary vasodilator). Endothelin receptor antagonists and phosphodiesterase inhibitors may also show improvement in symptoms.

> 💡 Pulmonary hypertension is associated with narrow splitting and accentuation of the second heart sound along with a systolic ejection click.

b. Heart–lung transplantation may be indicated if medical management is no longer effective.

c. Treatment of secondary pulmonary HTN consists of treating the underlying disorder in addition to those treatments mentioned earlier.

Restrictive Pulmonary Diseases

A. **Idiopathic fibrosing interstitial pneumonia (formerly idiopathic pulmonary fibrosis)**

1. General characteristics

a. This is the most common diagnosis among patients with interstitial lung disease.

b. Risk factors include cigarette smoking, exposure to metal and wood dust, and possibly exposure to certain viruses, diabetes, and gastroesophageal reflux disease (GERD).

c. More common in men aged 40 to 65 years

d. There are three histopathologic patterns with different natural histories and treatments: usual (most common) and nonspecific interstitial pneumonia; respiratory bronchiolitis–associated interstitial lung disease; cryptogenic organized pneumonia; and acute interstitial pneumonitis.

2. Clinical features

a. Symptoms include an insidious dry cough, exertional dyspnea, and constitutional symptoms (fatigue, malaise, etc.).

b. Examination may reveal clubbing of the fingers and inspiratory crackles.

3. Diagnostic studies

a. CXR demonstrates evidence of progressive fibrosis over several years.

b. CT shows diffuse, patchy fibrosis with pleural-based honeycombing.

c. Pulmonary function tests may show a restrictive pattern (decreased lung volume with a normal to increased FEV_1/FVC ratio).

d. Bronchoalveolar lavage, transbronchial biopsy, and surgical lung biopsy may also help to secure the diagnosis.

4. Management

a. Remains controversial; no therapeutic intervention has been shown to improve survival or quality of life compared to no treatment.

b. Definitive treatment is lung transplant.

B. **Pneumoconioses**

1. General characteristics

a. Pneumoconioses are chronic fibrotic lung diseases caused by the inhalation of coal dust or various inert, inorganic, or silicate dust.

b. Clinically important pneumoconioses include coal workers' pneumoconiosis, silicosis, berylliosis, and asbestosis.

2. Clinical features

a. In simple cases, pneumoconioses are usually asymptomatic.

b. In complicated cases, patients have dyspnea, inspiratory crackles, clubbing of the fingers, and cyanosis.

c. Table 2-14 provides a comparison of the most common pneumoconioses.

3. Diagnostic studies

a. Pulmonary function tests show restrictive dysfunction and reduced diffusing capacity.

> Restrictive lung disease is defined as a decreased lung volume with a normal to increased FIEV1/FVC ration.

Table 2-14 | Comparison of Pneumoconioses

Disease	Occupation	Diagnosis	Complications
Asbestosis	Insulation, demolition, construction, shipyard Agent: Asbestos	Bx: asbestos bodies CXR: linear opacities at bases and pleural plaques/calcifications	Increased risk of lung cancer and mesothelioma, especially if a smoker
Coal workers' pneumoconiosis	Coal mining Agent: Coal dust	CXR: nodular opacities at upper lung fields	Progressive massive fibrosis; Caplan's syndrome: necrobiotic rheumatoid nodules in lung periphery in RA patients
Silicosis	Mining, sandblasting, quarry work, stonework Agent: Free Silica	CXR: nodular opacities at upper lung fields; "eggshell" calcifications	Increased risk of tuberculosis; progressive massive fibrosis
Berylliosis	High-technology fields: aerospace, nuclear power, ceramics, foundries, tool and die manufacturing	CXR: diffuse infiltrates and hilar adenopathy	Requires chronic steroids

Bx, biopsy; CXR, chest radiography; RA, rheumatoid arthritis.

    b. CXR

        (1) Coal workers' pneumoconiosis: Small opacities are prominent in the upper lung fields.

        (2) Silicosis: Small rounded opacities are seen throughout the lung, and hilar lymph nodes may be calcified also known as "eggshell" calcifications.

        (3) Asbestosis: Interstitial fibrosis, thickened pleura, and calcified plaques appear on the diaphragms or lateral chest wall.

  4. Management

    a. Primarily supportive as no effective treatment is available. Supportive therapy includes oxygen, vaccinations (pneumococcal, influenza vaccine), and rehabilitation.

    b. Corticosteroids may relieve chronic alveolitis in silicosis.

    c. Smoking cessation is especially important for patients with asbestosis because smoking interferes with short asbestos fiber clearance from the lung. Smoking and asbestos are synergistically linked to lung cancer, especially mesothelioma.

C. Sarcoidosis

  1. General characteristics

    a. Sarcoidosis is a multiorgan disease of idiopathic cause. It is characterized by noncaseating granulomatous inflammation in affected organs (e.g., lungs, lymph nodes, eyes, skin, liver, spleen, salivary glands, heart, nervous system).

    b. Approximately 90% of patients have lung involvement.

    c. The incidence is highest in North American blacks (especially women) and Northern European whites.

    d. Onset is typically in the third or fourth decade.

  2. Clinical features

    a. Common respiratory symptoms include cough, dyspnea of insidious onset, and chest discomfort.

    b. Patients may present with malaise, fever, and symptoms consistent with the involvement of various organs.

    c. Extrapulmonary findings are common and include erythema nodosum, lupus pernio, or enlargement of parotid glands, lymph nodes, liver, or spleen.

  3. Diagnostic studies

    a. Serum blood tests may show leukopenia, eosinophilia, elevated erythrocyte sedimentation rate, hypercalcemia, and hypercalciuria.

> 90% of patients with sarcoid have lung disease; disease also develops in the skin, parotid glands, lymph nodes, liver and spleen.

   b. Angiotensin-converting enzyme levels are elevated in 40% to 80% of patients.

   c. Skin test anergy is present in 70% of patients.

   d. Chest x-ray findings demonstrate symmetric bilateral hilar and right paratracheal adenopathy and bilateral diffuse reticular infiltrates.

   e. Transbronchial biopsy of the lung or fine-needle node biopsy confirms the diagnosis. Biopsy shows noncaseating granulomas.

4. **Management**

   a. There is no cure.

   b. Approximately 90% of cases are responsive to corticosteroids and can be controlled with modest maintenance doses.

   c. Immunosuppressant cytotoxic drugs (methotrexate or infliximab) for patients refractory to corticosteroids

Other Pulmonary Diseases

A. **Acute respiratory distress syndrome (ARDS)**

1. General characteristics

   a. ARDS is defined as lung injury marked by acute onset of respiratory insufficiency with hypoxemia and bilateral radiographic infiltrates and without left atrial HTN.

   b. Three clinical settings account for 75% of ARDS cases: sepsis syndrome (the single most important), severe multiple trauma, and aspiration of gastric contents. Other causes include shock, toxic inhalation, near-drowning, and multiple transfusions.

   c. The underlying abnormality in ARDS is increased permeability of the alveolar-capillary membranes, which leads to the development of protein-rich pulmonary edema.

2. **Clinical features**

   a. Rapid onset of profound dyspnea occurring 12 to 48 hours after the precipitating event

   b. Physical examination shows tachypnea, intercostal retractions, frothy pink or red sputum, and diffuse crackles.

   c. Many patients are cyanotic with increasingly severe hypoxemia that is refractory to administered oxygen.

3. Diagnostic studies

   a. CXR may be normal at first. Infiltrates tend to be peripheral (spares the costophrenic angles) with air bronchograms present in 80% of patients. The heart is normal in size. Upper lung venous engorgement is uncommon. Pleural effusions are small to absent.

   b. Pulmonary capillary wedge pressure is normal.

   c. Multiple organ failure is common.

   d. Severity is determined by the level of oxygenation impairment:

   (1) Mild: P_{aO2}/F_{IO2} ratio between 200 and 300 mm Hg

   (2) Moderate: P_{aO2}/F_{IO2} ratio between 100 and 200 mm Hg

   (3) Severe: P_{aO2}/F_{IO2} ratio <100 mm Hg

4. **Management**

   a. Treatment includes identification and specific treatment of the underlying precipitating and secondary conditions.

   b. Supportive care is also required to compensate for the severe respiratory dysfunction. Oxygen should be delivered via endotracheal intubation with positive

> The abnormal permeability at the alveolar-capillary membrane leads to rapid edema and profound dyspnea with frothy pink or red sputum and diffuse crackles.

pressure ventilation and low levels of positive end-expiratory pressure (PEEP). Hypoxia is often refractory to treatment.

   c. The mortality rate associated with ARDS is high, which reflects the severity of the predisposing conditions.

   d. One-third of deaths occur within 3 days of the onset of symptoms. The remaining deaths occur within 2 weeks of diagnosis and are caused by infection and multiple organ failure.

B. **Aspiration of foreign bodies**

   1. General characteristics

   a. Unintentional inhalation of a foreign body into the airway. Most often occurring in children <3 years and adults older than 50

   b. Knowledge of the Heimlich maneuver is lifesaving.

   c. Aspiration may be of gastric contents, inert material, toxic material, or poorly chewed food. The degree of injury depends on the substance aspirated.

   2. **Clinical features**

   a. An episode of choking and coughing or unexplained wheezing or hemoptysis should raise the suspicion of foreign body aspiration.

   b. Asphyxia may result from the aspiration of obstructing material.

   c. Pneumonia may develop secondary to aspiration of toxic materials.

   d. Acute gastric aspiration is one of the most common causes of ARDS.

   3. Diagnostic studies: Expiratory radiography may reveal regional hyperinflation caused by a check valve effect.

   4. **Management**

   a. Bronchoscopy may help to establish the diagnosis but can also be the treatment of choice for removal of the object.

   b. Cultures should be obtained if postobstructive pneumonia is suspected.

C. **Respiratory distress syndrome (RDS)** (formerly called hyaline membrane disease)

   1. General characteristics

   a. RDS is the most common cause of respiratory disease in the preterm infant; it presents within the first minutes or hours after birth.

   b. It is caused by a deficiency of surfactant.

   2. **Clinical features**

   a. The infant will demonstrate typical signs of respiratory distress: tachypnea, nasal flaring, use of accessory respiratory muscles, expiratory grunting, retractions, or cyanosis.

   b. Decreased breath sounds on auscultation, diminished peripheral pulses, decreased urine output in the first 24 to 48 hours, and peripheral edema are ominous signs.

   3. Diagnostic studies: CXR demonstrates air bronchograms, diffuse bilateral atelectasis causing a ground-glass appearance, and doming of the diaphragm.

   4. **Treatment**

   a. Synchronized intermittent mandatory ventilation should be used.

   b. Administration of exogenous surfactants can be used in the delivery room as prophylaxis or as rescue in established hyaline membrane disease.

> Foreign body aspiration most commonly occurs in the very young or old and can present with unexplained wheezing, choking, or asphyxia.

Practice Questions

Directions: *Each of the numbered items or incomplete statements in this section is followed by a list of answers or completions of the statement. Select the ONE lettered answer or completion that is BEST in each case.*

1. A 60-year-old patient in the cardiac unit is 3 days post–percutaneous coronary intervention (PCI) for mild ischemia. He describes a sudden onset of acute chest pain, dyspnea, and hemoptysis. He had a fall last night but denies hitting his head. CT scan reveals a vascular obstruction in the right middle lobe. What is the most likely origin?
   A. Air emboli from central line
   B. Fat emboli secondary to fall from bed
   C. Deep vein in femur
   D. Deep vein in lower leg
   E. Right atrium of heart

2. A 51-year-old male presents with dyspnea that has worsened over 2 days. Examination reveals dullness in bilateral bases, especially in the lateral chest. CXR shows blunting of the costophrenic angles and loss of diaphragm demarcation. Thoracentesis obtains fluid with low protein and normal LDH. What is the likely underlying cause?
   A. Cirrhosis
   B. Infection of the pleural space
   C. Lung cancer
   D. Trauma to the chest
   E. Tuberculosis

3. A 9-year-old presents with a recurrence of chronic lung disease. History reveals several bouts of pneumonia and an episode of pancreatitis. What is the most likely etiology of the underlying disorder?
   A. Autosomal dominant disorder
   B. Autosomal recessive disorder
   C. Mitochondrial mosaicism
   D. Triploidy 13, 15, or 17
   E. X-linked disorder

4. A 53-year-old female with a history of smoking ½ ppd for > 30 years is concerned about her health; an older cousin just died of lung cancer. She has tried to quit smoking several times, lasting no longer than 10 days in any attempt. She describes dyspnea with exertion which occasionally interferes with her ability to function. She rarely produces any sputum. Which of the following would be most helpful at this time?
   A. CXR, PA and lateral
   B. Culture and sensitivity with cytology studies of sputum
   C. Methacholine challenge
   D. Pulmonary function tests
   E. Walk test

5. The asymptomatic, 6-year-old grandson of a family member hospitalized with acute TB disease has a TST of 6-mm induration. What is the recommended management?
   A. Repeat TST in 6 weeks, as this result is not >10 mm
   B. Obtain CXR; induce sputum and obtain three samples of the next several hours
   C. Start INH and apply BCG
   D. Begin INH, continue 6 to 12 months or until TST clear for 12 weeks after exposure
   E. Begin INH, RIF, PZA, and ETH for minimum 2 weeks

6. A 26-year-old patient has a solitary pulmonary nodule found on screening CXR. Which of the following descriptions would most strongly support a diagnosis of benign nodule?
   A. Rounded, 1.5 cm, with sharply defined margins
   B. Rounded, sharp margins, with enlarged pulmonary arteries
   C. Several small opacities in the upper lobe
   D. Oval shaped with thickened calcified plaque
   E. Rounded, diffuse reticular infiltrate

7. A 50-year-old is diagnosed with metabolic paraneoplastic syndrome. He describes multiple endocrine patterns along with a history of smoking 1 ppd for over 30 years. Chest imaging confirms a central lesion with enlarged hilar and peribronchial lymph nodes. What is the recommended management?
   A. Broad-spectrum antibiotics, induce sputum for culture and cytology
   B. Combination antituberculin medications
   C. Combination chemotherapies
   D. Preoperative radiation, followed by surgical excision
   E. Surgical excision followed by combination chemotherapy

8. An 8-month-old with harsh barking cough and inspiratory stridor presents to the emergency department. Physical examination reveals low-grade fever and rhinorrhea. What is the most likely etiology?
   A. Dilated bronchi and obstructed bronchial walls
   B. Group A β-hemolytic Streptococci
   C. Inflammation of airway and mucous overproduction
   D. *H. influenzae*
   E. Parainfluenza virus

9. A 62-year-old male with very little previous health care presents for examination. He is a migrant farmworker without any nearby family. He is thin, smokes ½ ppd, and has a cough productive of scant amounts of purulence. The cough has been present for months. It has interfered with his sleep; he occasionally wakes up sweaty. What is the next step in the workup of this patient?
   A. Tuberculin skin testing
   B. CXR
   C. Sputum culture and sensitivity
   D. Begin treatment with INH × 9 months
   E. Admit to hospital, isolation, sputum inducement, multiple medications

10. A 32-year-old otherwise healthy woman presents with acute cough productive of rust-colored sputum. She awoke this morning with a fever and chills with diffuse achiness. Examination reveals dullness and crackles (rales) heard in the left lower lobe posteriorly. What is the best treatment?
    A. Admission to hospital for combination respiratory fluoroquinolone and cephalosporin
    B. Azithromycin and supportive care
    C. Levofloxacin and supportive care
    D. Supportive care only
    E. Vancomycin empirically until cultures return

11. A patient diagnosed with HIV 4 months ago presents for follow-up. He is not on any medications; he denies allergies. A dry cough is noted during the interview. There is mild cervical and axillary adenopathy. Vitals: T99.2F, P100, R20, O_2 sat 94%. What will most likely be found on CXR?
   A. Bilateral perihilar infiltrates
   B. Branching solid tumor
   C. Cavitary lesions in apices
   D. Crowded bronchial markings
   E. Negative chest radiograph

12. A 21-year-old presents with low-grade fever and an annoying dry cough. She also describes fatigue and malaise. Lungs have a few diffuse wheezes and rales that clear with cough. Presence of which of the following findings would indicate a *Mycoplasma* infection?
   A. Bullous myringitis
   B. Coryza and photophobia
   C. Hepatosplenomegaly
   D. Pharyngeal petechiae
   E. Splinter hemorrhages

Practice Answers

1. C. *Pulmonology; Basic Science; Pulmonary Embolus*

The risk factors for deep vein thrombophlebitis include inactivity, hypercoagulable state, and vascular injury. More thromboses form in the lower extremity overall; however, the majority of those that lead to pulmonary embolus originate in the upper leg. A fat emboli is typical in a trauma setting. Other emboli originate from the heart, areas of trauma (IV line), or foreign body.

2. A. *Pulmonology; Diagnosis; Pleural Effusion*

A transudative pleural fluid (with low protein and normal LDH) is typically caused by atelectasis, congestive heart failure, or renal or liver disease (cirrhosis). Exudative fluid is defined as elevated protein and elevated LDH; common causes include cancer, trauma, and infection.

3. B. *Pulmonology; Basic Science; Cystic Fibrosis*

CF is an autosomal recessive disorder characterized by pulmonary and GI issues and infertility.

4. D. *Pulmonology; Diagnostic Studies; COPD*

This patient describes the early manifestations of COPD. Smoking is the strongest contributing factor. Pulmonary function tests (PFT), especially FEV_1, are sensitive to diagnose and monitor patients with progressive disease. The walk test is a crude method to estimate PFT. Chest x-ray may have some nonspecific findings. Sputum is scant and likely without findings.

5. D. *Pulmonology; Pharmacology; TB*

This patient was closely exposed to active TB, with a positive TST (of ≥5 mm) for this patient group and should be treated with INH for at least 6 months. The child is asymptomatic; therefore, further diagnostic testing is not warranted. A four-drug regimen is for active, symptomatic disease. The BCG vaccine is only for nonexposed individuals in endemic areas.

6. A. *Pulmonology; Diagnostic Studies; Solitary Pulmonary Nodule*

A nodule is more likely to be benign if found in younger individuals (<30 years), <3 cm, rounded, with sharply demarcated margins. It may be calcified. Malignant lesions occur in older individuals and smokers, are typically >2 cm, with indistinct margins, and are progressive. Enlarged pulmonary arteries may be seen in pulmonary HTN. Thick plaques, interstitial fibrosis, calcified plaque, and multiple lesions are more indicative of pneumoconiosis.

7. C. *Pulmonology; Clinical Intervention; SCLC*

SCLC is the described malignancy, with a tendency to originate in a central lesion. SCLC is not amenable to surgery or radiation. Combination chemotherapy is given with a goal of slowing growth and increasing survival time. Non-SCLC may be treated with surgery, radiation, and/or chemotherapy depending on size, site, and type. Tuberculous disease would cause apical cavitary lesions with or without nodes; patients usually have a fever and wasting.

8. E. *Pulmonology; Basic Science; Croup*

This child has croup; the diagnosis is made clinically based on presentation. Parainfluenza virus is by far the most common etiology; less common etiologies include RSV, adenovirus, influenza virus, and rhinovirus. Hemoptysis influenza is a bacterium; it was the primary cause of epiglottitis before the onset of widespread vaccination programs. Group A Streptococci is now the most common cause of epiglottitis. Dilated bronchial and obstructed walls are seen in bronchiectasis. Inflammation and mucous production are characteristic of asthma.

9. E. *Pulmonology; Clinical Intervention; TB*

This patient has signs and symptoms of TB. He should be admitted and put in isolation until the workup is complete. Sputum and blood samples are obtained, imaging is completed, and multiple antituberculin drugs are begun.

10. B. *Pulmonology; Pharmacology; Pneumonia*

This patient has CAP. Recommended outpatient treatment is a macrolide. Supportive care is important. A fluoroquinolone or a macrolide with a cephalosporin is recommended for patients with CAP and chronic disease. Cultures are not routinely obtained in outpatient care but should be investigated in atypical cases or those that do not respond to treatment.

11. A. *Pulmonology; Diagnostic Studies, CXR; Pneumocystis*

This patient likely has *Pneumocystis jiroveci* (nee *carinii*), the most common opportunistic infection in persons with HIV disease. The chest radiograph can take many forms; the most common forms are bilateral perihilar infiltrates or diffuse infiltrates. Cavitary lesions indicate TB. Crowded bronchial marking occurs in bronchiectasis. A branching solid tumor indicates carcinoid or bronchogenic carcinoma.

12. A. *Pulmonology; History and Physical Examination; Mycoplasma*

Bullous myringitis is a rare finding, but it is unique to *Mycoplasma*, in otherwise healthy young patients. Coryza and photophobia support a diagnosis of influenza. Hepatosplenomegaly, pharyngeal petechiae, and splinter hemorrhages indicate Epstein–Barr (mononucleosis).

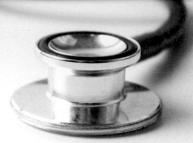

Cardiovascular Medicine | 3

Frank R. Giannelli

Major Principles of Cardiac Care

A. Three factors are needed to maintain adequate pressure in the cardiovascular system:

1. A functioning pump
2. Sufficient fluid volume
3. Vascular resistance

B. The majority of cardiac pathologies result from abnormalities of electrical or contractile functions of the heart muscle, fluid load, or vascular resistance.

C. Quantification and monitoring of severity of symptoms is important to management, such as with the New York Heart Association's (NYHA) functional classification system (Table 3-1).

D. The cardiovascular and pulmonary systems are intimately related. Symptoms suggestive of a problem in either system mandate a thorough evaluation of both.

Hypertension

A. General characteristics

1. **Primary (essential) hypertension (HTN)** causes 95% of cases of elevated blood pressure (BP). It has no specific identifiable cause; pathogenesis is multifactorial.

   a. Genetic predisposition and advanced age are important factors for determining the risk of developing HTN.

   b. Environmental factors may also be contributory and include excessive or increased salt intake and obesity.

   c. Other hypothesized factors are related to sympathetic nervous system hyperactivity, abnormal cardiovascular or renal development, imbalance in the renin–angiotensin system, defects in sodium excretion, and abnormalities in sodium and potassium exchange at the cellular level.

   d. Exacerbating factors include excessive use of alcohol, tobacco use, lack of exercise/sedentary lifestyle, polycythemia, use of nonsteroidal anti-inflammatory drugs (NSAIDs), and low potassium intake.

   e. The metabolic syndrome (truncal obesity, hyperinsulinemia and insulin resistance, hypertriglyceridemia, and HTN) is associated with the development of diabetes and increased risk of cardiovascular complications.

2. **Secondary causes of HTN** account for approximately 5% of all cases of HTN (see Table 3-2).

3. HTN plays a major role in the genesis and exacerbation of other forms of cardiovascular disease and causes numerous secondary disorders.

4. **Hypertensive urgencies** reflect BPs that must be reduced within hours: BP is persistently elevated >220 mm Hg systolic or >125 mm Hg diastolic or accompanied by complications (see Table 3-3).

Table 3-1 | New York Heart Association Functional Classification of Heart Disease

Class	Definition
I	No limitation of physical activity; ordinary physical activity does not cause undue fatigue, dyspnea, or anginal pain.
II	Slight limitation with moderate physical activity; ordinary physical activity results in symptoms
III	Marked limitation with limited physical activity; comfortable at rest, but less than ordinary activity causes symptoms
IV	Unable to engage in any physical activity without discomfort; symptoms may be present even at rest.

Adapted from Dolgin M, Association NYH, Fox AC, Gorlin R, Levin RI, Criteria Committee, New York Heart Association. *Nomenclature and Criteria for Diagnosis of Diseases of the Heart and Great Vessels*. 9th ed. Lippincott Williams and Wilkins; 1994. Original source: Criteria Committee, New York Heart Association, Inc. *Diseases of the Heart and Blood Vessels: Nomenclature and Criteria for Diagnosis*. 6th ed. Little, Brown and Co; 1964: 114. ©1994 American Heart Association, Inc. https://www.heart.org/en/health-topics/heart-failure/what-is-heart-failure/classes-of-heart-failure

Table 3-2 | Causes of Secondary Hypertension

System	Causes
Renal	Parenchymal renal disease Renal artery stenosis
Endocrine	Pheochromocytoma Cushing's syndrome Hyperthyroidism Primary hyperaldosteronism Chronic steroid use Estrogen
Pharmacology	Exogenous estrogens NSAID Decongestants
Obstructive	Sleep apnea Coarctation of the aorta

NSAIDs, nonsteroidal anti-inflammatory drugs.

Table 3-3 | Hypertensive Urgency and Hypertensive Emergency

Category	Goal needed	BP readings	Signs	Treatment
Hypertensive urgency	BP must be reduced within hours	BP persistently >220 systolic or >125 diastolic	± Associated complications	*First line*: nicardipine plus esmolol Nitroglycerin plus β-blocker (if myocardial ischemia is present) *Alternatives*: Enalapril Diazoxide Trimethaphan Loop diuretics *Preferred during pregnancy*: Nicardipine or labetalol *Outpatient*: Clonidine Captopril Nifedipine
Hypertensive emergency	BP must be reduced within 1 hour to prevent progression of end-organ damage or death	Strikingly elevated, >220/>130	Encephalopathy Nephropathy Intracranial hemorrhage Aortic dissection Pulmonary edema Unstable angina, MI Preeclampsia, eclampsia	
Malignant hypertension	Same	Strikingly elevated	Papilledema plus either nephropathy or encephalopathy	

BP, blood pressure; MI, myocardial infarction.

5. Hypertensive emergencies reflect elevated BP that must be reduced within 1 hour to prevent progression of end-organ damage or death. Encephalopathy, nephropathy, intracranial hemorrhage, aortic dissection, pulmonary edema, unstable angina (UA), or myocardial infarction (MI) in the presence of strikingly elevated pressure defines hypertensive emergency.

6. Malignant HTN is historically defined as elevated BP associated with papilledema and either encephalopathy or nephropathy; if untreated, progressive renal failure occurs.

7. Complications of untreated HTN include cardiovascular disease, cerebrovascular disease, dementia, renal disease, aortic dissection, and atherosclerotic complications.

> ⎯◯⎯ Stage 1 HTN is diagnosed with readings at two visits of 130 to 139/80 to 89 mm Hg; stage 2 HTN is >140/90 mm Hg.

B. **Clinical features** (Table 3-4)
1. Currently, **stage 1 HTN** is diagnosed when a patient has elevated BP reading of 130 to 139/80 to 89 mm Hg during at least two visits. Stage 2 HTN is >140/90 mm Hg. An elevated BP is defined as a BP reading of 120 to 129/ <80 mm Hg.

2. Most patients with mild to moderate HTN are asymptomatic; the most commonly voiced symptom is nonspecific headache.

3. Physical examination includes evaluation for evidence of end-organ damage or secondary causes (Table 3-5). This includes body mass index (BMI) and waist circumference measurements; BPs in both arms as well as comparison of radial and femoral pulses (rule out coarctation); cardiac examination for a displaced point of maximal impulse (PMI) or new murmur; auscultation for carotid, femoral, renal, or abdominal aorta bruits; examination for an abdominal aortic mass; and a careful funduscopic examination for hypertensive retinopathy or papilledema. End-organ damage in untreated HTN includes heart failure (HF), renal failure, stroke, dementia, aortic dissection, atherosclerosis, and retinal hemorrhage.

4. In **hypertensive urgencies**, the systolic pressure usually is >220 mm Hg or the diastolic pressure is >125 mm Hg, without life-threatening end-organ damage.

5. In **hypertensive emergencies**, the diastolic pressure is usually >130 mm Hg. Optic disc edema (papilledema) indicates the presence of end-organ damage. Complications include hypertensive encephalopathy, nephropathy, intracranial hemorrhage, aortic dissection, preeclampsia or eclampsia, pulmonary edema, cerebrovascular accident (CVA), and MI.

C. Diagnostic studies
1. Electrocardiogram (ECG) may reveal left ventricular hypertrophy (Fig. 3-1). A strain pattern is associated with advanced disease and a poorer prognosis.

2. Chest radiography may show cardiomegaly (Fig. 3-2); however, chest radiography is not considered to be necessary for the evaluation of uncomplicated HTN.

3. Decreased hemoglobin or hematocrit; elevations in blood urea nitrogen (BUN), creatinine, or glucose; and urinary glucose, urinary protein, and urine sediment may

Table 3-4 | Classification of Blood Pressure for Adults 18 Years of Age to <60 Years

Category	Systolic Pressure (mm Hg)	Diastolic Pressure (mm Hg)
Normal	<120	<80
Elevated blood pressure	120–129	<80
Hypertension		
Stage 1	130–139	80–89
Stage 2	≥140	≥90

Data from Whelton PK, Carey RM, Aronow WS, et al. 2017

ACC/AHA/AAPA/ABC/ACPM/AGS/APhA/ASH/ASPC/NMA/PCNA guideline for the prevention, detection, evaluation, and management of high blood pressure in adults: a report of the American College of Cardiology/American Heart Association Task Force on Clinical Practice Guidelines. *Hypertension*. 2018;71:e13–e115.

Table 3-5 | Hypertension Workup

Area of Evaluation	Findings, Studies
History	Usually asymptomatic Mild headaches
Physical examination	BMI, waist circumference BP in both arms, radial and femoral pulses PMI, murmur, bruit, aneurysm Retinopathy, papilledema
End-organ damage	Heart failure Renal failure Stroke Dementia Aortic dissection Atherosclerosis Retinal hemorrhage
Testing (lab, imaging)	ECG Hemoglobin, hematocrit BUN/creatinine, glucose Urinary glucose, protein, sediment Serum potassium, calcium, uric acid
Others (as indicated by above findings)	Chest radiography Plasma aldosterone concentration Plasma renin activity Plasma aldosterone to renin ratio Lip profile Brain CT/MRI Echocardiography Renal vessel imaging Ambulatory blood pressure monitoring

BMI, body mass index; BP, blood pressure; ECG, electrocardiogram; BUN, blood urea nitrogen; CT, computed tomography; MRI, magnetic resonance imaging; PMI, point of maximal impulse.

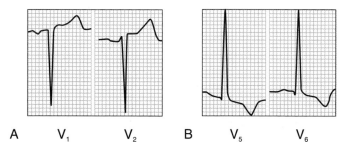

A   V₁   V₂   B   V₅   V₆

Figure 3-1 ▶ Electrocardiographic findings in left ventricular hypertrophy. **A:** Deep S waves in V_1 and V_2. **B:** Tall R waves in V_5 and V_6. (Reprinted with permission from Stein E. *Rapid Analysis of Electrocardiograms: A Self-Study Program*. 3rd ed. Lippincott Williams & Wilkins; 2000.)

indicate related renal disease or diabetes. Other parameters that should be measured include serum potassium, calcium, and uric acid. Plasma aldosterone concentration, plasma renin activity, and calculation of plasma aldosterone to renin ratio may also be helpful to evaluate renal function.

4. A lipid profile is important for ascertaining the associated risk of atherosclerosis.

5. In hypertensive urgencies and emergencies, diagnostic testing targets end-organ function. Studies include brain computed tomography (CT) scan/magnetic resonance imaging (MRI) in the setting of a neurologic disorder, cardiac vessel imaging and echocardiography in the setting of myocardial ischemia or congestive heart failure (CHF), and renal vessel imaging in the setting of renal failure (see Table 3-3).

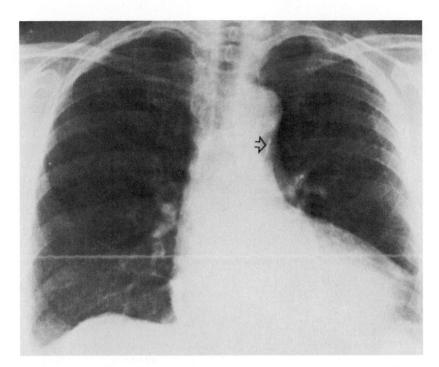

Figure 3-2 ▶ Hypertensive cardiovascular disease: frontal view. Note the left ventricular prominence and a slight increase in the tortuosity of the aorta at its arch. There is calcification in the descending aorta (*arrow*). (Reprinted with permission from Daffner RH, Hartman MS. *Clinical Radiology: The Essentials*. 4th ed. Lippincott Williams & Wilkins; 2014, Fig. 5.41.)

6. If "white coat" HTN is suspected, 24-hour ambulatory BP monitoring can be ordered. Home BP measuring is also an effective means of monitoring BP in this setting.

D. Treatment

> Patients with hypertension warrant an individualized approach, considering underlying comorbidities and lifestyle.

1. Once **primary HTN** is diagnosed, the treatment goal should be to achieve a BP reading of <130/80 mm Hg in nonelevated risk patients.

2. Nonpharmacologic therapies for essential HTN should be stressed and include following the DASH (Dietary Approaches to Stop Hypertension) diet (Table 3-6), weight loss, aerobic exercise, cessation of smoking, limitation of alcohol, and in some patients, limitation of sodium.

3. The threshold for initiating pharmacologic therapy in individuals with chronic diseases such as diabetes or chronic kidney disease should be low.

4. There are a number of different antihypertensive drugs available for use. Considerations for selection include clinical benefit, presence of other chronic diseases, adverse effects, and patient tolerance (Table 3-7).

a. Diuretics initially reduce plasma volume and chronically reduce peripheral resistance. They are currently recommended as initial therapy for essential HTN. Potassium supplements may be needed for some patients. Thiazide diuretics are most consistently effective; loop diuretics should be used only in those with renal dysfunction and when close electrolyte monitoring is assured.

b. β-Adrenergic antagonists are used to decrease heart rate and cardiac output. They tend to be more effective in younger white patients. They have also been shown to reduce mortality after MI and in patients with HF and are currently recommended in these patients unless contraindicated. They must be used with caution in patients with pulmonary disease or diabetes. Because of low efficacy in primary prevention of MI, traditional β-blockers are not generally considered first-line therapy for essential HTN.

Table 3-6 | DASH Diet: Dietary Approaches to Stop Hypertension

Food Group	Recommendation	Food Examples
Protein	Low saturated fat Low cholesterol Low total fat	Poultry, fish, little or no red meat (2 or less/day); nuts, beans (4–5 servings/week)
Fruits and vegetables	Increase; 8–10 servings/day	Leafy greens, fresh fruits
Dairy	Fat-free or low fat only; 2–3 servings/day	Milk, yogurt, cheese
Fiber	Increase; 6–8 servings per day	Whole grain bread or cereal
Sweets	Decrease; 5/week	Added sugar or sweetener, jelly/jam
Fats	Decrease; 2–3/day	Salad dressing, oils

From *Your Guide to Lowering Blood Pressure*. National Institutes of Health National Heart, Lung, and Blood Institute, NIH Publication No. 03-5232.

Table 3-7 | Common Antihypertensive Medications

Class	Mechanism	Comments
Diuretics (thiazides, loop)	Reduce plasma volume Reduce peripheral resistance	Monitor potassium, other electrolytes
β-Adrenergic antagonists	Decrease heart rate Reduce cardiac output Reduce mortality after MI, heart failure	Most effective in younger white patients Use with caution in diabetes or pulmonary disease
ACE inhibitors	Inhibit bradykinin degradation Stimulates synthesis of vasodilating prostaglandins Reduce mortality after MI and in heart failure	Initial drug of choice in diabetes or chronic kidney disease Cough is a common side effect
ARB agents	Block interaction of angiotensin II on receptors Beneficial in diabetes and chronic kidney disease	Does not increase bradykinins: no cough
Calcium channel blockers	Cause peripheral vasodilation	Preferable in blacks and elderly
Others	Aldosterone receptor antagonists	Useful in refractory hypertension
	α-Adrenergic antagonists (lower peripheral vascular resistance)	Initial drug of choice in men with symptomatic prostatic hyperplasia
	Central sympatholytics Arteriolar dilators Peripheral sympathetic inhibitors	Useful in refractory hypertension
	Renin inhibitor	For mono- or combination therapy

ACE, angiotensin converting enzyme; ARB, angiotensin II receptor blocking.

c. Angiotensin converting enzyme (ACE) inhibitors, which inhibit bradykinin degradation as well and stimulate the synthesis of vasodilating prostaglandins, are the initial drug of choice for hypertensive patients with diabetes and chronic kidney disease (must monitor potassium) as they have been shown to help preserve kidney function. They are increasingly the treatment of choice for mild or moderate HTN, especially in younger white patients, or when diuretics are insufficient. They have also been shown to reduce mortality after MI and in patients with HF and should be initiated in these patients unless contraindicated. The major side effect of ACE inhibitors is cough. Angioedema is also a possible side effect.

d. Angiotensin II receptor–blocking agents block the interaction of angiotensin II on receptors. Like ACE inhibitors, they have been shown to be beneficial in hypertensive patients with diabetes and chronic kidney disease as they have been shown to help preserve kidney function. They do not increase bradykinins and, therefore, do not cause cough.

e. Calcium channel blockers, which cause peripheral vasodilation, may be preferable in blacks and elderly patients.

5. Other agents are available for use in refractory cases or special situations.

   a. Aldosterone receptor antagonists, such as spironolactone, are increasingly used in refractory HTN as an addition to other antihypertensives. They have also been proven to be useful in combination with β-adrenergic antagonists and angiotensin II receptor–blocking agents after MI and in patients with HF.

   b. α-Adrenergic antagonists, which lower peripheral vascular resistance, may be the initial drug of choice in men with symptomatic prostatic hyperplasia.

   c. Central sympatholytics, arteriolar dilators, and peripheral sympathetic inhibitors also play a role in the treatment of refractory HTN.

   d. Aliskiren, a renin inhibitor, is approved for mono- or combination therapy. It is no longer recommended to be combined with ACE/angiotensin receptor blocker (ARB) in patients with diabetes.

6. Treatment of secondary causes of HTN targets the underlying cause.

7. Hypertensive urgencies and emergencies are treated with parenteral agents. Care must be taken not to decrease the BP too rapidly because this may lead to cerebral ischemia.

   a. A reasonable goal is to reduce BP by no >25% in the first hour and target a BP of 160/100 within 2 to 6 hours.

   b. Preferred agents include nicardipine plus esmolol and, if myocardial ischemia is present, nitroglycerin (NTG) plus a β-blocker. Other acceptable agents include enalapril, diazoxide, trimethaphan, and loop diuretics.

   c. Aortic dissection calls for esmolol plus nicardipine and urgent surgery.

   d. Fenoldopam, a dopamine-1 receptor agonist, appears to be useful in the setting of acute renal failure.

   e. Nicardipine or labetalol is the preferred agent during pregnancy.

   f. Oral agents for less severe urgencies or emergencies include clonidine, captopril, and nifedipine.

Heart Failure (HF)

A. General characteristics

1. HF is a complex clinical syndrome characterized by abnormal retention of water and sodium and pathologic changes in one or more of the following: myocardial contractility, structural integrity of the valves, preload or afterload of the ventricle, and heart rate. The resulting venous congestion causes typical symptoms such as dyspnea and edema.

2. HF may result from multiple causes including myocardial and pericardial disorders as well as valvular and congenital abnormalities. High-output failure has noncardiac causes (e.g., thyrotoxicosis, severe anemia).

3. HF may be right-sided, left-sided, or both. It may be associated with systolic and/or diastolic cardiac dysfunction.

4. HF is increasing in incidence and prevalence as the population ages; it occurs in 10% of persons older than 80 years.

5. HF is the final common condition of essentially every significant pathologic condition affecting the heart.

B. Clinical features

1. Left-sided failure causes exertional pulmonary vascular congestion leading to exertional dyspnea plus cough, fatigue, orthopnea, paroxysmal nocturnal dyspnea, basilar rales, gallops, and exercise intolerance.

2. Right-sided failure causes systemic vascular congestion and is characterized by distended neck veins, tender or nontender hepatic congestion, decreased appetite/

> Right-sided HF (with hepatomegaly, dependent edema, and distended neck veins) is often caused by left-sided failure (with exertional dyspnea, fatigue, orthopnea, and paroxsysmal nocturnal dyspnea [PND]).

nausea, and dependent pitting edema; it is most frequently caused by left-sided failure. Predominant features are peripheral edema and hepatomegaly.

3. Cardiac signs include parasternal lift; enlarged, displaced, or hyperdynamic apical impulse; diminished first heart sound; and an S_3 gallop. An S_4 gallop may be heard in diastolic failure.

4. Sympathetic activity produces pallor and cold, clammy skin.

5. Nocturia is a common symptom.

6. Hypotension and narrow pulse pressure are frequently present. Depending on the etiology of HF, BP can be low, elevated, or normal.

7. The New York Heart Association Functional Classification (NYHAFC) of Heart Disease delineates four classes of HF defined by the degree of limitation of daily activity (see Table 3-1).

C. Diagnostic studies

1. Labs: Patients may have anemia, renal insufficiency, hyperkalemia, hyponatremia, and elevated liver enzymes; those on diuretics may develop hypokalemia.

2. Chest radiography may show cardiomegaly and bilateral or right-sided pulmonary effusions, perivascular or interstitial edema (Kerley B lines), venous dilation and cephalization, and alveolar fluid (Fig. 3-3).

3. ECG may show either nonspecific changes (e.g., low voltage) or evidence of an underlying arrhythmia, intraventricular conduction defects, left ventricular hypertrophy, nonspecific repolarization changes, or new or old MI.

4. Echocardiography is the most useful imaging study because it is able to assess the size and function of the chambers, valve abnormalities, pericardial effusion, shunting, and segmental wall abnormalities. Echocardiography is also used to determine and monitor the ejection fraction—a key diagnostic and prognostic indicator in HF.

5. Serum B-type natriuretic peptide (BNP) or N-terminal pro-BNP is usually elevated in the acute setting. The sensitivity of BNP is reduced in the elderly and those with chronic obstructive pulmonary disease (COPD).

> Classic signs in HF include shortness of breath, edema, and nocturia.

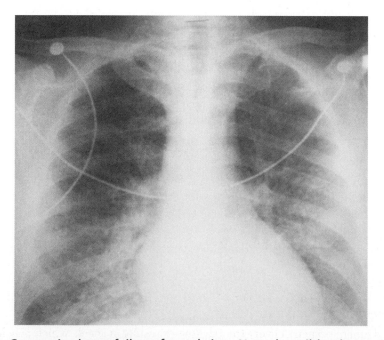

Figure 3-3 ▶ Congestive heart failure: frontal view. Note the mild pulmonary edema and pulmonary venous engorgement. (Reprinted with permission from Daffner RH, Hartman MS. *Clinical Radiology: The Essentials*. 4th ed. Lippincott Williams & Wilkins; 2014, Fig. 5.28A.)

6. Cardiac markers (creatine kinase MB [CK-MB] and troponins) should also be tested to evaluate for new MI.

7. Stress imaging or radionuclide angiography may be indicated to assess the cause or severity of the disease.

8. Cardiac catheterization is indicated if atherosclerosis is suspected. Catheterization can also visualize the ventricle and determine cardiac output.

9. Older patients should undergo thyroid function testing; iron studies are indicated in suspected cases of HF caused by hemochromatosis.

D. Treatment

1. The key management principle is the recognition and treatment of reversible underlying and contributing causes of HF.

2. Preventive and rehabilitative nonpharmacologic measures include progressive aerobic exercise, low-sodium diet, tobacco cessation, alcohol cessation, and stress reduction.

3. Initial therapy in most patients is based on the NYHAFC stage as well as ejection fraction.

4. For most patients, this includes early initiation of ACE inhibitors, which have been shown to decrease left ventricular wall stress and slow myocardial remodeling and fibrosis, and a diuretic (see D.5. below). If ACE inhibitors are not tolerated, angiotensin II receptor blockers can be used instead. For many patients, a β-blocker may also be useful as β-blockers have been shown to improve ejection fraction, reduce left ventricular dilation, and reduce the incidence of dysrhythmia. Aldosterone receptor antagonists have also been proven to be useful in combination with angiotensin II receptor–blocking agents and β-adrenergic antagonists in patients with HF.

5. As symptoms progress, right-sided HF with fluid retention, sodium retention, and edema may develop. In this case, a thiazide or loop diuretic will need to be added. Alternatives include potassium-sparing diuretics, direct inotropic agents (i.e., digitalis), and arterial and venous vasodilators. Diuretic therapy reduces fluid volume and produces relief of symptoms.

6. Calcium channel blockers, preferably amlodipine, are used only to treat associated angina or HTN.

7. Ivabradine inhibits the I_f channel in the sinus node and slows the progression of HF.

8. Patients may require antiplatelet therapy, anticoagulants, or antiarrhythmics, as dictated by the underlying disease.

9. Controlling the ventricular rate and restoring sinus rhythm (when possible) have been found to improve hemodynamics in patients with HF and atrial fibrillation.

10. Implantable cardioverter-defibrillators (ICDs) are indicated when the ejection fraction falls below 35%. Biventricular pacing is indicated to resynchronize the heart when the QRS becomes prolonged.

11. Coronary revascularization is indicated in the presence of reversible ischemia.

12. In severe cases refractory to therapy, mechanical support with a ventricular device or intra-aortic balloon pump may be used as a bridge to cardiac transplantation.

Shock

A. General characteristics

1. Shock is severe cardiovascular failure caused by poor blood flow or inadequate distribution of flow.

2. Inadequate oxygen delivery to body tissues results in shock, which may lead to organ failure and death unless a cause can be rapidly identified and treated.

3. The physical responses to shock are mediated by catecholamines, renin, antidiuretic hormone (ADH), glucagon, cortisol, and growth hormone.

> Shock is acute, severe cardiovascular failure and may be caused by hemorrhage, MI, pulmonary embolus (PE), sepsis, or spinal cord injury.

4. Shock may result from multiple causes (Table 3-8).

   a. **Hypovolemic shock** is caused by hemorrhage, loss of plasma, or loss of fluid and electrolytes, resulting in decreased intravascular volume. This may be caused by obvious loss or by "third-space" sequestration.

   b. **Cardiogenic shock** may arise from MI, dysrhythmias, HF, defects in the valves or septum, HTN, myocarditis, cardiac contusion, rupture of the ventricular septum, or cardiomyopathies.

   c. Causes of **obstructive shock** include tension pneumothorax, pericardial tamponade, obstructive valvular disease, and pulmonary problems, including massive pulmonary embolism.

   d. **Distributive shock** is shock caused by poorly regulated distribution of blood volume and includes septic shock, systemic inflammatory response syndrome (signs of systemic inflammation without end-organ damage), anaphylaxis, and neurogenic shock.

      (1) Septic shock is the most common cause, has a mortality rate of 20% to 50%, and is most often associated with Gram-negative and Gram-positive sepsis in persons at the extremes of age, persons with diabetes or immunosuppression, or those who have recently had an invasive procedure.

      (2) Causes of neurogenic shock include spinal cord injury or adverse effects of spinal or epidural anesthesia.

B. Clinical features

   1. Signs and symptoms of shock include low BP, orthostatic changes, tachycardia, peripheral hypoperfusion, altered mental status, oliguria or anuria, insulin resistance, and metabolic acidosis.

   2. The actual BP reading in shock is not as important as the decrease in BP compared to the usual BP for the individual patient.

   3. End-organ hypoperfusion usually results in cool or mottled extremities, diminished capillary refill, and weak ("thready") or absent peripheral pulses.

   4. Mental status may remain normal, or the patient can range from agitated, restless, confused, obtunded, to comatose.

Table 3-8 | Causes of Shock

Type	Mechanism	Examples
Hypovolemic shock	Decreased intravascular volume	Hemorrhage Loss of plasma Loss of fluid and electrolytes
Cardiogenic shock	Defective cardiac cycle or output	Myocardial infarction Dysrhythmias Heart failure Defects in valves or septum Hypertension Myocarditis Cardiac contusion Rupture of ventricular septum Cardiomyopathies
Obstructive shock	Blockage of blood flow into/out of heart	Tension pneumothorax Pericardial tamponade Obstructive valvular disease Pulmonary problems, massive PE
Distributive shock	Increased/excessive vasodilation	Septic shock (bacteremia) SIRS Neurogenic shock (SC injury) Anaphylaxis

PE, pulmonary embolus; SIRS, systemic inflammatory respiratory syndrome; SC, spinal cord.

C. Diagnostic studies

   1. All patients require a complete blood count (CBC), blood type and crossmatch, and coagulation parameters.

   2. Electrolytes, glucose, urinalysis, and serum creatinine will aid in determining the cause of shock.

   3. Pulse oximetry or serial arterial blood gases are needed to monitor oxygenation.

   4. ECG, chest radiograph (CXR), and cardiac biomarkers (troponins, brain natriuretic protein [BNP], N-terminal prohormone of BNP [NT-proBNP]) may be useful.

   5. Lactate levels can assist in identifying shock as well as monitoring treatment (Table 3-9).

D. **Treatment** must address both the specific cause and the manifestations of shock.

   1. The first step in treatment is attention to basic life support (airway, breathing, circulation).

   2. Specific treatments depend on the cause of shock.

   3. The Trendelenburg or supine position with legs elevated may maximize blood flow to the brain.

   4. Oxygen and intravenous (IV) fluids are essential.

   5. Urine flow should be monitored via indwelling catheter and sustained at 0.5 mL per kg per hour or more.

   6. Continuous cardiac monitoring is preferable to intermittent cardiac monitoring. Central venous pressure monitoring, pulmonary artery catheters, and capillary wedge pressure monitoring should be considered for critically ill patients. However, less invasive techniques to monitor cardiac output, such as transesophageal echocardiography, transthoracic bioimpedance, pulse contour techniques, capnography, and thermodilution techniques, are supplanting central venous monitoring in some patients.

   7. Inotropes (positive: dobutamine, dopamine, epinephrine; negative: labetalol, propranolol) increase cardiac output by increasing contractility; chronotropics alter heart rate (positive: adrenaline; negative: digoxin).

   8. Pressors (i.e., norepinephrine, vasopressin, dopamine, phenylephrine) improve pressure by increasing vascular tone.

> Early critical studies for evaluating shock: CBC, CMP, pulse ox, ECG, CXR, and lactate.

Hypotension

A. General characteristics

   1. Postural hypotension (Orthostatic) is a reversible cause of syncope and a significant cause of falls in the elderly.

     Postural hypotension may be related to reduced cardiac output; paroxysmal cardiac dysrhythmias; low blood volume; medications; and various endocrine, neurologic, and metabolic disorders.

   2. Vasovagal syncope ("fainting") is the result of an acutely stressful, painful, or claustrophobic experience.

Table 3-9 | Lactic Acid Values and Interpretation

Value (mmol/L)	Level	Interpretation
0.5–1.0	Normal level	Normal
2–4	Hyperlactatemia	Metabolic acidosis Anaerobic metabolism
>5.0	Lactic acidosis	75% mortality

B. **Clinical features**

   1. Postural hypotension is defined as >20 mm Hg drop in systolic BP or a drop of >10 mm Hg in diastolic BP between supine and sitting and/or standing measurements.

   2. If accompanied by a rise in pulse of >15 beats per minute (bpm), depleted circulating blood volume is the probable cause.

   3. If no change in pulse rate occurs, medications, central autonomic nervous system disease (e.g., Parkinson's disease or Shy–Drager syndrome), or peripheral neuropathies (e.g., diabetic autonomic neuropathy) should be considered.

C. Diagnostic studies for all causes of hypotension are directed at the suspected cause and often include CBC, basic metabolic panel including glucose, and ECG. A tilt test can be helpful in identifying the cause if clinical examination is unrevealing or symptoms are persistent or severe.

D. **Treatment**

   1. Postural hypotension treatment is directed at the suspected cause. The volume status and the medication list of the patient should be scrutinized first and foremost.

   2. Treatment for vasovagal hypotension includes reassurance and avoidance of known triggers.

Atherosclerosis

A. General characteristics

   1. Atherosclerosis is characterized by lipid deposition, fibrosis, calcification, and plaque formation in the intima of large and medium vessels.

   2. Atherosclerosis is associated with premature coronary and peripheral vascular morbidity and mortality.

      a. Atherosclerotic cardiovascular disease (ASCVD) is the most common cause of cardiovascular death and disability.

      b. Men are affected fourfold more often than women; however, by the age of 70 years, the ratio is 1:1.

   3. Smoking and hypercholesterolemia (elevated cholesterol levels) with total cholesterol levels >200 mg per dL and with high levels of low-density lipoproteins (LDLs) because of diet or familial dyslipidemias are major risk factors. Inflammation appears to play a role, and elevation of C-reactive protein (CRP) is often noted.

   4. Management of both blood glucose and BP is essential to the control of vascular disease.

   5. Obesity and physical inactivity must be addressed.

   6. The role of hypertriglyceridemia as a contributor to heart disease is up for debate.

B. **Clinical features**: These depend on the location of the vessels involved (e.g., cerebral occlusions lead to neurologic deficits, renal artery blockage leads to kidney failure, coronary blockage leads to myocardial ischemia and infarction).

C. **Treatment**

   1. Smoking cessation is essential.

   2. Control of HTN, treatment of diabetes, and treatment of dyslipidemia are also important.

   3. Patients who are overweight should be encouraged to achieve a BMI <25 kg per m^2 and a waist circumference of <40 inches (35 inches in women). Regular aerobic exercise, such as brisk walking for 30 to 60 minutes daily, should also be encouraged.

> Treatment of ASCVD is centered on smoking cessation, HTN control, weight control, lifestyle modification, and statin ± other pharmacologics for lipid management. *Refer to the Endocrine section of this text for a broader discussion of hypercholesterolemia.*

4. All patients should be encouraged to modify their diet to maintain a low-saturated-fat, low-trans-fat, and low-cholesterol diet high in fiber and rich in vegetables, fruits, and whole grains.

5. Statin therapy should be initiated in patients with clinical evidence of ASCVD, LDL >190 mg per dL, diabetics aged 40 to 75 years old without ASCVD and LDL between 70 and 189 mg per dL, and nondiabetics without ASCVD aged 40 to 75 years, LDL between 70 and 189 mg per dL, and a 10-year cardiovascular risk >7.5%.

6. Pharmacologic treatment for **hypertriglyceridemia** should aim to reduce the risk of developing pancreatitis.

Ischemic Heart Disease (Angina)

A. General characteristics

1. Ischemic heart disease is characterized by insufficient oxygen supply to cardiac muscle, most commonly caused by atherosclerotic narrowing and less often by constriction of coronary arteries. Rare causes include congenital anomalies, emboli, arteritis, and dissection.

2. Risk factors include HTN, diabetes mellitus, increased age, tobacco use, family history (cardiovascular disease in younger than 55 years for male relative and in older than 65 years for female relative), obesity (especially abdominal obesity), physical inactivity, dyslipidemias, increased alcohol intake, and low intake of fruits and vegetables. It is important to note that although male gender is considered a risk factor, in the United States, more women die of cardiovascular disease than men every year.

3. Metabolic syndrome is a major contributor to coronary heart disease and includes three or more of the following: abdominal obesity, triglycerides >150 mg per dL, high-density lipoprotein (HDL) <40 mg per dL for men and <50 mg per dL for women, fasting glucose >110 mg per dL, and HTN.

4. Patients are considered at high risk if they have the following medical conditions: cerebrovascular disease, peripheral arterial disease (PAD), abdominal aortic aneurysm (AAA), chronic or end-stage renal disease, or diabetes.

5. Cocaine use is associated with myocardial ischemia and infarction secondary to vasospasm. Patients are often much younger than typical cardiac patients.

B. **Clinical features**

1. Ischemia causes angina pectoris. Angina is characterized by paroxysmal chest "squeezing" or pressure, often accompanied by a sensation of smothering and a fear of impending death.

   a. Stable angina is predictably exacerbated by physical activity and is relieved by rest.

   b. Prinzmetal (or variant) angina is caused by vasospasm at rest, with preservation of exercise capacity.

   c. Unstable Angina (UA) is closely related to non–ST-segment elevation myocardial infarction (NSTEMI) and is a common manifestation of cardiovascular disease. There are three common patterns of presentation of UA: angina at rest, new onset of angina symptoms, or an increasing pattern of pain in previously stable patients. Of these three, the American Heart Association (AHA) reports that rest angina is the most common presentation of UA. UA is suspected when the pain is less responsive to NTG, lasts longer, and occurs at rest or with less exertion than previous episodes of angina.

2. Levine's sign, which is a clenched fist over the sternum and clenched teeth when describing chest pain, may be seen in patients with ischemia.

3. The pain of angina pectoris usually is midsternal but may radiate to the jaw, shoulders, arms, wrists, back of the neck, or some combination of these areas. Pain classically

> Angina is caused by ischemia and characterized by squeezing, pressure, and pain, which is often midsternal but can radiate to the jaw, shoulder, arm, and neck.

radiates to the left, but it may also radiate to the right or bilaterally. Women indicate right shoulder and back pain radiation more frequently than men.

4. Stable angina pectoris usually lasts for <3 minutes. Angina pectoris lasting for more than 30 minutes suggests UA, MI, or another diagnosis.

5. The pain of stable angina is significantly relieved by sublingual NTG. The sublingual NTG can be repeated every 5 minutes up to three times. If the pain is not completely resolved after three doses of the patient's usual sublingual NTG, UA, MI, or another diagnosis should be suspected.

C. Diagnostic studies

> Angina: Short-term treatment includes sublingual NTG; long-term treatment is focused on exercise, weight loss, and smoking cessation.

1. Horizontal or downsloping ST-segment depression on ECG during an anginal attack is among the most sensitive clinical signs, although the ECG will be normal in 25% of those with angina. Nonspecific T-wave changes (such as flattening or inversion) may be noted.

2. Exercise stress testing is the most useful and cost-effective noninvasive test. An ST-segment depression of 1 mm (0.1 mV) is considered to be a positive test. Pharmacologic stress testing can be performed in patients who are unable to exercise.

3. Myocardial perfusion scintigraphy, radionuclide angiography, and stress echocardiography are useful adjuncts to stress testing and can help determine the extent and location of ischemia.

4. Echocardiography is valuable in identifying wall-motion abnormalities associated with ischemia. It can also evaluate left ventricular function, an important prognostic indicator.

5. Positron emission tomography (PET), single-photon emission computed tomography (SPECT) cameras, CT angiography, electron beam computed tomography (EBCT), cardiac MRI, and ambulatory ECG monitoring may be indicated.

6. Coronary angiography is the definitive diagnostic procedure but should be used selectively because of cost and invasiveness.

D. **Treatment**

1. Preventive and rehabilitative treatment includes exercise; weight reduction; diet low in fat and cholesterol; smoking cessation; and aggressive control of diabetes, HTN, and hyperlipidemias.

2. Aggravating factors (e.g., HTN) must be identified and treated.

3. Sublingual NTG tablets or spray or sublingual isosorbide dinitrate is the primary pharmacotherapy for acute anginal attacks.

4. Long-acting nitrate (oral, ointment, or transdermal patches) therapy should include a daily 8- to 10-hour treatment-free interval to prevent drug tolerance. Major adverse effects of nitrates include headache, nausea, light-headedness, and hypotension.

5. β-Blockers prolong life in patients with coronary disease and are first-line therapy for chronic angina. They are indicated for treatment of ischemic symptoms.

6. Calcium channel blockers decrease cardiac muscle oxygen demand but are considered alternative therapy. They are indicated for treatment of ischemic symptoms in patients for whom β-blockers are contraindicated or have been maximized.

7. Platelet-inhibiting agents (e.g., aspirin, clopidogrel) reduce the possibility of infarction secondary to emboli and should be used in all patients unless a contraindication exists.

8. Ranolazine prolongs exercise duration and time to angina and is useful for symptom control. It is not recommended as monotherapy.

9. ACE inhibitors are also useful in the treatment of UA, particularly in patients who have symptoms of HF.

10. Revascularization via angioplasty or bypass grafting provides long-term relief of ischemia in suitable patients.

Acute Coronary Syndromes

A. General characteristics

1. Acute coronary syndromes (ACS) include a spectrum of problems, including UA, STEMI, and NSTEMI.

2. MI is defined as necrosis of myocardial tissue related to ischemia.

3. When a patient presents with symptoms of ACS, the 12-lead ECG is central to the decision pathway. If typical ST elevations are present, the patient is diagnosed with STEMI. If ST changes are absent or ST depressions and/or T-wave inversions are present, additional information including cardiac biomarkers, repeat ECG, and additional testing is needed because the patient may have NSTEMI, UA, a non-ACS cardiovascular condition, or a noncardiac condition. The AHA views UA and NSTEMI as a single entity—UA/NSTEMI—for initial treatment and intervention algorithms.

   a. Based on initial findings, patients can be triaged to acute reperfusion therapy if indicated. All patients with STEMI require reperfusion therapy.

   b. Diagnosis of acute MI is based on evolution of cardiac biomarkers.

   (1) MI is a result of prolonged myocardial ischemia, usually as a result of thrombus formation on a disrupted or eroded atherosclerotic plaque. Other causes include prolonged coronary vasospasm or vasoconstriction, reduced myocardial blood flow, excessive metabolic demand, embolic occlusion, vasculitis, aortitis, coronary artery dissection, and cocaine use. During a single event, more than one cause can be present.

   (2) Signs and symptoms, prognosis, and complications depend on the size and location of the infarct.

4. One-fifth of patients with acute MI will die, usually of ventricular fibrillation, before reaching a hospital.

5. About one-third of acute MIs are "silent" or accompanied by minor pain often attributed to the gastrointestinal (GI) tract. Women and patients with diabetes mellitus are more likely to present atypically. Elderly patients may have atypical symptoms such as generalized weakness, stroke, syncope, or a change in mental status.

B. Clinical features

1. Nontraumatic chest pain is the most common presenting factor in ACS. Other typical features include crushing retrosternal pain or pressure; heaviness or tightness; unexplained indigestion; or epigastric pain.

2. The patient with MI usually develops increasingly severe, prolonged ($>$30 minutes) anterior chest pain at rest, most often during the early morning hours. Ischemia can lead to arrhythmias, hypotension, shock, and HF.

3. Diaphoresis, dyspnea, nausea, vomiting, weakness, anxiety, restlessness, light-headedness, syncope, cough, orthopnea, and abdominal bloating are often present in patients with MI.

4. History should include documentation of prior coronary artery bypass graft (CABG), percutaneous coronary intervention (PCI), coronary artery disease (CAD), angina on effort, or MI. Risk factors, including family history, smoking, hyperlipidemia, HTN, diabetes mellitus, and cocaine or methamphetamine use, should also be assessed.

5. Patients may be bradycardic or tachycardic as well as hypotensive or hypertensive. The cardiovascular examination may be normal, or it may reveal jugular venous distention (JVD), soft heart sounds, a transient murmur of mitral regurgitation, and an S_4 gallop.

6. Lung fields may be clear, but basilar rales or other findings of pulmonary edema may be present.

7. Low-grade fever may develop after 12 hours and last for several days.

> Most common presenting features for ACS: nontraumatic chest pain, diaphoresis, and changes in HR and BP.

8. Pericardial friction rubs may appear after 24 hours.

9. Dressler syndrome (post-MI syndrome) includes pericarditis, fever, leukocytosis, and pericardial or pleural effusion, usually 1 to 2 weeks post-MI.

C. Diagnostic studies

1. ECG changes form the basis of an initial and ongoing evaluation of ACS.

a. STEMI must be rapidly identified. In STEMI, there are ST-segment elevations of ≥1 mm in two contiguous leads. The normal progression from peaked T waves to ST-segment elevations to Q waves to T-wave inversions classically occurs over hours to days. This is not present in all cases of MI (Fig. 3-4).

b. In STEMI, the location of cardiac damage may be determined by examining the location of the changes on the ECG (Table 3-10).

c. Patients with ST-segment depression are initially considered to have either **UA or NSTEMI**. If cardiac biomarkers become elevated during the evaluation, then NSTEMI will be diagnosed. NSTEMI patients will usually develop ECG evidence of non–Q-wave MI; however, as many as 25% will develop ECG evidence of Q-wave MI.

d. A patient who presents with transient ST-segment changes of ≥0.5 mm that develop during a symptomatic episode and resolve when the patient becomes asymptomatic is strongly suggested to have acute ischemia and CAD. A new **left bundle branch block** on ECG is also highly suspicious for a new MI.

> 💡 Diagnosing MI: elevated biomarkers and ECG findings with ST-segment elevations of ≥1 mm in two contiguous leads (for STEMI), or ST-segment depression (NSTEMI).

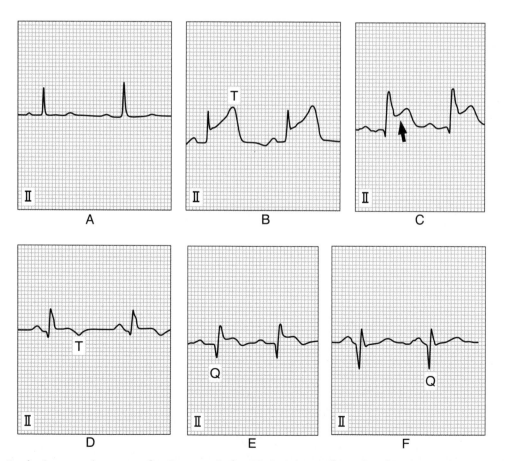

Figure 3-4 ▶ Evolutionary changes of a Q-wave infarction as seen from lead II. Examples are not necessarily from the same patient. **A:** Normal. **B and D:** T wave becomes tall then inverts symmetrically. **C:** ST-segment elevates (*arrow*). **E:** Significant Q waves develop. **F:** Healed infarction. Q waves persist, but ST-segment and T wave return to normal. (Reprinted with permission from Mulholland GC, Brewer BB. *Improving Your Skills in 12-Lead ECG Interpretation.* Lippincott Williams & Wilkins; 1990.)

Table 3-10 | Determining Location of Cardiac Damage by Examining ECG Changes

Ischemia Location	ECG Leads Most Likely to Exhibit Changes
Inferior	II, III, aVF
Posterior	V_1, V_2
Anteroseptal	V_1, V_2
Anterior	V_1, V_2, V_3
Anterolateral	V_4, V_5, V_6

aVF, augmented vector foot; ECG, electrocardiogram.

2. MI is further identified by the presence of elevations of cardiac biomarkers. Troponin T and/or troponin I is the most specific for myocardial damage. CK-MB is also a helpful biomarker, especially when reinfarction is suspected, but it is less sensitive and less specific for MI than the cardiac troponins (Table 3-11).

3. Echocardiography may show abnormalities of cardiac wall motion or mitral regurgitation. Doppler studies may show postinfarction ventricular septal defect (VSD).

4. Chest radiography may indicate pulmonary vascular congestion or signs of aortic dissection.

5. For stable patients with no acute ECG changes and no cardiac biomarker elevations during evaluation, exercise testing remains a useful and cost-effective noninvasive test.

6. Coronary angiography is the definitive diagnostic procedure but should be used selectively because of cost and invasiveness.

7. MRI with gadolinium contrast is one of the most sensitive tests to quantify the extent of infarction.

8. Scintigraphy and radionuclide angiography may be helpful in establishing the diagnosis.

Table 3-11 | Cardiac Markers in Acute Myocardial Infarction[a]

Marker	Timing of Initial Elevation (Hours)	Peak Elevation (Hours)	Return to Normal	Sampling Schedule
Myoglobin	1–4	6–7	24 hours	Often beginning 1–2 hours after onset of chest pain Reasonable to measure this biomarker, along with a cardiac troponin, if patient presents in <6 hours of symptom onset
Cardiac troponin I	3–12	24	5–10 days	12 hours after onset of chest pain Cardiac-specific troponins are the preferred biomarkers. They should be measured on all patients with symptoms consistent with ACS and repeated in 8–12 hours
Cardiac troponin T	3–12	12–48	5–14 days	12 hours after onset of chest pain
CK-MB	3–12	24	48–72 hours	Can be measured at presentation and repeated in 8–12 hours When evaluating possible reinfarction, sample at baseline when symptoms begin and repeat 6–12 hours later

[a]Repeat biomarker measurement in 8–12 hours if initial test is negative. Repeat biomarker measurement at 6- to 8-hour intervals two or three times or until the level peaks as an indication of infarct size. For patients presenting within 6 hours of symptoms, a 2-hour delta CK-MB mass in conjunction with a 2-hour delta troponin may be considered.

Creatine kinase (CK), lactate dehydrogenase (LDH), aspartate transaminase (AST), and alanine aminotransferase (ALT) should not be used for primary detection of myocardial injury. cardiac troponin T and I are cardiac-specific troponins.

ACS, acute coronary syndromes; CK-MB, isoenzyme of creatine kinase containing M and B subunits.

> 💡 Initiate oral beta blocker within 24 hours for patients with ACS—except in HF or bradycardia and heart block.

9. Hemodynamic studies may be useful in the management of cases with cardiogenic shock.

D. **Treatment**

1. All patients with ACS with ongoing discomfort should receive aspirin (162 to 325 mg chewed), IV fluids, oxygen, and NTG (0.4 mg sublingual every 5 minutes for up to three doses) and be placed on strict bed rest. Continuous cardiac monitoring, serial ECG, and pulse oximetry are important components of monitoring. Some patients will benefit from morphine sulfate for ischemic pain not controlled by NTG, and some may require sedation with a benzodiazepine.

2. Caution should be used in administering NTG to patients with suspected inferior wall MI owing to the risk of hypotension.

3. IV NTG is indicated in the first 48 hours for treatment of persistent ischemia, HF, or elevated BP.

4. An oral β-blocker should be initiated within the first 24 hours for all patients with ACS in the absence of contraindications including HF, bradycardia, and heart block. An oral ACE inhibitor should be initiated within the first 24 hours especially in the presence of HF. An ARB should be used for patients who cannot tolerate an ACE inhibitor.

5. Statin therapy should be started in most patients in the days following ACS.

6. A calcium channel blocker (verapamil or diltiazem) can be used to control persistent or frequently recurring ischemic symptoms in patients with contraindications to nitrates or β-blockers. It may be useful even after β-blockers and ACE inhibitors.

7. All patients with ACS (both STEMI and UA/NSTEMI) must undergo risk stratification. Rating systems aid in deciding which patients should undergo aggressive treatment. Several scoring systems are available based on the risk of reinfarction or death (Table 3-12).

   a. The TIMI (**T**hrombolysis **I**n **M**yocardial **I**nfarction) system is the quickest and easiest scoring system and can be completed easily at the bedside. One point is given for each of the following factors: age 65 years or older, three or more risk factors for CAD, use of aspirin within the last 7 days, known CAD with stenosis 50% or greater, more than one episode of rest angina within the last 24 hours, ST-segment deviation, and elevated cardiac markers. Scores of 3 or more are considered to be high risk.

   b. GRACE (**G**lobal **R**egistry of **A**cute **C**oronary **E**vents) is a somewhat more complex scoring method available through many digital resources. Age, gender, vital signs, ST-segment changes, and historical factors are included to predict a 6-month risk of death after discharge.

Table 3-12 | Risk Stratification

Calculator/Study	Factors	Results
TIMI Thrombolysis in Myocardial Infarction	Age ≥65 years 3 or more risk factors for CAD Use of aspirin within last 7 days Known CAD (stenosis 50% or more) Severe angina within last 24 hours ST-segment deviation Elevated cardiac markers	3 or more = higher risk Higher score reflects an increasing risk of percentage chance of event occurring within 14 days
GRACE Global Registry of Acute Coronary Events	Age Gender Vital signs ST-segment changes Historical factors	Complex schemata Results in hospital discharge risk assessment of death in a 6-month period

CAD, coronary artery disease.

8. **STEMI**: Patients with ACS and an acute STEMI should undergo immediate interventions to promote reperfusion.

   a. Aspirin and clopidogrel should be given at once.

   b. Immediate (within 90 minutes) coronary angiography and primary PCI are superior to thrombolysis in high-volume centers with experienced operators.

   c. Thrombolytic therapy within the first 3 hours of the onset of pain reduces mortality and limits the size of infarction. Some benefits may occur if therapy is initiated within the first 12 hours. In the United States, alteplase, reteplase, and tenecteplase are the most commonly used agents. Absolute contraindications include previous hemorrhagic stroke, any stroke within the past 1 year, known intracranial neoplasm, active internal bleeding, or suspected aortic dissection. Known bleeding diathesis, trauma within past 2 to 4 weeks, major surgery within past 3 weeks, prolonged or traumatic cardiopulmonary resuscitation (CPR), recent internal bleeding, noncompressible vascular puncture, active diabetic retinopathy, pregnancy, active peptic ulcer disease, current use of anticoagulants, and BP >180 systolic/>110 diastolic are relative contraindications.

9. **UA/NSTEMI**: ACS patients without ST-segment elevation should be evaluated, and a management strategy should be selected. Conservative management is appropriate for patients with low-risk features based on TIMI or GRACE scores; an invasive strategy should be chosen for patients with high-risk features.

   a. Conservative treatment includes antiplatelet therapy with both aspirin and clopidogrel. Anticoagulation should be initiated preferably with enoxaparin or fondaparinux. Consider initiating antiplatelet therapy with IV glycoprotein (GP) IIb/IIIa inhibitors, eptifibatide, or tirofiban.

   b. It is essential to carefully monitor UA/NSTEMI patients who are treated conservatively and intervene in cases of patients likely to progress to infarction. Symptom progression, echocardiography, and stress testing can be used on select patients to determine when diagnostic angiography should be initiated.

   c. Invasive treatment involves cardiac catheterization. Initial therapy includes antiplatelet therapy with aspirin and/or clopidogrel; anticoagulation should be initiated with unfractionated heparin, enoxaparin, fondaparinux, or bivalirudin. If coronary angiography will be delayed or ischemic discomfort recurs early, antiplatelet therapy with GP IIb/IIIa inhibitors may be initiated. Positive findings on angiography can often be treated with angioplasty and stenting.

Valvular Disorders

A. **Aortic and mitral valve disorders**

   1. General characteristics

      a. Aortic stenosis narrows the valve opening, impeding the ejection function of the left side of the heart. Aortic stenosis is the most common valvular disease in the United States and the second most frequent cause for cardiac surgery.

      b. Aortic insufficiency (regurgitation) results in volume overloading caused by the retrograde blood flow into the left ventricle.

      c. Mitral stenosis impedes blood flow between the left atrium and ventricle.

      d. Mitral insufficiency allows retrograde blood flow and volume overload of the left atrium.

      e. Mitral valve prolapse is usually asymptomatic, but it may be associated with mitral regurgitation.

      f. Valve-related progressive HF leads to pulmonary HTN and congestion.

> Valvular disorders are characterized by the resultant impedance of flow caused by the faulty valve.

g. The most frequent causes of mitral and aortic valve disorders are congenital defects (such as a bicuspid aortic valve); other causes include rheumatic heart disease, connective tissue disorders, infection, and senile degeneration.

h. Many patients present as adults after extended periods of asymptomatic conditions.

2. **Clinical features** (Table 3-13)

a. The most common presenting symptoms include dyspnea, fatigue, and decreased exercise tolerance.

b. Patients may also have cough, rales, paroxysmal nocturnal dyspnea or hemoptysis, and hoarseness.

c. Physical examination will usually demonstrate a heart murmur. In severe cases, a thrill may be palpable.

d. Carotid pulses typically are thready in aortic stenosis; aortic insufficiency produces bounding pulses and widened pulse pressures.

e. Most patients with mitral valve prolapse are thin females with minor chest wall deformities, midsystolic clicks, and late systolic murmur.

3. Diagnostic studies

a. ECG is not useful in establishing specific diagnoses but may demonstrate chamber hypertrophy.

b. Chest radiography

(1) With aortic valve disorders, chest radiography may show left-sided atrial enlargement and ventricular hypertrophy.

(2) With mitral valve disorders, chest radiography may show atrial enlargement alone.

c. Echocardiography, particularly transesophageal, and cardiac catheterization are the only definitive methods of identifying structural and functional abnormalities. Doppler ultrasonography is particularly useful for pressure gradient assessment.

4. **Treatment**

a. The only effective long-term treatment is surgical repair or replacement of the defective valve. Transcatheter aortic valve replacement (TAVR) may be used in

Table 3-13 | Comparison of Findings in Aortic and Mitral Valve Disorders

Valve Disorder	Murmur Location	Radiation	Intensity	Pitch/ Quality	Aids to Hearing	Associated Findings	Timing
Aortic stenosis	Second RICS	To neck and LSB	Often loud with a thrill (grades 4–6)	Medium pitch; harsh	Patient sitting and leaning forward		Midsystolic
Aortic regurgitation	Second–fourth LICS	To apex and RSB	Grades 1–3	High pitch; blowing	Patient sitting and leaning forward; full exhalation	Midsystolic or Austin Flint murmur suggests large flow; arterial pulses large and bounding	Systolic (soft) and diastolic decrescendo
Mitral stenosis	Apex	Little or none	Grades 1–4	Low pitch	Patient in left lateral position; full exhalation	S_1 accentuated; opening snap follows S_2	Middiastolic
Mitral regurgitation	Apex	To left axilla	Soft to loud	Medium to high pitch; blowing		S_2 often decreased; apical impulse prolonged	Pansystolic

RICS, right intercostal space; LSB, left sternal border; LICS, left intercostal space; RSB, right sternal border.

patients for whom open chest surgery is not an option. In selected cases, PCI such as balloon valvuloplasty may be effective.

b. Patients with good exercise tolerance may be treated medically with diuretics and vasodilators for pulmonary congestion and with digoxin or β-blockers for dysrhythmias.

c. Anticoagulant therapy may be indicated for the prevention of thromboemboli, particularly if atrial fibrillation occurs.

d. Antibiotics may be indicated for the prevention of endocarditis and recurrent rheumatic fever, especially in the presence of regurgitation.

B. **Tricuspid and pulmonic valve disorders**

1. General characteristics

a. Patients with congenital anomalies of these valves usually present during infancy or childhood; adults may present with stenosis resulting from rheumatic scarring or connective tissue disease.

b. Tricuspid regurgitation may be intrinsic or functional.

c. In all cases, right-sided pressure overload leads to right-sided cardiomegaly, systemic venous congestion, and right-sided HF.

2. **Clinical features**

a. Patients usually present with exercise intolerance (Table 3-14).

b. JVD, peripheral edema, and hepatomegaly suggest systemic venous congestion.

3. Diagnostic studies

a. Chest radiography may show a prominent right heart border with dilation of the superior vena cava.

b. ECG may show right-axis deviation, P-wave abnormalities associated with right atrial enlargement, or the prominent R and deep S waves of right ventricular hypertrophy.

c. Echocardiography and cardiac catheterization are the only definitive methods of identifying structural or functional abnormalities.

4. **Treatment**

a. Sodium restriction and diuretic therapy decrease fluid volume and right atrial filling pressure.

b. Underlying conditions causing pulmonary HTN are treated with arterial vasodilators or positive inotropic agents.

c. Definitive treatment includes surgical repair, valvuloplasty, or replacement with bioprosthetic valves, which is preferred.

> 💡 Patients with tricuspid regurgitation have right-sided HF, systemic venous congestion, JVD, peripheral edema, and hepatomegaly.

Table 3-14 | Comparison of Findings in Tricuspid Regurgitation and Pulmonic Stenosis

Valve Disorder	Murmur Location	Radiation	Intensity	Pitch/Quality	Aids to Hearing	Associated Findings	Timing
Tricuspid regurgitation	LLSB; holosystolic	To right sternum and xiphoid area	Variable	Medium; blowing	Increases slightly with inspiration	JVP often elevated	Pansystolic
Pulmonic stenosis	Second–third LICS; midsystolic crescendo–decrescendo	To left shoulder and neck	Soft to loud, possibly associated with thrill	Medium; harsh	—	Early pulmonic ejection sound common	Systolic

LLSB, left lower sternal border; JVP, jugular venous pressure; LICS, left intercostal space.

> 95% of cardiomyopathies are dilated type, which presents with dyspnea, pulmonary crackles, JVD, high diastolic pressures, and low cardiac output on echocardiogram.

Cardiomyopathies

A. General characteristics (Table 3-15)

   1. Cardiomyopathies are categorized by their presentation and pathophysiology.

   2. Dilated cardiomyopathy

   a. Dilated cardiomyopathies are the most common type (95%) and are associated with reduced strength of ventricular contraction, resulting in dilation of the left ventricle.

   b. Causes include genetic abnormalities (25% to 30%), excessive alcohol consumption, postpartum state, chemotherapy toxicity, endocrinopathies, and myocarditis; it may be idiopathic.

   c. It is more common in men.

   3. Takotsubo cardiomyopathy (also called stress-induced cardiomyopathy) occurs after a major catecholamine discharge and results in hypocontractility of the left ventricular apex. The clinical presentation can be indistinguishable from acute MI.

   4. Hypertrophic cardiomyopathy

   a. This cardiomyopathy demonstrates massive hypertrophy (particularly of the septum), small left ventricle, systolic anterior mitral motion, and diastolic dysfunction. Microscopic myocardial abnormalities promote the development of arrhythmia.

   b. It is transmitted genetically. The apical variety is more common in persons of Asian descent; hypertrophic cardiomyopathy in the elderly is a distinct form.

   c. Sudden cardiac death occurs in patients younger than 30 years of age at a rate of 2% to 3% yearly.

   5. Restrictive cardiomyopathy

   a. Restrictive cardiomyopathy results from fibrosis or infiltration of the ventricular wall because of collagen-defect diseases, most commonly amyloidosis, radiation, postoperative changes, diabetes, and endomyocardial fibrosis.

   b. The left ventricle is small or normal, with mildly reduced function.

Table 3-15 | Comparison of Cardiomyopathies

	Dilated	Hypertrophic	Restrictive
Causes	Idiopathic Alcohol related Major catecholamine discharge Myocarditis Endocrinopathies, genetic diseases	Hereditary syndromes Chronic hypertension	Amyloidosis Postradiation Post-open heart Diabetes Endomyocardial fibrosis
Symptoms	Left or biventricular heart failure	Dyspnea, chest pain, syncope	Dyspnea, fatigue, right-sided heart failure > left-sided
Examination	Cardiomegaly S_3, elevated JVP	Sustained PMI S_4 Variable systolic murmur Bisferiens carotid pulse	Elevated JVP Kussmaul's sign
ECG findings	S-ST changes Conduction abnormalities Ventricular ectopy	Left ventricular hypertrophy Exaggerated septal Q waves	ST-T changes Conduction abnormalities Low voltage
Echo results	Left ventricular dilation and dysfunction	Left ventricular hypertrophy Asymmetric septal hypertrophy Small left ventricular size Normal or supranormal function	Small or normal left ventricular size Normal or mildly reduced left ventricular function

Echo, echocardiography; ECG, electrocardiogram; JVP, jugular venous pressure; PMI, point of maximal impulse.

B. Clinical features

    1. Dilated cardiomyopathies result in signs and symptoms of left or biventricular congestive failure; the most common presentation is dyspnea. Patients may have an S_3 gallop, pulmonary crackles (rales), and increased jugular venous pressure.

    2. Takotsubo cardiomyopathy presents with retrosternal chest pain indistinguishable from acute MI.

    3. Hypertrophic cardiomyopathy

        a. Patients most commonly present with dyspnea and angina. Syncope and arrhythmias are common. It may be asymptomatic. Sudden death may be the initial presentation.

        b. Physical examination may show sustained PMI or triple apical impulse, loud S_4 gallop, variable systolic murmur, a bisferiens carotid pulse, and jugular venous pulsations with a prominent "a" wave.

    4. Restrictive cardiomyopathy

        a. Patients present with decreased exercise tolerance; in advanced disease, patients develop right-sided congestive failure.

        b. Pulmonary HTN is usually present.

> 💡 Hypertrophic cardiomyopathy MAY be asymptomatic and present with sudden death.

C. Diagnostic studies

    1. Dilated cardiomyopathies

        a. ECG may show nonspecific ST- and T-wave changes, conduction abnormalities, and ventricular ectopy.

        b. Chest radiography in long-standing disease shows cardiomegaly and pulmonary congestion.

        c. Echocardiography demonstrates left ventricular dilation and dysfunction, with high diastolic pressures and low cardiac output.

        d. Nuclear studies and cardiac catheterization also provide useful information.

    2. Takotsubo cardiomyopathy can demonstrate ECG changes and mild cardiac enzymes suggestive of MI. Cardiac catheterization reveals hypocontractility of the left ventricular apex and patent coronary arteries.

    3. Hypertrophic obstructive cardiomyopathy

        a. Chest radiography is often not remarkable.

        b. ECG abnormalities include nonspecific ST- and T-wave changes, exaggerated septal Q waves, and left ventricular hypertrophy.

        c. Echocardiography is the key to diagnosis. It demonstrates left ventricular hypertrophy, asymmetric septal hypertrophy, small left ventricle, and diastolic dysfunction.

        d. Myocardial perfusion studies, cardiac MRI, and cardiac catheterization can also be helpful.

    4. Restrictive cardiomyopathy

        a. Chest radiography may show a mildly to moderately enlarged cardiac silhouette.

        b. Echocardiography is the key to diagnosis; other low-voltage changes on ECG are typical. Cardiac MRI is distinctive, and cardiac catheterization may demonstrate normal or mildly reduced left ventricular function.

        c. Endomyocardial biopsy may be necessary to differentiate restrictive disease from other forms of cardiomyopathy or pericarditis.

D. Treatment

    1. Dilated cardiomyopathies

        a. Abstinence from alcohol is essential.

        b. Underlying disease should be treated.

        c. CHF requires supportive treatment.

2. Takotsubo cardiomyopathy is usually treated with supportive care. Inotropes should generally be avoided. Most patients return to baseline within 2 months.

3. Hypertrophic cardiomyopathies

   a. Initial treatment employs β-blockers or calcium channel blockers; disopyramide is used for its negative inotropic effects.

   b. Surgical or nonsurgical ablation of the hypertrophic septum may be required.

   c. Dual-chamber pacing, implantable defibrillators, or mitral valve replacement may be indicated as per underlying cause.

4. Diuretics may help patients with restrictive cardiomyopathies.

5. Cardiac transplantation may be indicated for severe disease.

Congenital Heart Anomalies

A. General characteristics

1. Congenital heart anomalies are the most common congenital structural malformations.

2. Congenital heart anomalies are classified as either cyanotic or noncyanotic.

   a. Cyanotic anomalies involve right-to-left shunts.

      (1) Tetralogy of Fallot (toF) consists of a ventricular septal defect, aortic origination over the defect, right ventricular outflow obstruction, and right ventricular hypertrophy.

      (2) Pulmonary atresia most often occurs with an intact ventricular septum. The pulmonary valve is closed; an atrial septal opening and patent ductus arteriosus (PDA) are present.

      (3) Hypoplastic left heart syndrome is actually a group of defects with a small left ventricle and normally placed great vessels.

      (4) Transposition of the great vessels most commonly is a complete transposition of the aorta and pulmonary artery.

   b. Noncyanotic types

      (1) Atrial septal defect (ASD) is an opening between the right and left atria. Of the four main types of ASD, ostium secundum is the most common.

      (2) Ventricular septal defects may be perimembranous (most common), muscular, or outlet openings between the ventricles.

      (3) Atrioventricular (AV) septal defect (AV canal) is caused by incomplete fusion of the endocardial cushions. It is common in Down syndrome.

      (4) Patent (persistent) ductus arteriosus is a failed or delayed closure of the channel bypassing the lungs, which allows placental gas exchange during the fetal state. Unlike other congenital anomalies, surgical treatment is usually not indicated as many patients respond to IV indomethacin.

      (5) Coarctation of the aorta involves narrowing in the proximal thoracic aorta.

B. **Clinical features**: See Table 3-16.

C. Diagnostic studies to evaluate cardiac anomalies may include ECG, echocardiography, Doppler ultrasonography, MRI, chest radiography, radionuclide flow studies, cardiac catheterization, and angiography.

D. **Treatment** of most congenital heart anomalies is early surgical repair. Interventions such as extracorporeal membrane oxygenation and alprostadil (prostaglandin E_1) to maintain a patent ductus can be helpful in stabilizing infants with cyanotic heart disease prior to surgery. Many anomalies may require staged procedures conducted as the patient grows.

Treatment for congenital anomalies involves early surgical repair and lifelong monitoring.

Table 3-16 | Comparison of Findings in Various Congenital Defects

Anomaly	Frequency	Murmur	Physical Findings	Important Clinical Information
Cyanotic defects				
Tetralogy of Fallot	6%–10% of significant congenital heart defects	Crescendo–decrescendo holosystolic at LSB, radiating to back	Cyanosis, clubbing, increased RV impulse at LLSB, loud S_2	Polycythemia usually present; tet (hypercyanotic) spells include extreme cyanosis, hyperpnea, and agitation—a medical emergency
Pulmonary atresia	1%–3% of congenital heart disease	Depends on presence of tricuspid regurgitation	Cyanosis with tachypnea at birth, tachypnea without dyspnea, hyperdynamic apical impulse, single S_1 and S_2	Sudden onset of severe cyanosis and acidosis requires emergency treatment
Hypoplastic left heart syndrome	7%–9% of significant congenital heart defects	Variable; not diagnostic	Shock, early heart failure, respiratory distress, single S_2; presentation varies with specific syndrome	Occurs more often in males; accounts for 25% of cardiac deaths before 7 days of age
Transposition of the great vessels	5%–7% of all congenital heart defects	Systolic murmur if associated with VSD; systolic ejection murmur if with pulmonary stenosis	Cyanosis in newborn is a most common sign; tachypnea without respiratory distress; if large VSD, symptoms of CHF and poor feeding; single loud S_2; absent LE pulses if with aortic arch obstruction	
Noncyanotic defects				
Atrial septal defect	7% of congenital heart disease; second most common	Systolic ejection murmur at second LICS; early to middle systolic rumble	Failure to thrive, fatigability, RV heave, wide fixed split S_2	
VSD	Most common of all congenital heart defects	Systolic murmur at LLSB; others depend on severity of defect	Depends on size of defect—from asymptomatic to signs of CHF	Outlet VSDs more common in Japanese and Chinese
PDA	12%–15% of significant congenital heart disease; higher in premature infants	Continuous (machinery) murmur in patients with isolated PDA	Wide pulse pressure, hyperdynamic apical pulse	
Coarctation of the aorta		Systolic, LUSB and left interscapular area; may be continuous	Infants may present with CHF; older children may have systolic hypertension or murmur or underdeveloped lower extremities	Differences between arterial pulses and blood pressure in UE and LE pathognomonic
Variable				
Atrioventricular canal defect (endocardial cushion defect, atrioventricular septal defect)	5% of all defects; more common in infants with Down syndrome (15%–20% of Down syndrome patients)	Depends on the degree of the defect	Cyanosis may be present; infants present with CHF if defect is large enough; first diagnosis may occur in adulthood with partial defects.	Because this refers to a constellation of defects, presentation is variable depending on whether the defect is complete, partial, or transitional.

LSB, left sternal border; RV, right ventricle; LLSB, left lower sternal border; VSD, ventricular septal defect; CHF, congestive heart failure; LE, lower extremity; LICS, left intercostal space; PDA, patent ductus arteriosus; LUSB, left upper sternal border; UE, upper extremity.

Rate and Rhythm Disorders

A. **Overview of arrhythmias**

   1. General characteristics

      a. The clinical significance of an arrhythmia depends on how much it impairs cardiac output or how likely it is to deteriorate into a more serious disturbance.

      b. Susceptibility is based on genetic abnormalities and acquired structural heart disease.

      c. Electrolyte abnormalities, hormonal imbalances, hypoxia, drug effects, and myocardial ischemia increase susceptibility.

      d. Classification of arrhythmias includes those caused by disorders of impulse formation or automaticity, abnormalities of conduction, reentry, and triggered activity.

   2. **Clinical features**

      a. Presentation ranges from asymptomatic to hemodynamic instability, shock, and death.

      b. Specific features depend on the individual arrhythmia (see supraventricular and ventricular arrhythmias, below).

   3. **Diagnostic studies** include ECG monitoring, event recording, measurements of heart rate variability, signal-averaged ECG, exercise stress testing, electrophysiologic testing, and autonomic testing.

   4. **Treatment**: Antiarrhythmic drugs are divided into four classes based on the mechanism of action (Table 3-17).

B. **Supraventricular arrhythmias (origins in atria or AV node)**

   1. General characteristics

      a. Sinus bradycardia (heart rate <60 bpm) may be normal in well-conditioned athletes; in others, it may represent sinus node pathology, with increased risk for ectopic rhythms. When bradycardia causes symptoms, the rate is usually <50 bpm.

      b. Sinus tachycardia (heart rate >100 bpm) occurs with fever, exercise, pain, emotion, shock, thyrotoxicosis, anemia, HF, and use of many drugs. Tachycardia normally does not cause clinically significant symptoms until the rate is ≥150 bpm.

Table 3-17 | Antiarrhythmic Drugs

Class	Action	Indications	Examples
Ia	Sodium channel blockers; depress phase 0 depolarization; slow conduction; prolong repolarization	Supraventricular tachycardia; V-tach; prevention of V-fib; symptomatic ventricular premature beats	Quinidine, procainamide, disopyramide
Ib	Shorten repolarization	V-tach; prevention of V-fib; symptomatic ventricular premature beats	Lidocaine, mexiletine
Ic	Depress phase 0 repolarization; slow conduction	Life-threatening V-tach or fibrillation, refractory supraventricular tachycardia	Flecainide, propafenone
II	β-Blockers; slow AV conduction	Supraventricular tachycardia; may prevent ventricular fibrillation	Esmolol, propranolol, metoprolol
III	Potassium channel blockers; prolong action potential	Refractory V-tach; supraventricular tachycardia; individual agents have specific indications	Amiodarone, dronedarone, sotalol, dofetilide, ibutilide
IV	Slow calcium channel blockers	Supraventricular tachycardia	Verapamil, diltiazem
V	Adenosine: slows conduction time through AV node, interrupts reentry pathways; digoxin: direct action on cardiac muscle and indirect action on cardiovascular system via ANS	Supraventricular tachycardia	Adenosine, digoxin

V-tach, ventricular tachycardia; V-fib, ventricular fibrillation; AV, atrioventricular; ANS, autonomic nervous system.

c. Sinus Arrhythmia is a cyclical irregularity of the heartbeat which corresponds with the patient's respiratory cycle. It is benign and requires no intervention.

d. Atrial premature beats are usually a benign finding requiring no treatment in the absence of symptoms.

e. Paroxysmal supraventricular tachycardia (PSVT) is the most common paroxysmal tachycardia and usually occurs in persons without structural problems. Patients typically complain of a "racing heart."

f. Atrial fibrillation is the most common chronic arrhythmia, and both incidence and prevalence increase with age. This arrhythmia can lead to a significant decrease in cardiac output and is the most common cause of embolic CVAs. It is called "holiday heart" when caused by excessive alcohol use or withdrawal.

g. Atrial flutter usually occurs in patients with chronic obstructive pulmonary disease, HF, ASD, or CAD.

h. Junctional rhythms occur in patients with normal hearts or those with myocarditis, CAD, or digitalis toxicity.

2. Clinical features

a. Patients may present with palpitations, angina, fatigue, and other symptoms of HF.

b. Patients may be asymptomatic only to have an arrhythmia noted on a screening ECG.

3. Diagnostic studies: Characteristic ECG findings assist in the diagnosis of supraventricular arrhythmias (Fig. 3-5).

4. Treatment depends on the specific supraventricular arrhythmia.

a. A key principle of arrhythmia treatment is that stable arrhythmias are treated with medicine and unstable rhythms are treated with electricity. Signs and symptoms of an unstable rhythm include chest pain, dyspnea, altered mental status, and hypotension.

b. All patients with significant bradycardia or tachyarrhythmia should be monitored with continuous cardiac monitoring, BP monitoring, and pulse oximetry. They should have an IV initiated and be given oxygen if hypoxic. If these patients do not demonstrate signs of instability, they can be safely monitored in order to determine the need for further treatment and the best course of management.

c. Patients with unstable bradycardia leading to hypotension, shock, altered mental status, angina, or HF should be treated with a vagolytic (i.e., atropine) or a positive chronotropic (i.e., epinephrine or dopamine). Transcutaneous or transvenous pacing is often indicated and may need to be followed by permanent pacing.

d. Patients with unstable tachycardia leading to hypotension, shock, altered mental status, angina, or HF should be treated with synchronized cardioversion. Antiarrhythmic therapy (i.e., amiodarone, a β-blocker such as esmolol, or procainamide) may also be indicated.

e. A regular, narrow-complex tachycardia, with an abrupt start and stop, usually represents an AV nodal reentry tachycardia such as PSVT.

f. In a stable patient, Valsalva maneuvers (bearing down, coughing, breath holding, carotid sinus massage) may be attempted. The initial medication of choice is adenosine administered via rapid IV push. If adenosine is ineffective, β-blockers or calcium channel blockers can also be used.

g. Patients with signs of instability are treated with synchronized cardioversion. Patients with sustained or recurrent PSVT should be referred for catheter ablative surgery.

h. If a patient with significant tachycardia is stable and the QRS complex is wide, an antiarrhythmic infusion of procainamide, amiodarone, or sotalol should be used. Antiarrhythmic selection has become increasingly complex and often requires consultation with a cardiologist.

Intervention aligns with arrhythmia: bradycardia treated with a vasolytic; tachycardia treated with cardioversion or antiarrhythmic.

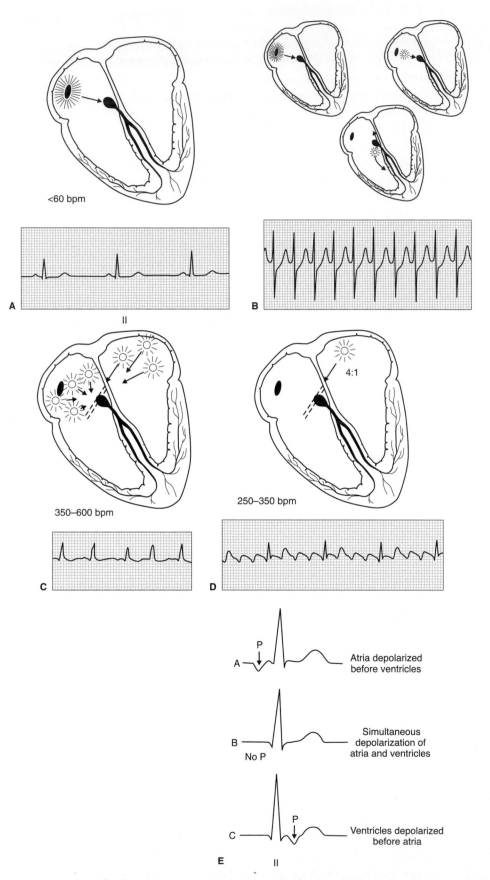

Figure 3-5 ▶ Electrocardiographic findings in supraventricular arrhythmias. **A:** Sinus bradycardia. **B:** Supraventricular tachycardia. **C:** Atrial fibrillation. **D:** Atrial flutter. **E:** Junctional rhythm, P waves. (Reprinted with permission from Stein E. *Rapid Analysis of Electrocardiograms: A Self-Study Program*. 3rd ed. Lippincott Williams & Wilkins; 2000.)

i. Treatment of acute atrial fibrillation depends on the presentation. In the absence of additional pathology, atrial fibrillation usually presents as a narrow-complex "irregularly irregular" rhythm. Atrial fibrillation with a rapid ventricular response is referred to as "uncontrolled" atrial fibrillation.

    (1) Treatment focuses on two objectives: maintaining a normal ventricular rate to decrease symptoms and restore normal sinus rhythm. Electric cardioversion with 100 to 200 J is the primary option in patients with hemodynamic or symptomatic instability.

    (2) The treatment of stable patients is guided by the presence or absence of a left atrial thrombus on echocardiography and the presence of HF.

        (a) Patients with a thrombus, or at high risk of thrombus formation including history of atrial fibrillation for >48 hours, should be treated with anticoagulants (with heparin or enoxaparin and warfarin or dabigatran) and rate control for 3 to 4 weeks prior to attempting conversion.

        (b) Patients with no thrombus and a low risk of thrombus formation can be treated with cardioversion, once anticoagulation with heparin is established.

    (3) Rate control methods in the presence of HF include use of digoxin, amiodarone, or dronedarone. In the absence of HF, rate control can be achieved with metoprolol or esmolol (β-blockers) or diltiazem or verapamil (calcium channel blockers).

    (4) Synchronized cardioversion is fast, safe, and efficient. Chemical conversion can be achieved with several agents including flecainide, propafenone, amiodarone, dronedarone, or ibutilide.

j. Treatment of atrial flutter is similar to treatment for atrial fibrillation in several ways. Electric cardioversion with 50 J is the primary option in patients with hemodynamic or symptomatic instability.

    (1) Stable patients should be treated with anticoagulants (with heparin, enoxaparin, and warfarin) and rate control prior to conversion.

    (2) Rate control can be achieved with metoprolol or esmolol (β-blockers) or diltiazem or verapamil (calcium channel blockers). Chemical conversion with IV ibutilide or synchronized cardioversion with 5 to 50 J can then be effective.

    (3) Patients with sustained or recurrent atrial flutter should be referred for catheter ablative surgery after anticoagulation with warfarin.

    (4) If antiarrhythmic therapy is chosen for chronic atrial flutter, dofetilide is the primary choice, but dronedarone, propafenone, amiodarone, sotalol, procainamide, and flecainide are also used.

> V-tach is associated with electrolyte abnormalities and acute MI.

C. **Ventricular arrhythmias (originate below the AV node)**

  1. General characteristics

    a. Ventricular premature beats (also referred to as premature ventricular complexes [PVCs]) are common and typically benign. They occur with increasing frequency if the myocardium is irritated by factors such as ischemia or an electrolyte disturbance.

    b. Ventricular tachycardia (V-tach)

      (1) V-tach is defined as three or more consecutive ventricular premature beats.

      (2) It may be sustained or nonsustained. Both forms are associated with electrolyte abnormalities. It can be stable or unstable and can even present without a pulse.

      (3) It is a frequent complication of acute MI and dilated cardiomyopathy.

    c. Torsades de pointes (polymorphic V-tach) is a V-tach in which the QRS complex twists around the baseline. The ECG exhibits a continuously changing axis ("turning of the points"). It may occur spontaneously or when the patient has hypokalemia or hypomagnesemia or following administration of drugs that prolong the QT.

d. Long QT syndrome may be congenital or acquired and is associated with recurrent syncope, a QT interval usually 0.5 to 0.7 seconds long, ventricular arrhythmias, and sudden death.

e. Brugada syndrome is a genetic disorder that causes syncope, ventricular fibrillation, and sudden death, often during sleep. It is more common in Asian men.

f. In ventricular fibrillation, no effective pumping action exists; without intervention, death ensues.

> Patients with V-tach may complain of palpitations, or dizziness and syncope.

2. Clinical features

a. Patients with ventricular premature beats may be asymptomatic or aware of skipped beats.

b. Patients with V-tach may be asymptomatic or complain of palpitations. If cardiac output diminishes, the patient may experience dizziness, syncope, or sudden death.

c. Ventricular fibrillation is associated with sudden unconsciousness and death, most often occurring in the early morning.

3. Diagnostic studies: Characteristic ECG findings assist in diagnosing ventricular arrhythmias (Fig. 3-6).

4. Treatment is based on hemodynamic compromise and duration of the dysrhythmia.

a. Ventricular premature beats and nonsustained V-tach without heart disease or electrolyte abnormalities are usually not treated. They may be treated with β-blockers or calcium channel blockers if the patient is symptomatic.

b. In V-tach with severe hypotension or loss of consciousness, synchronized cardioversion may be necessary; ventricular overdrive pacing may help. In pulseless V-tach, immediate defibrillation along with CPR is indicated.

c. The preferred pharmacologic interventions for acute V-tach include amiodarone, lidocaine, and procainamide, in that order (see Table 3-16).

d. In many types of ventricular arrhythmias, patients with an identifiable site of arrhythmic origin benefit from radiofrequency ablation.

e. An ICD may be indicated for recurrent sustained V-tach with structural heart disease or without a reversible cause, for congenital long QT syndrome, and for Brugada syndrome.

f. For acquired long QT syndrome, treatment includes treatment of electrolyte abnormalities and discontinuation of drugs that prolong the QT interval.

g. Torsades de pointes is treated with IV magnesium, correction of electrolyte abnormalities (hypokalemia or hypomagnesemia), and withdrawal of drugs that may have precipitated the event. Isoproterenol infusion and overdrive pacing may be indicated after initial therapy. Permanent pacemaker is indicated for recurrent torsades de pointes.

Conduction Disturbances

A. General characteristics

1. Sick sinus syndrome (SSS)

a. SSS encompasses physiologically inappropriate sinus bradycardia, sinus pause, sinus arrest, or episodes of alternating sinus tachycardia and bradycardia. It is most often found in the elderly. It is often caused by scarring of the heart's conduction system. It may occur in infants who have had heart surgery.

b. SSS may be caused or exacerbated by digitalis, calcium channel blockers, β-blockers, sympatholytic agents, antiarrhythmic drugs, and aerosol propellant

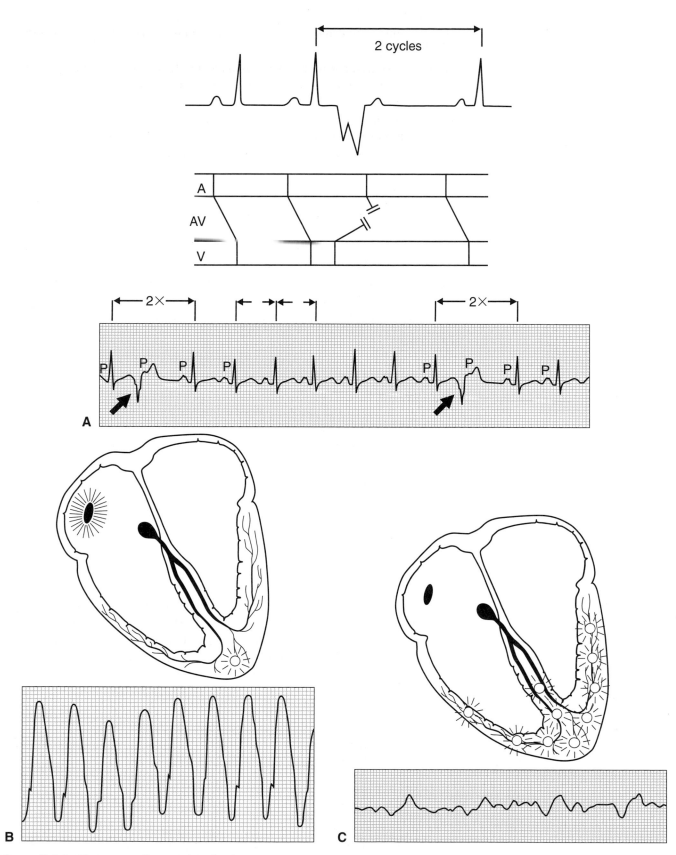

Figure 3-6 ▶ Electrocardiographic findings in ventricular arrhythmias. **A:** Premature ventricular contractions (*arrows*) are frequently identified by the accompanying compensatory pause. **B:** Ventricular tachycardia showing sustained tachycardia (it can also be intermittent). **C:** Ventricular fibrillation. (Reprinted with permission from Stein E. *Rapid Analysis of Electrocardiograms: A Self-Study Program*. 3rd ed. Lippincott Williams & Wilkins; 2000.)

abuse. It may also result from underlying collagen vascular or metastatic disease, surgical injury, or, rarely, coronary disease.

    c. It is reversible if caused by digitalis, quinidine, β-blockers, or aerosol propellants.

  2. AV block is characterized by refractory conduction of impulses from the atria to the ventricles through the AV node and/or bundle of His and is divided into first-degree, second-degree (subdivided into Mobitz type I [Wenckebach] and Mobitz type II), and complete or third-degree block (Table 3-18).

    a. First-degree heart block: All atrial beats are conducted to the ventricles, but the PR interval is >0.21 second.

    b. Second-degree heart block: Not all atrial beats are conducted to the ventricles.

      (1) Mobitz type I (Wenckebach) is a progressive lengthening of the PR interval with shortening of RR interval. Eventually, an atrial impulse will not be conducted to the ventricles. A typical pattern is a repeated cycle of normal PR interval, long PR, longer PR, even longer PR, and dropped beat. It is caused by abnormal conduction in the AV node.

      (2) Mobitz type II is intermittently nonconducted atrial beats. It is caused by a block within the His bundle system. It is almost always secondary to organic disease involving the infranodal system. It may progress to complete heart block.

    c. Third-degree (complete) heart block is a complete dissociation between atria and ventricles. It is caused by a lesion distal to the His bundle.

B. Clinical features

  1. Most patients with SSS are asymptomatic, but patients may have syncope, dizziness, confusion, HF, palpitations, or decreased exercise tolerance.

  2. First-degree AV conduction blocks are usually asymptomatic. Higher grade blocks may produce weakness, fatigue, light-headedness, and syncope.

C. Diagnostic studies: ECG changes associated with conduction disturbances are shown in Figure 3-7.

D. Treatment

  1. Most symptomatic patients with SSS require permanent pacing.

  2. AV Block

  3. First-degree AV conduction block requires no treatment.

  4. The only effective long-term treatment for other AV conduction disorders is permanent cardiac pacing. Temporary transthoracic or transvenous pacing should be followed by permanent pacing when Mobitz type II or complete heart block is diagnosed.

> 💡 Treatment for SSS: permanent cardiac pacing for Mobitz type II; no treatment for first-degree AV block.

Table 3-18 | Heart Block and Associated ECG Changes

Block	ECG Changes	Names/Notes
First degree (all atrial beats conducted to ventricles)	PR interval >0.21 seconds	
Second degree (not all atrial beats conducted to ventricles)	Progressive lengthening of RR interval Eventual loss of impulse Long, longer, longer, dropped	Mobitz I: Wenckebach
	Block within the bundle of His Secondary to organic disease in infranodal system	Mobitz II: intermittent nonconducted atrial beat
Third degree	Lesion distal to His bundle	Complete dissociation between atria and ventricles

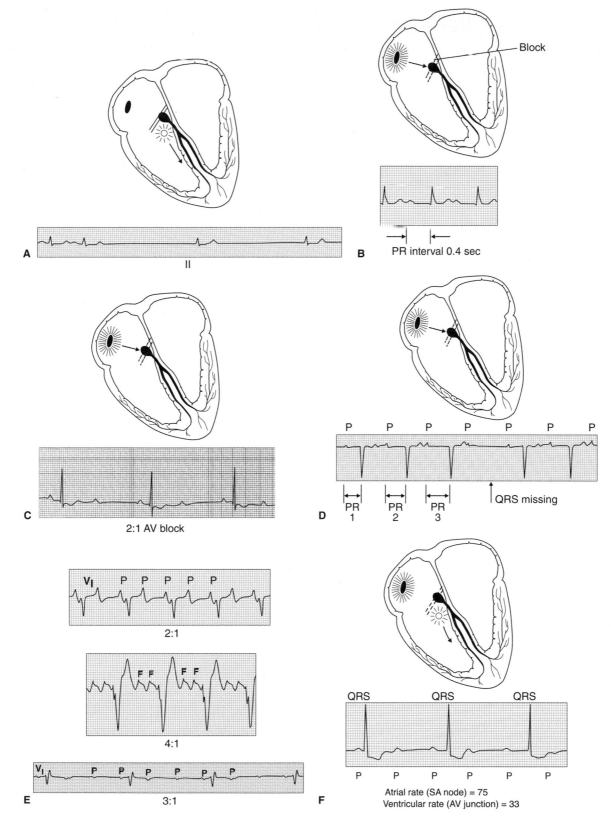

Figure 3-7 ▶ Electrocardiographic findings in conduction disturbances. **A:** Sinus arrest. **B:** First-degree atrioventricular (AV) block. **C:** Second-degree AV block. **D:** Second-degree AV block (Mobitz type I block). **E:** Second-degree AV block. **F:** Third-degree (complete) AV block. SA, sinoatrial. (Reprinted with permission from Stein E. *Rapid Analysis of Electrocardiograms: A Self-Study Program.* 3rd ed. Lippincott Williams & Wilkins; 2000.)

Pericardial Disorders

A. General characteristics

   1. Acute pericarditis is most commonly (90%) idiopathic or secondary to a viral infection. It can also be the result of bacterial infection, autoimmune or connective tissue disease, neoplasm, radiation therapy, chemotherapy or other drug toxicity, cardiac surgery, or myxedema; tuberculous pericarditis is common outside of developed nations. Pericarditis is more common in men and those younger than 50 years of age. Constrictive pericarditis is the result of scarring and loss of elasticity.

   2. Pericardial effusion (secondary to pericarditis, uremia, or cardiac trauma) produces restrictive pressure on the heart.

   3. Cardiac tamponade occurs when fluid compromises cardiac filling and impairs cardiac output.

B. **Clinical features**

   1. The primary presenting symptom of acute pericarditis is sharp, pleuritic substernal radiating chest pain often relieved by sitting upright and leaning forward; a cardiac friction rub is characteristic.

   2. Constrictive pericarditis presents with slowly progressive dyspnea, fatigue, and weakness, accompanied by edema, hepatomegaly, and ascites.

   3. Pericardial effusions may be painful or painless, often accompanied by cough and dyspnea.

   4. In infectious conditions, patients may be febrile.

   5. Post-MI pericarditis (Dressler syndrome) usually presents as a recurrence of chest pain with the presence of an audible rub.

   6. Cardiac tamponade typically presents with tachycardia, tachypnea, narrow pulse pressure, jugular vein distention, and pulsus paradoxus.

C. Diagnostic studies

   1. Elevated white blood cell (WBC) count indicates infection, necessitating blood and pericardial fluid cultures. Post-MI pericarditis shows a high erythrocyte sedimentation rate (ESR).

   2. Chest radiography or echocardiography is useful to determine the extent of cardiac effusion (Fig. 3-8) or pericardial calcification.

   3. ECG change most commonly associated with acute pericarditis is diffuse ST-segment elevation.

   4. ECG changes associated with effusion include nonspecific T-wave changes and low QRS voltage. Electrical alternans is pathognomonic of effusion.

   5. Echocardiography, Doppler ultrasonography, CT, and MRI may be helpful for more accurate diagnosis or before invasive procedures.

D. **Treatment**

   1. In the presence of hemodynamic compromise, pericardiocentesis is necessary to relieve fluid accumulation. Recurrent effusions may be treated surgically with a pericardial window.

   2. Conditions that are solely inflammatory may be treated with steroids or NSAIDs.

   3. Infectious conditions require antibiotic therapy only if bacterial infection is suspected.

   4. Pericardiectomy may be performed to relieve constrictive pericarditis.

> 💡 Acute pericarditis often presents with sharp, radiating chest pain which is relieved by leaning forward.

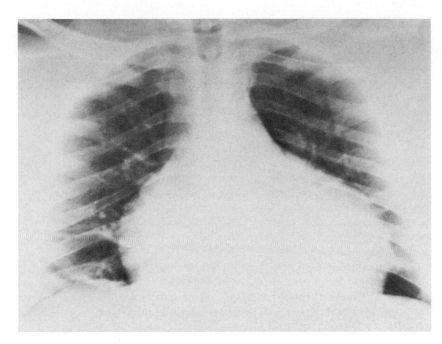

Figure 3-8 ▶ Pericardial effusion: frontal view. Note the massive enlargement of the patient's cardiac silhouette (water bottle heart). (Reprinted with permission from Daffner RH. *Clinical Radiology: The Essentials*. 3rd ed. Lippincott Williams & Wilkins; 2007, Fig. 5.53.)

Infective Endocarditis

A. General characteristics

   1. Most cases of native valve infective endocarditis (IE) are caused by *Streptococcus viridans*, *Staphylococcus aureus*, and enterococci and affect the left side of the heart.

   2. In patients who use IV drugs, *S. aureus* is the most common cause, and the tricuspid (right side) valve is frequently involved.

   3. Prosthetic valve endocarditis is most often caused by *S. aureus*, Gram-negative organisms, or fungi if disease develops during the first 2 months after implantation. Later disease is typically caused by streptococci or staphylococci.

   4. Most patients with endocarditis have an underlying regurgitant cardiac defect that provides a nidus for the development of vegetation.

   5. Infection may result from direct intravascular contamination or from bacteremia, which is common during dental, upper respiratory, urologic, and lower GI procedures.

B. **Clinical features**

   1. Most patients present with fever (although this may be absent in the elderly) and non-specific symptoms (e.g., cough, dyspnea, arthralgias, back or flank pain, GI complaints).

   2. Approximately 90% of patients will have a stable murmur, but this may be absent in right-sided infections. A changing murmur is rare but diagnostically significant.

   3. Classic features occur in 25% of patients and include palatal, conjunctival, or subungual petechiae; splinter hemorrhages; Osler nodes (painful, violaceous, raised lesions of the fingers, toes, or feet); Janeway lesions (painless red lesions of the palms or soles); and Roth spots (exudative lesions in the retina).

   4. Pallor and splenomegaly are common; strokes and emboli may occur.

> Patients with IE often present with stable murmur, fever, cough, dyspnea, petechiae, Osler nodes, Janeway lesions, or Roth spots.

C. Diagnostic studies

   1. Three sets of blood cultures at least 1 hour apart should be obtained, ideally before starting antibiotics.

   2. Echocardiography is essential to make the diagnosis of IE and identify the specific valve(s) involved. The presence of vegetation is diagnostic. Transesophageal echocardiography is particularly useful.

   3. Chest radiography may demonstrate underlying cardiac abnormality or reveal pulmonary infiltrates if the right side of the heart is involved.

   4. The ECG has no specific diagnostic features.

   5. The modified Duke criteria (Table 3-19) are used to establish the diagnosis of IE.

D. **Treatment**

   1. Empiric antibiotic treatment should include coverage of staphylococci, streptococci, and enterococci pending blood culture results. Vancomycin with ceftriaxone is appropriate initial therapy for patients with suspected IE. Gentamicin, vancomycin, plus cefepime—a fourth-generation cephalosporin—is appropriate for acutely ill patients with HF pending blood cultures. In order to minimize the negative side effects of therapy, antibiotics should be quickly adjusted based on the blood culture results.

   2. Antibiotic prophylaxis to prevent endocarditis is recommended before invasive dental work or surgical procedures in patients with prosthetic cardiac valves, previous IE, congenital heart disease, and cardiac transplant patients with valvulopathy. Amoxicillin is the usual drug of choice, with clindamycin, cephalexin, or azithromycin used in cases of Penicillin allergy (Table 3-20).

Table 3-19 | **Clinical Criteria (Modified Duke Criteria) for Infective Endocarditis**

Patient must have (1) two major, (2) one major and three minor, or (3) five minor criteria for the diagnosis to be made. IE is considered "possible" with (1) one major and one minor or (2) three minor

Major Criteria
- Two positive blood cultures of a typical causative microorganism
- Echocardiographic evidence of endocardial involvement
- New valvular regurgitation murmur

Minor Criteria
Predisposing factors such as
- Fever >100.4°F (38°C)
- Vascular phenomena (e.g., embolic disease or pulmonary infarction)
- Immunologic phenomena (e.g., glomerulonephritis, Osler nodes, Roth spots)
- Positive blood culture not meeting major criteria

For details, see Baddour LM, Wilson WR, Bayer AS, et al. Infective endocarditis: diagnosis, antimicrobial therapy, and management of complications: a statement for healthcare professionals from the Committee on Rheumatic Fever, Endocarditis, and Kawasaki Disease, Council on Cardiovascular Disease in the Young, and the Councils on Clinical Cardiology, Stroke, and Cardiovascular Surgery and Anesthesia, American Heart Association: endorsed by the Infectious Diseases Society of America. *Circulation.* 2005;111:e394–e434.

Table 3-20 | **Indications for Acute Rheumatic Fever Prophylaxis**

Cardiac Lesions	Procedures/Conditions
Prosthetic valve	Dental: manipulation of gingival tissue or periapical regional
Previous endocarditis	Respiratory: incision of respiratory mucosa
Selected congenital heart conditions:	Presence of infected skin or musculoskeletal tissue
Unrepaired cyanotic congenital defects	
Repaired defect with residual defect at site or adjacent	
Selected acquired valve disorders	
Cardiac transplantation	

Treatment: 2 g amoxicillin, 1 hour prior to the procedure (clindamycin, azithromycin, or clarithromycin as alternatives).

3. Valve replacement, especially of the aortic valve, may be necessary if the condition does not resolve with antibiotic therapy, if an abscess develops, or if a fungal infection is the cause.

4. Anticoagulants are not beneficial in patients with native valve infection and are controversial in patients with prosthetic valves.

Rheumatic Heart Disease

A. General characteristics

1. Rheumatic fever is a systemic immune response occurring usually 2 to 3 weeks following a β-hemolytic streptococcal pharyngitis. It most commonly affects the heart, joints, skin, and central nervous system.

2. It is a more common condition internationally, yet recent outbreaks have occurred focally in the United States. Children from 5 to 15 years of age are most often affected.

3. Rheumatic valve disease may be self-limited or lead to progressive deformity of the valve; the typical lesion is a perivascular granuloma with vasculitis.

4. The mitral valve is most often involved (75% to 80%), followed by the aortic valve (30%). Aortic or tricuspid involvement rarely occurs in isolation.

> Rheumatic fever can follow strep throat; rheumatic heart disease most often involves the mitral valve.

B. Clinical features (Table 3-21)

1. Two major or one major and two minor Jones criteria are required to establish the diagnosis of rheumatic fever.

   a. Major criteria: carditis (clinical or subclinical), erythema marginatum, subcutaneous nodules, chorea, and polyarthritis

   b. Minor criteria (for low-risk populations): fever, polyarthralgias, reversible prolongation of the PR interval, rapid ESR, or CRP

2. Supportive evidence includes positive throat culture or rapid streptococci test and elevated or rising streptococcal antibody (antistreptolysin O [ASO]).

C. Treatment

1. Strict bed rest is essential until the patient is stable.

2. Intramuscular (IM) penicillin is used for documented streptococcal infection; in patients who are allergic to penicillin, erythromycin is appropriate.

3. Salicylates reduce fever and relieve joint problems; corticosteroids relieve joint symptoms but do not prevent cardiac disease. Salicylates are also indicated for children with pericarditis.

4. Prevention includes early treatment of streptococcal pharyngitis. Prevention of recurrence is essential to prevent heart damage; benzathine penicillin every 4 weeks is a common prophylactic regimen.

Table 3-21 | Jones Criteria, Acute Rheumatic Fever

Criteria for diagnosis: Two major *or* one major plus two minor *and* evidence of recent streptococci infection	
Major criteria	Carditis (clinical or subclinical, diagnosed by echocardiogram) Erythema marginatum Subcutaneous nodules Chorea Polyarthritis
Minor criteria	Fever Polyarthralgias Reversible prolonged PR interval Rapid ESR C-reactive protein

ESR, erythrocyte sedimentation rate.

Peripheral Vascular Disorders

A. **Peripheral arterial disease (PAD)**

    1. General characteristics

        a. PAD is most commonly the result of atherosclerosis and is a significant independent risk factor for cardiovascular and cerebrovascular morbidity and mortality.

        b. Lower extremity atherosclerotic PAD is initially asymptomatic but typically progresses to claudication, ischemia, and pain with exercise, causing significant limitation of activity or disability. Further progression to critical or acute limb ischemia leads to pain at rest with skin ulceration, gangrene, or loss of limb.

        c. Acute arterial occlusion may be caused by **arterial thrombosis or embolism**.

        d. Thrombotic disease also may be a result of trauma, hypovolemia, inflammatory arteritis (including Takayasu arteritis and Buerger disease), polycythemia, dehydration, repeated arterial punctures, and hypercoagulable states.

    2. **Clinical features** (Table 3-22)

        a. Intermittent claudication, foot or lower leg pain with exercise that is relieved by rest, is usually the first symptom of PAD. Thigh or buttock pain with walking may also occur if atherosclerosis is present proximally in the arteries of the legs. As the condition progresses, pain at rest develops.

Table 3-22 | Comparison of Peripheral Vascular Conditions

	Peripheral Arterial Disease	Varicose Veins	Phlebitis	Chronic Venous Insufficiency
Symptoms	Intermittent claudication Foot or lower leg pain with exercise, relieved with rest Erectile dysfunction	Asymptomatic Aching and fatigue	Superficial: dull pain, erythema Deep: swelling, heat, redness	Progressive edema Itching, dull pain Ulceration
Signs	Weak or absent distal pulses Arterial bruits Loss of hair, shiny atrophic skin, pallor with dependent rubor	Dilated, tortuous veins Greater saphenous most common Flat reticular veins Telangiectasias Spider veins	Superficial: erythema, tenderness, induration Deep: heat, edema, Homans' sign	Shiny, thin, atrophic skin
Severe disease	Numbness, tingling, ulcerations Pain, pallor, pulselessness, paresthesias, poikilothermia, paralysis	Chronic distal edema Abnormal pigmentation Fibrosis, atrophy Skin ulceration	Vascular compromise	Ulceration (stasis ulcer, dermatitis)
Diagnostics	Doppler ultrasonography Ankle–brachial index ≤ 0.9 Angiography	Duplex ultrasonography	Duplex ultrasonography Venography D-dimer	Clinical Duplex ultrasonography
Management	Risk factor modification: discontinue tobacco, control diabetes, hypertension, hyperlipidemia	Weight loss Control of risk factors Graduated compression stockings	Superficial: bed rest, local heat, elevation, NSAIDs Deep: anticoagulation Prevention is key	Prevention Elevation Avoid extended standing or sitting Compression hose
Medications	β-Blocker ACE inhibitor Statins			
Interventions	Exercise program Antiplatelet therapy	Exercise programs Elevation Radiofrequency or laser ablation Compression sclerotherapy Surgical stripping	Surgical intervention	Wet compresses Compression boots or stockings Skin grafting

ACE, angiotensin converting enzyme; NSAIDs, nonsteroidal anti-inflammatory drugs.

b. Femoral and distal pulses will be weak or absent; an aortic, iliac, or femoral bruit may be present. Skin changes to the lower extremity include loss of hair, shiny atrophic skin, and pallor with dependent rubor.

c. Erectile dysfunction may occur with iliac artery disease (Leriche's syndrome).

d. Severe, chronic disease results in numbness, tingling, and ischemic ulcerations, which may lead to gangrene.

e. Symptoms of occlusion depend on the artery, the area it supplies, and the collateral circulation.

f. Acute arterial occlusion (whether embolic or thrombotic) threatens limb viability and results in the "6 Ps": pain, pallor, pulselessness, paresthesias, poikilothermia, and paralysis.

3. Diagnostic studies

a. Doppler ultrasound flow studies can be used to determine systolic pressures in the peripheral arteries.

b. An ankle–brachial index (ABI), which uses Doppler measures to compare the BP in the upper and lower extremities, is a highly sensitive and specific test. An ABI of ≤0.9 indicates significant disease and, together with signs and symptoms, may negate the need for more invasive studies.

c. Angiography remains the gold standard study. CT or magnetic resonance angiography is also useful for locating stenotic sites and for accurate diagnosis of thrombosis or embolism, especially if planning surgery.

d. Although not regularly used for screening, elevated homocysteine has a strong association with incidence and progression of PAD.

4. Treatment

a. Aggressive risk factor modification: Tobacco use must be discontinued; diabetes, HTN, and hyperlipidemia must be controlled.

b. β-Blockers, ACE inhibitors, statins, progressive exercise, and supervised exercise programs have been shown to be helpful at reducing symptoms of claudication. Adherence to behavior change is crucial.

c. Antiplatelet therapy, with aspirin and/or clopidogrel, should be used routinely in all patients who do not have a contraindication. Symptom relief, primarily improved pain-free walking distances, can be achieved with the addition of cilostazol.

d. If these interventions fail, revascularization using either endovascular or surgical techniques should be considered. This must be preceded by a thorough cardiac evaluation as well as evaluation of the arterial anatomy.

e. Erectile dysfunction may require revascularization or treatment with a phosphodiesterase, such as sildenafil.

> Treatment for PAD includes lifestyle modification, smoking cessation, HTN and diabetes management, lipid management, and antiplatelet therapy.

B. Varicose veins

1. General characteristics

a. Approximately 15% of adults, particularly women who have been pregnant, develop varicosities. Other risk factors include obesity, family history, prolonged sitting or standing, and history of phlebitis.

b. The main mechanisms are superficial venous insufficiency and valvular incompetence; inherited defects in vein walls or valves also play a role.

2. Clinical features

a. Dilated, tortuous veins develop superficially in the lower extremities, particularly in the distribution of the great saphenous vein. Smaller blue-green, flat reticular veins; telangiectasias; and spider veins are further evidence of venous dysfunction.

b. Varicosities may be asymptomatic or associated with aching and fatigue.

    c. Chronic distal edema, abnormal pigmentation, fibrosis, atrophy, and skin ulceration may develop in severe or prolonged disease.

    d. Duplex ultrasonography locates incompetent valves/venous reflux before surgery. In most cases, reflux arises from the greater saphenous vein.

3. Treatment

    a. Graduated compression stockings provide external support.

    b. Leg elevation and regular exercise provide symptomatic relief.

    c. Small venous ulcers heal with leg elevation and compression bandages; larger ulcers may require compression boot dressing (Unna boot) or skin grafts.

    d. Interventional techniques include endovenous radiofrequency or laser ablation, compression sclerotherapy, and sometimes surgical stripping of the saphenous tree.

    e. More aggressive preventive measures, such as intermittent compression stocking, may be needed if the patient is to be on prolonged rest or inactive.

C. **Thrombophlebitis and deep venous thrombosis (DVT)**

    1. General characteristics

        a. Thrombophlebitis involves partial or complete occlusion of a vein and inflammatory changes. Virchow triad of stasis, vascular injury, and hypercoagulability predispose a vein to development of thrombophlebitis.

        b. Superficial thrombophlebitis may occur spontaneously or following trauma and occurs frequently at the site of IV or peripherally inserted central catheter (PICC) lines.

        c. DVT most often occurs in the lower extremities and pelvis.

        d. DVT is associated with major surgical procedures (especially total hip replacement), prolonged bed rest, lower extremity trauma, use of oral contraceptives and hormone replacement therapy, and inherited (e.g., factor V Leiden, protein C, protein S, or antithrombin deficiencies) and cancer-associated hypercoagulable states.

        e. Other risk factors include advanced age, obesity, long-distance air travel, multiparity, inflammatory bowel disease, and lupus erythematosus.

    2. Clinical features

        a. Superficial thrombophlebitis may present with dull pain, erythema, tenderness, and induration of the involved vein or with no symptoms. It is most common in the great saphenous vein. A cord may be palpable following resolution of acute symptoms.

        b. Half of patients with DVT have no early signs or symptoms. Classic findings of DVT include swelling of the involved area with heat and redness over the site; Homans' sign is unreliable.

    3. Diagnostic studies

        a. Duplex ultrasonography is the preferred study for DVT. Negative results in a patient highly suspicious for DVT indicate the need for further study.

        b. Venography is the most accurate method for definitive diagnosis of DVT, but it is associated with increased risk and should be reserved for those with high suspicion and negative ultrasound.

        c. Dimerized plasmin fragment D (D-dimer) is a fibrin degradation product that is elevated in the presence of thrombus. An elevated D-dimer does not sufficiently diagnose thrombophlebitis; most hospitalized patients will have an elevated level. A negative D-dimer test (<500 ng/dL), however, suggests that ultrasonography may be omitted.

> For DVT, remember the Virchow triad of stasis (such as travel), vascular injury (perhaps trauma, infection, inflammation), and hypercoagulability (e.g., hormone use or cancer), which predisposes a vein to development of thrombophlebitis.

d. If PE is suspected, pulmonary angiography remains the gold standard study but is rarely performed. If the facility is equipped, CT angiography is the study of choice. Ventilation–perfusion scanning may be used if CT is contraindicated or unavailable.

4. Treatment

a. Superficial thrombophlebitis is usually treated with bed rest, local heat, elevation of the extremity, and NSAIDs. Antibiotics may be required if evidence of infection exists. More serious disease may require surgical intervention.

b. Prevention of DVT in bedridden patients is accomplished by elevation of the foot of the bed, leg exercises, compression hose, and intermittent compression devices; in high-risk patients, anticoagulation may be appropriate.

c. Prevention of perioperative and travel-associated DVT includes early or frequent ambulation, leg exercises, and compression hose.

d. Preferred treatment is anticoagulation with enoxaparin (a low-molecular-weight heparin) or unfractionated heparin followed by warfarin.

D. Chronic venous insufficiency

1. General characteristics

a. Chronic venous insufficiency is characterized by loss of wall tension in veins, which results in stasis of venous blood and is often associated with a history of DVT, leg injury, or varicose veins.

b. Prevention is accomplished by early aggressive treatment of venous reflux states, such as acute thrombophlebitis or varicose veins, use of compression hose, and weight reduction and exercise.

> Chronic venous insufficiency is often associated with history of DVT; progressive edema is seen clinically.

2. Clinical features

a. Progressive edema starting at the ankle is followed by skin and subcutaneous changes.

b. Itching, dull pain with standing, and pain with ulceration are common.

c. Skin is shiny, thin, and atrophic with dark pigmentary changes and subcutaneous induration. Pruritus is a common symptom.

d. Ulcers most commonly occur just above the ankle (stasis ulcer).

3. Treatment

a. General therapeutic measures include elevation of the legs, avoidance of extended sitting or standing, and compression hose. Pneumatic compression is used in refractory cases.

b. Stasis dermatitis should be treated with wet compresses and hydrocortisone cream; chronic dermatitis may require addition of zinc oxide with ichthammol and an antifungal cream.

c. Ulcerations may be treated with wet compresses, compression boots or stockings, and, occasionally, skin grafting.

d. Progressive exercise and avoidance of risk factors are essential to stabilization of disease.

E. Arteriovenous (AV) Malformation

1. AV malformations are congenital malformations resulting in inappropriate AV communication.

2. In approximately 10%, there is an aneurysm.

3. They are clinically significant when they rupture causing stroke.

Please refer to the Neurology Chapter for a detailed discussion on AV Malformations and stroke.

Giant Cell Arteritis

A. General characteristics

1. Giant cell arteritis is a systemic inflammatory condition of medium and large vessels. It primarily affects those older than 50 years and frequently coexists with polymyalgia rheumatic and probably represents a spectrum of one disease.

2. It most frequently involves the temporal artery and other extracranial branches of the carotid artery.

3. If not treated aggressively, it can cause blindness.

4. Large-vessel problems (e.g., thoracic aortic aneurysm) occur in 15% of patients within 7 years.

B. Clinical features

1. Patients are typically elderly and complain of unilateral temporal headache. Additional signs and symptoms include scalp tenderness, jaw claudication, throat pain, diplopia, and elevated inflammatory markers.

2. Symptoms of polymyalgia rheumatica (pain and stiffness mainly of shoulder and pelvic girdle) are present in 50% of patients.

3. Nonclassic symptoms include respiratory tract problems, mononeuritis multiplex, fever of unknown origin, or unexplained neck and head pain.

4. The temporal artery examination is usually normal but may be nodular, enlarged, tender, or pulseless.

C. Diagnostic studies

> To diagnose giant cell arteritis, ESR and CRP will be elevated; temporal artery biopsy is the gold standard.

1. ESR and CRP are markedly elevated.

2. Most patients have a normochromic normocytic anemia and thrombocytosis; some have elevated alkaline phosphatase.

3. Temporal artery biopsy should be performed promptly for definitive diagnosis. Temporal artery ultrasonography may show thickening (halo sign), stenosis, or occlusion.

D. Treatment is high-dose prednisone (1 to 2 months before tapering) and/or low-dose aspirin. Treatment should be initiated immediately and not delayed for biopsy results. The role of immune modulators is emerging to reduce the duration of steroid use.

Aortic Aneurysms

A. General characteristics

1. An aortic aneurysm is a weakness and subsequent dilation of the vessel wall, usually caused by genetic defect or atherosclerotic damage to the vessel intima.

2. Atherosclerosis is the most common cause, although some exist as congenital defects or as a result of syphilis, giant cell arteritis, vasculitis, trauma, Marfan syndrome, or Ehlers–Danlos syndrome.

3. Males are eight times more likely to have an aneurysm; the classic picture is an elderly male smoker with CAD, emphysema, and renal impairment.

4. Aneurysms may occur in the abdomen (AAA, 90%, most of which originate below the renal artery) or thoracic (10%) aorta.

5. The mortality rate for rupture (dissection) of an aneurysm approaches 90%.

B. Clinical features

1. AAA may be asymptomatic or present as a pulsating abdominal mass, sometimes accompanied by abdominal or back pain.

2. Renal or lower extremity occlusive disease is present in 25% of patients.

3. Thoracic aortic aneurysms may be asymptomatic or cause substernal, back, or neck pain; dyspnea, stridor, and cough; dysphagia; hoarseness; or symptoms of superior vena cava syndrome.

4. Severe symptoms such as "ripping" or "tearing" chest pain radiating to the back often indicate thoracic aortic dissection.

5. AAA rupture causes severe back, abdominal, or flank pain as well as hypotension and shock.

C. Diagnostic studies

1. Abdominal ultrasonography is the study of choice for abdominal aneurysms. The current recommendation for screening includes a single abdominal ultrasound for men older than 65 years who have ever smoked; this may be followed by contrast-enhanced CT (Fig. 3-9).

2. Thoracic aneurysms may require aortography for diagnosis; CT and MRI are preferred over ultrasonography.

D. Treatment

1. The only effective treatment is endovascular or open surgical repair.

2. Five-year survival after repair is >60%.

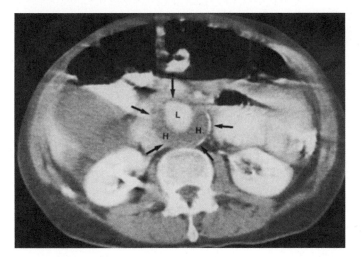

Figure 3-9 ▶ A CT scan through the abdomen showing a large abdominal aortic aneurysm (*arrows*). Note the central enlarged lumen (*L*), the more peripheral hematoma (*H*), and the calcification of the wall on the left side. (Reprinted with permission from Daffner RH. *Clinical Radiology: The Essentials*. 3rd ed. Lippincott Williams & Wilkins; 2007, Fig. 1.23A.)

Practice Questions

Directions: Each of the numbered items or incomplete statements in this section is followed by a list of answers or completions of the statement. Select the ONE lettered answer or completion that is BEST in each case.

1. A 41-year-old involved in a bicycle accident complains of abdominal pain and light-headedness. BP is 94/60 supine and 86/48 standing; pulses are weak but symmetric. Extremities are cool. Pulse oximetry supports low oxygenation. Which of the following will best assist in diagnosis and prognosis at this time?
   A. Cardiac biomarkers (troponins)
   B. Chest radiography
   C. Lactic acid levels
   D. Serum creatinine
   E. Serial glucose levels

2. A 45-year-old overweight male undergoes screening examination. BP is 126/79, waist circumference 40 inches. PMI is displaced, no bruits, funduscopic examination without findings. He is a nonsmoker and does not exercise regularly. What is the best recommendation?
   A. He has elevated BP; lifestyle modifications strongly suggested.
   B. Weight loss and daily diuretic therapy to prevent worsening pressure

C. He has HTN stage 1; start a β-blocker; refer to weight loss management ± surgery.

D. Short-term corticosteroids plus antihypertensive medication as titrated

E. He is normotensive, although at risk; recommend low-fat, low-fiber diet.

3. A 43-year-old female returns for follow-up care of diabetes, diagnosed 2 years ago. Last month, her BP was 144/92 and 144/96. She was counseled regarding dietary changes necessary to control her BP. She was begun on an unknown oral antihypertensive agent but stopped after 10 days because of a nagging cough. Today her BP is 148/96. She has lost 2 pounds in 1 month and has increased her walking from none to two short walks per week at lunchtime. Which of the following is the best recommendation at this time?

A. Start an ACE inhibitor to lower BP and preserve kidney function.

B. Begin a low-dose β-adrenergic antagonist and titrate up to the level tolerated by the patient.

C. Suggest a trial of a thiazide diuretic with close monitoring of electrolytes.

D. Add an aldosterone receptor antagonist and increase the exercise program to double the current walking time total per week.

E. Restrict fluid intake and total sodium intake per day.

4. An infant born at 33 weeks 4 days is in mild respiratory distress. She has a loud, continuous, machinery-like murmur. Apical pulse is hyperdynamic; there is wide pulse pressure. What is the most likely diagnosis?

A. ASD

B. PDA

C. toF

D. Transposition of the great arteries

E. VSD

5. An infant born at 33 weeks 4 days is in mild respiratory distress. She has a loud, continuous, machinery-like murmur. Apical pulse is hyperdynamic; there is wide pulse pressure. ECG is normal. What is the best next step in the workup of this patient?

A. Cardiac catheterization

B. Doppler carotid ultrasonography

C. Chest radiography

D. MRI of the heart and mediastinum

E. Echocardiography

6. A 68-year-old male is day 3 post–anterior wall MI treated successfully with PCI with two stents. His BMI is 29.1; he is a nonsmoker, denies diabetes. The stenosis was 60% preintervention and 40% postintervention. Troponins are trending down. According to TIMI, what is the patient's risk stratification for further cardiac events?

A. Low

B. Intermediate

C. High

D. Very high

7. A patient experiences acute chest pain and diaphoresis. Emergency medical technician (EMT) in the field records ST-segment elevations in three leads. The patient is given an aspirin to chew. An IV line placed, saline started, NTG provides some relief. What is the most common cause of death in patients presenting such as this?

A. Third-degree heart block

B. PE

C. Ruptured aneurysm

D. Ruptured chordae tendineae

E. Ventricular fibrillation

8. A patient experiences acute chest pain and diaphoresis. EMT in the field records ST-segment elevations in three leads. The patient is given an aspirin to chew. An IV line placed, saline started, NTG provides some relief. What is the most sensitive means to confirm the suspected diagnosis?

A. ECG showing left bundle branch block

B. ECG showing ST elevations >1 mm in two leads

C. Elevated CK-MB

D. Elevated troponin

E. Hypoxia per pulse oximetry

9. A 53-year-old female, G4 P3104, describes chest pain as squeezing pressure which is worse with activity and relieved with rest. The pain is fairly predictable with walking briskly or going upstairs. Which of the following statements is likely true in this patient?

A. β-Blocker is essential if there is a history of hormone replacement therapy.

B. Exercise stress testing will max out at 80% of the goal within 60 seconds.

C. Nonspecific T-wave changes will be seen on ECG.

D. A predictable relief with NTG sublingual makes the diagnosis.

E. ST-segment elevations will be visible between attacks.

10. A 26-year-old female complains of sharp chest pain which is relieved when sitting up and leaning forward. She had a viral upper respiratory illness last week that resolved without issue. ECG in the emergency department shows diffuse ST-segment elevations. What is likely present on physical examination?

A. Bounding distal pulses

B. Carotid bruit

C. Displaced PMI

D. Continuous machinery murmur

E. Friction rub

11. A 54-year-old male presents to the emergency department with dyspnea. Examination reveals an S_3 gallop, elevated jugular venous pressure, and diffuse crackles. Chest radiography shows cardiomegaly; ECG reveals nonspecific ST- and T-wave changes. What is the likely cause of this patient's condition?

A. Alcohol binge

B. Atherosclerosis

C. Catecholamine discharge

D. Collagen vascular disease

E. Genetic valve abnormality

12. A 28-year-old with history of injection drug use (IDU) presents to the emergency department with fever and fatigue. He is cachectic and diaphoretic. Pulse is regular, rate 110, Temp 101.0°F, BP 128/68. There is a high-pitched murmur along the left lower sternal border (LLSB). Small painless hemorrhages are noted on conjunctivae, palate, and palms. What is the recommended initial treatment?

A. Begin an aminoglycoside with penicillin and cefepime.

B. Begin vancomycin, adjust per blood culture returns.

C. Follow lactic acid, begin antibiotics if the level rises above 2.5 mmol per L.

D. High-speed fluid resuscitation while awaiting blood culture results

E. IM penicillin once

Practice Answers

1. C. *Cardiovascular Medicine; Hypovolemic Shock; Diagnostic Studies*

Lactic acid is a fairly sensitive marker for the diagnosis and monitoring of hypovolemic shock, identified by the orthostatic BP. Lactic acid of 2–4 mmol per L indicates hyperlactatemia; above 4–5 mmol per L indicates metabolic acidosis. Biomarkers support ischemic changes. Creatinine and glucose will aid in identifying underlying disease.

2. A. *Cardiovascular Medicine; Clinical Intervention; Hypertension*

This gentleman meets the criteria for elevated BP: systolic 120–139 and/or diastolic <80 mm Hg. Lifestyle modification including DASH diet, exercise, avoiding tobacco and alcohol, low salt, high fiber, stress reduction/mindfulness, should be strongly recommended. Stage 1 HTN is defined as systolic 130–139 and/or diastolic 80–89 mm Hg on at least two separate occasions.

3. C. *Cardiovascular Medicine; Pharmacology; Hypertension*

This patient meets the criteria for HTN: systolic 130–139 and/or diastolic 80–89 mm Hg. She likely had a reaction to an ACE inhibitor as indicated by the dry cough. A trial of thiazide diuretic and close monitoring of potassium and other lytes is recommended at this time. Further lifestyle modification is always encouraged.

4. B. *Cardiovascular Medicine; Diagnosis; PDA*

A continuous, machinery-like murmur indicates a PDA. The apical pulse is hyperdynamic against the obstruction, contributing to a wide pulse pressure. ASD is associated with a systolic ejection murmur with an early to midsystolic rumble. Tetralogy of Fallot is associated with a holosystolic, crescendo–decrescendo murmur at the left sternal border with radiation to the back. VSD is associated with a systolic murmur at the LLSB.

5. E. *Cardiovascular Medicine; Diagnostic Studies; PDA*

This infant likely has a PDA. An echocardiography will provide strong supportive evidence of the anatomical defect and help to plan an approach. Most close spontaneously. If not closing or if causing dysfunction or hemodynamic instability, indomethacin or ibuprofen can be given to hasten closure. It is effective up to 10–14 days of life. Further studies, including catheterization, are not necessary unless surgery is necessary.

6. C. *Cardiovascular Medicine; Health Maintenance; CAD*

The patient is awarded a point for: age >65 years; overweight; stenosis >50%; cardiac markers elevated—4 points. Scores of 3 or higher place the individual at the high risk for cardiac events. He should be treated with NTG, aspirin, a β-blocker, ACE inhibitor, and likely a statin.

7. E. *Cardiovascular Medicine; Diagnosis; MI*

The most common cause of death in patients with acute MI is ventricular fibrillation, especially if witnessed prior to arrival at the hospital. Patients with suspected MI should be treated aggressively with fluids, aspirin, a β-blocker, and ACE inhibitor. Close monitoring and quick arrival to emergency care are keys to survival.

8. D. *Cardiovascular Medicine; Diagnostic Studies; MI*

Cardiac markers, indicated infarction of cardiac muscle, are the most sensitive method to diagnose an acute MI. Troponin I, T, and C are the earliest markers to rise. CK-MBs rise later but are the better test for recurrent ischemia. ECG provides strong support, but less definitive.

9. D. *Cardiovascular Medicine; Clinical Intervention; Angina*

This patient describes the classic pain of stable angina. A predictable swift response to NTG will make the diagnosis. ECG changes, if present at all, will occur as ST-segment elevations during the painful episodes; inter-event rhythm is normal. An exercise stress test will help support the diagnosis and plan treatment.

10. E. *Cardiovascular Medicine; History and PE; Pericarditis*

Sharp chest pain that is relieved with sitting up and leaning forward is characteristic of pericarditis. The inflamed pericardium causes a friction rub which is audible on examination. Post-viral pericarditis does not cause vasculitis. Displaced PMI indicates cardiomegaly. A continuous machinery murmur is classic for PDA.

11. A. *Cardiovascular Medicine; History and PE; Dilated Cardiomyopathy*

The most common underlying cause of dilated cardiomyopathy is alcohol excess. Atherosclerosis leads to coronary ischemic events. Takotsubo cardiomyopathy is associated with events linked to a major catecholamine release. Genetic structural defects and collagen vascular disease are associated with hypertrophic cardiomyopathy.

12. B. *Cardiovascular Medicine; Pharmacology; Infective Endocarditis*

The empiric treatment for suspected bacterial endocarditis is vancomycin. Once cultures return and sensitivities are known, antibiotic regimen should be adjusted. Lactic acid levels above 2 mmol per L indicate heightened risk for sepsis. Antibiotics should not be delayed.

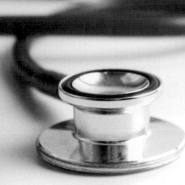

4 | Hematology

Allan Platt

Red Cell Disorders

A. General characteristics

1. Red blood cells (RBCs) transport the protein hemoglobin (Hgb) responsible for oxygen, carbon dioxide, carbon monoxide, and nitric oxide gas exchange.

   a. Anemia is defined as a low Hgb level, RBC count, or hematocrit (Hct; the percentage of RBCs to total blood volume) compared to normal age and gender controls.

   b. Polycythemia is an elevated Hgb, RBC count, or Hct.

   c. The best first tests to assess RBC disorders are the complete blood count (CBC) and peripheral smear that assesses cell morphology.

2. RBCs are manufactured from bone marrow stem cells under the hormonal influence of erythropoietin (epo) secreted by the kidney.

   a. Renal failure may cause anemia from lack of epo production. This can be measured and supplemented with recombinant epo.

   b. Dietary intake and absorption of iron, folic acid, vitamin B_{12}, and protein must be adequate to supply the bone marrow.

3. While in the bone marrow, RBCs have nuclei. The nuclei are extruded after all the Hgb is manufactured. The RBC leaves the marrow with some remaining RNA that stains as a reticulocyte. The reticulocyte develops into a mature RBC in 2 days and normally circulates for 120 days.

   a. The reticulocyte count is the best indicator of how the bone marrow is responding to a decrease in RBCs.

   b. The reticulocyte count must be corrected for the degree of anemia in the patient (raw reticulocyte count × patient Hgb/normal Hgb). This is the corrected reticulocyte percentage; levels >3% indicate bone marrow response.

   c. An anemic patient with corrected reticulocyte count over 2.0 indicates a working marrow and RBC loss from bleeding or hemolysis. A corrected reticulocyte count under 2.0 indicates bone marrow failure to produce RBCs from lack of epo or nutrients or because of damaged nonfunctioning marrow.

4. Normal RBCs are hemolyzed after 120 days, usually in the spleen, and the Hgb is degraded into heme and globin. Heme is processed into indirect bilirubin and transported to the liver to be conjugated into direct bilirubin for storage in the gallbladder.

   a. High indirect bilirubin could be from hemolysis or hereditary Gilbert's syndrome.

   b. High indirect bilirubin, high corrected reticulocyte count, high lactate dehydrogenase (LDH), and hemoglobinuria indicate hemolysis.

5. Pathophysiology: Hgb is a protein composed of a genetic sequence of amino acids containing two α-chains coded on each chromosome 16 and two β-, δ-, or γ-chains coded on each chromosome 11 enclosing four iron-containing heme groups.

   a. Everyone has at least three types of Hgb in each RBC: Hgb A (two α, two β), Hgb F (two α, two γ), and Hgb A_2 (two α, two δ).

> Anemia with reticulocytosis = loss or destruction of RBCs; anemia without reticulocytosis = failure to produce RBCs.

b. The predominant Hgb in utero is fetal hemoglobin (Hgb F) because of its strong affinity for placental oxygen. After birth, Hgb A becomes predominant.

c. Decreased α-chain production causes α-thalassemia and decreased β-chain production results in β-thalassemia.

d. There are over 900 β-chain mutations causing hemoglobinopathies of varying clinical manifestations; the most common is sickle hemoglobin (Hgb S).

e. The following laboratory tests are used to identify hemoglobinopathies: Hgb electrophoresis, isoelectric focusing (IEF), high-performance liquid chromatography (HPLC), or capillary zone electrophoresis (CZE).

B. Clinical features of red cell disorders

1. Anemia is clinically suspected by the presenting symptoms and signs of weakness, fatigue, palpitations, increased heart rate, dyspnea, positional dizziness, syncope, bleeding from any site, or increased or new-onset angina. It may be suspected when the physical findings of tachycardia, tachypnea, orthostasis, pallor, or jaundice are observed. Anemia may also be discovered during routine screening CBC.

2. Tachycardia, dyspnea, altered mental status, orthostatic hypotension, syncope, and shock may indicate severe uncompensated anemia, and a rapid workup with possible RBC transfusion is indicated.

> Careful history (melena, pica, bleeding; and weakness, dyspnea, positional dizziness) and thorough physical examination (tachycardia, pallor, jaundice) will unlock the clues to diagnosis.

3. Clues from the patient history may include the following:

a. History of melena, abdominal pain, aspirin or nonsteroidal anti-inflammatory drug (NSAID) use, anticoagulant use, or past peptic ulcer disease (PUD): Consider gastrointestinal (GI) bleeding or platelet dysfunction.

b. In females, the menstrual history quantifying the amount of blood loss or possible pregnancy should be obtained.

c. History of pica (an abnormal craving for ice, clay, or starch) or complaints of dysphagia: Consider iron deficiency.

d. Poor diet history: Consider iron, vitamin B_{12}, or folate deficiency, or general malnutrition.

e. History of gastric bypass surgery, distal paresthesias, gait problems, memory issues, or metformin use: Consider vitamin B_{12} deficiency.

f. History of alcohol abuse: Consider folate deficiency or liver disease. If moonshine use or lead paint/pipe exposure, consider lead toxicity.

g. Family history of blood cell disorder: Consider sickle cell disease, glucose-6-phosphate dehydrogenase (G6PD) deficiency, or thalassemia.

h. History of jaundice, transfusion, new medication, or infection: Consider a hemolytic process including (G6PD) or delayed transfusion reaction.

i. History of weight loss, low back or bone pain: Consider cancer, multiple myeloma, HIV, rheumatoid arthritis, thyroid disease, or renal disease.

j. History of fever and chills, tick exposure, foreign travel, cat scratch, rash, cough, and dyspnea: Consider infection with malaria, *Babesia*, or parvovirus B19.

k. History of prolonged bleeding, epistaxis, gum bleeding, heavy menses, and easy bruising: Consider thrombocytopenia or von Willebrand disease (vWD).

l. History of headaches, vertigo, pruritus, nosebleeds, deep vein thromboses (DVTs), chronic obstructive pulmonary disease (COPD), or high-altitude exposure: Consider polycythemia.

4. Clues from the physical examination may include the following:

a. General inspection: pallor of skin or conjunctiva, spoon nails, or palmar creases: Consider iron deficiency. Lindsey's nails in renal disease and low epo.

b. Weight loss: Consider cancer, HIV, chronic disease. Weight gain: Consider hypothyroidism.

    c. Skin: Petechiae or purpura may indicate low platelets or vWD.

    d. Vital signs: tachycardia from increased cardiac output in anemia; tachypnea from decreased Hgb–oxygen transport; orthostatic changes if volume depleted or acute bleeding; fever in infections and drug/transfusion reactions; hypothermia in severely hypothyroid state

    e. Eye: pallor in palpebral conjunctivae; jaundice in hemolysis

    f. Mouth: glossitis and angular stomatitis in iron, folate, or vitamin B_{12} deficiency

    g. Neck: thyroid enlargement or nodules

    h. Heart: increased output/murmur, S_3 gallop, and displaced point of maximal impulse (PMI) in high-output heart failure secondary to anemia

    i. Lung: Consider infection, cancer; rales in heart failure.

    j. Abdomen: liver/spleen size, masses, tenderness, surgical scars (gastric bypass, ileal resection as cause of vitamin B_{12} deficiency)

    k. Rectal: stool guaiac positive in GI bleeding; enlarged or stony prostate indicates malignancy

    l. Pelvic/breast: uterine abnormality as cause of menorrhagia; breast mass in breast cancer

    m. Lymph nodes, consistency, and size: Consider lymphoma, leukemia, infection, and connective tissue disease if enlarged.

    n. Neurologic: decreased vibratory and position sense in vitamin B_{12} deficiency

> Anemia = deficiency of Hgb and/or Hct.

C. Laboratory studies for the initial workup of anemia and polycythemia

    1. CBC: See Table 4-1 for normal adult values.

    2. Peripheral smear for red cell morphology: Table 4-2 illustrates some of the common RBC morphologies and possible etiologies.

    3. Reticulocyte count: The corrected reticulocyte count or reticulocyte production index over 2.0 in the presence of anemia suggests bleeding or hemolysis. Below 2.0 indicates a bone marrow production problem.

    4. Urinalysis: Proteinuria or hematuria may be clues to renal disease as the cause of blood loss or decreased epo production. Hemoglobinuria without RBCs in the sediment could indicate hemolysis.

Table 4-1 | The Complete Blood Count—Adult Normal Values

Parameter	Normal Adult Lab Values		Low Levels	High Levels
Hgb	**Male** 15.5 ± 2 mg/dL	**Female** 13.5 ± 2 mg/dL	Anemia	Polycythemia
Hct	**Male** 46.0% ± 6%	**Female** 41.0% ± 6%	Anemia	Polycythemia
RBC count	**Male** 4.3–5.9 million/µL	**Female** 4.0–5.2 million/µL	Anemia	Polycythemia
WBC count	4.5–11.0 k/µL		Leukopenia	Leukocytosis
Platelet count	150–400 k/µL		Thrombocytopenia	Thrombocytosis
Reticulocyte (retic) count	0.5%–1.5% 25–85 k/µL		Low in anemia (<2)	High in hemolysis or RBC loss (>2)
Red Cell Indices				
MCV	80–100 fL		Microcytosis	Macrocytosis
MCH	27–32 pg		Hypochromic	Hyperchromic
MCHC	30–36 g/dL		R/O Fe deficiency	R/O spherocytosis
RDW	11.5%–14.5%		Variation in RBC size	

R/O Fe deficiency, rule out iron deficiency; Hgb, hemoglobin; Hct, hematocrit; RBC, red blood cell; WBC, white blood cell; MCV, mean corpuscular volume; MCH, mean corpuscular hemoglobin; MCHC, mean corpuscular hemoglobin concentration; RDW, red cell distribution width.

Table 4-2 | Red Cell Morphology

Red Cell Morphology	Associated Conditions
Burr cells	Uremia Low K Artifact Cancer of stomach Peptic ulcer disease
Spur cell	Postsplenectomy
Stomatocyte	Hereditary Alcoholic liver disease
Spherocyte	Hereditary Immune hemolytic anemia Water dilution Posttransfusion
Schistocyte (helmet)	Thrombotic thrombocytopenia Disseminated intravascular coagulation Vasculitis Glomerulonephritis Heart valve Burns
Elliptocyte (ovalocyte)	Hereditary Thalassemia Iron deficiency Myelophthisic Megaloblastic anemias
Teardrop	Iron deficiency Myelophthisic Megaloblastic
Sickle cells	Sickle cell disease
Target cells	Thalassemias Hemoglobinopathies
Parasites	Malaria Babesiosis
Basophilic stippling	Lead toxicity
Bite cells	G6PD deficiency
Anisocytosis	Red cells are of unequal size (high RDW) Iron deficiency
Poikilocytosis	Red cells are of different shapes.
Rouleaux formation	Multiple myeloma Hyperviscosity
Howell–Jolly bodies	Postsplenectomy Sickle cell disease
Heinz bodies	Hemolytic anemia Thalassemia

G6PD, glucose-6-phosphate dehydrogenase; RDW, red cell distribution width.

5. Basic metabolic panel (BMP): Elevated indirect bilirubin and LDH indicate hemolysis. Elevated blood urea nitrogen (BUN) and creatinine indicates renal disease. Elevated aspartate aminotransferase (AST), alanine aminotransferase (ALT), alkaline phosphatase (ALP), and direct bilirubin implicate liver disease. Elevated protein and calcium may indicate multiple myeloma.

6. Diagnostic pathway for anemia: If the corrected reticulocyte count is over 2.0 and there is elevated indirect bilirubin and LDH, workup for hemolysis is indicated. If the corrected reticulocyte count is under 2.0, the mean corpuscular volume (MCV) will provide a

> 💡 Reticulocytosis + elevated indirect bilirubin and LDH → hemolysis.

> 💡 For microcytic anemias, remember the mnemonic **TICS**: **T**halassemias, **I**ron deficiency, **C**hronic inflammatory block, and **S**ideroblastic (lead toxicity until proven otherwise).

> 💡 Consider α-thalassemia when a patient fails to respond to treatment for suspected iron deficiency or with a normal ferritin level in microcytic anemia.

measure of red cell size. An MCV >100 fL should prompt a macrocytic workup, an MCV of 80 to 100 fL should prompt a normocytic path, and an MCV under 80 fL suggests a microcytic differential diagnosis. Figure 4-1 is a summary of the diagnostic pathway.

D. Microcytic anemias (MCV < 80 fL) (Table 4-3)

1. Microcytic anemias are the most common anemias found in clinical practice.

   a. Diagnostic testing includes serum ferritin, iron, total iron-binding capacity (TIBC; the amount of transferrin available to transport iron), and percent saturation (the percentage of transferrin saturated with iron).

   b. Inflammation can be detected by an elevated C-reactive protein (CRP) or elevated Westergren erythrocyte sedimentation rate (ESR).

   c. If iron deficiency and the anemia of chronic inflammation are excluded, Hgb electrophoresis with quantification of Hgb A_2 and Hgb F will aid the diagnosis of β-thalassemia.

   d. The most common sideroblastic anemia is caused by lead toxicity; a lead level should be ordered followed by bone marrow biopsy if the diagnosis remains unknown.

2. **Thalassemia syndromes**

   a. General characteristics

      (1) Thalassemia is genetic underproduction of α- or β-globin chains resulting in deficient Hgb synthesis and RBC hemolysis.

      (2) α-Thalassemia is more common in people of Southeast Asian or Chinese origin; β-thalassemia is more common in African and Mediterranean populations.

      (3) Thalassemia should be suspected in a person with a positive family history or a personal history of lifelong microcytic anemia with normal iron stores.

   b. **Clinical features**

      (1) Deficits range from silent carrier status to profound anemia.

      (2) α-Thalassemia

         (a) Patients may have mild symptoms or none (thalassemia trait [two normal α-chains]; carriers [three normal α-chains]).

         (b) Patients with one α-globin chain (instead of the normal four) have Hgb H disease, which is variably symptomatic; when all four chains are deleted, stillbirth occurs from hydrops fetalis.

      (3) β-Thalassemia major (Cooley's anemia)

         (a) Symptoms begin at 4 to 6 months of age, when the switch from Hgb F to adult hemoglobin (Hgb A) occurs. Manifestations include severe anemia, growth retardation, abnormal facial structure, pathologic fractures, osteopenia, bone deformities, hepatosplenomegaly, and jaundice.

         (b) Before effective iron chelation and allogeneic stem cell transplantation, patients usually died from cardiac failure by 30 years of age.

   c. Diagnostic studies

      (1) Table 4-4 differentiates the thalassemias per typical Hct, Hgb electrophoresis, reticulocyte count, and peripheral smear.

      (2) Serum iron and ferritin levels are characteristically normal or elevated.

      (3) Hgb level is usually between 3 and 6 g/dL.

      (4) Thalassemia produces more marked microcytosis for degree of anemia than does iron deficiency; red cell morphologic changes occur earlier.

      (5) Diagnosis is confirmed by Hgb electrophoresis for β-thalassemia and DNA analysis for α-thalassemia.

   d. **Treatment**

      (1) Patients with the mild disease should not receive iron if ferritin is normal because of the risk of iron overload.

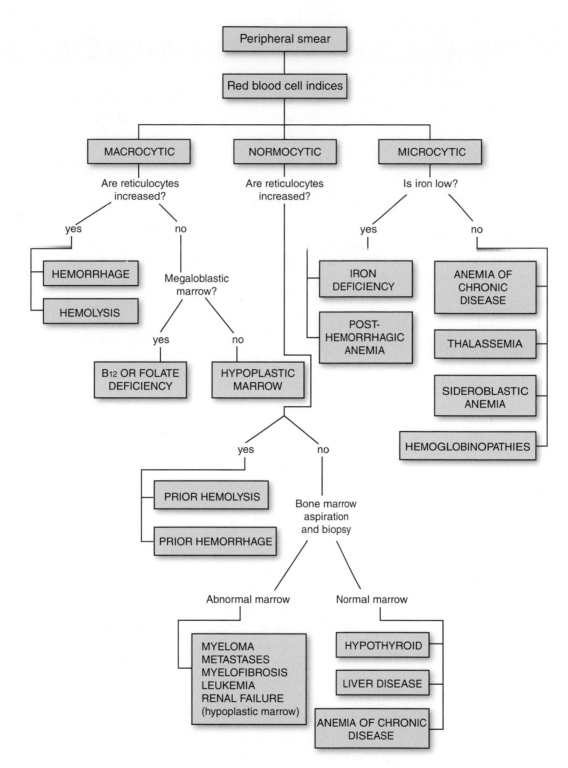

Figure 4-1 ▶ Diagnostic pathway. (Reprinted with permission from Nirula R. *High-Yield Internal Medicine*. 3rd ed. Lippincott Williams & Wilkins; 2007, Fig. 9-1.)

Table 4-3 | Summary of Findings in Microcytic Anemia

	Iron Deficiency	Chronic Inflammation	Sideroblastic Lead	Thalassemia
Red cells	Microcytic hypochromic	Normocytic microcytic	Dimorphic stippling	Microcytic target cells
Serum iron	Decreased	Decreased	Normal or increased	Normal or increased
TIBC	Increased	Decreased	Normal	Normal
Saturation	<16%	10%–20%	50%–100%	30%–100%
Serum ferritin	Decreased	Increased	Increased	Normal or increased
Hgb ELP	Normal	Normal	Normal	Abnormal
Indirect bilirubin LDH	Normal	Normal	Normal	Elevated

TIBC, total iron-binding capacity; Hgb ELP, hemoglobin electrophoresis; LDH, lactate dehydrogenase.

Table 4-4 | Differentiation of Thalassemias per Laboratory Parameters

Type	Hematocrit	Hemoglobin Electrophoresis	Peripheral Smear	Reticulocyte Count
α-Thalassemia minor (trait)	28%–40%	Normal	Target cells Acanthocytes	Normal
α-Thalassemia H	22%–32%	Hemoglobin H	Target cells Poikilocytes	Increased
β-Thalassemia minor or carrier	28%–40% B/B° or B/B⁺	Hemoglobin A₂ Hemoglobin F	Target cells Basophilic stippling	Normal or increased
β-Thalassemia major (severe, transfusion dependent)	As low as 10% B°/B° or B°/B⁺	Hemoglobin F Hemoglobin A₂	Target cells Poikilocytes Basophilic stippling Nucleated RBCs	Increased

RBCs, red blood cells.

(2) Persons with Hgb H disease (single α-chain) need folic acid supplements and should avoid iron supplements and oxidative drugs (e.g., dapsone, primaquine, quinidine, sulfonamides, nitrofurantoin).

(3) Treatment for β-thalassemia major consists of transfusions to keep Hgb concentrations at least 12 g per dL; however, iron overload may result in hemosiderosis, heart failure, cirrhosis, and endocrinopathies. Parenteral deferoxamine or oral deferasirox is administered to treat or postpone hemosiderosis.

(4) Allogeneic bone marrow transplantation is also used with increasing success, and gene therapy is now in clinical trials; splenectomy may also be required.

(5) Genetic counseling, testing, and prenatal diagnosis for severe forms are essential.

3. **Iron deficiency anemias**

   a. General characteristics

   (1) Iron deficiency is the most common cause of anemia worldwide.

   (2) In adults, GI blood loss secondary to PUD, NSAID use, or cancer is the likely cause; heavy menstrual blood loss may cause iron deficiency; however, GI bleeding must be ruled out.

   (3) Low dietary intake of iron may occur in children, impoverished persons, and pregnant women.

   (4) Other causes include decreased absorption of iron, increased requirements, hemoglobinuria, blood donation, iron sequestration, trauma, and intravascular hemolysis.

> Iron deficiency anemia in a postmenopausal woman demands a workup for occult colorectal cancer.

b. Clinical features

(1) Lack of iron causes few specific complaints. General complaints in moderate to severe iron deficiency include pallor, easy fatigability, irritability, anorexia, tachycardia, tachypnea on exertion, and poor weight gain in infants.

(2) Pica and anemia are hallmarks of iron deficiency.

(3) Severe deficiency (Hct < 25%) may cause brittle nails, cheilosis, smooth tongue, and formation of esophageal webs (Plummer–Vinson syndrome).

c. Diagnostic studies

(1) Hgb and Hct are decreased.

(2) Peripheral smear

    (a) Initially, there are no changes in red cell size.

    (b) Later, the peripheral smear shows hypochromic microcytic red cells, anisocytosis, and poikilocytosis.

(3) A plasma ferritin level of <20 µg per L reliably indicates iron deficiency anemia.

(4) Serum iron is decreased to <30 µg per dL, and TIBC is elevated. Transferrin saturation decreases to <15%.

d. Treatment

(1) Ferrous sulfate, 325 mg three times orally, should be given in a slowly escalating dose. It is best absorbed on an empty stomach but is frequently given with meals because of intolerability. Supplemental vitamin C may enhance absorption. Constipation is a common side effect; treatment with stool softener is advised to improve medication compliance.

(2) Although Hgb/Hct will be within the normal range in 2 months, therapy should be continued for up to 6 months or longer to replenish tissue stores measured by ferritin.

(3) Iron supplementation during pregnancy and lactation is essential.

(4) Parenteral iron is appropriate for patients with intolerance to oral iron, GI disease, and continuing blood loss. Sodium ferric gluconate is less likely than iron dextran to cause anaphylaxis.

(5) Workup for occult blood loss is imperative.

(6) Treatment failures may be caused by noncompliance, poor absorption, incorrect diagnosis, or ongoing blood loss.

> Iron supplements include ferrous sulfate, ferrous gluconate, and ferrous fumarate. They are equally effective but with varying side effects.

4. Chronic inflammation

a. Chronic infections, neoplastic diseases, and autoimmune inflammatory processes (e.g., rheumatoid arthritis, systemic lupus erythematosus [SLE]) increase hepcidin levels, which block the iron absorption from the gut and the release of iron from the bone marrow leading to chronic anemia.

b. Laboratory findings

(1) Thirty percent are microcytic, 70% are normocytic.

(2) Elevated CRP or Westergren ESR is characteristic of chronic inflammation.

(3) A normal or elevated ferritin level with a high percent saturation is typical.

> Most anemias of chronic disease are normocytic anemia; about a third are micryocytic.

c. Treatment

(1) Treating the underlying cause will reduce inflammation and the anemia will improve.

(2) Transfusion may be required if symptomatic.

(3) Patients do not respond to epo or iron supplements.

5. Sideroblastic anemias

a. General characteristics

> **(1)** Sideroblastic anemias are acquired disorders with reduced Hgb synthesis causing iron accumulation, especially in the mitochondria. Prussian blue staining of bone marrow cells shows ringed sideroblasts.
>
> **(2)** Causes include myelodysplasia, chronic alcoholism, and lead poisoning.

b. Laboratory findings

> **(1)** Hct is usually 20% to 30%. MCV varies.
>
> **(2)** Peripheral smear shows normal and hypochromic cells.
>
> **(3)** In lead poisoning, basophilic stippling of red cells may be present.
>
> **(4)** Bone marrow evaluation and serum lead levels are necessary to establish the diagnosis.

c. Treatment

> **(1)** Chelation therapy is needed for symptomatic lead toxicity.
>
> **(2)** Transfusion may also be required if the patient is symptomatic. Monitor for iron overload.
>
> **(3)** Removal of toxins is warranted.
>
> **(4)** Treatment with pyridoxine (vitamin B_6) may result in reticulocytosis and improved Hgb levels.

> Peripheral blood smear provides data on the number and shape of RBCs.

E. Normocytic anemias (MCV = 80 to 100 fL)

1. General characteristics

a. These anemias are caused by organ failure (kidney, endocrine, or liver), impaired marrow function, acute blood loss, or chronic systemic disease elevating hepcidin in response to inflammation.

b. The impaired marrow function causing aplastic anemia may be associated with infection (parvovirus B19 is common), medications, chemotherapy, toxins, radiation, myelodysplasia, and infiltrative marrow disease (myelophthisic syndromes).

2. Clinical features

a. Acute blood loss from GI bleeds or trauma can present with normocytic indices.

b. Clinical features are consistent with the underlying organ failure or chronic disease.

c. Patients with aplastic anemia and pancytopenia have weakness, fatigue, dyspnea, increased infection, pallor, purpura, and petechiae. Hepatosplenomegaly, lymphadenopathy, or bone tenderness suggests a neoplastic, autoimmune, or infectious cause.

3. Laboratory studies

a. Anemia of chronic inflammatory disease is normochromic normocytic 70% of the time and hypochromic microcytic 30%. The CRP or Westergren ESR is typically elevated.

b. Anemia of chronic disease has normal or increased bone marrow iron stores and serum ferritin and normal or low TIBC.

c. Red cell morphology and reticulocyte count are unremarkable or mildly abnormal.

d. Pancytopenia or two cytopenias can be present in aplastic anemia, myelodysplasia leukemia, or myelofibrosis. This will require a bone marrow biopsy for diagnosis.

e. The BMP and urinalysis will help identify renal or hepatic causes.

4. Treatment

a. In anemia of chronic inflammatory disease, the underlying disease must be treated and inflammation reduced.

b. Recombinant epo is effective in treating anemia of renal failure or anemia secondary to chemotherapy.

c. Symptomatic aplastic anemia is treated with RBC transfusions. Severe disease is treated with bone marrow transplantation or immunosuppression.

F. Macrocytic anemias (MCV > 100 fL)

    1. General characteristics (Table 4-5)

        a. The most common causes are folate and vitamin B_{12} deficiency.

        b. Laboratory studies: Obtain serum vitamin B_{12}, folate, and RBC folate levels. Consider methylmalonic acid (MMA) and homocysteine levels. Consider thyroid-stimulating hormone (TSH) if all other tests are normal, then a bone marrow biopsy.

    2. **Folic acid deficiency anemia**

        a. General characteristics

            (1) Folic acid deficiency is most often caused by poor dietary intake. Other causes include defective absorption, pregnancy, chronic hemolytic anemias, alcohol abuse, and folic acid antagonists (e.g., phenytoin, trimethoprim–sulfamethoxazole, sulfasalazine).

            (2) Inadequate intake is common in alcoholics, persons with anorexia, and those whose diet is low in fruits and vegetables.

            (3) Malabsorption is a rare cause as folic acid is absorbed throughout the GI tract.

            (4) The daily requirement of folic acid is 50 to 100 mg per dL and is usually met by a balanced diet.

            (5) Pregnancy, chronic hemolytic anemias, and exfoliative skin disease increase daily requirements and may necessitate supplementation.

        b. **Clinical features**

            (1) Sore tongue (glossitis)

            (2) Vague GI symptoms

            (3) No neurologic symptoms

        c. Laboratory findings

            (1) Howell–Jolly bodies (nuclear DNA remnants) are typical.

            (2) RBC folate level of <150 ng per mL is diagnostic.

            (3) Serum vitamin B_{12} level is normal.

            (4) Serum homocysteine levels are elevated. MMA is not elevated.

        d. **Treatment**

            (1) Oral replacement (1 mg/day) with folic acid is the first-line treatment.

            (2) Avoid alcohol and folic acid metabolism antagonists (e.g., trimethoprim, seizure medications).

    3. **Vitamin B_{12} (cobalamin) deficiency**

        a. General characteristics

            (1) Pernicious anemia is the most common cause because of a lack of intrinsic factor (produced in the stomach) that is necessary for vitamin B_{12} absorption.

            (2) Other causes include a strict vegan diet, gastric bypass surgery, blind loop syndrome, pancreatic insufficiency, metformin use, and Crohn's disease.

> In macrocytic anemia with neuropsychiatric symptoms, think B_{12}; without neuropsychiatric symptoms, think folate deficiency.
> Folate is from plant sources; B_{12} is mainly from animal sources.

Table 4-5 | Folate and Vitamin B_{12} Results

Test	Vitamin B_{12} Deficiency	Folate Deficiency
Serum vitamin B_{12}	Low	Normal or low
Serum folate	Normal	Low
RBC folate	Normal	Low
Methylmalonic acid	High	Normal
Homocysteine	High	High

RBC, red blood cell.

(3) Irreversible neurologic damage can be caused by uncorrected deficiency. Folate administration can mask the deficiency but does not correct it.

(4) Foods of animal origin supply vitamin B$_{12}$.

(5) Absorption occurs in the terminal ileum and storage is in the liver.

b. Clinical features

(1) Examination of the mouth may reveal smooth tongue, glossitis, or cheilosis.

(2) Neurologic findings may include stocking-glove paresthesias; loss of position, fine touch, and vibratory sensation; balance problems and ataxia; or dementia.

(3) Abdominal surgical scars may indicate gastrectomy or bariatric surgery, which may lead to impaired vitamin B$_{12}$ absorption as a contributing factor.

c. Diagnostic studies

(1) Hypersegmented neutrophils (more than six lobes) are seen on the peripheral smear. Anisocytosis, poikilocytosis, and macro-ovalocytosis may be seen as well.

(2) Serum LDH and indirect bilirubin can be elevated if hemolysis is present.

(3) Serum vitamin B$_{12}$ is abnormally low.

(4) Schilling test (a 24-hour urine collection of radioactive vitamin B$_{12}$) is rarely used today.

(5) Anti-intrinsic factor antibodies can be present.

(6) Both serum MMA and homocysteine levels are increased in anemia because of vitamin B$_{12}$ deficiency.

d. Treatment

(1) Lifelong supplemental vitamin B$_{12}$ (1,000 μg monthly) is usually given intramuscularly (IM) for pernicious anemia.

(2) Daily (1,000 μg) oral cobalamin may be effective, especially after an adequate parenteral loading. A nasal spray or gel is also available.

(3) Reversible causes of malabsorption should be treated.

(4) Strict vegans; patients with gastric bypass, gastrectomy, or resection of the ileum; and those with blind loop syndrome require vitamin B$_{12}$ supplementation.

(5) Neurologic signs and symptoms are reversible if treated within 6 months.

G. Hemolytic anemias

1. General characteristics

a. Hemolytic anemias are characterized by decreased RBC survival and increased cell lysis.

(1) Hereditary causes are intrinsic (problem within the RBC) and include hereditary spherocytosis and elliptocytosis, G6PD deficiency, thalassemias, and sickle cell syndromes.

(2) Causes external to the erythrocyte include immune attack and trauma to RBCs caused by thrombotic thrombocytopenic purpura (TTP), hemolytic uremic syndrome (HUS), disseminated intravascular coagulation (DIC), valvular hemolysis, metastatic adenocarcinoma, vasculitis, infections, hypersplenism, transfusion reactions, and burns.

2. Clinical features

a. Symptoms of anemia and jaundice that develop rapidly with no source of bleeding indicate hemolysis. Chronic hemolysis causes bilirubin gallstones and bone marrow expansion visible on x-rays.

b. Dark urine is seen with intravascular hemolysis.

> The mnemonic HIT is a memory tool to classify the causes into Hereditary, Immune attack, and Trauma to the RBCs.

    c. Hepatosplenomegaly may be the cause of RBC lysis.

    d. Petechiae and purpura may indicate thrombocytopenia caused by TTP; DIC; HUS; and hemolysis, elevated liver enzymes, and low platelets (HELLP) syndrome (see Table 4-6).

3. Diagnostic studies

    a. An elevated corrected reticulocyte count (over 2.0) in the presence of a falling Hgb, elevated indirect bilirubin, and elevated LDH are the hallmarks of hemolytic anemia.

    b. Peripheral smear may reveal immature red cells, nucleated red cells, or morphologic changes.

    c. A direct Coombs or direct antiglobulin test (DAT) may identify antibodies on the RBCs. An indirect Coombs test may identify antibodies in the patient's serum.

    d. Other helpful tests include an Hgb electrophoresis for hemoglobinopathies; Heinz body stain for G6PD deficiency; osmotic fragility for spherocytosis and elliptocytosis; D-dimer; prothrombin time (PT); activated partial thromboplastin time (aPTT); and a pregnancy test if thrombocytopenia is present.

4. Treatment depends on the underlying disorder.

5. **Sickle cell disease**

    a. General characteristics

       (1) Sickle cell disease is a family of autosomal recessive inherited hemoglobinopathies (SS, SC, SD, SO Arab, S β^+ thalassemia, and S β^0 thalassemia).

       (2) RBCs containing primarily Hgb S sickle under hypoxia, dehydration, acidosis, and extreme temperature conditions

       (3) In the United States, this disease is most often seen in blacks (1 in 400 births); 8% carry the Hgb S gene as the sickle cell trait.

    b. **Clinical features**

       (1) Problems begin about 6 months after birth when protective Hgb F levels fall to adult levels.

       (2) Patients with sickle cell disease present with a spectrum of mild to severe complications including vascular occlusions, painful crises, strokes, chest syndrome, bone infarctions, avascular necrosis (AVN), splenic sequestration, and delayed growth/puberty.

> Hemolytic anemia = falling Hgb plus rising indirect bilirubin and LDH.

> Sickling is precipitated by hypoxia, dehydration, acidosis, and extreme temperature conditions.

Table 4-6 | Hemolysis and Thrombocytopenias

Issue/Disease	TTP	HUS	DIC	HELLP— Eclampsia	HIT
Age/gender	Adults	Children	Any	Pregnant females	Any
Cause	ADAMTS 13 and big vWF	Infections: *Escherichia coli* O157:H7	Sepsis, burns, trauma	Eclampsia	Heparin exposure PF4 activates + HIT assay
PT/aPTT	Normal	Normal	Abnormal	±	PTT abnormal with unfractionated heparin
Fever	Yes	Yes	Depends	±	Depends
Bleeding or clotting	Both	Both	Both	Both	Clotting
Organ failure	CNS > renal	Renal > CNS	All possible	Liver	All possible
Treatment	Plasma exchange, no platelets	Support, no platelets	FFP, cryoprecipitate, platelets	Deliver (MgSO₄)	Stop heparin—use other anticoagulants

TTP, thrombotic thrombocytopenia; HUS, hemolytic uremic syndrome; DIC, disseminated intravascular coagulation; HELLP, hemolysis, elevated liver enzymes, and low platelets; HIT, heparin-induced thrombocytopenia; vWF, von Willebrand factor; PF4, platelet factor 4; PT, prothrombin time; aPTT, activated partial thromboplastin time; PTT, partial thromboplastin time; CNS, central nervous system; FFP, fresh frozen plasma; MgSO₄, magnesium sulfate.

(3) Sickle complications can be precipitated by red cell dehydration, acidosis, or hypoxemia as well as stress, menses, and temperature changes. Patients should avoid high altitudes (above 7,000 feet) and deep-sea diving.

(4) Patients with sickle cell anemia are at increased risk for cholelithiasis, splenomegaly, leg ulcers, infection with encapsulated organisms (e.g., *Streptococcus pneumoniae*), strokes, AVN, priapism, retinopathies leading to blindness, and osteomyelitis.

(5) Hemolytic or aplastic crises may be life-threatening.

(6) AVN of the femoral and humeral head is more common in type SC.

(7) Life expectancy for type SS is 40 to 50 years of age but has been increasing over the past few decades because of advancements in monitoring and treatment.

(8) Sickle cell trait may result in difficulty concentrating urine and hematuria.

  c. Diagnostic studies

(1) Electrophoresis demonstrates the level of different Hgbs in the red cell. Hgb S is 50% or greater in sickle cell disease. The MCV is low in S β^+ thalassemia and S β^0 thalassemia.

(2) Peripheral smear may reveal sickled cells (5% to 50%) and target cells, nucleated RBCs, and Howell–Jolly bodies.

(3) Reticulocyte count, indirect bilirubin, and LDH are elevated when hemolyzing.

(4) White blood cell (WBC) count is elevated; thrombocytosis may be present.

  d. Treatment

(1) Symptomatic treatment of pain episodes includes administration of analgesics, hypotonic fluids, and rest.

(2) Stroke, sequestration, acute chest syndrome, and multiorgan failure may require transfusion or exchange transfusion.

(3) Patients should receive low-dose daily penicillin from birth until 6 years of age, pneumococcal vaccine (booster vaccine every 10 years), transcranial Doppler (TCD) screening for stroke prevention, pulmonary function testing (PFT) for restrictive disease screening, and chronic folate supplementation.

(4) Daily lifelong oral hydroxyurea therapy should be considered for all SS and S β^0 thalassemia patients as young as 1 year old to increase Hgb F production, prevent complications, and increase life span. L-Glutamine is a Food and Drug Administration (FDA)-approved treatment to use independently or add to hydroxyurea for added benefits of reduced pain events. Stem cell transplant is curative, and now gene therapy is in clinical trials.

(5) For patients who cannot tolerate or who have reduced response to hydroxyurea, there are two new treatments. Crizanlizumab-tmca is a monthly IV infusion of humanized IgG2 kappa monoclonal antibody that binds to P-selectin preventing blood cell adhesion and reducing pain events. Voxelotor is a daily oral Hgb S polymerization inhibitor that regulates the affinity of hemoglobin for oxygen improving red cell survival and decreases pain events.

(6) Genetic counseling for patients with either the disease or trait is recommended. Prenatal testing is available.

6. G6PD deficiency—hereditary

  a. General characteristics

(1) G6PD deficiency is an X-linked recessive disorder commonly seen in American black males (10% to 15%) and some Mediterranean populations.

(2) Oxidative drugs (e.g., aspirin, dapsone, primaquine, quinidine, sulfonamides, nitrofurantoin), fava bean ingestion, and infection cause episodic hemolysis.

(3) Severe deficiency may cause chronic hemolysis.

> In G6PD, remember Heinz bodies and bite cells in peripheral smear.

b. Clinical features

(1) Patients with episodic hemolysis are usually healthy and have no splenomegaly.

(2) Female carriers are rarely affected.

c. Laboratory findings

(1) During hemolytic episodes, reticulocytes and serum indirect bilirubin increase.

(2) Peripheral smear reveals bite cells and Heinz bodies (denatured hemoglobin).

(3) G6PD levels will be low between hemolytic episodes; in severe cases, G6PD levels will always be low.

d. Treatment

(1) In most cases, hemolytic episodes are self-limited as red cells are replaced as soon as the offending agent is stopped.

(2) Oxidative drugs and fava beans should be avoided.

7. RBC membrane problems

a. Spherocytosis and elliptocytosis can be diagnosed from the peripheral smear and the osmotic fragility test.

b. Paroxysmal nocturnal hemoglobinuria (PNH) is caused by lysis of red cells by complement causing dark first voided urine from hemoglobinuria.

c. Lack of RBC surface CD55 or CD59 detected by flow cytometry is diagnostic.

8. Immune hemolysis and transfusion issues

a. A history of a recent blood transfusion or new medication should suggest an immune cause. Table 4-7 describes the Coombs test results when positive.

b. Coombs positive: transfusion reaction, immunoglobin M (IgM) only—cold antibody because of infections, immunoglobin G (IgG) warm antibody—may be drug induced or because of malignancy or other autoimmune disorder.

c. Transfusion reactions can occur immediately as blood is being transfused, acutely within 24 hours, or delayed up to two weeks after transfusion. Immediate reactions include dyspnea, flushing, pruritis, tachycardia, wheezing, fever, hypotension, anxiety-impending doom, and hemoglobinuria. The transfusion should be stopped and supportive measures implemented.

d. Transfusion-related acute lung injury (TRALI) presents with dyspnea, hypoxemia, bilateral lung infiltrates on the chest radiograph, without signs of acute cardiogenic pulmonary edema and fever. Supportive therapy is required.

e. Delayed transfusion reaction is usually caused by RBC alloantibodies not detected in the type and cross. Signs of hemolysis are present, and supportive therapy is required.

f. A nonimmune complication of multiple RBC transfusions (usually over 20 units) is iron overload or hemochromatosis. Iron deposits in the heart causing conduction problems, the liver causing cirrhosis, and endocrine organs causing failure.

(1) Early symptoms include severe fatigue, impotence, and arthralgias. The most common signs at the time of presentation are hepatomegaly, jaundice, bronze skin pigmentation, diabetes, hypogonadism, hypothyroid, and arthritis.

Table 4-7 | Coombs Test Results

Antibody Type	IgG	Complement C3d	Causes
Warm IgG	Positive	Positive or negative	CLL, NHL, Hodgkin, SLE, ulcerative colitis drugs, transfusion reactions
Cold IgM	Negative	Positive	Infections (EBV, CMV, mononucleosis, *Mycoplasma*), drugs (antibiotics), transfusion reactions

IgM, immunoglobin M; IgG, immunoglobin G; CLL, chronic lymphocytic leukemia; NHL, non-Hodgkin's lymphoma; SLE, systemic lupus erythematosus; EBV, Epstein–Barr virus; CMV, cytomegalovirus.

(2) Serum ferritin levels over 200 μg /L in premenopausal women and 300 μg /L in men and postmenopausal women with a transferrin saturation over 50% indicates iron overload.

(3) The genetic cause of hemochromatosis is the *HFE* gene mutations C282Y and H63D. This is a common mutation with 1 case in 200 to 500 individuals. This causes low levels of hepcidin, allowing too much iron absorption from the GI tract. Excessive iron can be removed by regular phlebotomy and oral or parenteral iron chelation therapy. Patients should avoid iron-rich foods, iron supplements, alcohol, and raw seafood.

9. Trauma to RBCs

a. Splenomegaly and prosthetic heart valves can cause hemolysis by external mechanical breaking of cells.

b. Red cell parasites such as *Plasmodium* (malaria), *Bartonella*, and *Babesia* cause destruction of the red cell from within.

c. Microangiopathic destruction of red cells can occur when the clotting system is activated, as evidenced by an elevated D-dimer, and fibrin threads shear red cells as they flow by. The CBC reveals thrombocytopenia, and the peripheral smear has helmet cells or schistocytes.

d. PT and aPTT will help diagnose TTP, HUS, DIC, HIT, or the pregnancy-related variant of eclampsia with HELLP. Table 4-6 has a comparison of these conditions.

H. Polycythemia vera

1. General characteristics

a. Polycythemia vera is a slowly progressive bone marrow disorder characterized by increased numbers of RBCs and increased total blood volume. The presence of the JAK2 mutation and low epo levels are diagnostic for the primary (genetic) cause.

b. Increased red cell mass causes hyperviscosity, leading to decreased cerebral blood flow and hypercoagulability.

c. Secondary causes of polycythemia include chronic hypoxia, cigarette smoking, living at high altitudes, and renal tumors.

d. Morbidity and mortality most commonly result from thrombosis; other complications include bleeding, PUD, and GI bleeding.

e. Median age at presentation is 60 years, and 60% of patients are male. Median survival time for patients with polycythemia vera is 11 to 15 years.

f. Polycythemia vera may convert to myelofibrosis or chronic myeloid leukemia and, rarely, to acute myeloid leukemia.

2. Clinical features

a. Clinical features include headache, dizziness, fullness in the head and face, weakness, fatigue, tinnitus, blurred vision, pruritus, burning, pain, and redness of the extremities. Epistaxis may be the presenting complaint. Generalized pruritus after bathing is characteristic.

b. Incidence of PUD is high.

c. Plethora, systolic hypertension, engorged retinal veins, and splenomegaly may be found on physical examination.

d. Thrombosis is the most common complication and the cause of most morbidity and mortality; increased bleeding also occurs.

e. Absence of splenomegaly suggests secondary polycythemia.

3. Diagnostic studies

a. At sea level, Hct levels in polycythemia vera are typically >54% in males and >51% in females.

Pruritus after bathing is the hallmark of polycythemia vera.

b. Patients with primary polycythemia vera have low epo levels, thrombocytosis, and leukocytosis. Peripheral smear shows neutrophilic leukocytosis, increased basophils and eosinophils, and increased number of large platelets. Patients with secondary polycythemia only have an increased red cell count and a high epo level.

c. Red cell morphology is usually normal.

d. Hyperuricemia can also develop.

4. Treatment

    a. Serial phlebotomy is the treatment of choice.

    b. Myelosuppressive therapy with hydroxyurea may be indicated.

    c. Low-dose aspirin reduces the risk of thrombosis.

    d. The JAK1/2 inhibitor ruxolitinib is approved for refractory patients.

White Cell Disorders

A. Leukopenia and leukocytosis

    1. General characteristics

        a. Leukopenia can be caused by infections, toxins, medications, chemotherapy, leukemia, myeloma, or myelodysplasia.

        b. Leukocytosis can be caused by infections, leukemia, or chronic hemolytic anemias.

    2. Clinical features

        a. Leukopenia, especially neutropenia, may present with fever, chills, opportunistic infections, or signs of malignancy.

        b. Leukocytosis may present with signs of infection (fever, chills, night sweats, tachycardia, productive cough, dysuria, pharyngitis, lymphadenopathy, or splenomegaly) or leukemia or hemolysis.

    3. Diagnostic studies

        a. A WBC count below 4.5 k/μL is leukopenia and above 11.0 k/μL is leukocytosis.

        b. The WBC differential gives great clues to the diagnosis of leukocytosis (Table 4-8).

        c. Peripheral WBC blasts are always abnormal and should prompt a referral for bone marrow biopsy.

B. Leukemias

    1. General characteristics

        a. Leukemias are characterized by increased production of abnormal leukocytes and leukocyte precursors in the circulation and bone marrow.

        b. Leukemias are classified according to cell type, either myelocytic (ML) or lymphocytic (LL), and whether acute (acute myelogenous leukemia [AML], ALL) or chronic (chronic myelocytic leukemia [CML], CLL).

        c. Risk factors include genetics and exposures to ionizing radiation, benzene, and certain alkylating agents.

    2. Acute leukemias (ALL and AML)

        a. General characteristics

            (1) There are two types of acute leukemias: ALL and AML.

            (2) The incidence increases with age. In children 3 to 7 years old, ALL (80%) is more common than AML.

            (3) AML is primarily a disease of adulthood (median age at onset is 60 years).

        b. Clinical features

            (1) Most clinical findings (pallor, dyspnea, tachycardia, infections, bleeding, bone pain) are related to the replacement of normal bone marrow with abnormal cells.

> Chronic lymphocytic leukemia (CLL) is the most common leukemia overall; acute lymphocytic leukemia (ALL) is the most common leukemia in children.

Table 4-8 | Leukocytosis Differentials

Cell Type	Normal Values	Causes of Elevated Level
Neutrophils (segs)	54%–62%	Bacterial infections
Neutrophils (bands)	3%–5%	Acute bacterial infections and sepsis
Lymphocytes	25%–33%	Viral infections
Monocytes	3%–7%	Chronic infections such as tuberculosis and subacute bacterial endocarditis, mononucleosis
Eosinophils	1%–3%	Allergies, parasitic infections, autoimmune disease
Basophils	0%–0.75%	Allergies
Atypical lymphocytes	Usually none	Epstein–Barr virus (mononucleosis)

(2) Gingival bleeding, epistaxis, and menorrhagia may be the presenting complaints in patients with thrombocytopenia.

(3) Neutropenia predisposes to infections, most commonly those caused by Gram-negative bacteria or fungi.

(4) Children and young adults present with fatigue, abrupt onset of fever, lethargy, headache, and bone and/or joint pain, especially in the sternum, tibia, and femur.

(5) Older adults have a slow, progressive onset, with lethargy, anorexia, and dyspnea.

(6) Symptoms of anemia, thrombocytopenia, gingival hyperplasia, rashes, or cranial nerve palsies may occur.

(7) Lymphadenopathy and hepatosplenomegaly are more common in ALL than in AML.

> In acute leukemias, CBC shows pancytopenia and Auer rods in AML; and TdT in ALL.

c. Diagnostic studies

(1) CBC reveals pancytopenia with circulating blasts; bone marrow biopsy demonstrates over 20% blasts.

(2) Hyperuricemia may be present.

(3) A bone marrow biopsy is indicated.

(4) Auer rods (rod-shaped structures in cell cytoplasm) can be seen in AML.

(5) Terminal deoxynucleotidyl transferase (TdT) is diagnostic for ALL.

(6) Cytogenetic studies and flow cytometry are the most powerful prognostic factor and can guide targeted therapy.

d. **Treatment**

(1) Induction (remission-inducing) chemotherapy is targeted toward eradication of most of the leukemic cells.

(2) Consolidation therapy destroys the remainder of the leukemic cells.

(3) Treatment often causes increased serum urate levels. Allopurinol and diuretics may be needed to prevent uric acid stones.

(4) Allogeneic bone marrow transplantation is used in patients with adverse cytogenetics or poor response to treatment.

(5) Children with ALL have an overall survival of approximately 80%, with some groups having a 98% cure rate (induction plus consolidation therapy). Prognosis is related to age and WBC count at diagnosis.

(6) Greater than 70% of adults younger than 60 years of age achieve a complete remission with treatment for AML; further chemotherapy leads to cure in 30% to 40% of patients.

3. **Chronic leukemias (CML and CLL)**

a. General characteristics

(1) CLL is a clonal malignancy of B lymphocytes.

(2) CML is a myeloproliferative disorder.

(3) CLL is the most prevalent of all leukemias. It is twice as common in men as in women. Incidence increases with advancing age; median age at presentation is 65 years.

(4) The B-cell form accounts for 95% of CLL cases.

b. Clinical features

(1) CML

(a) CML presents in young to middle-aged adults (median age at presentation is 55 years). Greater than 80% are alive 6 years later.

(b) It occurs in three phases: chronic, accelerated, and acute (blast crisis, defined as >30% blast cells in the blood or bone marrow).

(c) Symptoms

i. Fatigue, anorexia, weight loss, low-grade fever, and excessive sweating are common.

ii. Most patients also have abdominal fullness caused by splenomegaly.

iii. Rare presentations include blurred vision, respiratory distress, and priapism.

(d) The symptoms of CML develop gradually. CML generally runs a mild course until the blast-crisis phase, which indicates accelerated disease and short survival.

(2) CLL

(a) CLL usually has an indolent course, with a median survival time of 6 years. Patients with stage 0 or I have a median survival of 10 to 15 years. It is often harmless but is resistant to cure. A variant, polylymphocytic leukemia, is more aggressive.

(b) Clinical manifestations of CLL include peripheral lymphocytosis and lymphocytic invasion of bone marrow, liver, spleen, and lymph nodes.

(c) Patients may have recurrent infections, splenomegaly, and lymphadenopathy.

> Hallmark labs for chronic leukemias are: Philly chromosome for CML; and isolated lymphocytosis for CLL.

c. Diagnostic studies

(1) The hallmark of CLL is isolated lymphocytosis, with a leukocytosis of >20,000 per μL.

(2) The hallmark of CML is leukocytosis, with a median WBC count of 150,000 per μL. The Philadelphia chromosome is identified in 95% of cases.

(3) Identification of the *BCR-ABL* gene by polymerase chain reaction has replaced the search for the Philadelphia chromosome to establish the diagnosis.

(4) Peripheral smear

(a) CML may show anemia and thrombocytosis.

(b) CLL shows increased mature small lymphocytes; smudge cells are pathognomonic.

(5) Bone marrow biopsy is hypercellular with a left shift.

d. Treatment

(1) CML

(a) Tyrosine kinase inhibitors (imatinib, nilotinib, dasatinib, or bosutinib) are standard therapy. It is very effective during the chronic phase.

(b) Allogeneic bone marrow transplantation may be the initial treatment and is the only therapy proven to be curative. A cure rate of 80% is achieved in those younger than 40 years with transplantation from human leukocyte antigen (HLA)–matched siblings. Bone marrow transplantation is reserved for patients with severe disease which progresses after initial treatment.

(2) CLL: Treatment of CLL is watchful waiting until symptomatic, then includes fludarabine, cyclophosphamide, and rituximab.

Lymphomas and Myeloma

A. Hodgkin's disease

1. General characteristics

   a. Hodgkin's disease refers to a group of cancers characterized by enlargement of lymphoid tissue, spleen, and liver and the presence of Reed–Sternberg cells in lymph node biopsy tissue.

   b. The Epstein–Barr virus also appears to be an important factor; it can be found in 40% to 50% of cases.

   c. It is most common between the ages of 15 and 45 years, peaking in the 20s, and again after 50 years of age. It is rare in children younger than 5 years of age.

2. **Clinical features**

   a. Patients usually present with painless cervical, supraclavicular, and mediastinal lymphadenopathy. Pain in the affected node after ingestion of alcohol may occur.

   b. Stages I through IV are based on the number and location of involved lymph nodes. Nodes on both sides of the diaphragm indicate stage III or above. Stage A designation indicates a lack of constitutional symptoms. One-third of patients present with constitutional (stage B) symptoms (fever, night sweats, weight loss, pruritus, and fatigue), which are associated with a poorer prognosis.

3. Diagnostic studies

   a. Other causes of lymphadenopathy should be excluded, such as syphilis, HIV, and mononucleosis.

   b. Lymph node biopsy is definitive.

   c. Reed–Sternberg cells confirm the diagnosis.

   d. Basic staging includes CT of neck, chest, abdomen, and pelvis as well as biopsy of the bone marrow; laparotomy is no longer routine.

4. **Treatment**

   a. Combination chemotherapy cures most patients, even those with advanced-stage disease.

   b. Radiation therapy is the initial treatment of choice for patients with low-risk stage IA and IIA disease; the 5-year survival rate exceeds 80%.

   c. Most other patients receive adriamycin, bleomycin, vinblastine, and dacarbazine (ABVD) chemotherapy; shorter, intensive treatments are under study.

B. Non-Hodgkin's lymphoma

1. General characteristics

   a. About 90% of cases are derived from B lymphocytes.

   b. The incidence of B-cell lymphomas is higher in patients with HIV disease and other immunodeficiencies.

   c. Peak incidence occurs between 20 and 40 years of age.

   d. These lymphomas are divided into clinically indolent and aggressive groups.

> Hodgkin's lymphoma can present with stage "B symptoms": fever, night sweats, weight loss, pruritus, and fatigue; and Reed–Sternberg cells on smear.

(1) Indolent lymphomas tend to convert to aggressive disease.

(2) One-third of aggressive lymphomas are curable with chemotherapy.

2. Clinical features

   a. Diffuse or isolated, painless, persistent lymphadenopathy is the most common presentation; bone marrow involvement is frequent.

   b. Common extra-lymphatic sites are the GI tract, skin, bone, and bone marrow. Burkitt's lymphoma is likely to present with abdominal fullness.

   c. Fever, night sweats, weight loss, pruritus, and fatigue are less likely than with Hodgkin's disease but do occur in intermediate- and high-grade disease.

3. Diagnostic studies

   a. Rule out other causes of lymphadenopathy.

   b. Persistent, unexplained, enlarged nodes should be excised for histologic study.

   c. Staging is accomplished by chest radiography, CT of the abdomen and pelvis, bone marrow biopsy, and possibly lumbar puncture.

4. Treatment is based on the stage of disease and the patient's clinical status.

   a. Patients with indolent lymphoma with one or two involved nodes may be treated with radiation alone.

   b. Intermediate- or high-grade lymphomas are treated with chemotherapy, immunotherapy, and autologous stem cell transplantation.

C. Multiple myeloma

1. General characteristics

> Pathologic fracture → think multiple myeloma.

   a. Multiple myeloma is a malignancy of plasma cells, producing an abundance of monoclonal paraprotein (M protein).

   b. Replacement of bone marrow leads to pancytopenia, osteolysis with bone pain, osteoporosis, hypercalcemia, and pathologic fractures. Plasmacytomas may cause spinal cord compression.

   c. Patients are prone to recurrent infections, particularly with encapsulated organisms, because of neutropenia and failure of antibody production.

   d. Paraprotein levels are increased (IgG or IgA may cause hyperviscosity; light-chain components may lead to renal failure).

2. Clinical features

   a. Median age at diagnosis is 65 years.

   b. The most common presenting complaints include anemia, bone pain (particularly in the low back or ribs), and infection. Less common presenting complaints include renal failure, spinal cord compression, and hyperviscosity syndrome.

3. Diagnostic studies

   a. Patients will be anemic, with normal cell morphology; rouleaux formation (RBCs stacking like coins) is common.

> Hallmark labs for multiple myeloma: Bence-Jones urinary protein.

   b. The hallmark of myeloma is a monoclonal spike on serum protein electrophoresis. Positive Bence-Jones protein in the urine is also typical.

   c. Lytic lesions are present on radiography of the axial skeleton; generalized osteoporosis may be present.

   d. Other laboratory findings: hypercalcemia and increased serum protein; elevated BUN/creatinine if with renal involvement. Hypercalcemia is a late finding.

   e. Bone scans are not helpful because multiple myeloma does not have an osteoblastic component.

4. Treatment involves referral for specialist care with combination chemotherapy and transplant options. Bisphosphonates are important adjunctive therapy.

Platelet and Bleeding Disorders

A. General characteristics

1. An intact and healthy endothelium, adequate functioning platelets, von Willebrand factor (vWF) to adhere platelets to damaged blood vessels, and adequate clotting/anticlotting factors are necessary to keep blood flowing in the vasculature and prevent leaking. Bleeding and platelet disorders present with excessive or repetitive bleeding, bruising, or bleeding at unusual sites.

   a. Platelet problems and vWD present with skin petechiae, bruising, and increased mucosal bleeding (e.g., epistaxis, gum bleeding, and menorrhagia).

   b. Hemarthroses and deep tissue hematomas are found in coagulation defects such as hemophilia.

   c. Purpura can be from vasculitis.

B. Differential diagnosis: The mnemonic "PVC Pipes" is helpful:

1. P—Platelets

   a. Not enough (usually below 50,000/μL): may be because of decreased production, destruction, or sequestration.

   b. Not working: may be secondary to aspirin, NSAIDs, uremia, or genetic causes.

2. V—vWD (type 1 is most common) results in decreased platelet adhesion and lack of stabilized factor VIII.

3. C—Clotting factors (most commonly factors VIII and IX), vitamin K deficiency (vitamin K is required for factors X, IX, VII, II, and I), liver disease (manufactures clotting factors), and presence of factor inhibitors

4. P—Pipes: vasculitis, scurvy (vitamin C deficiency), Ehlers–Danlos syndrome, hereditary hemorrhagic telangiectasias, steroids, and palpable purpura (sepsis, meningococcemia, Henoch–Schönlein purpura, drugs)

C. Diagnostic studies

1. CBC with platelet count and peripheral smear is done to identify and quantify cellular changes.

2. PT is an assessment of the extrinsic clotting pathway; it is usually reported as international normalized ratio (INR). aPTT assesses the intrinsic clotting pathway. If either is prolonged, a mixing study for inhibitor detection and thrombin time (TT) is indicated.

3. TT measures the rate of conversion of fibrinogen to fibrin in the presence of thrombin to assess the common pathway.

4. Platelet function analysis (PFA) measures the ability of platelets to activate and aggregate. It also tests the function of vWF to assist platelet adhesion.

5. A metabolic profile is recommended to assess kidney and hepatic function.

6. D-dimer is indicated for thrombosis detection in suspected TTP, HUS, DIC, HELLP, and HIT (see Table 4-6).

D. **Thrombocytopenia**

1. General characteristics

   a. Mild thrombocytopenia (low platelets) is 100,000 to 150,000 per μL. Moderate thrombocytopenia, where caution is needed for surgery or procedures, is 50,000 to 100,000 per μL. Severe thrombocytopenia, where spontaneous bleeding can occur, is <50,000 per μL.

   b. Thrombocytopenia may be caused by impaired marrow production (e.g., vitamin B_{12} or folate deficiency; congenital; or marrow damage from drugs, leukemia, infections), increased destruction (e.g., immune-mediated HIT, immune thrombocytopenic purpura [ITP], HIV, SLE, or nonimmune-mediated in DIC, TTP, and HELLP), and hepatosplenic sequestration.

> Diagnostic labs include: CBC with smear, PT, PTT, PFA, CMP, and possibly D-dimer (if indicated).

(1) Acute ITP is a self-limited, autoimmune (IgG) disorder found most commonly in children of both sexes. It is associated with a preceding viral upper respiratory infection.

(2) Chronic ITP may occur at any age (peak incidence is from 20 to 50 years) and is more common in women; it often coexists with other autoimmune diseases, HIV, and hepatitis C.

(3) Thrombotic thrombocytopenia (TTP) is rare but often fatal. It is found in previously healthy people, most commonly between the ages of 20 and 50 years. It occurs more often in women than in men and in patients with HIV disease. TTP may be precipitated by estrogen use, pregnancy, and drugs such as quinine, clopidogrel, and ticlopidine.

(4) HUS is similar to TTP but is found primarily in children and adults exposed to toxigenic *Escherichia coli* O157:H7.

(5) DIC causes generalized hemorrhage in patients with severe underlying systemic illness such as sepsis, tissue injury, burns, obstetric complications, cancer, and in severe transfusion reactions.

2. **Clinical features**

   a. Thrombocytopenia below 50,000 per μL (severe) is characterized by petechiae, purpura, and bleeding (nose, gums, GI tract, menorrhagia).

   b. TTP, HELLP, HIT, HUS, and DIC cause severe thrombocytopenia and microangiopathic hemolytic anemia. Table 4-6 documents the differences. TTP can cause abnormal neurologic signs.

   c. HUS is similar to TTP but has more renal problems. It affects primarily children younger than 10 years of age, particularly after infection with *E. coli* O157:H7, *Shigella* sp., *Salmonella* sp., and various viruses.

   d. HELLP—The variant of eclampsia includes hemolysis, elevated liver enzymes, and low platelets.

3. Diagnostic studies

   a. Acute ITP shows decreased platelets (10,000 to 20,000/μL), eosinophilia, and mild lymphocytosis.

   b. Chronic ITP shows a platelet count of 25,000 to 75,000 per μL.

   c. Platelet antibodies may detect an autoimmune cause of ITP.

   d. Anemia, red cell fragmentation (schistocytes), normal leukocytes, high LDH, high indirect bilirubin, elevated D-dimer, and reticulocytosis may all be present in TTP, HUS, DIC, HELLP, and HIT.

   e. Autoantibodies against ADAMTS 13 (also known as vWF–cleaving protease) lead to excessive platelet aggregation and, thus, TTP.

   f. HIT assay (PF4 heparin antibody enzyme-linked immunosorbent assay [ELISA] test) is positive in HIT.

4. **Treatment**

   a. Acute ITP usually resolves spontaneously; some patients require corticosteroids or splenectomy. Second-line therapy is IV immunoglobulin (IVIG) or in Rh(D)-positive patients with ITP and intact spleens, IV Rho immunoglobulin (RhIG) is an option.

   b. Patients with chronic ITP, TTP, HUS, DIC, HELLP, and HIT should be referred to expert care.

   c. TTP and HUS are treated with emergent plasma exchange.

   d. Platelet transfusions may be used for life-threatening bleeding but not in immune causes.

   e. Platelet antagonists (e.g., aspirin, NSAIDs) should be avoided.

   f. Thrombopoietin receptor analogs are now available for treatment.

> Acute ITP treatment is corticosteroids or IVIG.

E. **Disorders of platelet function**

1. General characteristics

a. Congenital abnormalities are varied; most result in normal counts and morphology but prolonged bleeding time or abnormal PFA.

b. Acquired platelet dysfunction is more common than congenital.

(1) The most common causes of acquired platelet dysfunction are aspirin and other NSAIDs.

(2) Acquired platelet dysfunction is also seen with the use of certain other drugs, herbals, uremia, alcoholism, myeloproliferative diseases, hypothermia, various vitamin deficiencies, and other conditions.

2. **Clinical features** are prolonged PFA and skin and mucosal bleeding.

3. Laboratory findings indicate a normal number of platelets, but PFA results are abnormal.

4. **Treatment**

a. In drug-related cases, the drug should be discontinued.

b. Dialysis may help patients with uremia.

c. Transfusion with platelets is necessary for serious bleeding.

F. vWD and clotting factor deficiencies (hemophilia)

1. **von Willebrand disease**

a. General characteristics

(1) vWD is an autosomal dominant, congenital bleeding disorder. It is the most common congenital coagulopathy found in 1% of the population. Most cases are mild.

(2) vWF stabilizes factor VIII, and low levels can cause pseudohemophilia A with prolonged aPTT.

(3) Both men and women may be affected.

(4) vWD has six major types, all characterized by deficient or defective vWF. Type I accounts for 75% to 80% of cases.

b. **Clinical features**

(1) Bleeding occurs in nasal, sinus, vaginal, and GI mucous membranes. It is a common cause of menorrhagia.

(2) Spontaneous hemarthrosis and soft-tissue bleeds are less common than in hemophilia A.

(3) Bleeding is exacerbated by aspirin or NSAIDs and decreases with use of estrogen or pregnancy.

c. Laboratory findings

(1) PT is generally normal, aPTT may be prolonged (low factor VIII), and the PFA is usually prolonged (Table 4-9).

(2) vWF is low.

d. **Treatment** varies according to the type of disease.

(1) Desmopressin acetate (DDAVP nasal spray) is useful in type I for bleeding prevention prior to procedures.

(2) Factor VIII concentrates are preferred if factor replacement is necessary.

2. **Hemophilia A (factor VIII deficiency or classic hemophilia)**

a. General characteristics

(1) Hemophilia A is a hereditary disease characterized by excessively prolonged coagulation time.

> vWD presents with bleeding, often exacerbated by NSAIDs or aspirin, and with a prolonged aPTT.

(2) It is the most severe bleeding disorder and the most common congenital coagulopathy after vWD.

(3) It is X-linked recessive and occurs in about 1/7,500 male births.

b. Clinical features

(1) Severely affected patients have repeated spontaneous hemorrhagic episodes with hemarthroses, epistaxis, intracranial bleeding, hematemesis, melena, microscopic hematuria, and bleeding into the soft tissue and gingiva.

(2) Less severely affected patients may experience excessive bleeding following trauma or surgery.

c. Diagnostic studies

(1) PTT is prolonged.

(2) PT, PFA, fibrinogen level, and platelet count are normal.

(3) Factor assay shows reduced factor VIII levels; vWF is normal (see Tables 4-9 and 4-10).

d. Treatment

(1) Infusion of recombinant factor VIII concentrates is the standard treatment.

(2) Desmopressin (DDAVP) may elevate factor VIII levels in patients with mild to moderate disease.

(3) Patients should avoid aspirin; pain management should be accomplished with celecoxib, acetaminophen, or opioids.

(4) Gene therapy is now in clinical trials.

Table 4-9 | Clotting/Platelet Tests

Test/Disease	PT	aPTT	PFA	Platelet Count
vWD	Normal	Increased (VIII)	Abnormal	Normal
Hemophilia A/B	Normal	Increased	Normal	Normal
DIC	Increased	Increased	Abnormal	Low
Uremia	Normal	Normal	Abnormal	Normal
Aspirin NSAIDs	Normal	Normal	Abnormal	Normal
Liver failure—early	Increased	Normal	Normal	Normal
Liver failure—late/severe	Increased	Increased	Abnormal	Low
ITP, TTP, HUS, HIT	Normal	Normal	Normal	Low

PT, prothrombin time; aPTT, activated partial thromboplastin time; PFA, platelet function analysis; vWD, von Willebrand disease; DIC, disseminated intravascular coagulation; NSAIDs, nonsteroidal anti-inflammatory drugs; ITP, immune thrombocytopenic purpura; TTP, thrombotic thrombocytopenic purpura; HUS, hemolytic uremic syndrome; HIT, heparin-induced thrombocytopenia.

Table 4-10 | Clotting Studies

Test/Disease	PT	aPTT	Mixing Study	TT
Inhibitor of factors VIII, IX, XI, XII, Lupus–aPL antibodies	Normal	Increased	Abnormal	Normal
Hemophilia A VIII Hemophilia B IX	Normal	Increased	Normal	Normal
DIC	Increased	Increased	Normal	Increased
Heparin	Normal	Increased	Abnormal	Increased Reptilase time normal
Low fibrinogen	Increased	Increased	Normal	Increased
Factor VII deficiency	Increased	Normal	Normal	Normal

PT, prothrombin time; aPTT, activated partial thromboplastin time; TT, thrombin time; aPL, antiphospholipid; DIC, disseminated intravascular coagulation.

3. Hemophilia B, also known as factor IX deficiency or Christmas disease, is a heterogeneous group of disorders similar to hemophilia A but occurring less frequently. It is an X-linked recessive disorder affecting males (1/25,000 incidence). Treatment is factor IX replacement.

4. Hemophilia C is factor XI deficiency in both males and females (1/100,000 incidence). It is usually milder than hemophilia A and B. Treatment is factor XI replacement, DDVAP, and fresh frozen plasma (FFP).

5. Factor inhibitors may be present when the PFA or aPTT do not correct with a mixing study (normal plasma factors added back in). Factor VIII inhibitors are seen not only in hemophilia A patients receiving factor VIII replacement but also in patients with autoimmune diseases and lymphoma and in pregnant (postpartum) or elderly patients. Refer these patients to expert care.

6. **Vitamin K deficiency**

   a. General characteristics

      (1) Vitamin K deficiency is the most common acquired coagulopathy.

      (2) Deficiency may be secondary to poor diet, liver failure, malabsorption, malnutrition, and use of some drugs, especially broad-spectrum antibiotics.

   b. **Clinical features**

      (1) The typical patient is postoperative, not eating well, and receiving broad-spectrum antibiotics that suppress colonic bacteria.

      (2) Soft-tissue bleeding may occur.

   c. Laboratory findings

      (1) PT is prolonged, and PTT may be prolonged.

      (2) Fibrinogen, TT, PFA, and platelet count are normal.

      (3) Liver enzymes may be elevated.

      (4) Levels of vitamin K and factors II, VII, IX, and X are decreased.

   d. **Treatment**

      (1) Treatment is directed at the underlying cause.

      (2) Oral or parenteral vitamin K (phytonadione) rapidly restores factor production if there is no hepatic dysfunction.

      (3) Treat hemorrhage with FFP.

      (4) Prevention includes a diet high in leafy vegetables.

G. **Vasculitis (leaking pipes)**

   1. Purpura may be caused by vitamin C deficiency (scurvy), Ehlers–Danlos syndrome, hereditary hemorrhagic telangiectasias, and steroid use.

   2. Palpable purpura is seen in sepsis, meningococcemia, Henoch–Schönlein purpura, and drug reactions.

> The most common acquired coagulopathy is vitamin K deficiency, with soft tissue bleeding, often post-op; treatment with parenteral replacement.

Thrombotic Disorders and Hypercoagulable Conditions

A. General characteristics

   1. Hypercoagulable conditions present with recurrent unprovoked DVTs, pulmonary embolism (PE), fetal loss, thrombotic stroke, and myocardial infarction (MI). There is no reliable hypercoagulable screening panel to predict clotting risk, but diagnostic testing should be performed after the patient presents with excessive clotting.

   2. The differential diagnosis can be remembered with the mnemonic PVCS:

      a. P—Platelets: too many (usually more than 1 million/high-power field [hpf]) or overactive (TTP, HIT, HUS, and HELLP)

b. V—Vascular injury from plaques, trauma, or burns

c. C—Clotting factors: anticlotting factors protein C, protein S, or antithrombin III deficient or not working

d. S—Stasis and surgery

3. Virchow triad is blood stasis, hypercoagulable state, and vascular injury.

4. Acquired hypercoagulable states are associated with malignancy (Trousseau syndrome), pregnancy, nephrotic syndrome, ingestion of certain medications (especially estrogen), immobilization, myeloproliferative disease, ulcerative colitis and Crohn's disease, Behçet's syndrome, polycythemia vera, intravascular devices, DIC, hyperlipidemia (particularly familial type II hyperbetalipoproteinemia), PNH, TTP–HUS, hyperviscosity syndrome, anticardiolipin antibodies, HIT, and antiphospholipid syndrome (APS).

5. Heparin therapy (unfractionated heparin [UFH] or low-molecular-weight heparin [LMWH]) can cause HIT, causing a decrease in platelets (usually in half), followed by platelet activation causing clotting and infarction.

6. Genetic causes include antithrombin III deficiency, factor V Leiden deficiency, protein C deficiency, protein S deficiency, dysfibrinogenemia, and abnormal plasminogen.

7. APS formerly known as Lupus anticoagulant. This IgM or IgG immunoglobulin is seen in 5% to 10% of patients with SLE but is more common in persons without lupus or in those taking phenothiazines.

B. Diagnostic studies

1. Hypercoagulation panel includes protein S, protein C, antithrombin III assay, factor V Leiden assay, fasting homocysteine level, anticardiolipin antibodies, antiphospholipid antibody, prothrombin 20210 mutation test, fibrinogen level, and HIT assay.

2. Russell's viper venom time is specific to detect antiphospholipid.

3. CBC reveals increased Hct and RBC count in polycythemia vera. Thrombocytopenia occurs with HIT, TTP, DIC, HUS, and HELLP.

4. D-dimer is elevated in active thrombosis.

5. Metabolic panel will uncover hepatic or renal dysfunction or hyperglycemia in diabetes.

6. Lipid panel to assess for hyperlipidemia

7. Antinuclear antibody (ANA) and CRP in SLE

8. HIT assay if exposed to heparin

9. Venous Doppler ultrasound to detect DVT

C. **Treatment**

1. To prevent or treat thrombotic stroke or MI, use antiplatelet therapy: aspirin, clopidogrel, prasugrel, ticagrelor, vorapaxar, or dipyridamole/aspirin combination.

2. To prevent or treat DVT, PE, or arterial thrombosis, use anticoagulants such as parenteral UFH or LMWH or non-heparinoids (if there is a history of HIT) fondaparinux or danaparoid.

3. Oral anticoagulant is preferred for long-term use; choices include vitamin K antagonist, warfarin, direct thrombin inhibitor dabigatran, or factor Xa blockers rivaroxaban, apixaban, and edoxaban.

4. Parenteral tissue plasminogen activator (tPA) is used to lyse clots in an attempt to reperfuse tissue.

5. Prednisone is used for lupus anticoagulant autoimmune causes.

6. At-risk persons with previous thrombotic events should be anticoagulated for prolonged periods until the D-dimer values return to baseline. Those with a genetic predisposition and unprovoked clot should be anticoagulated indefinitely.

Practice Questions

Directions: *Each of the numbered items or incomplete statements in this section is followed by a list of answers or completions of the statement. Select the ONE lettered answer or completion that is BEST in each case.*

1. A 15-year-old healthy male has been mildly anemic all his life. Today his hemoglobin is 12 g/dL (13.5 to 18 g/dL), and his MCV is low at 75 (80 to 100 fL); ferritin is normal at 35 (20 to 250 ng/mL). Which of the following is the most appropriate diagnostic test?
   A. Serum folate levels
   B. Heinz body stain
   C. Hemoglobin electrophoresis
   D. Epo level
   E. Peripheral smear

2. A 50-year-old male has a hemoglobin of 10 g per dL (13.5 to 18 g/dL) and an MCV of 72 (80 to 100 fL); ferritin is 10 (20 to 250 ng/mL). His vital signs are normal. Treatment is initiated with oral ferrous sulfate 325 mg three times a day. Which of the following is the most appropriate next step in diagnostic workup?
   A. Routine 6-month follow-up
   B. Referral for colonoscopy
   C. Referral to dietitian
   D. Referral for bone marrow biopsy
   E. Admit for transfusion

3. A 20-year-old healthy male was treated 4 days ago for a methicillin-resistant *Staphylococcus aureus* (MRSA) skin infection with sulfamethoxazole-trimethoprim (Bactrim). The infection is improving, but he is increasingly weak and his sclera have turned yellow. Today his hemoglobin is 11 g per dL (13.5 to 18 g/dL), and his MCV is 85 fL (80 to 100 fL); the corrected reticulocyte count is elevated. What is the best test for the most likely diagnosis?
   A. Homocysteine level
   B. Heinz body stain
   C. Hemoglobin electrophoresis
   D. Epo level
   E. Iron studies

4. A 16-year-old male with sickle cell disease hemoglobin type SS is in the emergency department for his third pain crisis this year. He is not on any medication except folic acid 1 mg daily for red cell production. What is the best preventive therapy to recommend?
   A. Daily low-dose aspirin
   B. Daily hydroxyurea
   C. Daily iron supplementation
   D. Monthly blood transfusions
   E. Plasmapheresis monthly

5. A 5-year-old boy has a history of recurrent knee hemarthroses and excessive nosebleeds. The clotting time/PFA is normal and the PT is normal. The aPTT is prolonged but corrects with a mixing study. Which of the following tests will be most revealing of his diagnosis?
   A. Factor VIII assay
   B. Factor X assay
   C. Platelet count
   D. TT (thrombin time)
   E. Hemoglobin electrophoresis

6. A 6-year-old boy has 2 days of excessive nosebleeds. The child had a viral illness 2 weeks ago that resolved and now he is active, is afebrile, and seems healthy to the parents. The CBC reveals normal hemoglobin, Hct, and WBC count but a low platelet count of 40,000 (normal 200,000 to 400,000). The PT and aPTT are normal. What is the most likely diagnosis?
   A. HUS
   B. Henoch–Schönlein purpura
   C. TTP
   D. ITP
   E. vWD

7. A 30-year-old female admitted with a DVT and PE has been treated with UFH IV for 3 days. The CBC on day 4 reveals a normal hemoglobin, Hct, and WBC count, but a low platelet count of 70,000 (normal 150,000 to 400,000). What is the most likely reason for the drop in platelets?
   A. HUS
   B. TTP
   C. HIT
   D. ITP

8. A 25-year-old female is 1 week postpartum after a normal vaginal delivery. She now has increased vaginal bleeding. The clotting time/PFA is normal and the PT is normal. The aPTT is prolonged and does not correct with a mixing study. What is the most likely cause?
   A. Spontaneous antibodies to factor VIII
   B. Factor VIII deficiency—Hemophilia A
   C. Factor IX deficiency—Hemophilia B
   D. vWD type 1

9. A patient with suspected type 1 vWD would have an abnormal PFA and which other abnormal coagulation study?
   A. PT
   B. aPTT
   C. TT
   D. Reptilase time—RT

10. A 60-year-old male with increasing fatigue and low back pain for 3 months has a normocytic anemia with a low reticulocyte count. He has increased calcium, total serum protein, and proteinuria. What is the most likely diagnosis?
   A. Anemia secondary to renal failure
   B. Multiple myeloma
   C. Monoclonal gammopathy of undetermined significance (MGUS)
   D. Renal carcinoma
   E. Hyperparathyroidism

11. A 23-year-old female was treated for gonococcal cervicitis with IM ceftriaxone and oral doxycycline 2 days ago. She now has jaundice and fatigue. Labs reveal corrected reticulocytosis, normocytic anemia, elevated indirect bilirubin, and elevated LDH, and she is Coombs positive for IgG. What is the most likely diagnosis?
   A. G6PD deficiency
   B. Warm antibody drug-induced hemolysis

C. Allergic reaction to ceftriaxone
D. Cold antibody hemolysis
E. Disseminated intravascular coagulopathy

12. A 20-year-old male patient presents after 2 weeks of fever, chills, fatigue, and night sweats. He has enlarged unilateral cervical and supraclavicular lymph nodes that are rubbery in texture. A node is excised. What cells are most likely to be seen?

A. Auer rods
B. Reed–Sternberg cells
C. Lymphocytic blast cells
D. Proliferation of mature lymphocytes
E. Eosinophilia

Practice Answers

1. C. *Hematology; Diagnostic Studies; Thalassemia*

Thalassemia is the most common hereditary anemia causing a microcytic cell size and normal ferritin, which also indicates this is not iron deficiency. A peripheral smear would confirm the microcytic anemia but lend no additional information. A hemoglobin electrophoresis would be the next step. Heinz body stain-positive G6PD deficiency causes hemolytic anemia when the patient is exposed to oxidant medications, like sulfa or antimalarials, or eating fava beans. Folate deficiency causes macrocytic anemia. Epo would be decreased in chronic renal failure which would cause normocytic anemia.

2. B. *Hematology; Clinical Intervention; Iron Deficiency Anemia*

Ferrous sulfate 325 mg per day is the correct replacement therapy for iron deficiency. Colonoscopy is the correct next step to search for the most common cause of iron deficiency anemia in older males and postmenopausal males: GI blood loss.

3. B. *Hematology; Diagnostic studies; G6PD deficiency*

G6PD deficiency causes hemolytic anemia when the patient is exposed to oxidant medications, like sulfa or antimalarials, or eating fava beans. Heinz body stains for G6PD deficiency. Folate and B$_{12}$ deficiencies cause elevated homocysteine levels. Hemoglobin electrophoresis quantifies proteins. Epo levels are low in chronic renal disease. Iron studies are warranted in microcytic anemia.

4. B. *Hematology; Pharmacology; Sickle Cell Anemia*

Hydroxyurea is an FDA-approved preventive treatment for sickle cell type SS. It reduces pain events by half. Acetaminophen treats acute pain but will not prevent pain crisis. Blood transfusions are not recommended for pain crisis prevention and can lead to iron overload and alloimmunization. Plasmapheresis is the treatment for thrombotic thrombocytopenia.

5. A. *Hematology; Diagnostic Studies; Hemophilia*

Factor VIII deficiency or hemophilia A is the most common genetic factor deficiency. Recurrent hemarthrosis indicates a factor deficiency. Factor X deficiency is rare. Low platelets usually cause mucous membrane bleeding, not hemarthrosis, and the bleeding time PFA would be normal. The TT measures factors in the common pathway; the normal PT indicates a normally functioning common pathway. Hemoglobin electrophoresis quantifies the different types of hemoglobin present.

6. D. *Hematology; Diagnosis; ITP*

ITP is usually a self-resolving thrombocytopenia that appears after a viral illness. It is typically benign. TTP would present with evidence of multiorgan failure. HUS would present with acute renal and hepatic failure with red cell hemolysis. Henoch–Schönlein purpura would present with palpable purpura. vWD does not affect platelet count.

7. C. *Hematology; Diagnosis; Hemolytic Uremic Syndrome*

This patient is exhibiting signs of HIT, which would be the most likely cause and confirmed with a HIT assay. HUS presents with acute renal and hepatic failure with red cell hemolysis. TTP presents with evidence of multiorgan failure. ITP is usually a benign self-resolving thrombocytopenia after a viral illness.

8. A. *Hematology; Diagnosis; Factor VIII Antibodies*

Factor VIII antibodies can occur postpartum, causing a prolonged aPTT that does not correct; the mixing study does not correct the aPTT. The clotting time/PFA is normal, excluding vWD.

9. B. *Hematology; Diagnostic Studies; von Willebrand*

aPTT will be prolonged because vWF stabilizes and transports factor VIII; without enough vWF, the aPTT will be prolonged because of low FVIII. Factor VII is the common pathway for PT. TT and RT do affect the common pathway.

10. B. *Hematology; Diagnosis; Multiple Myeloma*

Multiple myeloma is associated with the described findings. Anemia secondary to renal failure would not explain the hypercalcemia and elevated serum protein. MGUS is asymptomatic but may progress to multiple myeloma. Renal carcinoma does not fit this profile. Hyperparathyroidism causes increased calcium, but total serum protein is normal and there is no protein in the urine.

11. B. *Hematology; Diagnosis; Hemolytic Anemia*

This patient most likely exhibits warm antibody drug-induced hemolysis secondary to ceftriaxone. An allergic reaction would not cause hemolysis or be Coombs positive. A G6PD deficiency hemolysis is not precipitated by these medications and Coombs should be negative. Babesiosis is a red cell parasite and does not cause a Coombs reaction. Disseminated intravascular coagulopathy presents with bleeding, petechiae, and purpura caused by consumption of clotting factors.

12. B. *Hematology; Basic Science; Hodgkin's Lymphoma*

Reed–Sternberg cells are seen in the lymph nodes in Hodgkin's lymphoma and make the diagnosis. Auer rods are seen in the WBCs in AML. Lymphocytic blasts cells are seen in ALL. Proliferation of mature lymphocytes is seen in CML. Eosinophils are increased in parasitic infections, allergies, and autoimmune disorders.

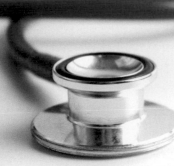

5 | Gastroenterology

Susan LeLacheur

Diseases of the Esophagus

A. Gastroesophageal reflux disease (GERD; reflux esophagitis)

1. General characteristics

   a. Reflux esophagitis is the result of recurrent reflux of gastric contents into the distal esophagus owing to mechanical or functional abnormality of the lower esophageal sphincter.

   b. GERD is present in an estimated 10% of the population; up to 40% of the population experiences heartburn at some point in their lives. In infants, about 50% have reflux, but less than 10% have evidence of esophagitis.

   c. Factors that protect the esophagus include gravity, lower esophageal sphincter tone, esophageal motility, salivary flow, gastric emptying, and tissue resistance.

   d. In a minority of patients, reflux causes erosion of the esophagus that leads to Barrett's esophagitis (replacement of normal squamous epithelium with metaplastic columnar epithelium), which can predispose to malignancy.

   e. Medications may cause or worsen symptoms of GERD, including antibiotics (tetracycline), bisphosphonates, iron, nonsteroidal anti-inflammatory drugs (NSAIDs), anticholinergics, calcium channel blockers, narcotics, benzodiazepines, and others.

   f. Foods that may aggravate GERD include chocolate, peppermint, onions, alcohol, and coffee.

   g. Other predisposing factors include obesity, pregnancy, diabetes, hiatal hernia, and some connective tissue disorders.

2. **Clinical features**

   a. Heartburn is the most common presenting feature of GERD. Heartburn is generally worse after meals and when lying down and may be relieved with antacids. Regurgitation or dysphagia may occur.

   b. Hoarseness, halitosis, cough, hiccupping, sore throat, laryngitis, and atypical chest pain are less common symptoms of reflux.

   c. More severe disease, generally caused by a severe impairment of lower esophageal sphincter tone, occurs spontaneously when supine, whereas less severe disease is associated with a pattern of heartburn following meals but not associated with nighttime symptoms.

3. Diagnostic studies

   a. Most often, a clinical diagnosis is made based on a history of heartburn and regurgitation of gastric contents, especially if relieved by antacids. More severe symptoms warrant endoscopy to confirm the diagnosis and to assess for epithelial damage.

   b. Endoscopy is also warranted in patients older than 45 years with a new onset of symptoms, long-standing or frequently recurring symptoms, and failure to respond to therapy or symptoms indicating more severe conditions such as anemia, dysphagia, evidence of gastrointestinal (GI) bleed, or recurrent vomiting.

> Manifestations of GERD are a result of abnormal relaxation of the lower esophageal sphincter, resulting in proximal misplacement of gastric fluids.

c. Electrocardiography (ECG) and appropriate cardiac workup should be considered as symptoms may be caused by myocardial ischemia.

d. Barium swallow, esophageal manometry, and ambulatory 24-hour pH monitoring may be indicated in more severe or refractory cases or when surgical intervention is planned.

e. Consider complete blood count (CBC) to evaluate for anemia if there is suspicion or evidence of esophageal bleed.

4. Treatment

a. Implement lifestyle modifications on presumptive diagnosis, with further workup if symptoms persist. Appropriate lifestyle modifications include cessation of smoking, avoidance of eating at bedtime, avoidance of large meals, avoidance of alcohol and foods that cause irritation (tomatoes, fried foods, caffeine, etc.), and raising the head of the bed.

b. Pharmacotherapy

(1) Antacids or alginic acid may be used for mild symptoms.

(2) Histamine (H_2) blockers (cimetidine, ranitidine, famotidine, nizatidine) may be used for relief of mild symptoms.

(3) An acid-suppressant PPI is the most powerful anti-GERD medication. PPIs (omeprazole, rabeprazole, esomeprazole, lansoprazole, dexlansoprazole, pantoprazole) are first-line treatment in moderate to severe disease or in patients who are unresponsive to H_2 blockers or have evidence of erosive gastritis. They bring symptomatic relief and promote healing of eroded tissue. Consider the benefits of long-term PPI use relative to potential risks.

(4) A combination of an H_2 blocker at bedtime and a PPI in the daytime may be helpful in patients with significant nighttime symptoms.

(5) β-Agonists, α-adrenergic antagonists, nitrates, calcium channel blockers, anticholinergics, theophylline, morphine, meperidine, diazepam, and barbiturate agents decrease lower esophageal sphincter pressure and, therefore, should be avoided.

c. Surgical and endoscopic techniques are available for refractory cases but have not been shown to prevent complications of the disease.

> GERD treatment includes lifestyle modifications for all; plus an H_2 blocker for mild or intermittent symptoms, and proton pump inhibitor (PPI) for severe symptoms.

B. Infectious esophagitis

1. General characteristics

a. Infectious esophagitis is rare, except in immunocompromised persons.

b. Causes

(1) Fungal: *Candida* sp. is the most likely cause in patients with HIV, especially if oral thrush is present.

(2) Viral: Herpes simplex virus (HSV) and cytomegalovirus (CMV) are common causes.

(3) *Mycobacterium tuberculosis*, Epstein–Barr virus (EBV), *Mycobacterium avium–intracellulare*, and direct inflammation caused by HIV are additional but uncommon causes of infectious esophagitis.

2. Clinical features: The main clinical feature is odynophagia (painful swallowing) or dysphagia (difficulty swallowing) in an immunocompromised patient. Physical examination may reveal signs of underlying immune deficiency, such as fever, lymphadenopathy, or rashes.

3. Diagnostic studies

a. Test for HIV; evaluate for underlying immunodeficiency.

b. In an immunocompromised patient with thrush and symptoms of esophagitis, empiric treatment with fluconazole is appropriate with further evaluation only if the treatment is ineffective.

> The most common cause of infectious esophagitis is *Candida*; treatment is fluconazole.

    c. Endoscopy in patients with CMV or HIV reveals large, deep ulcers. Infection with HSV is characterized by multiple shallow ulcers. Candidal infection shows white plaques.

    d. Cytology or culture from endoscopic brushings provide definitive diagnosis.

4. Treatment

    a. Treatment is specific to the type of infection.

    b. Fluconazole is recommended for *Candida* sp.

    c. Acyclovir is recommended for HSV.

    d. Intravenous (IV) ganciclovir for CMV; valganciclovir or foscarnet are options in cases of poor tolerability or poor response.

    e. Treatment of the underlying immunodeficiency, where possible, will aid in both resolution and prevention of esophageal infection.

C. Esophageal dysmotility

1. General characteristics

    a. Disorders of esophageal motility include neurogenic dysphagia, Zenker's diverticulum, esophageal stenosis, achalasia, diffuse esophageal spasm, and scleroderma.

    b. Dysmotility can be caused by neurologic factors, intrinsic or external blockage, or malfunction of esophageal peristalsis.

2. Clinical features

    a. Dysphagia is the most common presenting symptom for all motility disorders. Its descriptive presentation can help to determine the underlying cause.

    b. Neurogenic dysphagia causes difficulty with both liquids and solids and is caused by injury or disease of the brain stem or the cranial nerves involved in swallowing (IX, X).

    c. Zenker's diverticulum is an outpouching of the posterior hypopharynx that can cause regurgitation of undigested food and liquid into the pharynx several hours after eating.

    d. Esophageal stenosis causes dysphagia for solid foods. Slow progression of solid food dysphagia indicates a more benign process (e.g., webs or rings), and rapid progression indicates malignancy.

    e. Achalasia is a global esophageal motor disorder in which peristalsis is decreased and lower esophageal sphincter tone is increased, causing slowly progressive dysphagia with episodic regurgitation and chest pain.

    f. Diffuse esophageal spasm is characterized by dysphagia or intermittent chest pain that may or may not be associated with eating.

    g. Scleroderma eventually progresses to involve the esophagus in most patients with the disease, causing decreased esophageal sphincter tone and peristalsis, predisposing the patient to the symptoms and complications of reflux esophagitis.

3. Diagnostic studies

    a. Endoscopy (esophagogastroduodenoscopy) should be done to allow direct observation and biopsy of abnormalities and rule out mechanical obstruction or malignancy.

    b. Barium swallow can reveal both structural and motor abnormalities of the esophagus that may cause dysphagia. Achalasia typically has a "parrot beak" appearance (i.e., a dilated esophagus tapering to the distal obstruction).

    c. Esophageal manometry can be used to assess the strength and coordination of peristalsis. Manometric studies are typically done after structural and motor defects have been ruled out.

> Zenker's diverticulum is just above the cricopharyngeal muscle and causes dysphagia and regurgitation with cough and halitosis, but rarely pain.

> Dysphagia is the common presenting symptom for motility issues of any etiology; endoscopy and barium swallow are initial workup.

4. Treatment

    a. Neurogenic dysphagia must be managed by treating the underlying disease.

    b. Strictures

        (1) Most benign strictures can be managed by dilation.

        (2) Malignant strictures must be resected.

    c. Diverticula, achalasia, and stenosis may be managed surgically (endoscopic dilation, resection) if the condition is severe enough to warrant intervention. Medical therapies such as calcium channel blockers, nitrates, and botulinum may provide some symptomatic relief in patients unable to undergo dilation or surgery; results are mixed.

D. Esophageal neoplasms

    1. General characteristics

        a. Squamous cell carcinomas and adenocarcinomas are the most common types.

        b. Barrett's esophagitis is associated with adenocarcinomas in the distal third of the esophagus, whereas squamous cell lesions tend to occur in the proximal two-thirds.

        c. Local spread to the mediastinum is common because the esophagus has no serosa.

        d. Esophageal cancers are frequently related to cigarette smoking and chronic alcohol use. Contributing factors include exposure to other caustic agents (e.g., nitrosamines, fungal toxins, and other carcinogens), spicy foods, mucosal abnormalities, poor oral hygiene, and human papillomavirus (HPV).

    2. Clinical features: The main clinical feature of esophageal cancer is progressive dysphagia for solid food associated with marked weight loss. Heartburn, vomiting, and hoarseness may occur.

    3. Diagnostic studies

        a. Endoscopy or biopsy is the best initial evaluation. Double-contrast barium esophagography may be used in patients unable to undergo endoscopy.

        b. Endoscopic sonography and computed tomography (CT) imaging are used for staging.

        c. Endoscopic screening is recommended for those at high risk—patients with Barrett's esophagus, achalasia, tylosis (a rare genetic disorder with hyperkeratosis of palms and soles and squamous cell carcinoma of the esophagus), history of radiation, or caustic injury.

    4. Treatment

        a. Treatment of esophageal cancer is generally surgical. Radiotherapy and adjunctive chemotherapy have been used in various combinations with or without surgery.

        b. Prognosis depends on the stage of disease at diagnosis, ranging from 4% to 60% 5-year survival.

E. Mallory–Weiss tear

    1. A Mallory–Weiss tear is a linear mucosal tear in the esophagus, generally at the gastroesophageal junction, that occurs with forceful vomiting or retching, causing hematemesis. It accounts for 5% to 10% of upper GI bleeds.

    2. A Mallory–Weiss tear is often associated with alcohol use, but it should be considered in all cases of upper GI bleed.

    3. Diagnosis may be established by endoscopy.

    4. Most episodes resolve without treatment. Antiemetics and PPI may be used. Endoscopic injection of epinephrine or thermal coagulation may be required if bleeding does not resolve on its own.

> Progressive dysphagia, first with solids and then including liquids, is indicative of esophageal cancer.

> Patients with Barrett's esophagus should be treated with PPIs and continue with endoscopic surveillance every 3 to 5 years.

F. **Esophageal varices**

1. General characteristics

   a. Esophageal varices are dilations of the veins of the esophagus, generally at the distal end.

   b. The underlying cause in adults is portal hypertension, most commonly caused by cirrhosis from nonalcoholic steatohepatitis (NASH), alcohol abuse, or chronic viral hepatitis. Use of NSAIDs can exacerbate bleeding.

   c. Budd–Chiari syndrome is an uncommon cause of thrombosis of the portal vein, leading to esophageal varices.

   d. Patients generally present with painless upper GI bleed that can be bright red frank bleeding or coffee ground in appearance. Melena may occur. Large bleeds may cause hypovolemic shock.

2. Diagnosis

   a. Diagnosis is generally established clinically when a patient with signs of portal hypertension presents with hematemesis. Endoscopy will localize the bleeding.

   b. Varices are generally asymptomatic until they bleed, at which point they are frequently life-threatening.

3. **Treatment**

   a. Patients with cirrhosis should be screened for varices at the time of diagnosis and monitored on a targeted basis thereafter.

   b. Prevention of variceal bleeding in patients with cirrhosis may be accomplished with β-blockers with or without isosorbide mononitrate, along with discontinuation of hepatotoxic agents especially alcohol.

   c. Hemodynamic support with high-volume fluid replacement and vasopressors and immediate control of bleeding are necessary because bleeding varices have high mortality (~15% to 25% with the first bleed).

   d. Use IV vasoconstriction (e.g., octreotide) in conjunction with endoscopic ligation (preferred) or sclerotherapy to control the bleed.

   e. Pharmacologic or surgical (transjugular intrahepatic portosystemic shunt [TIPS]) management of portal hypertension is used to prevent rebleed.

> Consider esophageal varices in a case of liver disease with portal hypertension and painless upper GI bleed.

Diseases of the Stomach

A. **Gastritis and duodenitis**

1. General characteristics

   a. Gastritis and duodenitis are defined as inflammation of the stomach or duodenum.

   b. Protective factors include mucus, bicarbonate, mucosal blood flow, prostaglandins, alkaline state, hydrophobic layer, and epithelial renewal. Any imbalance in protective factors can lead to inflammation.

   c. Causes

      (1) Autoimmune disorders (e.g., pernicious anemia) and other noninfectious factors cause type A gastritis, which involves the body of the stomach.

      (2) *Helicobacter pylori* is a Gram-negative, spiral-shaped bacillus. It is implicated in almost all non-NSAID-induced GI mucosal inflammation.

         (a) *H. pylori* causes type B gastritis, which involves the antrum and body of the stomach.

         (b) *H. pylori* tolerates well the acidity of a normal stomach and is also associated with peptic ulcer, gastric adenocarcinoma, and gastric lymphoma.

> Gastric defenses include mucous barrier, bicarbonate, prostaglandins, and increased blood flow.

(3) NSAIDs can cause gastric injury by diminishing prostaglandin production in the stomach or duodenum.

(4) Stress from central nervous system injury, burns, sepsis, or surgery can lead to diffuse erosion of the stomach or duodenum.

(5) Alcohol use is another leading cause of gastritis.

2. **Clinical features**

   a. The clinical features of gastritis generally reflect the underlying syndrome rather than the gastric injury itself.

   b. Dyspepsia and abdominal pain of varying degrees are common indicators of gastritis.

3. Diagnostic studies

   a. Endoscopy with biopsy reveals the location and extent of gastritis as well as the presence of *H. pylori*.

   b. A urea breath test can be used to detect *H. pylori*; urea is a product of bacterial metabolism. Fecal antigen testing or serology for *H. pylori* is also helpful.

   c. Specific tests for underlying conditions (e.g., vitamin B_{12} level, CBC for pernicious anemia) should be assessed as indicated by history.

4. **Treatment**

   a. Remove the causative factor (e.g., NSAIDs, alcohol).

   b. Treat the underlying cause.

B. **Peptic ulcer disease (PUD)**

1. General characteristics

   a. PUD describes any ulcer of the upper digestive system (e.g., gastric ulcer, duodenal ulcer).

   b. Causes

      (1) Any discreet break in mucosa caused by injury, NSAIDs, stress, alcohol, or other irritants will lead to an ulcer.

      (2) *H. pylori* is the most common cause of PUD. When *H. pylori* is the cause, the ulcer disease can be eradicated with treatment.

   c. The lifetime risk of ulcer disease is 5% to 10%. Men and women are equally affected.

   d. Both gastric ulcers and *H. pylori* are highly associated with gastric malignancy. Although most patients with *H. pylori* or a gastric ulcer will not get gastric cancer, almost all patients with gastric cancer have had *H. pylori* or a gastric ulcer.

2. **Differential diagnosis:** Dyspepsia, abdominal pain, discomfort, or nausea is often associated with gastric or duodenal ulcers but can also occur in a variety of other conditions including gastritis, malignancy, and ischemic heart disease.

3. **Clinical features**

   a. Abdominal pain or discomfort is the primary clinical feature.

      (1) The pain may be described as burning or gnawing and often radiates to the back.

      (2) The pain of a duodenal ulcer often improves with food, whereas the pain of a gastric ulcer typically worsens, which leads to anorexia and associated weight loss. It is often difficult to localize the site until endoscopy is performed.

   b. Dyspepsia (belching, bloating, distention, heartburn) or nausea is also reported.

   c. Complications include bleeding, perforation, and penetration. Bleeding typically manifests as melena.

H. pylori is implicated in most non-NSAID-related mucosal inflammation and is associated with gastric cancer.

H. pylori is the most common cause of PUD; PUD is the most common cause of GI bleeds.

4. Diagnostic studies

    a. Endoscopy is best for detecting small or healing ulcers. It differentiates gastritis from ulcer disease, provides samples for culture or urease testing, and allows immediate biopsy of gastric or suspicious ulcers to rule out malignancy.

    b. Various tests may be used to detect *H. pylori*. Urea breath test, serum or urine antibody test, stool antigen test, polymerase chain reaction (PCR), or culture may all be used but false-negative results may occur if the patient is taking bismuth, antibiotics, PPIs, or high-dose histamine-2 (H_2) blockers.

5. Treatment

    a. Irritating factors (smoking, NSAIDs, alcohol) should be avoided.

> *H. pylori* is treated with combination therapy to eradicate the bacteria and heal the mucosa.

    b. Combination therapy for *H. pylori* regimen should be taken for 2 to 4 weeks. Options include the following:

        (1) Bismuth subsalicylate plus tetracycline, metronidazole, and PPI

        (2) PPI with clarithromycin and amoxicillin or metronidazole

    c. Prophylactic treatment with misoprostol or a PPI should be considered in patients with a history of ulcer who require daily NSAID use; a history of complications such as a bleed; a need for chronic steroids or anticoagulants; or significant other comorbidities.

C. Gastric neoplasm

    1. Zollinger–Ellison syndrome (ZES)

        a. General characteristics

            (1) In ZES, a gastrin-secreting tumor (gastrinoma) causes hypergastrinemia, which results in refractory PUD.

            (2) Only 1% of cases of PUD is caused by ZES.

            (3) Most gastrinomas are found in the pancreas or duodenum, but they may be found anywhere or may metastasize.

            (4) About one-third of gastrinomas are part of multiple endocrine neoplasia type I (MEN1), an autosomal dominant condition; check for family history of ulcer.

        b. Clinical features

            (1) Most commonly, the clinical presentation is indistinguishable from that of PUD, although ZES is usually more advanced or refractory to treatment.

            (2) Abdominal pain may be accompanied by secretory diarrhea that improves with H_2 blockers (ranitidine, cimetidine) or PPIs (omeprazole, lansoprazole).

            (3) Occult or frank bleeding, causing anemia, may be present.

        c. Diagnostic studies

            (1) A fasting hypergastrinemia along with gastric hyperchlorhydria (gastric pH $<$ 2).

            (2) A secretin provocation test may be used if the results are unclear.

            (3) Endoscopy, CT, or magnetic resonance imaging (MRI) may help to localize the tumor.

> Zollinger-Ellison is treated with PPIs unless the tumor is localized and can be resected.

        d. Treatment

            (1) Use of PPIs controls gastrin secretion.

            (2) Surgical resection of the gastrinoma should be attempted when possible.

    2. Gastric adenocarcinoma

        a. General characteristics

            (1) Gastric adenocarcinoma is among the most common types of cancer worldwide but is less common in the United States.

            (2) Gastric adenocarcinoma is almost twice as common in men than in women.

            (3) It almost never occurs in a patient younger than 40 years.

(4) With early diagnosis, an 80% cure rate can be accomplished. If the muscularis propria is involved, the cure rate is 50%, but if there is lymphatic spread, the cure rate is 10%.

(5) There is a strong association of gastric adenocarcinoma with *H. pylori*, although genetic factors are involved in some types. Cigarette smoking also increases risk.

b. Clinical features

(1) Dyspepsia and weight loss associated with anemia and occult GI bleeding or melena in a patient older than 40 years are the typical presenting complaints.

(2) Progressive dysphagia may be caused by a neoplasm impinging on the esophagus.

(3) Postprandial vomiting may be caused by a neoplasm near the pylorus.

(4) Signs of metastatic spread include left supraclavicular lymphadenopathy (Virchow's node) and an umbilical nodule (Sister Mary Joseph's nodule).

c. Diagnostic studies

(1) Iron deficiency anemia is the most common laboratory finding.

(2) Liver enzymes may be elevated with hepatic metastases.

(3) After the diagnosis has been established, abdominal CT is used to determine the extent of the disease.

> For gastric cancer evaluation, endoscopy with cytology should be done on any patient older than 40 years with dyspepsia who is unresponsive to therapy.

d. Treatment

(1) Treatment is either curative or palliative resection of the tumor.

(2) Chemotherapy or radiation may provide some palliative benefit or may be used preoperatively for some tumors.

3. Carcinoid tumors of the stomach rarely occur in response to hypergastrinemia and are generally benign and self-limited.

4. Gastric lymphoma

a. General characteristics

(1) Gastric lymphomas account for less than 2% of gastric malignancies, but the stomach is the most common extranodal site for non-Hodgkin's lymphoma.

(2) The risk of gastric lymphoma is greater by sixfold if *H. pylori* infection is present.

b. Clinical features: Clinical features are the same as those for gastric adenocarcinoma.

c. Diagnostic studies: Findings differ from those of gastric adenocarcinoma only in the pathology of the lesion.

d. Treatment: Treatment is resection with or without radiation or chemotherapy.

Diseases of the Small Intestine and Colon

A. Diarrhea

1. General characteristics

a. Diarrhea is increased frequency or volume of stool (e.g., three or more liquid or semisolid stools daily for at least 2 to 3 consecutive days).

b. Causes of diarrhea may be infectious (Table 5-1), toxic, dietary (e.g., laxative use), or other GI disease.

c. Patient history: The history should include all current medications as well as illnesses among others who have shared meals with the patient. A travel history is also pertinent.

d. *Clostridium difficile*–associated diarrhea can be prevented by careful handwashing; alcohol-based sanitizers are ineffective in preventing transmission of spores.

> The majority of cases of diarrhea are infectious, toxic, or related to dietary intake.

Table 5-1 | Foodborne and Waterborne Causes of Diarrhea

Agent	Source	Onset	Nausea and Vomiting	Diarrhea	Fever	Duration	Therapy
Norovirus	Food, water, person to person	1–3 days	Yes	Watery	Low grade	1–2 days	Hydration (prevention: handwashing)
Rotavirus	Person to person	1–3 days	Yes	Watery	Low grade	5–8 days	Hydration (prevention: handwashing)
Staphylococcus aureus (toxin)	Food, after cooking	1–7 hours	Yes, rapid onset	Cramping, some diarrhea	Uncommon	Acute (4–6 hours); total (1–2 days)	Supportive
Clostridium perfringens (toxin)	Food, before cooking	8–14 hours	Uncommon	Cramping, watery	Rare	24 hours	Supportive
Vibrio spp. (cholera)	Water	2–3 days	Some	Profuse, watery	Rare	Days	Hydration
Enterotoxic *Escherichia coli*	Food	5–15 days	Some	Cramping, watery	Low grade	1–5 days	Hydration, bismuth/loperamide
Giardia lamblia	Water, person to person	5–25 days	Nausea	Diarrhea, bloating	None possible	Until treated	Metronidazole, 250 mg twice a day for 10 days
Cryptosporidium	Water, outbreaks	2–10 days	Yes	Watery	Possible	30 days (unless HIV)	Supportive, HIV treatment
Cyclospora	Imported, uncooked foods	7 days	Nausea, anorexia	Watery	Low grade	Weeks	Trimethoprim–sulfamethoxazole twice a day for 7 days
Salmonella (invasive)	Poultry	6–72 hours	Nausea, some vomiting	Purulent	Yes, septicemia common	4–7 days	Hydration
Enterohemorrhagic *E. coli* (invasive)	Undercooked ground beef	12–60 hours	No	Purulent, bloody, cramping	Yes	5–10 days	Supportive unless severe
Shigella (invasive)	Fecal–oral	1–6 days	No	Purulent, bloody, cramping	Yes	1–7 days	Supportive
Campylobacter (invasive)	Undercooked poultry	2–5 days	Some	Purulent, bloody, cramping	Yes	2–5 days	Supportive

2. Clinical features

    a. Secretory diarrhea (large volume without inflammation) indicates infection, pancreatic insufficiency, ingestion of preformed bacterial toxins, or laxative use.

    b. Inflammatory diarrhea (bloody diarrhea with fever, dysentery) indicates invasive organisms or inflammatory bowel disease.

    c. Antibiotic-associated diarrhea is frequently caused by *C. difficile* colitis, which in the most severe cases causes the classic pseudomembranous colitis.

> Differentiate between secretory or inflammatory diarrhea to help determine the etiology.

3. Diagnostic studies

    a. Acute diarrhea is generally self-limited; no specific testing is warranted.

    b. White blood cells (WBCs) in stool denote an inflammatory process.

    c. Cultures for bacterial agents, microscopy for parasites, or toxin identification (if enterotoxic *Escherichia coli* or *C. difficile* is suspected) can identify infectious agents in stool.

4. Treatment

    a. Supportive therapy is sufficient for most patients with viral or bacterial diarrhea.

    b. Antibiotics may be indicated for patients with severe diarrhea and systemic symptoms (e.g., *Shigella* sp., *Campylobacter* sp., severe cases of *C. difficile* infection). Oral vancomycin, metronidazole, or fidaxomicin are the antibiotics of choice for antibiotic-induced *C. difficile* colitis.

    c. Treatment of the underlying cause is required for noninfectious diarrhea.

B. Constipation

    1. General characteristics

        a. Normal bowel function ranges from three stools per day to three stools per week. Constipation is a decrease in stool volume and an increase in stool firmness accompanied by straining.

        b. Patients older than 50 years with new-onset constipation should be evaluated for colon cancer.

    2. Treatment

        a. In most cases, an increase in insoluble fiber (up to 10 to 20 g/day), fluid intake (up to 1.5 to 2 L/day), and exercise will resolve the problem.

        b. A patient with constipation lasting for more than 2 weeks or with constipation refractory to modifications in diet, exercise, and fluid intake should undergo further investigation to detect the underlying cause. If a treatable underlying cause is found, constipation will resolve with treatment of the disease process.

C. Bowel obstruction

    1. General characteristics

        a. Most small bowel obstructions are caused by adhesions or hernias; other causes include neoplasm, inflammatory bowel disease, and volvulus.

        b. Large bowel obstructions are more likely caused by neoplasm; other causes include strictures, hernias, volvulus, intussusception, and fecal impaction.

        c. Complete strangulation of bowel tissue leads to infarction, necrosis, peritonitis, and death.

> Constipation that does not respond to fiber therapy after 2 weeks warrants further investigation.

    2. Clinical features

        a. Small bowel obstruction presents with abdominal pain, distention, vomiting of partially digested food, and obstipation.

        b. In small bowel obstruction, bowel sounds are high pitched and come in rushes. Later in the process, the bowel becomes silent.

        c. Large bowel obstruction presents with distention and pain. Dehydration and electrolyte imbalance are common.

        d. Patients may be febrile and tachycardic. Shock may ensue.

3. Diagnostic studies

    a. Evaluate for electrolyte abnormalities.

    b. Upright radiographs may illustrate air–fluid levels and multiple dilated loops of the bowel.

    c. If radiography is inconclusive, abdominal CT with contrast should be obtained.

4. Treatment

    a. Treatment includes bowel rest (nothing by mouth [NPO]), nasogastric suctioning, IV fluids, and monitoring.

    b. Partial obstruction in a hemodynamically stable patient may be managed with IV hydration and nasogastric decompression.

    c. Urgent surgical consultation is necessary when mechanical obstruction is suspected, especially of the large bowel. Without intervention, the bowel is at risk for perforation or ischemia.

    d. Pain management is necessary for patients with bowel obstruction.

> 💡 First-line treatment for small bowel obstruction: bowel rest, nasogastric suctioning, IV fluids, and pain management.

D. Volvulus

1. Volvulus is twisting of any portion of the bowel on itself, most commonly in the sigmoid or cecal area of the bowel, requiring emergent decompression to avoid ischemic injury.

2. Clinical features

    a. Patients present with cramping abdominal pain and distention, nausea, vomiting, and obstipation.

    b. Ischemia can lead to gangrene, peritonitis, and sepsis.

    c. Abdominal tympany will be found on examination, along with tachycardia, fever, and severe pain if ischemia is present.

3. Diagnosis is generally confirmed by abdominal plain film, which will show colonic distension.

4. Treatment

    a. Endoscopic decompression is possible in many cases.

    b. Surgical evaluation and treatment are required urgently if volvulus fails to quickly resolve by nonsurgical means.

E. Malabsorption

1. General characteristics

    a. Malabsorption may involve a single nutrient, as with pernicious anemia (vitamin B_{12}) or lactase deficiency (lactose), or it may be global, as with celiac disease or HIV/AIDS.

    b. Malabsorption may be caused by problems in digestion, absorption, or impaired blood and lymph flow.

2. Clinical features

    a. Diarrhea is usually the primary complaint and may be accompanied by bloating and abdominal discomfort.

    b. Weight loss and edema may also develop.

    c. Steatorrhea (fatty stools) may occur and is indicated by a history of stools that are foul smelling and float.

    d. Specific deficiencies may cause bone demineralization, tetany, bleeding, or anemia.

> 💡 Malabsorption most commonly presents with diarrhea, weight loss, and edema.

3. Diagnostic studies

    a. If a 72-hour fecal fat test is normal, specific defects, such as pancreatic insufficiency and abnormal bile salt metabolism, should be considered.

    b. A D-xylose test will distinguish maldigestion (e.g., pancreatic insufficiency, bile salt deficiency) from malabsorption. A normal result rules out malabsorption.

    c. Specific tests may be used to detect vitamin B_{12}, calcium, or albumin deficiency.

4. Therapeutic trials of the following can help in both diagnosis and treatment

    a. Lactose-free diet for lactase deficiency

    b. Gluten-free diet for celiac disease

    c. Pancreatic enzyme replacement for pancreatic insufficiency

    d. Antibiotics may be indicated for specific bacterial infections if the agent is known.

F. Celiac disease (celiac sprue)

  1. General characteristics

    a. Celiac disease is among the most common genetic conditions in Europe and the United States (multifactorial inheritance) present in between 0.5% and 1% of the population.

    b. It is characterized by inflammation of the small bowel secondary to the ingestion of gluten-containing foods such as wheat, rye, and barley, leading to malabsorption.

    c. Clinical presentation is highly variable, often leading to a delay in diagnosis in milder cases.

  2. Clinical presentation

    a. Diarrhea, steatorrhea, flatulence, weight loss, weakness, and abdominal distension are common.

    b. Infants and children may present with failure to thrive.

    c. Older patients may present with iron deficiency, coagulopathy, and hypocalcemia.

  3. Diagnostic studies

    a. IgA antiendomysial (EMA) and anti-tissue transglutaminase (anti-tTG) antibodies are the serologic screening tests.

    b. Small bowel biopsy is needed to confirm the diagnosis.

  4. Treatment

    a. Treatment involves a gluten-free diet. Patients should be referred to a nutritionist for assistance because of the pervasive nature of gluten in the North American diet. A lactose-free diet may also be needed initially until the intestinal inflammation resolves.

    b. Supplementation may be needed to correct nutritional deficiencies in iron, vitamin B_{12}, folic acid, calcium, and vitamin D.

    c. Prednisone may be required in refractory cases.

> Presenting symptoms of celiac disease reflect the global malabsorption that occurs: diarrhea, steatorrhea, flatulence, weight loss, weakness, and abdominal distension.

G. Crohn's disease (regional enteritis)

  1. General characteristics

    a. Crohn's disease is an inflammatory bowel disease for which there is some genetic predisposition, although the cause is unknown. Males and females are equally affected. Peak incidence is between 15 and 35 years of age. Crohn's disease must be differentiated from ulcerative colitis (UC) (Table 5-2).

    b. Crohn's disease may involve both the small and large bowels as well as the mouth, esophagus, and stomach. Most commonly, the terminal ileum and right colon are involved, but the rectum is frequently spared. Skip areas are characteristic.

    c. Complications include fistulas, abscesses, aphthous ulcers, renal stones, and predisposition to colonic cancer.

    d. The success or failure of treatment is variable. The disease usually waxes and wanes throughout life.

  2. Clinical features

    a. Abdominal cramps and diarrhea in a patient younger than 40 years are the most common presenting complaints.

    b. Low-grade fever, polyarthralgia, anemia, and fatigue are frequently encountered.

    c. Blood is often present in the stool.

> Crohn's disease can occur anywhere along the GI tract whereas ulcerative colitis is confined to the large intestine.

Table 5-2 | Differentiation of Crohn's Disease and Ulcerative Colitis

Characteristic	Crohn's Disease	Ulcerative Colitis
Onset	Gradual	Sudden or gradual
Distribution	Mouth to anus, predominantly right-sided; skip areas	Distal to proximal, continuous
Depth of lesions	Transmural	Mucosal surface
Symptoms	Diarrhea and pain	Bloody, pus-filled diarrhea; tenesmus
Complications	Fistulas (common), toxic megacolon, colon cancer	Toxic megacolon, colon cancer

   3. Diagnostic studies

      a. Colonoscopy is the most valuable tool for establishing the diagnosis, determining the extent and severity of disease, and guiding the treatment.

      b. Contrast studies and endoscopic procedures should be avoided in patients with fulminant disease because of the possibility of inducing toxic megacolon or perforation.

      c. Biopsy will reveal involvement of the entire bowel wall in Crohn's disease. Granulomas are frequent.

      d. Tests for inflammation may include increased sedimentation rate, C-reactive protein, or fecal calprotectin.

      e. Evaluate for anemia, nutritional deficits, and electrolyte imbalances.

   4. **Treatment**

      a. Treatment recommendations vary with disease severity and include corticosteroids, thiopurines, methotrexate, and biologics.

      b. For patients with malabsorption, supplementation may be needed especially for vitamin B_{12}, folic acid, and vitamin D.

      c. Smoking cessation is critical for reducing the frequency and severity of attacks.

      d. Surgery is not curative in Crohn's disease and is reserved for treatment of complications such as bleeding, abscess, or obstruction. Segmental resection is the approach of choice.

H. **Ulcerative colitis (UC)**

   1. General characteristics

      a. UC must be differentiated from inflammatory infectious conditions (see Table 5-1) and Crohn's disease (see Table 5-2).

      b. The disease generally starts distally, at the rectum, and progresses proximally. Disease is continuous, and skip areas are not seen as in Crohn's disease.

      c. Onset is generally gradual but can also be abrupt.

   2. **Clinical features**

      a. Tenesmus and bloody, pus-filled diarrhea are the most common symptoms.

      b. Pain is less common but may occur, typically in the lower-left quadrant.

      c. Weight loss, malaise, and fever may occur in more severe disease.

      d. Toxic megacolon and malignancy are more likely in UC than in Crohn's disease.

      e. Other complications include scleritis and episcleritis, arthritides, sclerosing cholangitis, and skin manifestations (erythema nodosum and pyoderma gangrenosum).

      f. As opposed to Crohn's disease, where smoking increases disease, ironically, smoking seems protective in UC. Smokers who have recently quit will often have a disease flare.

> 💡 The pathology of ulcerative colitis begins distally and progresses proximally in the colon.

3. Diagnostic studies

a. Anemia, vitamin D deficiency, and decreased serum albumin are common. Evaluation for inflammation with sedimentation rate, C-reactive protein, or fecal calprotectin along with liver and renal function tests may also be helpful.

b. Stool studies can help to rule out infectious pathogens, including sexually transmitted infections, which may lead to exacerbations.

c. Abdominal plain-film radiography may show colonic dilation. Sigmoidoscopy or colonoscopy is the best method of establishing the diagnosis.

d. Colonoscopy and barium enema should be avoided in acute disease because of the risks of perforation and toxic megacolon.

4. Treatment

a. Topical or oral aminosalicylates and corticosteroids are the mainstays of medical treatment. Immunomodulators are indicated for severe or refractory disease.

b. Induction of remission may be followed by lowering of pharmaceutical burden during maintenance.

c. Surgery can be curative in UC. Segmental resection is possible, but total proctocolectomy is the most common surgical cure.

> Clinical features of UC include tenesmus, bloody diarrhea, weight loss, and malaise.

I. **Irritable bowel syndrome (IBS)**

1. General characteristics

a. IBS is a functional disorder without a known pathology. It is thought to be a combination of altered motility, hypersensitivity to intestinal distention, and psychological distress.

b. IBS is the most common cause of chronic or recurrent abdominal pain in the United States.

c. IBS generally remains an intermittent, lifelong problem. Symptoms typically begin during early to mid-adulthood.

d. IBS is more common in women than in men. Exacerbations may be associated with menses or stress.

e. IBS is a diagnosis of exclusion. The differential diagnosis includes lactose intolerance, cholecystitis, chronic pancreatitis, intestinal obstruction, chronic peritonitis, celiac disease, and carcinoma of the pancreas or stomach.

f. Diagnosis is based on the Rome IV criteria (symptoms including change of stool frequency and form, along with relief on defecation, occurring at least 1 day per week for the past 3 months).

g. Alarm features that indicate a diagnosis other than IBS include more than minimal rectal bleeding, unintentional weight loss, unexplained iron deficiency anemia, or nocturnal symptoms.

> IBS is a diagnosis of exclusion, presenting with abdominal pain relieved by defecation, changes in stool, and often dyspepsia.

2. Clinical features

a. Abdominal pain may occur anywhere or may be localized to the hypogastrium or left lower quadrant.

(1) Pain may be worsened by food intake and is typically relieved with defecation.

(2) Pain may be associated with bowel distention from the accumulation of gas and associated spasm of the smooth muscle; postprandial urgency is common.

b. Physical examination is generally normal but may include a tender, palpable sigmoid colon and hyperresonance on percussion over the abdomen.

c. IBS is strongly identified with changes in stool frequency and character. Constipation, diarrhea, or alternating constipation and diarrhea may occur.

d. Dyspepsia is common.

e. Urinary frequency and urgency are common in women.

3. Diagnostic studies

    a. Laboratory findings are generally normal. The stool should be tested for blood, bacteria, parasites, and lactose intolerance.

    b. Colonoscopy, barium enema, ultrasonography, or CT should be performed to rule out other pathology.

    c. Endoscopic studies are indicated in patients with persistent symptoms, weight loss or anorexia, bleeding, or history of other GI pathology.

4. **Treatment**

    a. Reassurance and a strong provider–patient relationship are key. Avoidance of any known triggers is important.

    b. A high-fiber diet and bulking agents, such as psyllium hydrophilic mucilloid, are the mainstays of treatment.

    c. Antispasmodics, antidiarrheals, prokinetics, or antidepressants can be used if indicated by the patient's symptoms or course of illness.

    d. Constipation-predominant IBS that does not respond to osmotic laxatives can be treated with lubiprostone (prostaglandin-E analog) or linaclotide (guanylate cyclase agonist).

> Treatment of IBS must be individualized according to symptoms and response.

J. Intussusception

1. General characteristics

    a. Intussusception is the invagination of a proximal segment of the bowel into the portion just distal to it.

    b. It occurs most commonly in children (95% of cases), generally following a viral infection.

    c. In adults, intussusception almost always is caused by a neoplasm.

2. **Clinical features**

    a. Children will exhibit signs of severe colicky pain. Stool, if passed, will contain mucus and blood (currant jelly stools). A sausage-like mass may be felt on abdominal examination.

    b. Adults may present with a more indolent course of crampy abdominal pain. Bloody stool and abdominal mass are rare.

3. Diagnostic studies

    a. For children, barium or air enema may be both diagnostic and therapeutic, although ultrasonography is often the initial diagnostic test in children who are stable.

    b. For adults, barium enema should not be used, and abdominal plain-film radiography shows nonspecific obstruction. CT is the best means of establishing the diagnosis, but many cases are diagnosed only at surgery.

> Intussusception commonly occurs in children presenting with "currant jelly stools" and a mass in the abdomen.

4. **Treatment**

    a. All patients with suspected intussusception should be hospitalized.

    b. Air or barium enema may be curative for children; if not, surgery is needed.

    c. Adults generally require surgery.

K. Diverticular disease

1. General characteristics

    a. Diverticulosis is defined as large outpouchings of the mucosa in the colon.

    b. Diverticulitis is defined as inflammation of the diverticula caused by obstructing matter.

    c. Approximately 60% of people older than 60 years of age have diverticula; of these, 20% become symptomatic.

    d. Approximately 20% of patients with acute diverticulitis are younger than 40 years.

e. In patients with diverticulosis, diverticulitis and its complications can be prevented with a high-fiber diet and avoidance of obstructing or constipating foods.

2. Clinical features

a. Diverticulitis

(1) It generally presents with sudden-onset abdominal pain, usually in the left lower quadrant or suprapubic region, with or without fever.

(2) Symptoms may range from mild disease to severe infection with peritonitis.

(3) Altered bowel movements as well as nausea and vomiting are common.

b. Diverticular bleeding generally presents as sudden-onset, large-volume hematochezia. It resolves spontaneously, although continuous or recurrent bleeding is an indication for surgery.

3. Diagnostic studies

a. Occult blood in the stool and mild to moderate leukocytosis may occur with diverticulitis.

b. Plain-film radiography should be done to rule out free air.

c. CT is warranted if patients do not respond to therapy.

d. Barium enema and endoscopy should be avoided during an acute episode because it may lead to perforation and peritonitis.

> For mild diverticulitis, treatment includes antibiotics and low-residue diet.

4. Treatment

a. Low-residue diet and broad-spectrum antibiotics are appropriate for patients with mild diverticulitis.

b. Hospitalization for IV administration of antibiotics, bowel rest, and analgesics is often required. A nasogastric tube is inserted if ileus develops.

c. Surgical management may be necessary in severe cases, including peritonitis, large abscesses, fistulae, or obstruction.

d. Patients with diverticulosis should maintain a high-fiber diet to prevent diverticulitis. Evidence has negated the need to recommend global avoidance of nuts, seeds, and popcorn.

L. Ischemic bowel disease

1. General characteristics

a. Mesenteric ischemia (MI) can be acute (AMI) or chronic (CMI). In chronic ischemia, the blood supply is present but insufficient to meet the needs of the intestine.

b. For both AMI and CMI, patients will generally be older than 50 years and have other signs of cardiovascular or collagen vascular disease.

c. AMI

(1) AMI may be caused by arterial embolus, arterial thrombosis, or venous thrombosis, with differing risk factors and prognosis for each.

(2) AMI represents an emergency. Mortality remains high despite advances in treatment.

> Postprandial pain disproportionate to exam findings indicates ischemia.

d. Intestinal infarction is more common in the small bowel than in the large bowel. Shock is common.

2. Clinical features

a. CMI presents as abdominal angina, with pain occurring 10 to 30 minutes after eating, which is relieved somewhat by squatting or lying down. Physical examination is normal.

b. AMI presents with sudden onset of severe abdominal pain out of proportion to examination findings. Later in the process, involuntary guarding, rebound, and heme-positive stool may develop.

3. Diagnostic studies

    a. Plain-film radiography and CT are performed to rule out other causes of abdominal pain or to show areas of edema or dilation.

    b. All patients should have duplex ultrasonography of the mesenteric arteries, which may be confirmed by angiography if necessary prior to surgery.

4. Treatment for AMI or CMI is surgical revascularization. Hydration is also a critical factor.

M. Toxic megacolon

> 💡 Toxic megacolon is most often seen in patients with IBD; it is often fatal.

    1. General characteristics

        a. Toxic megacolon is extreme dilation and immobility of the colon and represents a true emergency.

        b. Hirschsprung's disease is a congenital aganglionosis of the colon, leading to functional obstruction in the newborn.

        c. In adults, toxic megacolon occurs as a complication of UC, Crohn's colitis, pseudomembranous colitis, and specific infectious causes (particularly amebiasis, *Shigella* sp., *Campylobacter* sp., and *C. difficile*).

    2. Clinical features

        a. Symptoms include fever, prostration, severe cramps, and abdominal distention.

        b. A rigid abdomen and localized, diffuse, or rebound abdominal tenderness are found on physical examination.

    3. Diagnostic studies: Abdominal plain-film radiography will show colonic dilation.

    4. Treatment

        a. Decompression of the colon is required. In some cases, colostomy or even complete colonic resection may be required.

        b. Careful attention must be paid to fluid and electrolyte balance.

N. Colonic polyps

    1. General characteristics

        a. Colonic polyps are common in the industrialized world and can be either benign or malignant.

        b. Removal of polyps can reduce the occurrence of colon cancer.

        c. Inherited polyposis syndromes (familial adenomatous polyposis, hamartomatous polyposis syndromes, Peutz–Jeghers syndrome, familial juvenile polyposis, PTEN multiple hamartoma syndrome) convey genetic predisposition to multiple colonic polyps with a near-100% risk of developing colonic cancer. Up to 5% of colorectal cancers are found in individuals with one of these syndromes.

> 💡 Bleeding polyps can lead to anemia; removal can reduce development of colon cancer.

    2. Clinical features

        a. Polyps generally are asymptomatic, although constipation, flatulence, and rectal bleeding may occur.

        b. Bleeding polyps may lead to iron deficiency anemia.

    3. Diagnostic studies

        a. Heme-positive stool is common.

        b. Barium enema, flexible sigmoidoscopy, and colonoscopy can detect polyps.

        c. Histologic evaluation is needed to determine dysplasia. Hyperplastic polyps have the lowest risk of dysplasia; tubular polyps carry an increased risk; villous polyps carry the highest risk of malignancy.

        d. Family members of those with familial polyposis syndrome should be evaluated every 1 to 2 years beginning at 10 to 12 years of age. Elective colectomy may be an option for high-risk individuals.

4. **Treatment** depends on the size and histology of polyps. Larger and dysplastic polyps should be removed and frequent follow-up arranged. Generally, a single distal hyperplastic polyp requires the same follow-up as someone without polyps—every 10 years. Having multiple hyperplastic polyps, hyperplastic polyps at sites rather than distal, or tubular polyps requires a 5-year follow-up. Villous polyps require follow-up colonoscopy at 3 years. In addition to these general guidelines, surveillance becomes more frequent with increased numbers and larger sizes of polyps.

O. **Colorectal cancer**

1. General characteristics

   a. Colorectal cancer is the third leading cause of cancer death in the United States after lung cancer and skin cancers.

   b. Approximately 90% of cases occur in people older than 50 years.

   c. Screening colonoscopy (every 10 years) or flexible sigmoidoscopy (every 5 years) is recommended starting at age 50 for those without risk factors (hereditary risk or history of inflammatory bowel disease).

   d. Hereditary nonpolyposis colorectal cancer (HNPCC or Lynch syndrome) also leads to an extremely high risk of colon cancer. This is an autosomal dominant condition accounting for 3% of colorectal cancers.

   e. Individuals with familial polyposis have a virtually 100% risk of developing the disease.

   f. Prognosis

      (1) Prognosis is good in early disease.

      (2) When the cancer involves only the mucosa (Dukes A or stage I), the 5-year survival rate is >90%.

      (3) Penetration through the wall or involvement of regional lymph nodes (Dukes B or stage II) has a 5-year survival rate of 70% to 80%.

      (4) When there is metastasis (Dukes C or stage III [lymph node positive] and Dukes D or stage IV [distant metastases]), the 5-year survival rate drops to 5%.

2. **Clinical features**

   a. Colorectal cancer is slow growing, and symptoms often appear late in the disease. Abdominal pain, change in bowel habits, occult bleeding, and intestinal obstruction are common presentations.

      (1) Right-sided lesions typically cause chronic blood loss and iron deficiency anemia. Obstruction is uncommon.

      (2) Left-sided lesions are often circumferential, causing change in bowel habits and obstructive symptoms.

   b. Fatigue and weakness may occur if chronic blood loss has led to anemia.

   c. Changes in stool size and shape may be noted; frank blood may be seen in the stool.

3. Diagnostic studies

   a. Screening guidelines vary, but for average risk Americans, it should begin at ages 45 to 50 and continue through ages 75 to 85 using colonoscopy every 10 years, fecal immunochemical testing every 1 to 3 years. Alternative schedules include other modalities such as stool guaiac or flexible sigmoidoscopy. Patients at higher risk require earlier and more intensive screening.

   b. Carcinoembryonic antigen (CEA) may be used to monitor, although not to detect, colorectal cancer.

   c. Sigmoidoscopy, colonoscopy, or barium enema may all be used to visualize suspected colonic masses; chest radiography and CT are used to detect metastases.

> Endoscopic screening for colorectal cancer has an A grade from the U.S. Preventive Services Task Force (UPSTF).

> Change in bowel habits or occult bleeding may present with colorectal cancer, and colonoscopy or barium enema is indicated for diagnosis.

4. Treatment

  a. Treatment is by surgical resection, which is accompanied by chemotherapy in patients with stage III (Dukes C or higher) or higher (and sometimes in stage II [Dukes B]) lesions.

  b. Radiation may be used for rectal tumors.

Diseases of the Rectum and Anus

A. Anorectal abscess/fistula

  1. General characteristics

  a. Anorectal abscess is a result of infection, whereas fistula is a chronic complication of abscess.

  b. Fistula is an open tract between two epithelium-lined areas and is most commonly associated with deeper anorectal abscesses.

  2. Clinical features

  a. Perirectal and perianal abscesses are most common and produce painful swelling at the anus as well as painful defecation. Examination reveals localized tenderness, erythema, swelling, and fluctuance; fever is uncommon.

  b. Deeper abscesses may produce buttock or coccyx pain and rectal fullness; fever is more likely.

  c. Fistulae will produce anal discharge and pain when the tract becomes occluded. The tract should not be explored on examination because this may open new tracts.

  3. Treatment

  a. Treatment of abscess requires surgical drainage, followed by warm-water cleansing, analgesics, stool softeners, and high-fiber diet (WASH regimen).

  b. Fistulae must be treated surgically.

> Fistulae are abnormal tracts or tunnels that must be treated surgically.

B. Anal fissure

  1. Anal fissures are linear lesions in the rectal wall most commonly found on the posterior midline.

  2. Patients describe severe tearing pain on defecation, often accompanied by hematochezia; bright red blood is often noted on the stool or tissue paper.

  3. Treatment includes bulking agents and increased fluids to avoid straining. Sitz baths will relieve acute pain. Topical nitroglycerin ointment or topical styptic, such as silver nitrate (1% to 2%) or gentian violet solution (1%), may help with healing.

C. Hemorrhoids

  1. General characteristic: Hemorrhoids are varices of the hemorrhoidal plexus.

  2. Clinical features

  a. External hemorrhoids are visible perianally.

  b. Stage I internal hemorrhoids are confined to the anal canal and may bleed with defecation.

  c. Stage II internal hemorrhoids protrude from the anal opening but reduce spontaneously. Bleeding and mucoid discharge may occur.

  d. Stage III internal hemorrhoids require manual reduction after bowel movements. Patients may develop pain and discomfort.

  e. Stage IV internal hemorrhoids are chronically protruding and risk strangulation.

> Hemorrhoid staging is helpful for treatment choices: fiber, laxatives, and fluids for early stage; suppositories for larger hemorrhoids; and ligation or sclerotherapy for severe cases.

3. Treatment

a. Stages I and II disease can be managed with a high-fiber diet and increased fluids. Bulk laxatives are helpful.

b. Higher stage hemorrhoidal disease may benefit from suppositories with anesthetic and astringent properties.

c. Surgical treatment is indicated for those unresponsive to conservative treatment and all stage IV hemorrhoids. Choices include injection, rubber band ligation, or sclerotherapy.

D. Pilonidal disease

1. General characteristics

a. Pilonidal cyst is an abscess in the sacrococcygeal cleft associated with subsequent sinus tract development.

b. Pilonidal cysts are four times more likely in males than in females, are more common in hirsute and obese individuals, and are rare in those older than 40 years.

2. Clinical presentation is a painful, fluctuant area at the sacrococcygeal cleft.

3. Treatment

a. Treatment is surgical drainage, which may be supplemented with antibiotics.

b. Follicle removal may be required, with unroofing of sinus tracts.

E. Fecal impaction

1. General characteristics

a. Fecal impaction is a large mass of hard, retained stool. It generally occurs in the rectum but may also occur higher in the colon.

b. Complications

(1) Complications include urinary tract obstruction and infection, spontaneous perforation of the colon, and stercoral ulcer where the mass has pressed on the colon.

(2) Fecaliths may develop and cause appendicitis.

c. More proximal impaction generally indicates neoplasm.

2. Clinical features

a. Abdominal pain, rectal discomfort, anorexia, nausea, and vomiting are common but nonspecific.

b. Headache and a general sense of illness are common; acute confused state may occur.

c. Incontinence of small amounts of water and semi-formed stool may occur as leakage passes by a large impaction. Sometimes, this is confused for diarrhea, and patients will take antidiarrheal medicine, which compounds the problem.

d. Rock-hard stool in the rectal vault on examination is diagnostic. Abdominal mass may also be palpated. Sigmoidoscopy or barium enema may be needed to confirm a more proximal impaction.

3. Treatment

a. Treatment involves breaking up the impaction digitally, followed by a saline or tepid-water enema.

b. More proximal impaction can be broken up by sigmoidoscopic water irrigation and suction.

c. Subsequent attention must be paid to bowel habits and hydration.

F. Anal cancer

1. General characteristics: Anal cancer is caused by HPV and is a common finding among women with HPV and people with HIV infection, particularly men who have sex with men.

Pilonidal disease is most commonly diagnosed in males over the age of 40 years.

Acute management of fecal impaction requires digital evacuation plus saline enema.

2. **Clinical presentation** is generally asymptomatic, but screening is not yet routinely recommended. Some specialists recommend anal Pap smear for at-risk populations, with follow-up anoscopy for positive findings.

3. **Treatment** is surgical.

Appendicitis

A. General characteristics

1. Appendicitis occurs when obstruction of the appendix leads to inflammation and infection.

   a. The most common cause is a fecalith. In children, lymphoid hyperplasia is also a common cause.

   b. Less common causes include infection (CMV, adenovirus, Histoplasma, etc.), collagen vascular disease, and inflammatory bowel disease.

2. Patients are usually between 10 and 30 years of age.

3. Appendicitis affects 10% of the U.S. population, making it the most common abdominal surgical emergency.

4. Perforation and peritonitis occur in about 20% of patients with appendicitis, causing high-grade fever, generalized abdominal pain, and increased leukocytosis.

B. **Clinical features**

1. The initial symptom is intermittent periumbilical or epigastric pain.

2. In about 12 hours, pain typically localizes to the right lower quadrant (McBurney's point), becomes constant, and is worsened by movement, leading to rebound tenderness on examination.

3. Nausea and anorexia are common. Vomiting may occur but is generally isolated and begins subsequent to the onset of pain.

4. Diarrhea may occur but is not common.

5. A low-grade fever is common; a high-grade fever is unlikely.

6. Psoas sign (patient is supine and attempts to raise the leg against resistance) and obturator sign (patient is supine and attempts to flex and internally rotate the right hip with the knee bent) are generally positive, indicating inflammation adjacent to those muscles.

7. Variability in anatomy can cause unusual presentations of appendicitis, with symptoms reflecting the location of the appendix. A patient with retrocecal appendicitis is more likely to have pain on rectal examination.

> Appendicitis presentation most commonly includes right lower quadrant (RLQ) abdominal pain, low fever, and leukocytosis.

C. Diagnostic studies

1. Leukocytosis (usually 10,000 to 20,000/μL) is characteristic. Higher levels suggest perforation and peritonitis.

2. Some microscopic hematuria and pyuria may be seen.

3. Abdominal ultrasonography is the preferred initial imaging (no exposure to radiation), although CT is more sensitive in confirming the diagnosis. CT will also help to locate an abnormally placed appendix.

D. **Treatment**

1. Treatment is appendectomy. A laparoscopic approach is preferred.

2. Broad-spectrum antibiotics are administered before and after surgery.

Diseases of the Pancreas

A. **Acute pancreatitis**

1. General characteristics

   a. Causes

      (1) The most common causes are cholelithiasis or alcohol abuse, but hyperlipidemia (especially hypertriglyceridemia), trauma, drugs, hypercalcemia, and penetrating PUD may also cause pancreatitis.

   b. The range of presentation is wide, from mild episodes of deep epigastric pain with nausea and vomiting to the sudden onset of severe pain with shock.

2. **Clinical features**

   a. Epigastric abdominal pain is a presenting complaint; nausea and vomiting are common.

   b. Fever, leukocytosis, and sterile peritonitis may occur.

   c. Severe hypovolemia, adult respiratory distress syndrome, and tachycardia of >130 beats per minute (bpm) indicate a grave prognosis.

   d. Hemorrhagic pancreatitis may cause bleeding into the flanks (Grey Turner's sign) or umbilical area (Cullen's sign).

3. Diagnostic studies

   a. Elevation of serum amylase occurs but may be transient and can return to normal after 48 to 72 hours.

   b. Serum lipase is more sensitive and specific than amylase for acute pancreatitis, but only with elevations of threefold or greater.

   c. WBC count is generally elevated, and hemoconcentration may occur with third spacing of fluid.

   d. Liver enzymes may increase as a result of biliary obstruction.

   e. Mild hyperbilirubinemia and bilirubinuria, hyperglycemia, and hypocalcemia may occur.

   f. Poor prognosis is indicated by Ranson's criteria (Table 5-3). Risk of mortality rises with each additional factor.

   g. Ultrasound may be helpful to look for gallstones. Plain films may reveal a sentinel loop indicating localized ileus.

4. **Treatment**

   a. Oral intake must be stopped to prevent continued secretion of pancreatic juices.

   b. Fluid volume must be restored and maintained. Parenteral hyperalimentation should be started early to prevent nutritional depletion.

   c. Pain is managed with an opioid. Antibiotics should be considered.

> The classic presentation of acute pancreatitis is epigastric pain radiating to the back, which lessens when the patient leans forward or lies in a fetal position.

Table 5-3 | Ranson's Criteria for Poor Prognosis for Pancreatitis

Leukocyte count	>16,000/µL
Blood glucose level	>200 mg/dL
Lactate dehydrogenase	>350 IU/dL (normal, <20–50 IU/dL)
AST	>250 IU/dL (normal, <120 IU/dL)
Arterial PO$_2$	>60 mm Hg
Base deficit	>4 mEq/L
Calcium	Falling
BUN	Rising

AST, aspartate aminotransferase; BUN, blood urea nitrogen.

Most cases of chronic pancreatitis are caused by alcohol use and will resolve with abstention.

d. The patient must be monitored closely for complications, including pancreatic pseudocyst, renal failure, pleural effusion, hypocalcemia, and pancreatic abscess.

B. **Chronic pancreatitis**

1. General characteristics

   a. Between 60% and 90% of cases of chronic pancreatitis in the United States are caused by alcohol abuse; other causes include cholelithiasis, PUD, hyperparathyroidism, and hyperlipidemia.

   b. Some chronic cases can resolve if alcohol consumption is decreased.

   c. The classic triad of pancreatic calcification, steatorrhea, and diabetes mellitus occurs in only 20% of patients.

2. **Clinical features** are the same as those of acute pancreatitis, with the addition of fat malabsorption and steatorrhea late in the disease. Fecal fat will be elevated if malabsorption is present.

3. Diagnostic studies

   a. The amylase level may be elevated early but will decrease with each episode of pancreatitis and cease to be a useful marker.

   b. Abdominal plain-film radiography reveals calcification in 20% to 30% of patients. Gallstones may also be seen.

4. **Treatment**

   a. Treatment is as for acute pancreatitis. A low-fat diet should be recommended at discharge.

   b. Surgical removal of part of the pancreas can control pain.

   c. The only definitive treatment for chronic pancreatitis is to address the underlying cause, which most commonly is alcohol.

C. **Pancreatic neoplasm**

1. General characteristics

   a. Pancreatic cancer is the fifth leading cause of cancer death in the United States.

   b. Risk factors include increased age, obesity, tobacco, chronic pancreatitis, previous abdominal radiation, and family history.

2. **Clinical presentation**

   a. Abdominal pain occurs in most patients and, depending on the location of the tumor, can radiate.

   b. Jaundice and a palpable gallbladder (Courvoisier's sign) may be seen in patients with cancer of the pancreatic head.

Courvoisier's sign is a palpable gallbladder seen in cancer of the pancreatic head.

3. **Diagnostic studies** include CT to delineate disease and search for metastases and angiography to look for vascular invasion.

4. **Treatment**

   a. Treatment is surgical resection (modified Whipple procedure) in those without metastases. Complete resection has the potential to prevent recurrence.

   b. Subsequent radiation and chemotherapy are controversial.

   c. Prognosis is poor.

Diseases of the Biliary Tract

A. **Cholelithiasis and choledocholithiasis**

1. General characteristics

   a. Cholelithiasis denotes gallstones in the gallbladder and choledocholithiasis in the common bile duct.

   b. By age 75 years, 35% of women and 20% of men have gallstones.

   c. Only 30% of people with gallstones develop symptomatic disease.

2. Treatment

   a. Generally, only the complications of choledocholithiasis should be treated because most people with gallstones will never develop the disease.

   b. Complications include cholecystitis, pancreatitis, and acute cholangitis.

B. Acute cholecystitis

1. Acute cholecystitis is caused by obstruction of the bile duct, generally by a stone, leading to chronic inflammation.

2. Clinical presentation

   a. Colicky epigastric or right upper quadrant (RUQ) pain becomes steady and increases in intensity. It often occurs after a high-fat meal.

   b. Right shoulder or subscapular pain may occur because of irritation of the phrenic nerve.

   c. Nausea, vomiting, and low-grade fever are common.

   d. Constipation and mild paralytic ileus may occur.

> Acute cholecystitis classically presents with nausea/vomiting, RUQ pain after a fatty meal, increased bilirubin, and leukocytosis.

3. Diagnostic studies

   a. After 24 hours, bilirubin levels increase in blood and urine.

   b. Leukocytosis is common.

   c. Gallstones are found in 95% of patients with cholecystitis. Only 20% are radiopaque, the remainder generally are visible by sonography.

   d. Sonography is the primary imaging technique used but CT, MRI, hepatoiminodiacetic acid (HIDA) scintigraphy can be used for confirmation of the diagnosis or exclusion of other causes or of complications.

   e. Endoscopic retrograde cholangiopancreatography (ERCP) can identify the cause, location, and extent of biliary obstruction.

4. Treatment is surgical.

C. Acute cholangitis

1. General characteristics

   a. This is a potentially deadly condition of common bile duct obstruction combined with ascending infection most commonly caused by *E. coli*, *Enterococcus*, *Klebsiella*, and *Enterobacter* that can lead to sepsis and death.

   b. It is most often caused by choledocholithiasis, although neoplasms, postoperative strictures, or other causes of obstruction may be involved.

2. Clinical presentation

   a. Presentation varies from mild to fulminant.

   b. RUQ tenderness, jaundice, and fever (Charcot's triad) are present in 50% to 70% of cases.

   c. In addition to Charcot's triad, altered mental status and hypotension may be present (Reynolds' pentad) and indicate sepsis. If present, the disease can become rapidly fatal.

   d. Elderly patients may present with confusion, falls, and incontinence.

> Charcot's triad of ascending cholangitis: RUQ tenderness, jaundice, and fever

3. Diagnostic studies

   a. RUQ ultrasonography will generally show biliary dilation or stones and is a good initial test.

   b. Leukocytosis with left shift along with increased bilirubin and mildly increased transaminase levels support the diagnosis.

   c. ERCP is the optimal procedure both for diagnosis and for treatment but, unless urgent decompression is necessary, should not be done until the patient is stable.

4. Treatment

a. Antibiotics (generally a fluoroquinolone, a cephalosporin, ampicillin, or gentamicin with metronidazole), fluid and electrolyte replacement, and analgesia are the initial treatment.

b. ERCP for drainage, sphincterotomy, and stone removal and stent placement can be done when the patient is stable. Percutaneous transhepatic biliary drainage or surgical biliary drainage may be required.

c. Cholecystectomy should be performed after the acute syndrome is resolved when choledocholithiasis is present.

D. Primary sclerosing cholangitis (PSC)

1. General characteristics

a. PSC is a chronic thickening of the bile duct walls of unknown etiology, although 80% of cases are associated with inflammatory bowel disease, generally UC (although only 10% of patients with UC will develop PSC).

b. PSC is strongly associated with cholangiocarcinoma (10% to 30% of patients) as well as with an increased risk of pancreatic and colorectal carcinoma.

c. Male to female ratio is 7:3, and the age at diagnosis is between 21 and 67 years (mean 39 years).

> Consider PSC when evaluating cases of IBD with associated jaundice and pruritus.

2. Clinical presentation

a. Jaundice and pruritus are the most common presenting features, with fatigue, malaise, and weight loss seen in many patients.

b. Hepatomegaly and/or splenomegaly may be found on examination.

3. Labs are the same as for acute cholangitis.

4. Treatment

a. Localized strictures may be relieved with balloon dilation and stent placement. Long-term stenting increases the risk of cholangitis.

b. Liver transplant is the only treatment with a known survival benefit.

Diseases of the Liver

A. Hepatitis

1. General characteristics

a. Hepatitis can describe acute or chronic hepatocellular damage.

b. The most common cause of acute hepatitis is viral; toxins (e.g., alcohol) are the second most common cause.

c. Chronic hepatitis most often results from viral infection (hepatitis B, C, D) but is often caused by inherited disorders (e.g., Wilson's disease, α_1-antitrypsin deficiency), autoimmune disease of the liver, or hepatic effects of systemic disease.

> Almost all hepatitis in the United States is caused by infection or alcohol.

2. Viral hepatitis

a. General characteristics

(1) The severity of the disease is highly variable, ranging from asymptomatic to fulminant (generally fatal) infection.

(2) Hepatitis A and E are transmitted by fecal–oral contamination and can be prevented by maintaining a sanitary water supply and handwashing.

(3) Hepatitis B, C, and D are transmitted parenterally or by mucous membrane contact.

(4) Of those with chronic hepatitis C, only 20% to 30% will progress to serious liver disease, which occurs most often when alcohol is involved or the patient is coinfected with hepatitis B or HIV.

b. Clinical features

(1) Fatigue, malaise, anorexia, nausea, tea-colored urine, and vague abdominal discomfort are common presenting complaints.

(2) Hepatitis A and E are self-limited and mild, without long-term sequelae.

(3) Hepatitis B and C can have a highly variable presentation, ranging from asymptomatic to fulminant. Chronic hepatitis B or C causing liver damage may require treatment.

(4) Hepatitis D is seen only in conjunction with hepatitis B and is associated with a more severe course.

(5) All individuals born between 1945 and 1965 should be screened for hepatitis C.

(6) Hepatitis C and HIV are frequent coinfections, as are hepatitis B and HIV, necessitating specialist care if treatment of the hepatitis is indicated.

> Aminotransferase elevations are seen in all types of acute hepatitis, indicating hepatocellular damage.

c. Diagnostic studies

(1) Bilirubin of >3.0 mg per dL will be associated with scleral icterus, if not frank jaundice.

(2) Immunoglobulin M antibody to hepatitis A virus (anti-HAV) can be detected with the onset of clinical disease (after a 15- to 40-day incubation period), but it disappears after several months. HAV IgG indicates resolved hepatitis A.

(3) Hepatitis B surface antigen (HBsAg) indicates ongoing infection of any duration; antibody against hepatitis B surface antigen (anti-HBs) indicates immunity by past infection or vaccination (Figure 5-1).

(4) Hepatitis B core antibody (anti-HBc) is present between the disappearance of HBsAg and the appearance of anti-HBs, indicating acute hepatitis.

(5) Hepatitis B envelope antigen (HBeAg) indicates active infection that is highly contagious, whereas hepatitis B envelope antigen–antibody (anti-HBe) indicates a lower viral titer.

(6) Hepatitis B may exist in a carrier state or a chronic infection. Both exhibit positive HBsAg, but in chronic infection, liver damage is demonstrated by elevated aspartate aminotransferase (AST) and alanine aminotransferase (ALT) and by hepatocellular damage on biopsy. In chronic infection, the viral DNA load will be >10^5 copies. HBeAg seroconversion (to negative) tends to occur with a reduction in viral DNA.

> The presence of HBsAg indicates ongoing infection.

(7) Hepatitis C is detected by its antibody followed by a hepatitis C viral load. About 15% of those infected with hepatitis C will clear the infection without therapy as indicated by a positive antibody but negative viral PCR.

(8) A positive hepatitis C antibody does not protect against reinfection once the virus is cleared naturally or by treatment.

(9) Those with hepatitis C may benefit from viral typing by genotype testing to guide therapy.

(10) Hepatitis D antibody indicates ongoing infection if hepatitis B infection is ongoing.

(11) Sonography helps evaluate for neoplasm as is MRI of the liver. The level of fibrosis may be evaluated using transient ultrasound elastography or magnetic resonance elastography or estimated with serum tests including FibroSURE or the AST to platelet ratio (APRI), calculated using the AST and platelet count.

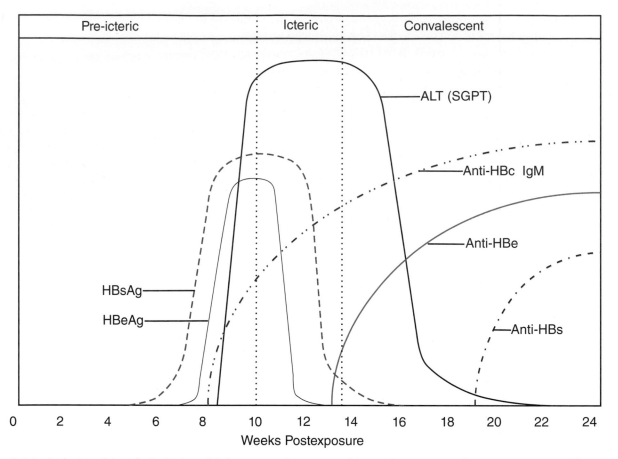

Figure 5-1 ▶ Relationship of clinical and laboratory features of hepatitis B. ALT, alanine aminotransferase; Anti-HBc, hepatitis B core antibody; Anti-HBe, hepatitis B envelope antigen–antibody; Anti-HBs, hepatitis B surface antigen–antibody; HbeAg, hepatitis B envelope antigen; HBsAg, hepatitis B surface antigen; IgM, immunoglobulin M; SGPT, serum glutamic-pyruvic transaminase.

- **d. Treatment**
    - **(1)** Treatment of acute viral hepatitis is supportive. Patients with hepatitis A must be cautious about transmission to others by not sharing food or dishes and by frequent handwashing.
    - **(2)** All patients with acute or chronic hepatitis should avoid alcohol and other hepatotoxins.
    - **(3)** All HIV-positive patients with chronic hepatitis B should be treated for HIV with therapies that cover both infections. Tenofovir disoproxil fumarate or tenofovir alafenamide with either emtricitabine or lamivudine will cover hepatitis B, and the additional antiretroviral medication will cover the HIV infection.
    - **(4)** Patients with hepatitis C should be vaccinated against hepatitis A and B.
    - **(5)** The standard of care for the treatment of hepatitis C virus (HCV) infection involves a combination of oral therapies that may differ depending on the serotype of the virus. The goal of therapy is the reduction of viral RNA to undetectable at 6 months posttherapy.
- **3. Toxic hepatitis**
    - **a.** Toxic hepatitis may be caused by numerous agents, including alcohol, acetaminophen, carbon tetrachloride, isoniazid, halothane, phenytoin, and many others. The maximum daily acetaminophen dose should not exceed 4 g; maximum dose for children is based on age.

b. Both diagnosis and treatment are accomplished by discontinuing the suspected agent. Acetylcysteine can be used for acetaminophen toxicity.

c. Toxic hepatitis may be reversible, depending on the amount of the toxin. If the patient survives the acute episode, the prognosis is good.

B. Nonalcoholic fatty liver disease (NAFLD)

   1. General characteristics

      a. NAFLD is defined as fat in more than 5% of hepatocytes not caused by heavy alcohol use or other cause after clinical and laboratory evaluation.

      b. NAFLD is a hepatic manifestation of metabolic syndrome that can range from hepatic steatosis to steatohepatitis to progressive fibrosis and cirrhosis.

      c. NASH is a type of NAFLD where inflammation is present along with fibrosis and cirrhosis.

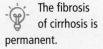 NAFLH is often found incidentally in those with central adiposity, and treatment centers on minimizing fibrosis.

   2. Clinical presentation

      a. Usually asymptomatic unless fibrosis has developed; often found on incidental transaminase elevation.

      b. Most patients will have a history of obesity with a high waist to hip ratio, glucose elevation, hypertension, and dyslipidemia.

      c. Individuals of normal weight may have other aspects of metabolic syndrome including elevated glucose, triglycerides, and low high-density lipoprotein (HDL) cholesterol.

      d. Painless hepatomegaly may be present.

   3. Diagnostic studies

      a. Diagnosis begins with the rule out alcohol or other causes with a careful history and lab evaluation for viral agents, autoimmune or Wilson's disease.

      b. Obtain biomarkers to predict fibrosis (prothrombin time [PT]/international normalized ratio [INR], platelet, albumin, alkaline phosphatase); AST to platelet ratio index or other composite scores are used.

      c. Elastography maps the elastic properties and stiffness of liver tissue; it may be sufficient for diagnosis although liver biopsy remains the definitive diagnostic study.

      d. Those with cirrhosis require screening for hepatocellular carcinoma every 6 months with ultrasound or MRI.

   4. Treatment

      a. Weight loss is the optimal therapy.

      b. Antioxidants (vitamin E), ω-3 fatty acids, or pioglitazone may be considered for some patients.

C. Cirrhosis

   1. General characteristics

      a. Cirrhosis is irreversible fibrosis and nodular regeneration throughout the liver.

      b. In the United States, more than 45% of cases are alcohol related, with the remainder associated with hepatitis B or C or with congenital disorders.

The fibrosis of cirrhosis is permanent.

   2. Clinical presentation

      a. Weakness, fatigue, and weight loss are common.

      b. Nausea, vomiting, and anorexia are usually present.

      c. Menstrual changes (generally amenorrhea), impotence, loss of libido, and gynecomastia occur.

      d. Abdominal pain and hepatomegaly are generally present.

      e. Late-stage disease includes ascites, pleural effusions, peripheral edema, ecchymoses, esophageal varices, and signs of hepatic encephalopathy (e.g., asterixis, tremor, dysarthria, delirium, and, eventually, coma).

     f. Spontaneous bacterial peritonitis presents with fever, chills, worsening ascites, and abdominal pain. It may lead to diarrhea and renal failure.

   3. Diagnostic studies

     a. Anemia is common, as are mild elevations of AST and alkaline phosphatase, increased γ-globulin, decreased albumin, and abnormal coagulation studies.

     b. Ultrasonography, CT, or MRI can confirm the size and number of nodules and is helpful in guiding biopsy.

     c. Cirrhotic patients must be screened every 6 months for hepatic carcinoma regardless of successful treatment of the underlying cause.

> In cirrhotic patients, laboratory values are often minimally abnormal until late-stage disease.

   4. Treatment

     a. Abstinence from alcohol is the key feature of treatment.

     b. Treatment of viral causes is required.

     c. Salt restriction and bed rest may be sufficient treatment for ascites, although spironolactone, 100 mg daily, may be added as a diuretic.

     d. Liver transplant is indicated in selected patients.

     e. Spontaneous bacterial peritonitis is treated with antibiotics.

D. Liver abscess is generally caused by *Entamoeba histolytica* or coliform bacteria. It may occur either after travel or secondary to an intra-abdominal infection and presents with fever and abdominal pain. Treatment includes antibiotics and percutaneous drainage or surgical excision.

E. **Liver neoplasm**

   1. General characteristics

     a. Liver neoplasms may be malignant or benign, and malignant neoplasms may be primary or metastatic.

     b. Benign liver neoplasms include cavernous hemangioma, hepatocellular adenoma, and infantile hemangioendothelioma.

     c. The liver is a common site of metastasis for other primary cancers, especially lung and breast cancers. If the primary tumor is silent, liver manifestations may be the presenting complaints.

     d. Primary hepatocellular carcinoma is associated with hepatitis B, hepatitis C, aflatoxin B1 exposure (produced by *Aspergillus* spp. and found in contaminated vegetation and contaminated food), and cirrhosis.

   2. Clinical characteristics

     a. Presenting complaints include malaise, weight loss, abdominal swelling, weakness, jaundice, and upper abdominal pain. Clinical manifestations typically occur late in the disease.

     b. Hepatomegaly, splenomegaly, hepatic bruit, ascites, jaundice, wasting, and fever may be detected on examination.

   3. Diagnostic studies

> Alpha-fetoprotein is a tumor marker that can be used to monitor risk in those at greatest risk for hepatic carcinoma.

     a. α-Fetoprotein may be elevated in hepatic carcinoma. It is also elevated in chronic hepatitis C and cirrhosis.

     b. Imaging with sonography, CT, MRI, or hepatic angiography can show the lesion.

     c. Needle biopsy should generally not be performed if the tumor is resectable for fear of seeding.

   4. Treatment

     a. Benign neoplasms should be treated if the tumor size indicates a danger of rupturing the hepatic capsule.

     b. Treatment of metastatic disease involves treatment of the primary lesion.

    c. Surgical resection of hepatic carcinoma may be attempted if the cancer is confined to one lobe and there is no concurrent cirrhosis. Liver transplant can also be considered. The overall prognosis is poor.

Hernias

A. General characteristics

    1. A hernia is a protrusion of an organ or structure through the wall that normally contains it.

    2. Hernias of various types can entrap the intestines and cause intestinal blockage.

B. Types

    1. Umbilical hernia is generally congenital and appears at birth. Many umbilical hernias resolve on their own, but surgery may be indicated.

    2. Diaphragmatic or hiatal hernia involves protrusion of the stomach through the diaphragm via the esophageal hiatus. It can cause symptoms of GERD; acid reduction may suffice, although surgical repair can be used for more serious cases.

    3. Incisional hernias are associated more commonly with vertical incisions, especially in patients with concurrent obesity or wound infection.

    4. Inguinal hernias can be indirect (most common; passage of intestine through the internal inguinal ring down the inguinal canal, may pass into the scrotum), direct (passage of intestine through external inguinal ring at Hesselbach's triangle, rarely enters the scrotum), or femoral (least common; passage through femoral ring).

    5. Ventral hernia occurs when there is a weakening in the anterior abdominal wall and may be either incisional or umbilical.

C. Treatment of hernias is surgical correction.

> Most common hernia is a direct inguinal hernia; may pass into the scrotum in males; surgical correction is treatment.

Congenital Abnormalities

A. Esophageal atresia is commonly associated with tracheoesophageal fistulae.

    1. Atresia presents in newborns as excessive saliva and choking or coughing with attempts to feed.

    2. Inability to pass a nasogastric tube will establish the diagnosis.

    3. Treatment is surgical; pulmonary aspiration should be prevented in the interim by suction and withholding of oral feedings.

B. Diaphragmatic hernia causes immediate respiratory distress in the newborn because the affected lung is compressed by pressure from abdominal contents.

    1. Immediate intubation and ventilation is required, along with suction of the stomach by nasogastric tube.

    2. Diagnosis can be made if bowel sounds are heard in the chest.

    3. Radiography shows loops of bowel in the involved hemithorax, with displacement of the heart and mediastinal structures.

    4. Treatment is surgical.

C. **Pyloric stenosis**

    1. General characteristics

        a. The gastric outlet is obstructed by pyloric hypertrophy.

        b. Males are affected about five times more often than females.

> Pyrloric stenosis is 5 times more frequent in male babies than female babies.

    2. Clinical features

        a. Progressive, nonbilious, often projectile vomiting occurs in a child who remains hungry, generally presenting between 4 and 6 weeks of age.

        b. Weight loss and dehydration are common.

        c. An olive-shaped mass may be felt to the right of the umbilicus in most cases, especially shortly after vomiting.

    3. Laboratory findings: Ultrasonography will generally demonstrate the lesion, although barium swallow, showing delayed emptying and a "string sign," may be required in some cases.

    4. Treatment is surgical.

  D. Bowel atresia can occur in the ileum (most common), duodenum, jejunum, or colon and presents with signs of obstruction within the first few days of life.

  E. Hirschsprung's disease (congenital megacolon) is caused by congenital absence of Meissner and Auerbach's autonomic plexuses enervating the bowel wall.

    1. Symptoms may include constipation or obstipation, vomiting, and failure to thrive.

    2. Treatment is surgical resection of the affected bowel.

Nutritional Deficiencies

See Table 5-4.

Table 5-4 | **Nutritional Deficiencies**

Vitamin	Sources	Function(s)	At-Risk Groups	Deficiency Presentation	Toxicity Presentation
Vitamin A	Liver, fish oils, fortified milk, eggs	Vision, epithelial cell maturity, resistance to infection, antioxidant	Elderly, alcoholics, liver disease	Night blindness, dry skin	Skin disorders, hair loss, teratogenicity
Vitamin D	Fortified milk	Calcium regulation, cell differentiation	Elderly, shut-ins with low sun exposure	Rickets, osteomalacia	Hypercalcemia, kidney stones, soft-tissue deposits
Vitamin E	Plant oils, wheat germ, asparagus, peanuts, margarine	Retard cell aging, vascular and red cell wall integrity, antioxidant	Rare	Hemolytic anemia, degenerative nerve changes	Inhibition of vitamin K, myalgia, headache, weakness
Vitamin K	Liver, green leafy vegetables, broccoli, peas, green beans	Clotting	Rare	Bleeding	Anemia, jaundice
Thiamin	Pork, grains, dried beans, peas, brewer's yeast	Carbohydrate metabolism, nerve function	Alcoholism, poverty	Beriberi (nervous tingling, poor coordination, edema, weakness, cardiac dysfunction)	
Riboflavin	Milk, spinach, liver, grains	Energy		Oral inflammation, eye disorders	
Niacin	Bran, tuna, salmon, chicken, beef, liver, peanuts, grains	Energy, fat metabolism	Poverty, alcoholism	Flushing	
Pantothenic acid	Liver, broccoli, eggs	Energy, fat metabolism	Alcoholism	Tingling, fatigue, headache	
Biotin	Cheese, eggs, cauliflower, peanut butter, liver	Glucose production, fat synthesis	Alcoholism	Dermatitis, tongue pain, anemia, depression	
Vitamin B_6 (pyridoxine)	Animal protein, spinach, broccoli, bananas, salmon	Protein metabolism, neurotransmitter synthesis, hemoglobin	Adolescents, alcoholism	Headache, anemia, seizures, flaky skin, sore tongue	Nerve destruction

Table 5-4 | Nutritional Deficiencies *(Continued)*

Vitamin	Sources	Function(s)	At-Risk Groups	Deficiency Presentation	Toxicity Presentation
Folate	Green leafy vegetables, orange juice, grains, organ meats	DNA synthesis	Alcoholism, pregnancy	Megaloblastic anemia, sore tongue, diarrhea, mental disorders	
Vitamin B$_{12}$ (cobalamin)	Animal foods	Folate metabolism, nerve function	Elderly, vegans	Megaloblastic anemia, poor nerve function	
Vitamin C	Citrus fruits, strawberries, broccoli, greens	Collagen synthesis, hormone function, neurotransmitter synthesis	Alcoholism, elderly men	Scurvy (poor wound healing, petechiae, bleeding gums)	Diarrhea

Adapted from Wardlaw GM. *Perspectives in Nutrition.* 4th ed. McGraw-Hill; 1999.

Metabolic Disorders

A. Lactose intolerance

1. Lactose is digested by lactase, which is produced in the small intestine.

2. The persistence of lactase production past the age of 12 years is common only in northern European populations. For most of the world's population, lactase does not persist, and lactose-containing products are not well digested.

3. Symptoms of lactose intolerance include nausea, bloating, flatulence, diarrhea, cramping, and, occasionally, vomiting.

4. Lactose intolerance is easily managed by avoiding milk and dairy products or use of lactase enzyme tablets or drops.

> Resolution of symptoms with avoidance of lactose-containing products is enough to diagnose lactose intolerance.

B. Phenylketonuria

1. Phenylketonuria is a rare autosomal recessive inability to metabolize the protein phenylalanine.

2. Phenylalanine and its metabolites accumulate in the central nervous system, causing mental retardation and movement disorders.

3. Screening at birth is simple and allows early detection and management; delay in diagnosis (after age 3 years) will lead to irreversible brain damage.

4. Management is by a low-phenylalanine diet and tyrosine supplementation. Breast milk is low in phenylalanine, and special formulas are available. Strict control of protein intake is required for life.

Practice Questions

Directions: Each of the numbered items or incomplete statements in this section is followed by a list of answers or completions of the statement. Select the ONE lettered answer or completion that is BEST in each case.

1. Your patient is a 42-year-old male complaining of intermittent, moderate burning chest pain over the past 6 months. It is worse at night and after a larger meal. The pain is relieved somewhat by antacids. He is a nonsmoker and has no significant medical history. What is the *next* best step?
A. Recommend eating at least 2 hours prior to bedtime.
B. Order an ECG.
C. Order upper endoscopy.
D. Prescribe a PPI.

2. A 34-year-old female presents with new-onset dysphagia accompanied by weight loss and oral irritation. On initial examination, you diagnosed thrush; an HIV test was positive with a CD4 count of 75. She was started on fluconazole for thrush and presumptive esophageal candidiasis. When she returns to begin antiretroviral therapy, she notes that while her mouth symptoms are resolved the dysphagia has continued unabated. What is the most likely cause of her symptoms?
A. Cryptosporidium
B. CMV
C. Esophageal cancer
D. EBV

3. A 36-year-old male has just completed treatment for *H. pylori* PUD. Which of the following is the best recommendation to confirm the success of treatment?
   A. Serum antibody test today
   B. Serum antibody test in 4 weeks
   C. Stool antigen test today
   D. Stool antigen test in 4 weeks

4. Two members of a family come to the primary care office complaining of nausea and vomiting which occurred last night several hours after the family ate dinner at a local restaurant. The other three family members are well and neither patient is experiencing fever. Both have had cramping and some diarrhea. What is the recommended treatment?
   A. Rest and hydration
   B. Trimethoprim–sulfamethoxazole
   C. Ciprofloxacin
   D. Metronidazole

5. A 68-year-old receives a positive hepatitis C (HCV) antibody result on screening. What is the next best step?
   A. Order elastography of the liver.
   B. Order ultrasonography of the liver.
   C. Determine viral load (via PCR) for HCV virus.
   D. Refer to infectious disease for treatment.

6. A 45-year-old female presents to the emergency department complaining of a deep boring epigastric pain that radiates to the back and is relieved somewhat by leaning forward. Vital signs are significant only for a slightly elevated pulse. In addition to a CBC and chemistry panel, which of the following should be ordered?
   A. *H. pylori* stool antigen
   B. Lipase and amylase
   C. Abdominal CT
   D. Barium swallow

7. A 75-year-old male presents to the primary care office complaining of gradually increasing fatigue and weight loss over the past 6 months. He notes he is also experiencing some constipation but was previously well. On examination, you note an ill-appearing thin male with pallor and tachycardia. His rectal examination shows a smooth, slightly enlarged prostate and positive occult blood in the stool. He is afebrile and his examination is otherwise benign. Which diagnosis should be at the top of your differential?
   A. Diverticulitis
   B. Colon cancer
   C. PUD
   D. Crohn's disease

8. An 18-year-old male presents to the emergency department with abdominal pain in the right lower quadrant increasing to severe over the past 4 hours. Which of the following would be the most helpful examination technique at this time?
   A. Have the patient place one hand vertically on his abdomen while you tap on one side feeling for the response on the other side.
   B. Flexing and internally rotating the supine patient's right knee
   C. Percussing from the umbilicus toward the pubic symphysis
   D. Evaluating for pain at the costovertebral angle (CVA)

9. A 66-year-old female was recently released from a 3-day hospitalization for pneumonia. She will complete her home antibiotics, ciprofloxacin, tomorrow but comes in today because she is now experiencing severe, foul-smelling diarrhea. What is the treatment for the most likely cause?
   A. Hydration and rest
   B. Trimethoprim–sulfamethoxazole
   C. Oral vancomycin
   D. Doxycycline

10. A 58-year-old female presents to the emergency department with RUQ tenderness, fever, and jaundice. Sonography shows biliary dilatation; initial labs show leukocytosis and elevated bilirubin and mild elevation of liver enzymes. What is the most likely diagnosis?
   A. Acute cholangitis
   B. Cholecystitis
   C. Choledocholithiasis
   D. Fulminant hepatitis

11. A 19-year-old male returned from a recent camping trip about a month ago and has, since that time, experienced dyspepsia and mild diarrhea. He admits to drinking some untreated water from mountain streams. No one else in his family is experiencing symptoms. What is the most likely diagnosis?
   A. *E. coli*
   B. *Giardia lamblia*
   C. *Staphylococcus aureus*
   D. *Shigella*

12. A new mother brings in her 5-week-old infant son because he is vomiting with increasing frequency. The vomitus is nonbilious and occurs shortly after feeding and the child is losing weight. On examination, you note a firm rounded mass in the epigastrium. What is the most likely diagnosis?
   A. Bowel atresia
   B. Esophageal atresia
   C. Hirschsprung's disease
   D. Pyloric stenosis

Practice Answers

1. A. *GI; Clinical Intervention; GERD*

Lifestyle changes including smoking cessation, avoiding foods that cause problems, raising the head of the bed, and avoiding large meals at bedtime are the initial therapy for gastric reflux. Endoscopy is recommended if symptoms are long-standing or with new onset in an older (over 45 years) patient. PPIs are recommended if lifestyle modifications are insufficient. ECG would be recommended in a patient in whom ischemia is likely.

2. B. *GI; Diagnosis; CMV Esophagitis*

CMV is a more common cause of esophagitis in patients with HIV and a low CD4 cell count. Epstein–Barr is an uncommon cause of esophagitis in patients with HIV. Esophageal cancer causes blockage but not pain; cryptosporidium causes diarrhea.

3. D. *GI; Diagnostic Studies; PUD*

Stool antigen test in 4 weeks is the recommended follow-up to assure treatment success. Either this or urea breath test may be used to confirm cure but neither is effective until 4 weeks after the completion of therapy. Serum antibody test will remain positive after cure and is not helpful for confirmation.

4. A. *GI; Clinical Intervention; Acute Gastroenteritis*

Rest and hydration is the correct answer. The description indicates a rapid onset toxin for which only symptomatic treatment is indicated. Antibiotics are only indicated in enteritis caused by bacteria that have invaded the GI tract.

5. C. *GI; Diagnostic Studies; HCV*

The next best step is to order direct HCV viral detection to confirm ongoing infection, as approximately 15% of those infected with HCV will clear the infection without therapy. Elastography, sonography, and treatment are only appropriate for those with ongoing infection. Elastography evaluates the level of hepatocellular damage (fibrosis) and sonography looks for hepatocellular carcinoma, both complications of long-standing ongoing HCV infection.

6. B. *GI; Diagnostic Studies; Pancreatitis*

It is imperative to evaluate lipase and amylase. The description of epigastric pain radiating to the back is typical of pancreatitis. *H. pylori* testing, CT, and barium swallow will not aid in diagnosing pancreatitis.

7. B. *GI; Diagnosis; Colon Cancer*

Colon cancer should be at the top of the differential. He has weight loss and change in bowel habits including occult blood. Although each of these options is associated with GI bleed, all are associated with significant pain and would likely occur at a much younger age.

8. B. *GI; History and PE; Appendicitis*

The patient is likely experiencing acute appendicitis. Checking for peritoneal signs is a must. The obturator sign evaluates for inflammation of the appendix and peritoneum. Fluid wave is helpful to identify ascites. The obturator sign (described in b) identifies peritonitis. Percussing from the symphysis pubic helps to identify bladder retention. CVA tenderness indicates nephrolithiasis or pyelonephritis.

9. C. *GI; Pharmacology; C Diff*

Presumptive diagnosis warrants empiric treatment with oral vancomycin to treat presumed *C. difficile*, which often occurs after antibiotic therapy. Hydration and rest will also help, but will not resolve the infection. Metronidazole might also be used but because of her recent hospitalization, oral vancomycin would be the preferred option. Trimethoprim–sulfamethoxazole might be used for traveler's diarrhea, and doxycycline would not be used for a GI infection.

10. A. *GI; Diagnosis; Cholangitis*

This patient is presenting with acute cholangitis. The presenting symptoms constitute Charcot's triad, the classic presentation for this disease. Choledocholithiasis refers to the presence of stones which is most often asymptomatic, cholecystitis presents more often with colicky pain after a high-fat meal, and hepatitis with high transaminase levels.

11. B. *GI; Diagnosis; Giardia*

Giardia lamblia is a parasite found in untreated water and causes mild to moderate GI symptoms. *E. coli* can cause a variety of GI syndromes ranging from mild to severe hemorrhagic disease but is generally of shorter duration. *Shigella* causes severe, purulent diarrhea and *S. aureus* causes immediate onset short-duration symptoms.

12. D. GI, Diagnosis, Pyloric stenosis

Pyloric stenosis commonly presents within the first 2 months of life and can be detected by finding a firm olive-shaped mass in the epigastrium on examination. Esophageal or bowel atresia will present within days of birth, and Hirschsprung's disease causes constipation and failure to thrive.

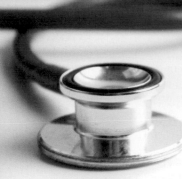

6 | Nephrology and Urology

Andrew M. Zolp

Renal Failure

A. **Acute kidney injury (AKI) (previously acute renal failure [ARF])**

1. General characteristics

   a. AKI refers to a syndrome of rapidly deteriorating glomerular filtration rate (GFR) with the accumulation of nitrogenous wastes (urea, creatinine) referred to as azotemia. Serum creatinine acutely increases by more than 0.5 mg per dL or more than 50% over baseline levels; the process develops in a time frame of <7 days.

   b. Criteria to define AKI vary widely; therefore, expert consensus opinion (Acute Dialysis Quality Initiative Group) developed the **RIFLE** classification of AKI in the critical care setting based on the GFR and urine output (UO). See Table 6-1.

   c. Two other modalities of classification exist as modifications to the RIFLE criteria

      (1) AKIN (Acute Kidney Injury Network). See Table 6-2.

      (2) KDIGO (Kidney Disease: Improving Global Outcomes). See Table 6-3.

   d. It is important to distinguish between an acute insult and worsening of a chronic state. Of the many conditions that can result in AKI, two conditions account for the majority of cases: reduced renal perfusion and acute tubular necrosis (ATN).

   e. Causes are classified into three categories: prerenal, intrinsic renal, and postrenal (Table 6-4).

   f. AKI occurs in 5% of hospitalized patients and in up to 30% of critical care patients. The overall mortality rate for AKI is 10% to 50%, depending on patient comorbidities and clinical setting.

2. **Clinical features**

   a. A thorough medical history can identify possible causes of AKI, such as procedures and medications as well as exposure to nephrotoxins; family history of renal

Table 6-1 | RIFLE Classification of Acute Kidney Failure

Risk of renal dysfunction	Increase serum creatinine 1.5-fold *or* decrease GFR >25%	Urine output <0.5 mL/kg/hour for 6 hours
Injury to kidney	Increase serum creatinine 2-fold *or* decrease GFR >50%	Urine output <0.5 mL/kg/hour for 12 hours
Failure of kidney function	Increase creatinine 3-fold *or* decrease GFR >75%	Urine output <0.3 mL/kg/hour for 24 hours *or* anuria for 12 hours
Loss of kidney function (persistent AKD)	Complete loss of function (need for renal replacement) for more than 4 weeks	
End-stage kidney disease (ESKD) (end-stage renal disease [ESRD])	Complete loss of kidney function for more than 3 months	

AKD, acute kidney disease; GFR, glomerular filtration rate.

Table 6-2 | Akin Classification of Acute Kidney Failure

Abrupt onset within 48 hours Increase serum creatinine ≥0.3 mg/dL	
Stage I (risk)	Increase serum creatinine 0.3 mg/dL or >50%
Stage II (injury)	Increase serum creatinine by 100%
Stage III (failure)	Increase serum creatinine by 200%

Table 6-3 | KDIGO Classification of Acute Kidney Failure

Increase serum creatinine 0.3 mg/dL developing over 48 hours *or* increase serum creatinine >50% developing over 7 days *or* urine volume <0.5 mL/kg/hour for 6 hours		
Stage I	Increase serum creatinine 0.3 mg/dL *or* >50%	Urine output <0.5 mL/kg/hour for 6–12 hours
Stage II	Increase serum creatinine 100%	Urine output <0.5 mL/kg/hour for ≥12 hours
Stage III	Increase serum creatinine 200%	Urine output <0.3 mL/kg/hour for ≥24 hours *or* anuria ≥12 hours *or* initiation of renal replacement therapy

Table 6-4 | Causes of Acute Renal Failure and Common Laboratory Findings

Type of AKI	Common Laboratory Findings
Prerenal Causes (60%–70%)	
Hypovolemia	Urine sodium <20 mEq/L
Hypotension	$FE_{Na} < 1\%$
Ineffective circulating volume (HF, cirrhosis, nephrotic syndrome, early sepsis)	Urine osmolality > 500 mOsm/kg *Elevated* BUN-to-plasma Cr ratio (20:1)
Aortic aneurysm	Urine specific gravity >1.020
Renal artery stenosis or embolic disease	Urinalysis normal
Intrinsic Renal Causes (25%–40%)	
Acute tubular necrosis	Increased urine sodium >40 mEq/L
Nephrotoxins (NSAIDs, aminoglycosides, radiologic contrast)	$FE_{Na} > 1\%–2\%$
Interstitial diseases (acute interstitial nephritis, SLE, infection)	Urine osmolality of 300–500 mOsm/kg
Glomerulonephritis	*Decreased* BUN-to-plasma Cr ratio (<15:1)
Vascular diseases (polyarteritis nodosa, vasculitis)	Urine specific gravity of 1.010–1.020
	Urinalysis + for granular casts, WBCs and casts, RBCs and casts, proteinuria, and tubular epithelial cells
Postrenal Causes (5%–10%)	
Tubular obstruction	Urine sodium, FE_{Na}, osmolality, and BUN-to-Cr ratio vary based on time frame of obstruction
Obstructive uropathy (urolithiasis, BPH, bladder outlet obstruction)	
	Urinalysis normal

AKI, acute kidney injury; BUN, blood urea nitrogen; HF, heart failure; NSAIDs, nonsteroidal anti-inflammatory drugs; SLE, systemic lupus erythematosus; BPH, benign prostatic hyperplasia; FE_{Na}, fractional excretion of sodium; WBCs, white blood cells; RBCs, red blood cells.

disease; urologic disease; or contributing factors such as hypertension, hypotension, volume loss, congestive heart failure (CHF), or diabetes.

b. General symptoms include nausea, vomiting, diarrhea, pruritus, drowsiness, dizziness, hiccups, shortness of breath, anorexia, and hematochezia.

c. Signs can reflect the underlying cause.

(1) Tachycardia and hypotension may indicate prerenal causes.

(2) A distended bladder, costovertebral angle tenderness, or enlarged prostate suggests postrenal causes.

(3) Other signs include anuria or oliguria, change in volume status (weight), change in mental status, edema, weakness, dehydration, rashes, jugular venous distention, uriniferous odor, and ecchymosis.

3. Diagnostic studies: see Table 6-4
   a. Prerenal causes
      (1) Urine sodium <20 mEq per L
      (2) Fractional excretion of sodium (FE_{Na}) <1%
      (3) Urine osmolality >500 mOsm per kg
      (4) Elevated blood urea nitrogen (BUN)-to-plasma Cr ratio (20:1)
      (5) Urine specific gravity >1.020
   b. Intrinsic renal causes
      (1) Increased urine sodium >40 mEq per L
      (2) FE_{Na} >1% to 2%
      (3) Urine osmolality of 300 to 500 mOsm per kg
      (4) Decreased BUN-to-plasma Cr ratio (<15:1)
      (5) Urine specific gravity of 1.010 to 1.020
   c. Postrenal causes: Urine sodium, FE_{Na}, osmolality, and BUN-to-Cr ratio can vary depending on how long the obstruction has been present.
   d. GFR is the key parameter to measure renal function. Serum creatinine or BUN is less reliable, although more easily measured; creatinine and BUN are helpful for monitoring renal insufficiency and provide clues to cause.
   e. BUN provides an estimate of renal function but is much more sensitive to dehydration, catabolism, diet, renal perfusion, and liver disease. Urea is reabsorbed in the nephron during stasis, which causes false elevations of BUN; therefore, this is not a reliable indicator of renal function.
   f. Urinalysis is essentially normal in prerenal and postrenal causes of AKI with only a few hyaline casts. Granular casts, white blood cells (WBCs) and casts, red blood cells (RBCs) and casts, proteinuria, and tubular epithelial cells indicate intrinsic renal causes of AKI.
   g. Serum cystatin C is a serum biomarker that can be used for detecting AKI.
      (1) Cystatin C is a low-molecular-weight protein, a member of the cystatin superfamily of cysteine protease inhibitors. It is filtered at the glomerulus and is not reabsorbed. Metabolism in the tubules prevents direct measurement of clearance.
      (2) When cystatin C is used in combination with serum creatinine, GFR may be better estimated than either alone. Cystatin C has good sensitivity (87% to 97%) and specificity (85% to 100%).
   h. Urine biomarkers for detecting AKI include interleukin-18 (IL-18), kidney injury molecule-1 (KIM-1), neutrophil gelatinase–associated lipocalin (NGAL), and liver-type fatty acid–binding protein (L-FABP). Urinary angiotensinogen may be useful as a prognostic marker in patients with severe AKI.
   i. Point-of-care tests for urinary insulin-like growth factor binding protein (IGFBP) and tissue inhibitor of metalloproteinases-2 (TIMP-2) can be used to predict AKI and long-term dialysis or death as well.
   j. If the presentation is unknown with respect to an acute episode versus a chronic problem, renal ultrasonography may be used to measure renal size. A kidney smaller than 10 cm indicates a chronic problem.
   k. Many other abnormal laboratory findings are associated with loss of renal function, including azotemia, decreased creatinine clearance, metabolic acidosis, hyperkalemia, and hypocalcemia. Other blood chemistries and hematologic tests may be abnormal, depending on the severity of the disease.
   l. Urine flow: The normal response to decreased effective intravascular volume and kidney perfusion is to concentrate the urine and increase sodium reabsorption.

In prerenal and postrenal causes of AKI, urinalysis may be normal or may reveal few hyaline casts; in intrinsic renal causes of AKI, urinalysis may be normal or may reveal few hyaline casts, WBCs, RBCs, proteinuria, and tubular epithelial cells.

Kidney size >10 cm indicates chronic pathology.

Decreased urine flow can provide helpful information about the cause of AKI, although accurate measures may be difficult.

4. Treatment

   a. Treatment involves correction of the underlying problem. Examples include the following:

      (1) Prerenal—achievement of normal hemodynamics (intravenous [IV] fluids, blood products, and improving cardiac output)

      (2) Intrarenal—adjustment and avoidance of medications and nephrotoxic agents

      (3) Postrenal—relief of urinary tract obstruction (ureteral stents, urethral catheter)

      (4) Consideration of early intervention under the supervision of a nephrologist or intensivist for management of potential renal replacement therapy

   b. Short-term dialysis should be implemented when serum creatinine exceeds 5 to 10 mg per dL. Other indications for dialysis include unresponsive acidosis, electrolyte disorders, fluid overload, or uremic complications.

B. Chronic kidney disease (CKD)

   1. General characteristics

      a. Definitions

         (1) CKD is a progression of ongoing loss of kidney function (GFR). The National Kidney Foundation (NKF) defines CKD as (1) GFR <60 mL per min per 1.73 m^2 or (2) presence of kidney damage (proteinuria [urine albumin excretion >30 mg/day], glomerulonephritis (GN), or structural damage from polycystic kidney disease [PKD]) for ≥3 months.

         (2) CKD is classified into five stages based on the estimated GFR. These stages have been developed by the NKF to help provide an intervention plan for evaluation and management of each stage. (1 and 2 only) Criteria for stage of CKD and general symptoms can be found in Table 6-5.

      b. Diabetes mellitus, hypertension, GN, and PKD are the most common causes of CKD (see Table 6-6).

> The majority of all CKD cases are a result of chronic diabetes and hypertension; strict control of these conditions will significantly reduce risk.

Table 6-5 | Stages of Chronic Kidney Disease

GFR Categories in CKD			
	Stage 1	Kidney damage with normal GFR >90 mL/min/1.73 m^2 BSA Persistent albuminuria	Generally asymptomatic No increase in BUN or creatinine Acid–base maintenance is adaptive through an increase in remaining nephron function
	Stage 2	Kidney damage with mild decrease in GFR 89–60 mL/min/1.73 m^2 BSA	Generally asymptomatic No increase in BUN or creatinine Acid–base maintenance is adaptive through an increase in remaining nephron function
	Stage 3a	Mild-moderate decrease in GFR 59–45 mL/min/1.73 m^2 BSA	May remain asymptomatic Serum BUN and creatinine increase
	Stage 3b	Moderate-severe decrease in GFR 44–30 mL/min/1.73 m^2 BSA	Other hormones (PTH), erythropoietin, calcitriol become abnormal
	Stage 4	Severe decrease in GFR 29–15 mL/min/1.73 m^2 BSA	Anemia, acidosis, hyperkalemia, hypocalcemia, hyperphosphatemia
	Stage 5	Kidney failure with GFR <15 mL/min/1.73 m^2 BSA	Candidate for renal replacement therapy
Albumin Categories in CKD	**A1**	<30 mg/day	Normal to mildly increased
	A2	30–300 mg/day	Moderately increased
	A3	>300 mg/day	Severely increased

BSA, body surface area; BUN, blood urea nitrogen; GFR, glomerular filtration rate; PTH, parathyroid hormone.

Table 6-6 | Causes of Chronic Renal Failure

Diabetes mellitus
Hypertension
Glomerulonephritis
Polycystic kidney disease
Other causes
Primary glomerular diseases (membranous nephropathy, minimal change disease, IgA nephropathy)
Secondary glomerular diseases (sickle cell anemia, SLE)
Tubulointerstitial renal diseases (nephrotoxins, infection, multiple myeloma, HIV)
Chronic pyelonephritis (tuberculosis)
Vascular diseases (renal artery stenosis or obstruction)
Obstructive nephropathies (nephrolithiasis, prostate disease, neurogenic bladder)

IgA, immunoglobulin A; SLE, systemic lupus erythematosus.

   c. Patients with CKD generally progress to chronic renal failure.

     (1) The rate of progression depends on the underlying cause, the effectiveness of treatments, and the individual patient.

     (2) The 5-year survival rate for chronic renal failure with patients on dialysis is about 40%.

2. Clinical features

   a. Uremic symptoms may develop (stages 3 to 5) insidiously and include fatigue, malaise, anorexia, nausea, vomiting, metallic taste, hiccups, dyspnea, orthopnea, impaired mentation, insomnia, irritability, muscle cramps, restless legs, weakness, pruritus, easy bruising, and altered consciousness.

   b. Signs include cachexia, weight loss, muscle wasting, pallor, hypertension, ecchymosis, sensory deficits, asterixis, and Kussmaul's respirations.

3. Diagnostic studies

   a. Measurement of GFR is the gold standard. The Cockcroft–Gault formula (requires the patient age, body weight, and serum creatinine) or the Modification of Diet in Renal Disease (MDRD) equation (requires serum albumin and BUN as well as patient age, body weight, and serum creatinine) will give a fairly accurate prediction of GFR. The MDRD is probably more accurate. The MDRD also takes into account gender and ethnicity. For children, use a pediatric GFR calculator.

> GFR is the gold standard of kidney function.

   b. Proteinuria is a marker for kidney damage. Albuminuria (formerly microalbuminuria) appears early in the disease.

   c. BUN and creatinine are elevated.

   d. Hemoglobin and hematocrit, serum electrolytes, and urinalysis are abnormal.

   e. Serum biomarker cystatin C is elevated when the GFR is <88 mL per min per 1.73 m^2 BSA; however, its clinical role has not been defined.

4. Treatment is aimed at slowing the progression of CKD and treating reversible causes of acute deterioration.

   a. Angiotensin-converting enzyme (ACE) inhibitors and angiotensin receptor blockers (ARBs) slow the progression of renal dysfunction, particularly in patients with proteinuria.

   b. Managing comorbid conditions improves the outcome: tight hypertensive control (blood pressure [BP] < 130/80), tight glycemic control in patients with diabetes (hemoglobin A$_{1c}$ [HbA$_{1c}$] <7.0%), cholesterol-lowering therapy (goals: low-density lipoprotein [LDL] <100 mg/dL, high-density lipoprotein [HDL] >50 mg/dL, and triglycerides <150 mg/dL), tobacco cessation, and weight control.

   c. Erythropoietin, iron supplements, and antiplatelet therapy should be considered to maintain hemoglobin (11 to 12 g/dL) and bleeding time as needed. Hemoglobin >13 g per dL shows an increased risk of stroke and adverse cardiovascular events.

d. Medical therapy requires careful drug dosing to adjust for decreased renal function.

e. Dietary management includes restriction of protein intake; adequate caloric intake; calcium and vitamin D supplements; and limitation of water, sodium, potassium, and phosphorus.

f. Need for hemodialysis, peritoneal dialysis, or kidney transplantation should be coordinated with nephrology service.

g. Pneumococcal vaccination is recommended.

h. Refer to nephrology for management of GFR stages 4 and 5.

Glomerular Disorders

A. Glomerulonephritis

1. **General characteristics**

   a. GN is an inflammation of the glomerulus caused by damage (primary or secondary glomerular injury) including immunologic responses, ischemia, free radicals, drugs, toxins, vascular disorders, and infection.

   b. About 60% of cases are in children 2 to 12 years of age.

   c. Prognosis is excellent in children and worse in adults, especially in those with preexisting renal disease.

2. **Causes**

   a. The major causes of GN are listed in Table 6-7.

   b. Causes are divided into focal GN, which is characterized by involvement of less than half the glomeruli, and diffuse GN, which affects most glomeruli.

3. **Clinical features**

   a. Hematuria is present; urine is often tea or cola colored.

   b. Oliguria or anuria is present.

   c. Edema of the face and eyes is present in the morning, and edema of the feet and ankles occurs in the afternoon and evening.

   d. Hypertension is also a common, but not an essential, clinical finding.

4. **Diagnostic studies**

   a. Antistreptolysin-O (ASO) titer is increased in 60% to 80% of cases and should be considered if there is a possibility of a recent streptococcal infection. A common cause of GN is streptococcal infection (poststreptococcal glomerulonephritis [PSGN]).

> Although the majority of cases occur in children, the majority of severe cases and sequelae occur in adults.

Table 6-7 | Causes of Glomerulonephritis

Type	Children	Adults
Focal	Benign hematuria Henoch–Schönlein purpura Mild postinfectious GN IgA nephropathy Hereditary nephritis	IgA nephropathy Hereditary nephritis SLE
Diffuse	Postinfectious GN Membranoproliferative GN	SLE Membranoproliferative GN Rapidly progressive GN Postinfectious GN Vasculitis

GN, glomerulonephritis; IgA, immunoglobulin A; SLE, systemic lupus erythematosus.

      b. Urinalysis reveals hematuria (>3 RBCs/high-power field [HPF]. RBCs will often be misshaped [acanthocytes] because of their passage through the glomerulus as opposed to a normal-shaped RBC that could represent bleeding from the bladder or urethra). RBC casts and proteinuria (1 to 2 g/24 hours) are also common.

      c. Serum complement (C3) levels are often decreased.

      d. Renal biopsy may be done to determine the exact diagnosis or severity of disease if diagnosis remains in doubt.

5. Treatment

      a. Steroids and immunosuppressive drugs may be used to control the inflammatory response, which is responsible for the damage. These are usually not needed in PSGN.

      b. Dietary management: Salt and fluid intake should be decreased.

      c. Dialysis should be performed if symptomatic azotemia is present.

      d. Medical therapy

          (1) ACE inhibitors or ARBs are renal protective (reduce urinary protein loss) in chronic GN.

          (2) Use medications as appropriate for hyperkalemia, pulmonary edema, peripheral edema, acidosis, and hypertension.

B. Nephrotic syndrome

> The criterion for diagnosis of nephrotic syndrome is >3.5 g of protein in 24 hours.

1. General characteristics

      a. Nephrotic syndrome is defined as the excretion of more than 3.5 g of protein per 1.73 m² of body surface in 24 hours. It manifests with hypoalbuminemia, lipiduria, hypercholesterolemia, and edema. It can predispose to thrombosis secondary to loss of proteins S and C and antithrombin III.

      b. It can affect adults and children, depending on the underlying cause. It can be primary (caused by renal disease) or secondary (Table 6-8).

      c. Prognosis depends on the specific cause and degree of renal damage. Complete remission is possible if the underlying disease is treatable.

2. Clinical features

      a. Symptoms include malaise, abdominal distention, anorexia, facial edema/puffy eyelids, oliguria, scrotal swelling, shortness of breath, and weight gain.

      b. Signs include ascites, edema, hypertension, orthostatic hypotension, retinal sheen, and skin striae.

3. Diagnostic studies

      a. Urinalysis reveals proteinuria, lipiduria, glycosuria, hematuria, and foamy urine.

      b. Microscopic examination of the urine shows RBC casts, granular casts, hyaline casts, and fatty casts. Key finding in microscopic urinalysis is the oval fat body

Table 6-8 | Causes of Nephrotic Syndrome

Primary Renal Disease	Secondary Renal Disease
Focal GN	Poststreptococcal GN
Focal glomerulosclerosis	SLE
IgA nephropathy	Malignancy
Membranoproliferative GN	Toxemia of pregnancy
Membranous glomerulopathy	Drugs and nephrotoxins
Mesangial proliferative GN	Lymphomas and leukemias
Minimal change disease	Diabetic glomerulosclerosis
Rapidly progressive GN	Amyloidosis
Congenital nephrotic syndrome	

GN, glomerulonephritis; IgA, immunoglobulin A; SLE, systemic lupus erythematosus.

(Maltese cross), which is a renal tubular cell that has reabsorbed some of the excess lipids in the urine.

   c. Blood chemistry shows hypoalbuminemia, azotemia, and hyperlipidemia. Hyperlipidemia is secondary to the liver producing increased lipoproteins because of hypovolemia from the loss of intravascular volume (edema).

   d. C3 levels can be low or normal, depending on the cause.

4. Treatment

   a. Medical therapy

      (1) ACE inhibitors or ARBs should be used early in the course of the disease.

      (2) Judicious use of diuretics is recommended to reduce fluid accumulations.

   b. Dietary management

      (1) Sodium and fluid intake may be restricted for the management of edema.

      (2) Dietary protein and potassium intake can be normal but not excessive.

   c. Infections should be treated aggressively.

   d. Anticoagulants should be used if thromboses are present.

   e. Nephrotoxic drugs (e.g., nonsteroidal anti-inflammatory drugs [NSAIDs], aminoglycoside antibiotics) should be avoided.

   f. Children with minimal change disease (the most common cause of nephrotic syndrome in children) respond to steroid therapy better than adults.

   g. Frequent relapse or steroid nonresponse may be treated with cyclophosphamide, cyclosporine, tacrolimus, or mycophenolate mofetil.

> Marked protein loss in nephrotic syndrome leads to hypoalbuminemia, which causes osmotic loss of fluid into any interstitial space.

Polycystic Kidney Disease

A. General characteristics

   1. PKD is characterized by growth of numerous cysts in the kidneys. The cysts are made of epithelial cells from the renal tubules and collecting system. The cysts replace the mass of the kidneys, reducing function and leading to kidney failure.

   2. Autosomal dominant polycystic kidney disease (ADPKD) is the most common form and almost always is bilateral. Symptoms typically develop during the fourth and fifth decades of life.

   3. The less common autosomal recessive polycystic kidney disease (ARPKD) begins in utero and can lead to fetal and neonatal death. Surviving infants have significantly reduced life expectancy, usually because of renal and hepatic failure.

   4. An acquired form of cystic kidney disease (ACKD) occurs in individuals with long-term renal disease or end-stage renal disease (ESRD). It is more common in African American men than in other ethnicities.

> The most common type of polycystic kidney disease (PCKD) is autosomal dominant; family members should be tested prior to clinical manifestations to provide supportive care and guidance.

B. Clinical features

   1. The most common symptoms of ADPKD are back and flank pain (secondary to the massive enlargement of the kidneys and/or liver) and headaches (greater risk of intracranial aneurysms). Nocturia is an early sign of abnormal renal function; it reflects the early impairment in urinary concentration.

   2. Hematuria, hypertension, recurrent urinary tract infection (UTI), weight loss, nephrolithiasis, and renal colic, as well as nausea and vomiting, may also be present.

   3. One or both kidneys may be palpable and feel nodular or tender. Cysts may also be present on the liver, pancreas, and other locations.

C. Diagnostic studies

   1. Anemia is commonly noted on complete blood count (CBC).

   2. Urinalysis shows proteinuria, hematuria, and, commonly, pyuria and bacteriuria.

3. Imaging studies
   a. The diagnostic method of choice is ultrasonography, which shows fluid-filled cysts.
   b. Plain-film radiography of the abdomen shows enlarged kidneys.
   c. Excretory infusion urography reveals multiple lucencies.
   d. Angiography shows bending of small vessels around cysts.
   e. Computed tomography (CT) shows large renal size and multiple thin-walled cysts.
4. Genetic studies for PKD 1 and PKD 2 can detect the presence of the mutation before symptoms develop. Early detection may allow affected individuals to forestall loss of kidney function through diet and BP control.

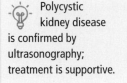

Polycystic kidney disease is confirmed by ultrasonography; treatment is supportive.

D. **Treatment**
1. There is no cure for ADPKD; treatment is supportive to ease symptoms and prolong life.
2. General measures should include management of pain (secondary to cyst hemorrhage), control of hypertension (goal of <130/80 mm Hg through use of an ACE inhibitor or ARB), high intake of fluids, and a low-protein diet, although no evidence of benefit has been shown in advanced renal dysfunction.
3. Infections should be treated vigorously with antibiotics (trimethoprim–sulfamethoxazole, fluoroquinolones, chloramphenicol, or vancomycin) that can penetrate the cyst wall.
4. Dialysis or transplantation should be considered when renal insufficiency becomes life-threatening. Transplantation has been successful, and non-PKD kidneys do not develop cysts.

Nephrolithiasis

A. General characteristics
1. Nephrolithiasis (renal calculi) occurs throughout the urinary tract and is common cause of pain, infection, and obstruction.
2. Pathogenesis
   a. Stones are caused by increased saturation (supersaturation) of urine with stone-forming salts (calcium, oxalate, and other solutes) or a possible lack of inhibitors (citrate) in the urine to prevent crystal formation. If either situation happens, then precipitation occurs and crystalluria develops.
   b. They are typically formed in the proximal tract and pass distally.
   c. They lodge at the ureteropelvic junction (UPJ: kidney stones), the ureterovesicular junction (UVJ: bladder stones), or the ureter at the level of the iliac vessels.
3. Nephrolithiasis commonly occurs during the third to fourth decade of life onward. The lifetime risk is about 19% in men and about 9% in women.
4. Four major types of stones exist (Table 6-9).
5. Patients usually have a complete return to health, but recurrences can occur. Frequency of recurrence is controversial but may be up to 30% to 50% in 5 years in uncontrolled studies or as low as 2% to 5% in controlled studies.

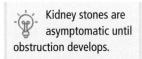

Kidney stones are asymptomatic until obstruction develops.

B. **Clinical features**
1. Nephrolithiasis is generally asymptomatic until inflammation or complete or partial ureteral obstruction develops.
2. Clinical features of nephrolithiasis include unilateral back pain and renal colic that waxes and wanes.

Table 6-9 | Types of Kidney Stones

Type	Mechanism	Incidence	Radiology	Notes
Calcium oxalate	Formation of calcium crystals	75%–85%	Radiopaque	Most common
Uric acid	Precipitation of uric acid	5%–10%	Radiolucent	Form in individuals with persistently acidic urine with or without hyperuricemia More common in men
Cystine	Impairment of cystine transport	<1%	Radiolucent	Occur only in autosomal recessive cystinuria
Struvite	Combination of calcium, ammonium, magnesium	10%–15%	Radiopaque	Formation increased by UTIs with urease-producing bacteria Common in patients with abnormal urinary tract anatomy and urinary diversions Common in patients who require frequent catheterization

3. Symptoms include hematuria, dysuria, urinary frequency, fever, chills, nausea, and vomiting.

4. Location can determine the direction of pain and its radiation.

   a. A stone in the upper ureter: The pain tends to radiate to the anterior abdomen.

   b. A stone in the lower part of the ureter: The pain tends to radiate to the ipsilateral groin, testicle in men, or labia in women.

   c. A stone lodged in the UVJ: Urinary frequency and urgency are noted, as well as lower pelvic pain.

   d. As the stone passes through the ureter, it may mimic other acute conditions, for example, acute cholecystitis, acute appendicitis, acute cystitis, and diverticulitis.

5. Signs include diaphoresis, tachycardia, tachypnea, restlessness, costovertebral angle tenderness, and abdominal distention because of ileus.

C. Diagnostic studies

   1. Serum chemistries are usually normal; however, there may be a leukocytosis from infection or stress.

   2. Urinalysis usually reveals microscopic or gross hematuria and may show leukocytes and/or crystals. Urine culture should be performed to rule out infection.

   3. Imaging modality of choice is the helical (spiral) CT. This does not require the use of radiocontrast and can detect stones as small as 1 mm. For children and pregnant patients, ultrasound is the imaging modality of choice; its improved sensitivity and lowered risk is making ultrasound first line where available.

   4. Plain-film radiography of the abdomen can identify radiopaque stones; unfortunately, it may miss a small stone even if radiopaque.

   5. Renal ultrasonography can identify stones in the kidney, proximal ureter, or UVJ.

   6. An intravenous pyelogram (IVP) is rarely indicated in the treatment and evaluation of a patient with nephrolithiasis. If an IVP is considered, remember to confirm that the patient has normal renal function before the procedure.

> Stones can be composed of calcium oxalate, uric acid, cystine, or struvite, and should be chemically analyzed to indicate further treatment.

D. **Treatment:** Size of stone indicates management. All stones should undergo chemical analysis as the type of stone may dictate additional treatment.

   1. Stones measuring <5 mm

      a. Many are likely to pass spontaneously and, in an otherwise healthy individual, may be managed on an outpatient basis.

      b. The patient should drink plenty of fluids.

      c. Strain urine to catch the stone and save it for analysis.

      d. Use an adequate supply of analgesics.

e. An α-blocker or calcium channel blocker may facilitate passage.

f. Follow up weekly or biweekly to monitor progress. Most stones that pass do so within 2 to 4 weeks of the onset of symptoms.

2. Stones measuring 5 to 10 mm

a. These are less likely to pass spontaneously; patients should be considered for early elective intervention if no other complicating factors (e.g., infection, high-grade obstruction, solitary kidney, anatomic abnormality preventing passage, and intractable pain) are present.

b. Increased fluids and analgesics are needed.

c. Elective lithotripsy or ureteroscopy with stone basket extraction may be used.

3. Stones measuring >10 mm

a. These are not likely to pass spontaneously; these patients are more likely to have complications.

b. The patients should be treated on an inpatient basis if they are unable to maintain adequate oral intake.

c. Vigorous hydration should be maintained.

d. Ureteral stent or percutaneous nephrostomy (gold standard) should be used if renal function is jeopardized.

e. Urgent treatment with extracorporeal shock wave lithotripsy (ESWL) can be used for renal stones of <2 cm or ureteral stones of <10 mm; ureteroscopic fragmentation may also be used. Ureteroscopy is more effective than ESWL for ureteral calculi. Percutaneous nephrolithotomy can be used for stones >2 cm.

4. Analgesics should be administered, including morphine, meperidine, or ketorolac. A combination of morphine and ketorolac is found to be more effective than single-agent use.

5. Pharmacologic intervention depends on patient status and stone makeup: Antibiotics if signs of infection are present, thiazide diuretics (such as chlorthalidone) to decrease urine calcium excretion, xanthine oxidase inhibitors (allopurinol) to decrease urine uric acid excretion, and alkali (potassium citrate or bicarbonate) to increase urine citrate excretion are options to consider.

> ☀ Kidney stones >10 cm require intervention.

> ☀ All patients post kidney stones should be encouraged to drink more fluids to help prevent recurrence.

Disorders of Salt and Water

A. Hyper- and hyponatremia reflect disturbances in water homeostasis. Serum sodium accurately reflects changes in serum osmolality and, therefore, changes in free water balance.

B. **Disorders of water deficiency: hypernatremia**

1. General characteristics

a. In hypernatremia, the water content of body fluid is deficient in relation to sodium content (serum sodium >145 mEq/L). There is either too much salt or not enough water.

b. Hypernatremia generally results from either inadequate fluid intake or excessive water loss. Causes include deficit of thirst, hypotonic fluid loss, urinary loss, gastrointestinal (GI) loss, insensible loss, burns, diuretic therapy, osmotic diuresis (hyperglycemia, mannitol administration), sodium excess, and diabetes insipidus (DI).

c. It occurs commonly in the elderly and may occur in infants with diarrhea.

2. **Clinical features**

a. Neurologic manifestations result from alterations in the brain water content and include thirst, restlessness, irritability, disorientation, lethargy, delirium, convulsions, and coma. Brain cell shrinkage may be substantial and can cause damage to the supporting vasculature.

b. Other findings include dry mouth and dry mucous membranes, lack of tears and decreased salivation, flushed skin, tachycardia, hypotension, fever, oliguria and anuria, hyperventilation, lethargy, and hyperreflexia. In children, use of the clinical dehydration scale may further distinguish the degree of dehydration.

3. Diagnostic studies

a. By definition, plasma sodium will be >145 mEq per L. Urine sodium is decreased if the hypernatremia is because of extrarenal losses and is elevated if the hypernatremia is because of renal losses or sodium excess. Urine is concentrated with extrarenal losses and diluted with DI.

b. Diabetes insipidus (see Diabetes Insipidus, below)

(1) Low urine sodium and polyuria usually indicate DI.

(2) Antidiuretic stimulation does not increase urine osmolality in nephrogenic DI.

c. Hyperosmolar coma may be indicated by elevated serum glucose, decreased UO, and increased urine osmolality.

4. Treatment

a. Hypernatremia should be treated on an inpatient basis.

b. Identify the underlying cause and treat accordingly.

c. Free water may be administered orally, which is the preferred route, or intravenously or subcutaneously (SQ), as a 5% dextrose solution in water (D5W) or half normal saline (D5 NS 0.45%).

d. Hypovolemia should be treated first (with isotonic saline or lactated Ringer's) and the hypernatremia second.

e. Dialysis should be implemented if sodium is >200 mEq per L.

f. Use caution during treatment because rapid correction of hypernatremia can cause pulmonary or cerebral edema, especially in patients with diabetes mellitus.

> Imbalance in sodium risks permanent brain injury and should be treated closely in an inpatient setting.

C. Disorders of water excess: hyponatremia

1. General characteristics

a. Hyponatremia is defined as a plasma sodium concentration of <135 mEq per L. Signs and symptoms may not occur until the concentration falls below 125 mEq per L.

b. Hyponatremia is the most common electrolyte disorder seen in the general hospital population secondary to the use of hypotonic fluid administration.

c. Type is determined by the serum osmolality and volume status.

(1) Hyponatremia with hypervolemia occurs in the setting of heart failure (HF), nephrotic syndrome, renal failure, and hepatic cirrhosis.

(2) Hyponatremia with euvolemia occurs with hypothyroidism, glucocorticoid excess, and syndrome of inappropriate secretion of antidiuretic hormone (SIADH).

(3) SIADH is defined as hypotonic hyponatremia; urine osmolality of >100 mOsm per kg; normal cardiac, hepatic, thyroid, adrenal, and renal function; and absence of extracellular fluid volume deficit. Urine sodium is usually >40 mEq per L.

(4) Hyponatremia with hypovolemia occurs with renal or nonrenal sodium loss.

(5) Table 6-10 provides an approach to the causes of hyponatremia.

2. Clinical features

a. Symptoms correlate to the sodium concentration and may include lethargy, disorientation, muscle cramps, anorexia, hiccups, nausea, vomiting, and seizures.

b. Signs include weakness, agitation, hyporeflexia, orthostatic hypotension, Cheyne–Stokes respiration, delirium, coma, or stupor.

Table 6-10 | Differential Diagnosis of Hyponatremia

1.	Is the plasma osmolality between 280 and 295 mOsm/kg? If yes, think isotonic hyponatremia (paraproteinemia, hypertriglyceridemia).
2.	Is the plasma osmolality >295 mOsm/kg? If yes, think hypertonic hyponatremia (hyperglycemia).
3.	Is the plasma osmolality <280 mOsm/kg? If yes, think hypotonic hyponatremia and measure the urine osmolality.
4.	Is the urine osmolality <100 mOsm/kg? If yes, think excessive water intake (primary polydipsia).
5.	Is the urine osmolality >100 mOsm/kg? If yes, think impaired renal diluting ability and assess the ECFV.
6.	Does the ECFV appear normal? If yes, think endocrinopathies (hypothyroidism, glucocorticoid insufficiency), SIADH (drugs, tumors, CNS disorders, nausea, pain, stress), a reset osmostat, potassium depletion, or thiazide diuretics.
7.	Is the ECFV decreased and the urine sodium increased (>20 mEq/L)? If yes, think renal solute loss (diuretics, osmotic diuresis, Addison's disease).
8.	Is the ECFV decreased and the urine sodium decreased (<10 mEq/L)? If yes, think extrarenal sodium loss.
9.	Is the ECFV increased and the urine sodium increased? If yes, think renal failure.
10.	Is the ECFV increased and the urine sodium decreased? If yes, think edematous disorders (CHF, cirrhosis, nephrotic syndrome).

CHF, congestive heart failure; CNS, central nervous system; ECFV, extracellular fluid volume; SIADH, syndrome of inappropriate secretion of antidiuretic hormone.

> In hyponatremia, if plasma osmolality is low, check urine osmolality. If urine osmolality is elevated, check extracellular fluid volume (ECFV) status.

3. Diagnostic studies

   a. Serum sodium of <135 mEq per L.

   b. Plasma osmolality is usually decreased, except in cases of fluid redistribution because of hyperglycemia or proteinemia.

   c. Urine sodium is either increased or decreased depending on the cause (see Table 6-10).

   d. If SIADH is suspected, brain CT may be done to rule out a central nervous system (CNS) disorder, and chest radiography may be done to rule out lung pathology.

4. **Treatment**

   a. Treat hypovolemia on an inpatient basis, especially if symptomatic or if serum sodium is <125 mEq per L. Also consider consultation with a nephrologist and/or endocrinologist.

   b. Treat the underlying cause, which usually requires fluid restriction except in hypovolemic hyponatremia where isotonic saline is the treatment.

   c. Monitor volume status.

   d. In severe symptomatic hyponatremia with sodium of <120 mEq per L, hypertonic (3%) saline may be used very cautiously.

      (1) Overly rapid correction can cause central pontine myelinolysis, resulting in neurologic damage.

      (2) Serum sodium levels should be checked hourly and neurologic status closely monitored.

   e. In chronic hyponatremia unresponsive to fluid restriction, demeclocycline may be used to induce nephrogenic DI but may cause nephrotoxicity in patients with cirrhosis. Vasopressin antagonists (conivaptan) may be considered in euvolemic or hypervolemic hyponatremia.

D. **Diabetes insipidus**

1. General characteristics

a. DI is a disorder of water.

b. Neurogenic (or central) DI is caused by deficient secretion of arginine vasopressin (antidiuretic hormone [ADH]) from the posterior pituitary.

c. Nephrogenic DI is caused by kidneys that are unresponsive to normal vasopressin levels.

d. Nephrogenic DI may be an inherited X-linked trait or acquired as a result of lithium therapy, hypokalemia, hypercalcemia, or renal disease.

2. **Clinical features**

a. Physical findings are associated with the primary cause.

b. Polyuria (50 to 60 mL/kg/day), nocturia, and polydipsia are the main symptoms. Seizures may develop related to the level of hypernatremia.

3. Diagnostic studies

a. Neurogenic (central) and nephrogenic DI can be distinguished by water deprivation and desmopressin (1-deamino-8-D-arginine vasopressin) testing. If the test results in reduced UO and resultant increase in urine osmolality, central DI is diagnosed. If little or no change in urine osmolality results, it is most likely nephrogenic DI.

b. Urine osmolality of <250 mOsm per kg, despite hypernatremia, indicates DI.

> In DI, if water deprivation testing results in reduced UO, the cause is neurogenic (central DI); if there is no change, it is renal.

4. **Treatment**

a. Neurogenic or central DI is best treated with parenteral or intranasal desmopressin.

b. Diuretics, chlorpropamide, or carbamazepine can be used in patients with mild disease.

c. Nephrogenic diabetes can be treated with hydrochlorothiazide or amiloride diuretics or indomethacin. Adequate water intake is essential to prevent dehydration.

d. Dietary measures, such as limiting salt and protein intake, can be helpful in nephrogenic DI.

E. **Volume depletion**

1. General characteristics

a. Volume depletion occurs when body fluids are lost from the extracellular compartment at a rate that exceeds intake.

b. Fluid can be lost from the GI tract, kidneys, or skin; from "third spacing" in the abdomen (i.e., ascites); or from injured tissues (i.e., burns).

2. **Clinical features**

a. Volume-depleted patients become thirsty, and urinary output decreases.

b. Mild volume depletion can cause increased heart rate, fatigue, and muscle cramps.

c. Moderate fluid loss causes dizziness and hypotension when standing.

d. Severe hypovolemia results in general hypotension, signs of ischemia and shock, and lethargy and confusion.

e. Decreased skin turgor and dry mucous membranes are unreliable signs of hypovolemia in older adults.

> Severe hypovolemia results in shock.

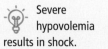

3. Diagnostic studies

a. Hematocrit and serum albumin may be increased.

b. Urinary sodium decreases.

c. Urea increases (secondary to urine stasis in the nephron), but there is little change in serum creatinine.

4. Treatment

   a. Mild hypovolemia can be treated by increasing salt and water intake.

   b. Moderate to severe volume depletion can be treated with oral fluids containing electrolytes, glucose, and amino acids.

   c. IV fluids should be used when patients cannot tolerate oral solutions. Isotonic fluids should be given until tissue perfusion has improved.

Electrolyte Disorders

A. Disorders of potassium

   1. Hyperkalemia

   a. General characteristics

   (1) Hyperkalemia refers to an elevated serum potassium level higher than 5.0 mEq per L.

   (2) It may result from cellular redistribution from the intracellular to the extracellular compartment, potassium retention, impaired potassium excretion, or elevations caused by increased tissue breakdown.

   (3) Hemolysis, thrombocytosis, or severe leukocytosis may cause spurious hyperkalemia (pseudohyperkalemia).

   (4) It is most commonly associated with renal failure, ACE inhibitors, hyporeninemic hypoaldosteronism, cell death, and metabolic acidosis.

   b. Clinical features

   (1) Severe hyperkalemia can result in dysrhythmias and cardiac arrest.

   (2) Neurologic symptoms include numbness, tingling, weakness, and flaccid paralysis.

   c. Diagnostic studies

   (1) Serum potassium level is >5.0 mEq per L; serum creatinine and BUN should be measured to assess renal function. Urine potassium, creatinine, and osmolality can reveal decreased fractional excretion of potassium.

   (2) Electrocardiography (ECG) changes evolve as potassium rises to >6 mEq per L.

   (a) Earliest ECG manifestation is peaking of the T waves (>6.5 mEq/L).

   (b) Flattening of the P wave, prolongation of the PR interval, and widening of the QRS complex are seen with more severe hyperkalemia (>7.0 mEq/L).

   (c) A final event is a sine wave pattern with cardiac arrest (8.0 to 10.0 mEq/L).

   d. Treatment

   (1) Potentially life-threatening hyperkalemia should be treated first and then the underlying cause discovered. Review the clinical situation, determine the acid–base status, and consider drug-induced conditions.

   (2) Potassium-sparing drugs and dietary potassium supplements should be discontinued. A low-potassium diet is recommended.

   (3) In severe hyperkalemia with ECG changes, calcium gluconate should be given IV to antagonize the effects of hyperkalemia on the heart. Strict monitoring of cardiac function and electrolytes is required.

   (4) Sodium bicarbonate, glucose (D_{50}), and insulin (10 units) may be administered to drive potassium back into the intracellular compartment. The onset of action is rapid, but the duration is short; therefore, serial potassium levels should be followed until correction is complete.

> The earliest EKG change in hyperkalemia (peaked T waves) can be seen at >6.5 mEq/L.

> Hyperkalemia causing arrhythmias must be treated with calcium gluconate to preserve cardiac function.

(5) Sodium polystyrene sulfonate (Kayexalate), a cation-exchange resin, is used to remove potassium from the body when levels are extremely high. Patiromer (Veltassa), an oral potassium binder, is another option. It is not indicated for life-threatening situations where emergency correction is required. Diuretics can be used if the patient has adequate renal function. Nebulized inhaled albuterol has been used to reduce serum potassium levels; however, the evidence is inconclusive. Hemodialysis may be required if the above therapies fail.

2. **Hypokalemia**

   a. General considerations

   (1) Hypokalemia is defined as a decreased serum potassium level (<3.5 mEq/L).

   (2) It can result from a shift of potassium into the intracellular compartment or from potassium losses of extrarenal or renal origin.

   (3) It most commonly occurs with the use of diuretics (most commonly loop diuretics), renal tubular acidosis, or GI losses (diarrhea).

   b. **Clinical features**

   (1) Cardiovascular manifestations are the most important, resulting in ventricular arrhythmias, hypotension, and cardiac arrest.

   (2) Neuromuscular manifestations also occur, including malaise, skeletal muscle weakness, cramps, and smooth muscle involvement, leading to ileus and constipation.

   (3) Other manifestations include polyuria, nocturia, hyperglycemia, and rhabdomyolysis.

   c. Diagnostic studies

   (1) Serum potassium is <3.5 mEq per L.

   (2) ECG may reveal flattened or inverted T waves, increased prominence of U waves, depression of the ST segment, and ventricular ectopy.

   (3) The most helpful tests for causal workup include blood acid–base parameters and urinary potassium and chloride levels.

   d. **Treatment**

   (1) Hypokalemia is usually not an emergency unless cardiac manifestations are present. In nonemergent conditions, oral potassium therapy is preferred, usually as potassium chloride.

   (2) For emergent situations (serum potassium <2.5 mEq/L or arrhythmias), IV replacement is indicated.

   (3) Hypokalemia potentiates the effects of cardiac glycosides on myocardial conduction and may lead to digitalis intoxication. More aggressive potassium replacement may be required in this situation.

B. Disorders of calcium and phosphorus

   1. General considerations

   a. Mechanisms for calcium and phosphorus homeostasis are complex and carefully maintained by several interrelated and interdependent mechanisms. These involve vitamin D, the small intestine, renal tubules, parathyroid hormone (PTH), and bone.

   b. Increased PTH levels result in increased serum calcium and decreased phosphorus. Conversely, decreased levels of PTH result in decreased serum calcium and increased phosphorus.

   c. Parathyroid disorders, chronic renal failure, and malignancy are the most common causes of disorders of calcium and phosphorus.

> The most common cause of hypokalemia is diuretic use.

> Oral potassium replacement is preferred unless the condition is severe.

2. **Hypercalcemia**

   a. General characteristics

      (1) Hypercalcemia is a significant elevation in serum calcium after adjustment for albumin level (see below).

      (2) This is one of the most common disorders of calcium and phosphorus, especially in hospitalized patients with malignancy (e.g., lung cancer; squamous cell carcinoma of the head, neck, and esophagus; female genital tract carcinoma; multiple myeloma; lymphoma; renal cell carcinoma [RCC]).

      (3) Other causes include vitamin D intoxication, hyperparathyroidism, and sarcoidosis.

   b. **Clinical features:** Severity of symptoms depends on calcium level. Most patients are asymptomatic until serum calcium is >12 mg per dL (normal = 8.5 to 12.5 mg/dL). Symptoms will also differ by the rapidity of onset of hypercalcemia, state of hydration, and underlying malignancy if any.

      (1) Symptoms include anorexia, nausea, constipation, polyuria, polydipsia, dehydration, and change in the level of consciousness (lethargy, stupor, and coma).

      (2) Signs of intravascular volume depletion (e.g., orthostatic hypotension and tachycardia) are frequent.

   c. Diagnostic studies

      (1) Serum calcium is high.

         (a) The calcium level must be corrected for albumin levels.

         (b) Corrected calcium = measured total calcium + $[0.8 \times (4 - \text{albumin})]$

      (2) Chest radiography may reveal an underlying pulmonary mass.

      (3) Perform urinalysis for hematuria, an early sign of RCC.

      (4) Erythrocyte sedimentation rate may be elevated in monoclonal gammopathy. Protein electrophoresis of serum or urine may be needed to confirm the diagnosis.

      (5) A 24-hour urine collection must be done for calcium determination.

         (a) An elevated urine calcium suggests malignant neoplastic or paraneoplastic process or secondary hyperparathyroidism.

         (b) A decreased urine calcium suggests primary hyperparathyroidism.

      (6) Elevations of serum vitamin D levels are consistent with vitamin D toxicity.

   d. **Treatment**

      (1) Isotonic saline (normal saline or Ringer's lactate) should be used for volume repletion. Loop diuretics should be used if the patient is hypervolemic after volume repletion.

      (2) Bisphosphonates alone or in combination with calcitonin or zoledronic acid can also be considered in severe hypercalcemia.

      (3) Manage the underlying cause.

3. **Hypocalcemia**

   a. General characteristics

      (1) Hypocalcemia is more common than hypercalcemia, and it can be found in a significant number of critically ill patients.

      (2) It often results from a chronic disease (the most common cause is CKD) or hypoparathyroidism. Although it typically presents in a mild, asymptomatic form, severe hypocalcemia can result in complete cardiovascular collapse.

> Patients with low albumin levels will have falsely elevated calcium unless it is corrected.

> Compared with hypercalcemia, hypocalcemia results in more dramatic signs including muscular and neurologic signs.

b. Clinical features

(1) Symptoms include dry skin, brittle nails, pruritus, muscle cramping, shortness of breath, and numbness and tingling in the extremities. Severe cardiovascular manifestations include syncope and angina.

(2) Signs include psoriasis, dry skin, and perioral numbness. Cardiovascular signs include wheezing, bradycardia, crackles, and a third heart sound.

(3) Classic neurologic findings include the Trousseau sign (carpal tunnel spasm after BP cuff applied for 3 minutes) and the Chvostek sign (spasm of facial muscle after tapping facial nerve in front of the ear). Other neurologic manifestations include irritability, confusion, dementia, and seizures.

c. Diagnostic studies

(1) Hypocalcemia is defined as a corrected serum calcium level of <8.5 mEq per L.

(2) Ionized calcium should also be measured. Magnesium, phosphate, albumin, liver function tests, and other electrolytes should be obtained to assist in the differential.

(3) BUN and creatinine should be measured to assess renal function.

d. Treatment

(1) Treat any emergent cardiovascular states.

(2) Severe hypocalcemia should be replaced (IV calcium gluconate or calcium chloride).

(3) Mild hypocalcemia can be treated on an outpatient basis with oral calcium and vitamin D supplements.

4. Hyperphosphatemia and hypophosphatemia

a. General characteristics

(1) Hyperphosphatemia is most commonly secondary to CKD or excessive use of phosphate-containing laxatives or enemas. Hypophosphatemia is secondary to diminished supply or absorption, increased urinary losses, or redistribution; common causes include vitamin D deficiency, respiratory alkalosis, burns, or hyperparathyroidism.

(2) Hypophosphatemia can be classified by the serum level. Moderate is a serum level of 1.0 to 2.5 mg per dL and is usually asymptomatic. Severe is a serum level of 1 mg per dL or less.

(3) Physical manifestations

(a) Hypophosphatemia may result in muscle weakness, hemolysis, and impaired platelet and WBC function.

(b) Severe hypophosphatemia may lead to rhabdomyolysis, paresthesia, and encephalopathy.

(c) Hyperphosphatemia is usually asymptomatic unless there is a reduction in serum calcium.

b. Treatment

(1) Hyperphosphatemia secondary to CKD should be treated with dietary phosphorus restriction and oral phosphate binders. Calcium carbonate tablets may also help to reduce phosphate absorption: 0.5 to 1.5 g three times daily with meals (500-mg tablets). Volume expansion and dialysis are other options.

(2) Hypophosphatemia of chronic origin can be treated with oral phosphate repletion.

> 💡 Signs of hypocalcemia include Chvostek (facial spasm with tapping in front of ear) and Trousseau (carpal spasm with BP cuff inflation) signs.

C. Disorders of magnesium

1. Hypermagnesemia

a. General characteristics

(1) Hypermagnesemia is defined as plasma magnesium levels of >2.2 mEq per L.

(2) Most magnesium is stored in bones and muscles.

b. **Clinical features**

(1) Symptomatic hypermagnesemia rarely occurs, except in patients with CKD who are given magnesium-containing products such as laxatives or antacids.

(2) Hypermagnesemia can be iatrogenically induced as part of treatment in eclampsia or preterm labor.

(3) Signs and symptoms reflect impaired neuromuscular transmission.

(a) Initially, deep tendon reflexes are reduced.

(b) Muscle weakness, hypotension, respiratory depression, and then cardiac arrest can follow with increasing magnesium levels.

(c) Nausea, vomiting, and flushing can also occur.

c. Diagnostic studies

(1) ECG shows widened QRS complex, prolonged PR interval, and prolonged QT interval.

(2) Bleeding and clotting times are increased.

d. **Treatment**

(1) Administer 10 to 20 mL of 10% calcium gluconate IV over 10 minutes.

(2) Saline diuresis and IV furosemide may increase excretion of magnesium.

(3) Dialysis is effective in severe hypermagnesemia.

2. Hypomagnesemia

a. General characteristics

(1) Hypomagnesemia is defined as plasma magnesium levels of <1.8 mEq per L. Plasma levels do not reflect total body stores.

(2) Hypomagnesemia usually presents when total body stores are severely depleted. Depletion usually results from diminished intake and impaired absorption.

(3) It is most commonly associated with chronic alcoholism, chronic diarrhea, hypoparathyroidism, hyperaldosteronism, diuretic therapy, osmotic diuresis, and nutritional deficiencies (e.g., prolonged parenteral feeding, malnutrition).

(4) Long-term use (>5 years) of proton pump inhibitors (PPIs) has been shown to cause hypomagnesemia.

b. **Clinical features:** Signs and symptoms include lethargy, anorexia, nausea and vomiting, weakness, tetany, and seizures.

c. Laboratory tests

(1) Hypokalemia, hypocalcemia, and hypocalciuria are commonly associated with states of magnesium depletion.

(2) ECG may show prolonged PR and QT intervals or widening of the QRS.

d. **Treatment**

(1) Administer oral magnesium oxide for chronic hypomagnesemia. Administer twice the estimated deficit over several days.

(2) In severe symptomatic hypomagnesemia, a magnesium sulfate solution (1 to 2 g) can be administered IV followed by an infusion of 6 g of magnesium sulfate over 1 L of fluids in 24 hours to replete magnesium stores. This may be repeated for up to 7 days.

Hypermagnesemia is seen in chronic kidney or iatrogenic overload.

Hypomagnesemia is caused by poor intake and/or diminished absorption.

(3) Magnesium sulfate may also be given intramuscularly (IM) in four divided doses (200 to 800 mg/day) if IV access is difficult.

(4) Serum levels should be monitored for the development of hypermagnesemia.

Acid–Base Disorders

A. General characteristics

1. Disturbances in the acid–base equilibrium are common, especially in patients who are critically ill.

2. Acid–base disorders may be respiratory (characterized by alterations in carbon dioxide [CO_2]) or metabolic (characterized by alterations in serum bicarbonate [HCO_3^-]). Table 6-11 summarizes the relationships.

3. Hydrogen ion concentration (pH)

a. The pH is usually considered to be normal between 7.36 and 7.44; however, for mixed acid–base problems, a pH of 7.40 should be considered as the absolute normal. When dealing with mixed acid–base disorders, variations from a pH of 7.40 in either direction will indicate whether there is an underlying acidosis or alkalosis present.

b. A pH of <7.35 represents acidemia. A pH of 7.2 or lower represents severe acidemia.

c. A pH of >7.45 represents alkalemia. A pH ≥7.6 or greater represents severe alkalemia.

4. Compensation for changes in the pH will always occur in the buffering system, the lungs, or kidneys. The degree of compensation depends on the duration of the disturbance and the functioning of the organ.

B. **Respiratory acidosis**

1. General characteristics

a. Respiratory acidosis is defined as a primary increase in the partial pressure of carbon dioxide (PCO_2) in the blood (hypercapnia) and decreased blood pH. The normal compensatory response is a gradual slow increase in plasma bicarbonate by the kidneys.

b. Respiratory acidosis results from the failure of the lung to excrete CO_2 that is generated through normal metabolism. It can be a result of alveolar hypoventilation leading to pulmonary CO_2 retention or of overproduction of CO_2 or a combination of both.

c. The primary cause of respiratory acidosis includes all disorders that reduce pulmonary function and CO_2 clearance, such as primary pulmonary disease, neuromuscular disease (myasthenia gravis), primary CNS dysfunction (severe brain stem injury), and drug-induced (opioids and other CNS depressants) hypoventilation.

> Approach acid–base disorders systematically: Check pH, check for a change in CO_2. If both are abnormal and in opposite direction, it's respiratory, if both are abnormal and in the same direction, it's likely metabolic.

Table 6-11 | Acid–Base Disorders

Disorder	pH	Carbon Dioxide (PCO_2)	Bicarbonate (HCO_3^-)
Respiratory acidosis	Decreased (↓)	Increased (↑)[a]	Increased (↑)
Respiratory alkalosis	Increased (↑)	Decreased (↓)[a]	Decreased (↓)
Metabolic acidosis	Decreased (↓)	Decreased (↓)	Decreased (↓)[a]
Metabolic alkalosis	Increased (↑)	Increased (↑)	Increased (↑)[a]

[a]Represents the primary disturbance.

> 💡 Common causes of respiratory acidosis (from reduced CO_2 clearance) are primary pulmonary disease, brain stem injury, CNS depressant drugs, and neuromuscular disease.

Other causes of respiratory acidosis include higher-than-normal carbohydrate loads and parenteral nutrition in critically ill patients.

2. Clinical features

   a. Metabolic encephalopathy, also known as hypercapnic encephalopathy, with headache and drowsiness is the most characteristic change. It should be remembered that with an ensuing hypercapnia, a resultant hypoxemia also ensues. It is difficult to determine if the symptoms are a result of hypercapnia or hypoxemia.

   b. If not corrected, initial CNS symptoms may progress to stupor and coma.

3. Laboratory findings (the pH is decreased and the P_{CO_2} is increased)

   a. Acute CO_2 retention leads to an increase in blood P_{CO_2} with a minimal change in plasma bicarbonate content. Serum electrolyte levels are close to normal.

   b. After 2 to 5 days, renal compensation occurs, leading to increased hydrogen ion secretion and bicarbonate production in the distal nephron, after which the plasma bicarbonate level steadily increases.

4. Treatment

   a. The underlying disorder must be identified and corrected.

   b. A blood P_{CO_2} of >60 mm Hg may indicate the need for assisted ventilation if CNS or pulmonary muscular depression is severe.

C. **Respiratory alkalosis**

1. General characteristics

   a. Respiratory alkalosis is defined primarily by decreased blood P_{CO_2} (hypocapnia) and increased blood pH.

   b. Respiratory alkalosis is the result of excessive elimination of CO_2 from increased ventilatory drive. The response of the kidneys is to gradually (hours to days) eliminate plasma bicarbonate.

   c. The causes of respiratory alkalosis include any disorders associated with inappropriately increased ventilatory rate and CO_2 clearance.

   d. Anxiety (psychogenic hyperventilation) is the most common cause of respiratory alkalosis. Other causes include salicylate intoxication, hypoxia, intrathoracic disorders, primary CNS dysfunction, Gram-negative septicemia, liver insufficiency, and pregnancy. Respiratory alkalosis may also result from inappropriate ventilatory settings on a mechanical ventilator.

> 💡 The most common setting of respiratory alkalosis is acute anxiety.

2. Clinical features

   a. Obvious hyperventilation is usually present, particularly when alkalosis is caused by cerebral or metabolic disorders.

   b. The breathing pattern in the anxiety-induced syndrome varies from frequent, deep, sighing respirations to sustained and obvious rapid, deep breathing.

   c. Acute alkalemia may produce a tetany-like syndrome, which may be indistinguishable from acute hypocalcemia. Paresthesia of the extremities, chest discomfort, light-headedness, and confusion may be present.

   d. Circumoral paresthesias, acroparesthesias (painful burning of hands and feet), giddiness, or light-headedness may occur.

3. Laboratory findings (the pH is increased and the P_{CO_2} is decreased)

   a. In acute alkalosis, increased respiratory rate leads to a loss of CO_2 via the lungs, which in turn increases the blood pH.

   b. Within hours after an acute decrease in arterial P_{CO_2}, hydrogen ion secretion in the distal nephron decreases, leading to a decrease in plasma bicarbonate (HCO_3^-). Serum chloride level becomes elevated to maintain electroneutrality.

4. Treatment

  a. The primary goal of therapy is to correct the underlying disorder. Reassurance and light sedation (with benzodiazepines) are effective and avoid the additional anxiety often brought about by rebreathing techniques. Rebreathing techniques, such as breathing into a paper bag, will quickly increase CO_2, although this technique is not recommended because the potential for hypoxemia exists in patients with underlying cardiovascular or respiratory disease.

  b. β-Blockers and selective serotonin reuptake inhibitors (SSRIs) may be beneficial as an adjunct treatment.

  c. Acetazolamide 250 to 500 mg can be used in altitude sickness (hypoxemia and respiratory alkalosis).

  d. Use of CO_2-enriched breathing mixtures or controlled ventilation may be required in cases of severe respiratory alkalosis (pH 7.6).

D. Metabolic acidosis

  1. General characteristics

  a. Metabolic acidosis is a reduction in the normal serum pH that is initiated either by the loss of bicarbonate or by the addition of hydrogen ions to the serum. Respiratory response is immediate with a compensatory increase in respiration.

  b. Several conditions may result in increased hydrogen ions in the serum.

  (1) These include lactic acidosis; diabetic ketoacidosis; starvation ketosis; and ethylene glycol, methanol, and salicylate intoxication. These conditions result in an increased anion gap (AG). This can be remembered with the mnemonic MUDPILES (methanol, uremia, diabetic ketoacidosis, propylene glycol, infection, lactic acidosis, ethylene glycol, and salicylates).

  (2) Hydrogen ions may also be retained in renal tubular acidosis, renal insufficiency, and adrenal insufficiency.

  c. Conditions that may result in the loss of bicarbonate include diarrhea, pancreatic or biliary drainage, and ureteral diversion; these conditions typically have a normal AG.

  2. Clinical features

  a. Hyperventilation is the earliest and most recognized sign, resulting from stimulation of the respiratory drive to blow off CO_2 (pulmonary compensation). Using Winter's formula ($P_{CO_2} = [1.5 \times HCO_3^-] + 8 \pm 2$) allows for the calculation of the expected P_{CO_2} compensation in metabolic acidosis.

  b. Ventricular arrhythmias may occur.

  c. Neurologic symptoms range from lethargy to frank coma.

  3. Laboratory studies (bicarbonate follows the pH in metabolic acid–base disorders; in acidosis, the pH and bicarbonate both decrease)

  a. Complete evaluation of a suspected acid–base disorder should include electrolytes, arterial blood gases, and serum albumin.

  b. Arterial blood gas measurements reveal a pH <7.38, decreased plasma bicarbonate, and decreased P_{CO_2} (owing to compensation).

  c. The AG should be calculated ($Na^+ - [HCO_3^- + Cl^-]$) to separate metabolic acidosis with an elevated AG from metabolic acidosis with a normal AG. The normal AG is 8 ± 4 mEq per L.

  (1) A normal AG acidosis can also be called hyperchloremic metabolic acidosis (chloride increases as bicarbonate decreases to maintain electroneutrality). Normal AG renal tubular acidosis can be divided into cases of the kidney failing

> Metabolic acidosis is the most common acid–base disorder in clinical medicine.

> The most common causes of metabolic acidosis are lactic acidosis, diabetic ketoacidosis, starvation ketosis, and intoxication.

to reabsorb bicarbonate or secrete acid. A mnemonic to remember common causes is USED CARP: ureteroenterostomy, small bowel fistula, endocrinopathies/extra chloride, diarrhea, carbonic anhydrase inhibitors, ammonium chloride, renal tubular acidosis, pancreatic fistula.

(2) When calculating the AG, it must be remembered that the negative charge of albumin can have an impact on the overall AG. If hypoalbuminemia is present, for each 1.0 g per dL decrease in serum albumin, the AG should be increased by 2.5 mEq per L.

(3) Common causes of elevated AG acidosis can be divided into four broad categories: lactic acidosis, ketoacidosis, toxins/drugs, and kidney failure.

> The anion gap may need to be adjusted in patients with hypoalbuminemia.

4. Treatment

a. Identify and, if possible, remove or correct the primary cause of the metabolic acidosis.

b. Insulin therapy and volume repletion are the mainstays of therapy for diabetic ketoacidosis.

c. Bicarbonate therapy can be considered if the pH is <7.20. Blood pH should be carefully monitored because ongoing acid production may increase bicarbonate requirements.

E. Metabolic alkalosis

1. General characteristics

a. Metabolic alkalosis is defined as an increase in serum bicarbonate with no change in Pco_2, causing an increase in extracellular pH to >7.42. Generally, the kidney fails to excrete the excess bicarbonate, thereby maintaining the alkalosis. The following formula allows calculation of expected CO_2 compensation: Expected Pco_2 = $(0.7 \times HCO_3^-) + 20 \pm 2$.

b. Metabolic alkalosis and increased serum bicarbonate can be caused by loss of hydrogen (vomiting), addition of bicarbonate (hyperalimentation therapy), or disproportionate loss of chloride (diarrhea).

c. Etiologies include vomiting, nasogastric tube suctioning, villous adenoma, chloride diarrhea, diuretics, hypercalcemia, milk–alkali syndrome, mineralocorticoid excess, Bartter and Gitelman syndromes, and chloride and potassium depletion secondary to excessive steroids.

2. Clinical features

a. Neurologic abnormalities are common. Symptoms reflecting low ionized calcium may be seen, which include paresthesias, carpopedal spasm, and light-headedness. Symptoms may occasionally progress to confusion, stupor, and coma.

> Metabolic alkalosis presents with neurologic abnormalities including paresthesias, lightheadedness, and carpopedal spams.

b. Symptoms arising from volume depletion are frequently present; weakness, muscle cramps, and postural dizziness may develop.

c. Abnormalities secondary to potassium depletion may lead to polyuria, polydipsia, and muscle weakness.

3. Laboratory studies (the pH is increased and the bicarbonate is also elevated)

a. Arterial blood gas measurements reveal pH >7.42, increased serum bicarbonate, and increased Pco_2 (pulmonary compensation).

b. Urine chloride concentrations can distinguish between hypovolemic hypochloremic patients with a decreased urine chloride concentration (<20 mEq/L) and volume-expanded patients with mineralocorticoid excess who have urine chloride concentrations of >30 mEq per L.

4. Treatment

a. Interventions to increase renal excretion of bicarbonate are the most effective therapy for metabolic alkalosis. Additional consideration should be given to the volume status of the patient as well.

b. Chloride-responsive conditions (e.g., gastric fluid loss, diuretic therapy) are treated with solutions containing sodium chloride to repair the sodium and chloride deficits.

c. Chloride-resistant conditions (e.g., mineralocorticoid excess) can be successfully treated by removing an adrenal adenoma, if present, or by using spironolactone, an aldosterone antagonist.

Urinary Tract Infection

A. Cystitis

  1. General characteristics

  a. Cystitis is an infection of the normal bladder most commonly caused by coliform bacteria (especially *Escherichia coli*, which accounts for 80% to 85% of cases) and occasionally Gram-positive bacteria (enterococci).

  b. The route of infection typically is ascending from the urethra. It is more common in women. UTI occurring in males should prompt further investigation.

  2. Clinical features

  a. Irritative voiding symptoms (frequency, urgency, dysuria) are common, as is suprapubic discomfort.

  b. Gross hematuria may occur. Symptoms in women often appear following sexual intercourse or the use of a diaphragm with spermicide.

  c. Physical examination may elicit suprapubic tenderness, but examination is often unremarkable, especially in elderly patients.

  3. Diagnostic studies

  a. Urinalysis shows pyuria, bacteriuria, and varying degrees of hematuria.

  b. Urine culture is positive ($>10^3$ CFUs/mL) for the offending organism.

  c. Imaging is warranted only if pyelonephritis, recurrent infections, or anatomic abnormalities are suspected.

  4. Treatment

  a. Uncomplicated cystitis in women can be treated with short-term antimicrobial therapy.

    (1) The suggested regimen is trimethoprim–sulfamethoxazole or nitrofurantoin for 3 to 5 days. Fluoroquinolones should be reserved for people with no alternative treatment options.

    (2) Resistant *E. coli* are common, but trimethoprim–sulfamethoxazole can be used as an alternative to a quinolone in susceptible strains.

    (3) Treatment selected should reflect regional prevalence of resistance.

  b. Uncomplicated cystitis is rare in men.

  c. Fluids should be encouraged. Preventive measures include proper hygiene, urine acidification, and voiding after intercourse.

  d. Hot sitz baths or urinary analgesics (phenazopyridine) may provide symptomatic relief. Patients should be warned that phenazopyridine will discolor the urine dark orange or reddish.

> Most UTIs are caused by *E. coli* and can be treated with a short-term antibiotic regimen and increased fluids.

B. Pyelonephritis

  1. General characteristics

  a. Acute pyelonephritis is an infectious inflammatory process involving the kidney parenchyma and renal pelvis. Bacteremia may occur in up to 10% of cases; however, this is more common in patients with diabetes and elderly women.

> The key to distinguishing clinical symptoms of UTI from pyelonephritis is the presence of fever and flank pain.

    b. Gram-negative bacteria are the most common causative agents including *E. coli* (85%), *Proteus* sp., *Klebsiella* sp., *Enterobacter* sp., and *Pseudomonas* sp. The infection usually ascends from the lower urinary tract.

    c. Chronic pyelonephritis is the result of progressive inflammation of the renal interstitium caused by bacterial infection. It occurs in patients with anatomic urinary tract abnormalities such as vesicoureteral reflux.

2. Clinical features

    a. Symptoms include fever, flank pain, shaking chills, and irritative voiding symptoms. Nausea, vomiting, and diarrhea are not uncommon.

    b. Young children may have fever and abdominal discomfort.

    c. Signs include fever and tachycardia. Costovertebral angle tenderness is usually pronounced.

3. Diagnostic studies

    a. CBC shows leukocytosis and left shift.

    b. Urinalysis shows pyuria, bacteriuria, and varying degrees of hematuria. WBC casts may be seen.

    c. Urine culture (which should be obtained before beginning antibiotics) will demonstrate heavy growth of the offending agent.

    d. In complicated pyelonephritis, renal ultrasonography may show hydronephrosis secondary to obstruction.

4. Treatment

    a. In the outpatient setting, treatment with a fluoroquinolone for 7 days is first-line therapy in uncomplicated disease, although trimethoprim–sulfamethoxazole for 14 days has also been shown to be effective in immunocompetent patients if the pathogen is susceptible. Immunocompromised patients should be treated for a longer duration.

    b. Hospital admission is required for patients with severe infections or complicating factors such as older age, comorbid conditions, signs of obstruction, or inability to tolerate oral antibiotics.

> Pyelonephritis requires antibiotic therapy for 7 to 14 days.

    c. IV fluoroquinolones, third- and fourth-generation cephalosporins, extended-spectrum penicillins, or gentamycin should be initiated while waiting for sensitivity results. IV antibiotics should be continued for 24 to 48 hours after the patient becomes afebrile; oral antibiotics are then given to complete a minimum of 2 weeks of therapy.

    d. Failure to respond warrants ultrasound imaging to exclude complicating factors such as nephrolithiasis or possible abscess formation that may require prompt intervention.

    e. Follow-up urine cultures are not mandatory following treatment in uncomplicated cases.

C. Prostatitis

1. General characteristics

    a. Acute bacterial prostatitis is caused by ascending infection of Gram-negative rods into the prostatic ducts.

    b. Chronic bacterial prostatitis may be associated with evolution or recurrence of an acute bacterial infection. Its route of infection is the same as for acute prostatitis. The same Gram-negative organisms are most commonly responsible. *Enterococcus* may be identified less often.

    c. Chronic nonbacterial prostatitis is the most common of the prostatitis syndromes, and its cause is unknown. It may represent a noninfectious inflammatory disorder, perhaps with an autoimmune origin, and is a diagnosis of exclusion. It is often associated with the term *chronic pelvic pain syndrome*.

    d. Prostatic abscess is an uncommon complication of acute bacterial prostatitis.

2. Clinical features

    a. Acute infection is characterized by sudden onset of high fever, chills, malaise, myalgias, and low back and perineal pain.

    b. Chronic infection has more variable symptoms, ranging from asymptomatic to acute symptomatology.

    c. All forms of prostatitis present with irritative bladder symptoms (frequency, urgency, dysuria) and some obstruction.

    d. The prostate is swollen and tender.

3. Diagnostic studies

    a. Urinalysis reveals pyuria. Hematuria and bacteriuria may also be found.

    b. Prostatic fluid will reveal leukocytosis; culture is typically positive for *E. coli* in acute infections. Other pathogens include *Proteus,* other Enterobacteriaceae species or *Pseudomonas.* Chronic infection is characterized by recurrence of the same organism or *Enterococcus.* In nonbacterial prostatitis, cultures are negative.

4. Treatment

    a. Antibiotics are the most effective treatment for bacterial infections. Hospitalization may be indicated in acute prostatitis. Treatment with parenteral antibiotics (fluoroquinolones or gentamicin and ampicillin) may be needed until culture results are available and the patient is afebrile for 24 to 48 hours.

        (1) Uncomplicated cases: ciprofloxacin 500 mg twice a day or levofloxacin 500 mg once a day for 2 to 6 weeks or trimethoprim–sulfamethoxazole 160 mg per 800 mg twice a day for 6 weeks. Culture urine 1 week after conclusion of therapy.

        (2) If fever is not resolved after 36 hours, suspect a prostatic abscess and consult a urologist for management.

        (3) In chronic prostatitis, a fluoroquinolone for 4 to 6 weeks is more effective than trimethoprim–sulfamethoxazole for 6 weeks to 3 months.

        (4) Antibiotics are not effective in nonbacterial prostatitis.

    b. NSAIDs are effective analgesics. α_1-Blockers may be helpful if lower urinary tract symptoms (LUTS) are present.

    c. Chronic, recurrent, or resistant prostatitis with or without prostatic calculi may require transurethral resection of the prostate (TURP) for ultimate resolution.

D. Orchitis

1. General characteristics

    a. Orchitis is commonly caused by ascending bacterial infection from the urinary tract.

    b. The most common cause of viral orchitis is mumps; orchitis occurs in 25% of postpubertal males who have mumps infection.

2. Clinical features

    a. Testicular swelling and tenderness, usually unilateral, occur.

    b. Fever and tachycardia are common.

3. Diagnostic studies

    a. Urinalysis reveals pyuria and bacteriuria with a bacterial infection.

    b. Cultures are positive for suspected organisms.

    c. Ultrasonography is useful if an abscess or tumor is suspected and to rule out testicular torsion. Carefully evaluate any scrotal masses.

> Vigorous prostate examination should be avoided in suspected acute prostatitis as it may cause septicemia.

> Orchitis is typically unilateral and presents with swelling and tenderness of the testicle; mumps virus is the most common cause.

> The cause of epididymitis changes with age owing to likely exposure. In men younger than 35 years, primary etiologies include *Chlamydia* and gonococcus; for those older than 35 years, *E. coli* is the predominant pathogen.

4. Treatment

a. If mumps is the cause, symptomatic relief with ice and analgesia should be provided.

b. If bacteria are the cause, the orchitis should be treated like epididymitis.

E. Epididymitis

1. General characteristics

a. Epididymitis is an infection of the epididymis acquired by retrograde spread of organisms through the vas deferens.

b. In men younger than 35 years, *Chlamydia* and gonococci are the most common organisms.

c. In men older than 35 years, *E. coli* is the most common organism.

2. Clinical features

a. Epididymitis presents with heaviness and dull, aching discomfort in the affected hemiscrotum, which can radiate up the ipsilateral flank. History of the patient may reveal heavy lifting, trauma, or sexual activity.

b. The epididymis is markedly swollen and exquisitely tender to touch, eventually becoming a warm, erythematous, enlarged scrotal mass. As the disease progresses, it may become difficult to distinguish the testes from the epididymis.

c. The patient may have fever and chills.

d. The Prehn sign (relief of pain with scrotal elevation) is a classic sign, but it is not very reliable.

3. Diagnostic studies

a. Urinalysis reveals pyuria and bacteriuria.

b. Cultures show positive results for suspected organisms.

> A test for cure after treatment of epididymitis is only recommended in patients younger than 35 years of age.

4. Treatment

a. In men younger than 35 years, ceftriaxone 250 mg IM in one dose, plus doxycycline 100 mg twice per day orally for 10 days or azithromycin 1 g orally in one dose, may be administered for gonococci or *Chlamydia*. A test for cure should be done 1 week after conclusion of therapy.

b. In men older than 35 years, ciprofloxacin 500 mg twice per day orally for 10 to 14 days may be used. Test for cure is not required.

c. Basis for treatment should be based on sexually transmitted infections (STI) risk (history, sexual practices, etc.) as well as age.

d. Supportive care may include bed rest, scrotal elevation, and analgesics.

Benign Prostatic Hyperplasia (BPH)

A. General characteristics

1. Proliferation of the fibrostromal tissue of the prostate can lead to compression of the prostatic urethra, creating an obstruction of the urinary outlet leading to LUTS.

2. BPH is a disease of older men. The mean age of onset is 60 to 65 years; however, LUTS can start as early as age 45 years.

B. Clinical features

1. The symptom complex is referred to as prostatism, which includes symptoms of obstruction and irritation. The American Urological Association (AUA) symptom index is beneficial to assess symptom severity prior to and throughout any treatment regimen (Table 6-12).

Table 6-12 | American Urological Association BPH Scoring Index

Over About the Past Month	Score					
	Never	**<1 in 5 Times**	**<50% of the Time**	**About 50% of the Time**	**>50% of the Time**	**Almost Always**
How often have you had a sensation of not emptying your bladder completely after you finish urinating?	0	1	2	3	4	5
How often have you had to urinate again <2 hours after you finished urinating?	0	1	2	3	4	5
How often have you stopped and started again several times when urinating?	0	1	2	3	4	5
How often have you found it difficult to postpone urination?	0	1	2	3	4	5
How often has your urinary stream been weak?	0	1	2	3	4	5
How often have you had to push or strain to begin urination?	0	1	2	3	4	5
How many times did you most typically get up to urinate between going to bed at night and waking in the morning?	None = 0	Once = 1	Twice = 2	3 times = 3	4 times = 4	≥5 times = 5
American Urological Association symptom score = total _____						

0 to 7 points: Symptoms are considered mild.

8 to 19 points: Symptoms are considered moderate.

20 to 35 points: Symptoms are considered severe.

Reprinted with permission from Barry MJ, Fowler FJ Jr, O'Leary MP, et al. The American Urological Association symptom index for benign prostatic hyperplasia. *J Urol.* 1992;148(5):1549–1557.

2. Obstructive symptoms include decreased force of urinary stream, hesitancy and straining, postvoid dribbling, and sensation of incomplete emptying.

3. Irritative symptoms include frequency, nocturia, and urgency.

4. Recurrent UTIs and urinary retention can also occur.

5. Digital rectal examination typically reveals an enlarged prostate.

C. Diagnostic studies

1. Prostate-specific antigen (PSA) is typically slightly elevated.

2. Other tests are done to evaluate for renal damage, infection, and prostate or bladder cancer, as indicated.

D. Treatment

1. Men with mild to moderate symptoms may choose watchful waiting and frequent monitoring.

2. Options for medical therapy include α-adrenergic antagonists (e.g., prazosin), 5α-reductase inhibitors (finasteride, dutasteride), and phosphodiesterase-5 (PDE-5) inhibitors (tadalafil, vardenafil), which may improve prostate symptom scores for LUTS caused by BPH. Anticholinergic agents may be appropriate and effective treatment alternatives for the management of LUTS secondary to BPH in men without an elevated postvoid residual and when LUTS are predominantly irritative. Tamsulosin plus tolterodine extended-release reduces symptoms in men with LUTS and overactive bladder. Intramuscular cetrorelix (60 mg, then 30 mg at 2 weeks) improves International Prostate Symptom Score in men with symptomatic BPH.

> First-line agents in BPH include alpha-adrenergic antagonists, 5-alpha reductase inhibitors, and phosphodiesterase-5 inhibitors.

3. Behavioral strategies include limiting fluids prior to bedtime.

4. Procedures that may be used to relieve obstruction include the use of balloon dilation, microwave irradiation, and stent placements.

5. Surgical treatment is transurethral resection of the prostate or transurethral incision of the prostate.

Incontinence

A. General characteristics

1. Urinary incontinence is defined as the unintentional leakage of urine at inappropriate times.

2. Women experience incontinence twice as often as men. Older women experience it more often than younger women.

3. Incontinence can be classified based on the underlying pathophysiologic mechanism.

   a. Urge incontinence results from bladder contractions that cannot be controlled by the brain.

   b. Stress incontinence is caused by dysfunction of the urethral sphincter, allowing urine to leak with increased intra-abdominal pressure.

   c. Overflow incontinence occurs when urinary retention leads to bladder distention and overflow of urine through the urethra.

   d. Functional incontinence is untimely urination caused by physical or cognitive disability, preventing a person from reaching a toilet.

   e. Mixed incontinence is a combination of elements of both stress and urge incontinence.

> Types of incontinence:
> Urge: strong desire followed by loss of urine
> Overactive: frequency, urgency, nocturia; with or without urge
> Stress: leakage with abdominal pressure
> Overflow: incomplete emptying

B. **Clinical features**

1. Reversible causes of incontinence, such as medication side effects, recent prostatectomy, excess fluid intake, atrophic vaginitis, fecal impaction, UTI, impaired mobility, and glycosuria, should be identified.

2. The principal symptom of urge incontinence is a strong desire to void, followed by loss of urine.

3. Overactive bladder disorder is a related symptom complex characterized by frequency of urination, urgency to urinate, and nocturia. Patients may present with or without urge incontinence.

4. The principal symptom of stress incontinence is leakage of urine with increased intra-abdominal pressure, such as with sneezing, coughing, or laughing.

5. Untreated overflow incontinence can lead to hydronephrosis and obstructive nephropathy secondary to bladder distention.

6. Incontinence is common with neurologic diseases (stroke, Parkinson's disease, or dementia), metabolic disorders (hypoxemia, diabetic neuropathy), and pelvic disorders (uterine prolapse).

C. Diagnostic studies

1. Urinalysis can identify diabetes-related glycosuria or acute UTI.

2. Postvoid residual urine volume should be measured to identify urinary retention.

3. Simple urodynamic studies such as cystometry (instillation of water into the bladder) can identify bladder contractions and should be considered.

4. Stress test, ultrasonography, cystoscopy, and cystographic studies may also be used to determine anatomic abnormalities.

> To be effective, Kegel exercises should be done in sets of 10 to 15 multiple times throughout the day.

D. **Treatment**

1. Pelvic floor muscle training (Kegel exercises), electrical muscle stimulation, biofeedback, and bladder training can be used to improve the strength and control of the pelvic muscles. Pessaries or implants can help decrease stress incontinence.

2. Anticholinergic medications, such as oxybutynin or tolterodine, are effective for urge incontinence. Vaginal estrogen can be used for stress incontinence. Oral estrogen may worsen urinary incontinence.

3. Tolterodine and oxybutynin can be used for overactive bladder.

4. Catheterization, either intermittent or indwelling, can be used for overflow incontinence.

5. Although surgical treatments are often the last resort, they are very effective for stress incontinence.

Neoplasms of the Urinary Tract

A. Prostate cancer

1. General characteristics

a. Prostate cancer is a common, generally slow-growing, malignant neoplasm of the adenomatous cells (>95% adenocarcinoma, <5% other types) of the prostate gland that can lead to urinary obstruction and metastatic disease.

b. The majority of prostate cancers (75%) originate in the peripheral zone (outer portion of the prostate palpable on rectal examination), followed by the transitional zone (20%) (portion of prostate surrounding the majority of the urethra [BPH symptomatology]), and lastly the central zone (5%) (portion of prostatic urethra with ejaculatory ducts).

c. A disease of aging, it is rarely seen in men younger than 40 years.

d. Risk factors may include genetic predisposition, hormonal influences, dietary and environmental factors, and infectious agents.

> Most prostate cancers are adenomas and arise in the peripheral zone

2. **Clinical features**

a. Many cases are not clinically apparent.

b. Symptoms of urinary obstruction or irritative voiding symptomatology may occur if the tumor has invaded into the urethra, bladder neck, or trigone of the bladder.

c. In advanced disease, patients may present with bone pain from metastases, possible spinal cord impingement if the vertebral bodies are involved.

d. The prostate may be enlarged, nodular, and asymmetric.

3. Diagnostic studies

a. PSA is usually elevated in patients with prostate cancer.

b. Screening, if indicated, should start at age 50. If at high risk for development of prostate cancer (African American men, family history of prostate cancer, known to have the *BRCA-1* or *BRCA-2* gene mutation), screen should start between 40 and 45 years of age. Discussion of the risk/benefit of screening is important.

c. Pathologic examination of tissue removed for treatment of obstructive prostatic hyperplasia reveals that 10% have malignancy.

d. Transrectal ultrasonography reveals hypoechoic lesions in the prostate (peripheral zone).

e. Biopsy confirms the diagnosis of adenocarcinoma and allows histologic grading which can provide prognostic information. The Gleason grading system, based on architectural pattern, adds together the primary and secondary grades of the tumor, resulting in a final score of 2 to 10. The total score can be used for prognostic purposes, with a higher score indicating a worse prognosis than a lower score.

> The U.S. Preventive Services Task Force assigned a grade of "C" for PSA screening in the general population; C indicates a recommendation to offer the test based on individual patient circumstances.

4. **Treatment**

a. Appropriate treatment depends on the staging, which is done by abdominal and pelvic CT or magnetic resonance imaging (MRI), pelvic lymphadenectomy, and bone scan.

b. Low-grade tumors that are well differentiated may not require any treatment, whereas higher grade tumors more typically are aggressive and, therefore, should be managed more aggressively. Active surveillance occurs with all stages.

c. Stages I and II disease (tumor confined to the prostate) may be treated with radical retropubic prostatectomy, brachytherapy, or external beam radiation therapy.

d. Stage III disease (tumor with local invasion) is treated similar to stages A and B disease but with reduced effectiveness.

e. Stage IV disease (distant metastases) is treated with hormonal manipulation using orchiectomy, antiandrogens, luteinizing hormone–releasing hormone agonists, or estrogens. Chemotherapy has limited usefulness, and palliative treatment is given for advanced disease. Surgery (TURP) may relieve symptoms of bleeding and urinary obstruction.

B. Bladder cancer

1. General characteristics

> Bladder cancer presents most commonly as painless hematuria.

a. Causal factors for bladder cancer include exposure to tobacco; occupational carcinogens from rubber, dye, printing, and chemical industries; schistosomiasis; exposure to cyclophosphamide; and chronic infections.

b. Uroepithelial tumors account for 3% of cancer deaths in the United States. Bladder carcinoma is three times more common in men than in women, and it usually occurs in patients 40 to 70 years of age.

c. Most (98%) are transitional cell carcinomas (TCCs).

2. Clinical features

a. Painless hematuria is the most common presenting symptom.

b. Bladder irritability, pain, voiding symptoms, and infection may also occur.

3. Diagnostic studies

a. CBC and blood chemistry should be done to evaluate for infection and renal function.

b. Cystoscopy with biopsy, which has an accuracy rate of nearly 100%, is the definitive diagnostic procedure. Biopsy confirms the histopathologic diagnosis.

c. Radiologic procedures include IV urography, pelvic and abdominal CT, chest radiography, bone scan, and retrograde pyelography for renal pelvic or ureteral tumors and staging.

4. Treatment

a. Treatment depends on the stage.

b. Superficial lesions are treated with endoscopic resection and fulguration, followed by cystoscopy every 3 months. Recurrent or multiple lesions can be treated with intravesical instillation of thiotepa, mitomycin C, or bacillus Calmette–Guérin (BCG).

c. Radical cystectomy is used for recurrent cancer, diffuse TCC in situ, and tumors that have invaded the muscle.

d. Combination chemotherapy has been used in bladder-sparing trials with or without radiation therapy. External beam irradiation therapy is typically reserved for those individuals who are not surgical candidates because of significant comorbid medical conditions.

C. Renal cell carcinoma

1. General characteristics

> The incidence of renal cell carcinoma is highest in Native American and Alaskan Native men.

a. RCC, also known as hypernephroma or renal adenocarcinoma, is the most common type of renal malignancy. It accounts for 3% of all adult cancers.

b. RCC is more common in men, usually affecting those older than 55 years. Incidence is higher in Native American/Alaskan Native men than in men of all other races.

c. The cause is unknown, but cigarette smoking is consistently linked to RCC.

d. There are forms of hereditary RCC, including von Hippel–Lindau disease and hereditary papillary renal carcinoma.

2. Clinical features

a. RCC is associated with a wide range of presenting signs and symptoms and is often called the "internists' tumor" because it is commonly discovered as an incidental finding on abdominal imaging.

b. The most common symptom is gross or microscopic hematuria, followed by pain or an abdominal mass. The classic triad of gross hematuria, flank pain, and a palpable mass, however, occurs only in a small percentage of patients.

c. RCC is associated with paraneoplastic syndromes, including erythrocytosis, hypercalcemia, hypertension, and hepatic dysfunction in the absence of hepatic metastases.

3. Diagnostic studies

a. Patients presenting with hematuria should undergo ultrasonography to rule out a stone.

b. CT scanning with and without contrast is the primary technique for diagnosing RCC. Other confirming studies can include MRI with contrast and arteriography.

4. Treatment

a. Treatment depends on the histology (Fuhrman grades 1, 2, 3, 4) and stage (TNM) of the tumor; therefore, a thorough evaluation is required.

b. Radical nephrectomy is the primary treatment for localized disease (stage T1 to T3a lesions). Neoadjuvant or adjuvant radiation therapy has not been shown to prolong survival for early-stage lesions.

c. Radiation therapy is an important method of palliation in patients with disseminated disease to the brain, bone, and lungs. Radical nephrectomy has little role in advanced disease.

d. Hormonal therapy and chemotherapy have shown little effect.

e. Medications, such as interferon-α and interleukin, have been successful in reducing the growth of some RCCs, including some with metastasis.

D. Wilms' tumor

1. General characteristics

a. Wilms' tumor, also known as nephroblastoma, is the most common solid renal tumor of childhood.

b. Most occur in healthy children; however, about 10% occur in children with recognized malformations.

c. Most cases of Wilms' tumor are curable, but in histologic study, about 5% of patients have anaplasia, which is associated with a poorer prognosis. The incidence of anaplasia increases with age.

2. Clinical features

a. The most common sign is an asymptomatic abdominal mass found by a caretaker or during physical examination.

b. Symptoms at presentation might include anorexia, nausea and vomiting, fever, abdominal pain, or hematuria.

c. Hypertension caused by elevated renin levels can occur.

3. Diagnostic studies

a. Urinalysis may show hematuria; anemia may be present.

b. Ultrasonography is the initial study of choice to evaluate abdominal masses.

c. Abdominal CT is performed in patients with suspected Wilms' tumor to assess tumor extension and regional lymph nodes. MRI also can provide information regarding tumor extension.

d. Chest radiography is used to evaluate the presence of metastases in the lungs.

> Wilms' tumor most often presents as an asymptomatic abdominal mass found by the child's caregiver.

4. Treatment

  a. The goal of therapy is to provide the highest possible cure rate with the lowest treatment-related morbidity.

  b. The most effective therapy is a multimodal approach that incorporates surgery, chemotherapy, and, in some patients, radiation therapy.

  c. Radical nephrectomy with lymph node sampling is the treatment of choice in surgically resectable tumors. Unresectable tumors should undergo preoperative biopsy followed by chemotherapy.

  d. Wilms' tumor is chemosensitive and responsive to dactinomycin, vincristine, and doxorubicin.

  e. Radiation therapy is added for higher stage tumors (stages III and IV) and for tumors with focal anaplasia.

E. <u>Testicular cancer</u>

  1. General characteristics

  a. Testicular cancer is the most common malignancy in young men (ages 15 to 35).

  b. Risk factors include history of cryptorchidism or a previous history of testicular cancer.

  2. Clinical features

  a. More than 90% of patients present with a painless, solid testicular swelling. Patients may also complain of heaviness in the testicle. Occasionally, patients with painful testicular masses are erroneously diagnosed as having epididymitis or orchitis.

  b. Para-aortic lymph node involvement can present as ureteral obstruction.

  c. Patients may also present with abdominal complaints from an abdominal mass or with pulmonary symptoms from multiple nodules.

  3. Diagnostic studies

  a. Scrotal ultrasonography may reveal a suspicious intratesticular echogenic focus.

  b. Radiologic studies for staging include radiography of the chest and CT of the chest, abdomen, and pelvis. CT scan of the chest remains controversial, as pulmonary metastasis is often detected by chest x-ray (CXR).

  c. Tumors are classified pathologically as seminomatous (35%) or nonseminomatous (65%). Subtypes of nonseminomatous include embryonal carcinoma (20%), teratoma (5%), mixed cell type (40%), and choriocarcinoma (<1%).

  d. Elevated blood levels of α-fetoprotein or β-human chorionic gonadotropin are diagnostic for nonseminomatous germ cell tumors; the majority of patients with seminoma have normal levels.

  4. Treatment

  a. Treatment depends on pathology and stage. Staging is based on the TNM system, degree of lymph node spread, and serum tumor markers.

  (1) Orchiectomy is performed for diagnostic and therapeutic reasons.

  (2) Seminomatous tumors are radiosensitive; nonseminomatous tumors are radioresistant.

  b. Nonseminomatous tumors

  (1) Stage I disease limited to the testis can be treated with nerve-sparing retroperitoneal lymph node dissection or rigorous surveillance without surgery or chemotherapy.

  (2) Stage II tumors can be treated with surgery or chemotherapy.

  (3) Stage III disease should be treated with surgery and chemotherapy.

Testicular cancer is rare after the age of 35 years.

Testicular cancers are either seminomatous (radiosensitive) or nonseminomatous (radioresistant).

c. Seminomatous tumors

(1) The mainstay of therapy for stage I disease isolated to the testis is radiation therapy to the para-aortic and ipsilateral iliac nodal areas.

(2) Therapy for stages IIa and IIb adds increased radiation to the affected nodes.

(3) Therapy for stages IIc and III is chemotherapy.

Male Reproductive Disorders

A. Phimosis

1. General characteristics

a. Phimosis is characterized by the inability to retract the foreskin over the glans penis.

b. It may be congenital or acquired.

(1) Congenital phimosis is identified in children and adolescents and is usually physiologic.

(2) Acquired phimosis is more typical in adults and is usually caused by poor hygiene and chronic balanitis. Consider evaluation for possible diabetes in men with chronic infections.

2. Clinical features

a. Erythema with tenderness and possible purulent drainage around the glans/foreskin

b. Inability to retract the foreskin over the glans penis

c. Obstructed urinary stream, hematuria, or pain of the prepuce can indicate more severe constriction.

3. Diagnostic studies: none usually required

4. Treatment

a. As long as it is asymptomatic, a congenital phimosis should be left alone, as the preputial opening will gradually widen as the child gets older.

b. If symptomatic, referral for circumcision is usually necessary.

c. Broad-spectrum antibiotics are indicated if infection is present. Steroidal creams or nonsteroidal ointments may be of benefit.

> Phimosis: inability to retract.
> Paraphimosis: inability to reduce

B. Paraphimosis

1. General characteristics

a. Paraphimosis is defined as entrapment of (inability to reduce) the foreskin behind the glans penis.

b. Frequent catheterizations without reducing the foreskin can lead to paraphimosis.

c. Forcibly retracting a constricted foreskin (phimosis) for cleaning or catheterization can lead to paraphimosis.

d. Vigorous sexual activity can predispose men to paraphimosis.

2. Clinical features

a. Pain, edema, tenderness, and erythema of the glans and foreskin are present.

b. Identification of any encircling foreign bodies, such as hair, clothing, rubber bands, or metallic objects, is important.

3. Diagnostic studies: none required

4. Treatment

    a. Paraphimosis should be reduced emergently.

        (1) Manual reduction should be tried initially. Firmly squeeze the glans for 5 minutes to reduce the tissue edema and decrease the size of the glans and then try to bring the foreskin back over the glans.

        (2) Surgical techniques (dorsal slit) to incise the restricted foreskin can be used if manual reduction fails.

    b. Inability to reduce paraphimosis requires emergent urologic referral.

    c. After reduction, referral for circumcision is necessary because the condition is likely to recur.

C. Erectile dysfunction (ED)

    1. General characteristics

        a. ED is defined as the consistent inability to maintain an erect penis with sufficient rigidity to allow sexual intercourse. It is part of a broader classification of sexual dysfunctions.

        b. Normal erections require intact parasympathetic and somatic nerve supply, unobstructed arterial inflow, adequate venous constriction, hormonal stimulation, and psychological desire. Disorders of any of these systems may result in impotence.

        c. Most cases of ED have a primary organic rather than a psychogenic cause. Nearly all cases have a secondary psychogenic component.

        d. ED affects millions of American men, and its incidence is age related.

        e. Major predictors of ED include hypertension, diabetes mellitus, hyperlipidemia, and cardiovascular disease.

> The prevalent chronic diseases of our time contribute to risk of erectile dysfunction: hypertension, diabetes mellitus, and hyperlipidemia.

    2. Clinical features

        a. The medical history must be adequately evaluated. Medications such as some antihypertensives (e.g., β-blockers) may be the cause of ED; switching to another antihypertensive agent may resolve the problem. SSRI medications can also cause ED.

        b. A sexual history should be taken, including detailed information on timing and frequency of sexual relations, partners, presence of morning erections, ejaculation, and the ability to masturbate. The International Index of Erectile Function (IIEF) is a validated questionnaire useful to determine baseline erectile function.

        c. Past medical history should document presence of hypertension, diabetes, vascular disease, endocrine disease, medications, pelvic surgery, or trauma.

        d. Physical examination should look for penile deformities (e.g., Peyronie's disease [fibrous plaque causing penile curvature]), testicular atrophy, hypertension, peripheral neuropathy, and other signs of endocrine, vascular, or neurologic abnormalities.

    3. Diagnostic studies

        a. CBC, urinalysis, lipid profile, thyroid function tests, serum testosterone, glucose, and prolactin screening should be done, depending on the suspected cause.

        b. Measurement of follicle-stimulating hormone and luteinizing hormone may be required for patients with abnormalities of testosterone or prolactin.

        c. Nocturnal penile tumescence testing will differentiate organic from psychogenic impotence. Patients with psychogenic impotence have normal nocturnal erections of adequate frequency and rigidity.

        d. Direct injection of vasoactive substances into the penis induces erections in men with intact vascular systems.

> Normal nocturnal tumescence testing supports a psychogenic cause of erectile dysfunction.

e. Patients who do not achieve erections with injections may undergo studies to evaluate the arterial and venous vasculature, such as ultrasonography of the cavernous arteries, pelvic arteriography, and cavernosonography.

4. Treatment

a. True psychogenic causes can be treated with behaviorally oriented sex therapy. Patients with organic causes of impotence may also benefit from counseling.

b. Hypogonadism may benefit from testosterone replacement therapy, but the evidence is limited.

c. Weight loss for body mass index (BMI) >30 kg per m² may help with ED. Control of underlying conditions is important.

d. PDE-5 inhibitor therapy is considered the mainstay of treatment for ED. Sildenafil, vardenafil, and tadalafil are the drugs currently indicated for ED. Side effects of PDE-5 therapy can include headache, flushing, dyspepsia, rhinitis, and visual disturbances and possible priapism. PDE-5 should be avoided in patients taking nitrates, as the combination may cause a significant drop in BP.

> Avoid PDE-5 inhibitors in patients taking nitrates; the combination can cause a severe drop in blood pressure.

e. For men in whom PDE-5 therapy is ineffective or inappropriate, there are other treatments, including use of vacuum constriction devices, injected or inserted vasoactive substances, and penile prostheses. Patients with disorders of the arterial system are candidates for arterial reconstruction.

D. Scrotal masses

1. Hydrocele

a. General characteristics: A hydrocele is a mass of the fluid-filled congenital remnants of the tunica vaginalis, usually resulting from a patent processus vaginalis.

b. Clinical features

(1) Hydrocele presents as a soft, nontender fullness of the hemiscrotum that transilluminates.

(2) The mass may wax and wane in size; an indirect hernia may be concurrently present.

> A hydrocele develops in the tunica vaginalis of the scrotum.

c. Diagnostic studies: Few studies are warranted for hydrocele.

(1) Urinalysis with microscopic analysis is negative.

(2) Ultrasonography is rarely indicated but can distinguish between hydrocele, spermatocele, and testicular tumors.

d. Treatment: elective repair as clinically indicated

2. Spermatocele

a. General characteristics

(1) A spermatocele is typically a painless cystic mass containing sperm.

(2) Most spermatoceles are <1 cm in size.

(3) They lie superior and posterior and are distinct from the testes.

(4) Some may simulate a solid tumor.

b. Clinical features: palpable, round, firm cystic mass with distinct borders, free floating above the testicle, which transilluminates. The mass may be tender.

c. Diagnostic studies

(1) Needle aspiration should not be performed.

(2) Scrotal ultrasonography provides a very accurate diagnosis.

> Spermatoceles develop in the epididymis; it can be palpated distinct from the testis, situated above.

d. Treatment

(1) No medical treatment is required.

(2) Large spermatoceles can be surgically removed or sclerosed.

E. Testicular torsion

1. General characteristics

   a. The testis becomes abnormally twisted on its spermatic cord, thus compromising arterial supply and venous drainage of the testis, leading to testicular ischemia.

   b. This condition is most common in prepubertal and postpubertal young males (12 to 18 years of age), especially with a history of cryptorchidism (late descent of the testes).

   c. Risk factors include age, previous history of torsion, family history of torsion. It may occur spontaneously or after vigorous activity, minor injury to the testis, cold temperatures, or prolonged sleeping.

2. **Clinical features**

   a. Sudden onset of severe unilateral pain and scrotal swelling are present.

   b. Testis is painful to palpation; testicle and scrotum are edematous. There is no relief with elevation of the testicle (negative Prehn sign).

3. Diagnostic studies

   a. Testicular torsion is a clinical diagnosis.

   b. If the diagnosis is equivocal, do not wait for laboratory studies.

   c. Doppler ultrasonography demonstrates decreased blood flow to the affected spermatic cord and testis.

   d. Radioisotope scan demonstrates decreased uptake in the affected testes.

4. **Treatment**

   a. Mild analgesics may be administered once the diagnosis is made.

   b. This is a surgical emergency. Manual detorsion (twisting the testes outward and laterally) may be attempted by experienced clinicians, but whether this is successful or not, surgery will be required. If the affected testicle is corrected within a 6-hour time frame, there is a greater chance of salvaging the testicle. Surgical detorsion with orchiopexy is the definitive therapy.

   c. Emergent surgical intervention on the affected testis must be followed by elective surgery (orchiopexy) on the contralateral testis, which is also at risk of torsion.

F. Varicocele

1. General characteristics

   a. Varicocele is the formation of a venous varicosity within the spermatic vein (pampiniform plexus).

   b. The left spermatic vein has an increased incidence of varicosity because the vein is longer than the right and joins the left renal vein at right angles.

2. **Clinical features**

   a. A chronic, nontender mass that does not transilluminate is seen, usually on the left side.

   b. The lesion has the consistency of a "bag of worms," increases in size with Valsalva, and decreases in size with elevation of the scrotum or supine position.

3. Diagnostic studies

   a. No laboratory studies are required.

   b. If the diagnosis is inconclusive, Doppler sonography is the diagnostic method of choice.

4. **Treatment:** Surgical repair (left spermatic vein ligation) can be performed if the varicocele is painful or if it appears to be a cause of infertility.

> Sudden, severe, unilateral testicular pain signals testicular torsion; it is a surgical emergency.

> Varicocele is varicosity of the spermatic vein, presenting as "bag of worms."

Practice Questions

Directions: Each of the numbered items or incomplete statements in this section is followed by a list of answers or completions of the statement. Select the ONE lettered answer or completion that is BEST in each case.

1. According to the RIFLE classification, risk of kidney failure begins with a reduction of the patient's GFR by greater than what percentage?
   A. 10%
   B. 25%
   C. 50%
   D. 60%

2. A 41-year-old male involved in a motor vehicle accident and sustained a fractured pelvis and a ruptured spleen. He underwent surgery and was admitted to the intensive care unit (ICU). He required 4 units of blood. The next day, his UO dropped to 10 cc per hour; plasma expanders did not improve output. Laboratory findings reveal an elevation in urinary sodium excretion; BUN, 70 mg per dL; and serum creatinine, 5.9 mg per dL. Urinalysis reveals granular casts. What is the most likely cause?
   A. ATN
   B. Bladder outlet obstruction
   C. Cirrhosis
   D. Hypovolemia
   E. Renal artery stenosis

3. A 10-year-old boy is brought to the clinic for evaluation of dark urine. The urine is in the color of cola; urinalysis reveals hematuria, acanthocytes, and RBC casts. His face and eyes are puffy. What is likely in this child's history?
   A. Abdominal trauma
   B. Antibiotic exposure
   C. Congenital bladder defect
   D. Diarrheal disease
   E. Streptococcal infection

4. A 44-year-old female complains of swelling of her face, eyes, and hands. Urinalysis shows moderate proteinuria and mild glycosuria. Microscopic findings include RBC casts, granular casts, and oval fat bodies. What is the initial treatment?
   A. ACE inhibitor
   B. Kayexalate
   C. Cyclophosphamide
   D. High-protein diet
   E. Sodium replacement

5. A 65-year-old male presents to the emergency department with penile pain. He is uncircumcised, and the foreskin is trapped behind the glans. The area is red, swollen, and very tender. After manual compression for 5 minutes, the foreskin was released. What is most likely in this patient's history?
   A. Benign prostatic hypertrophy
   B. Chronic balanitis
   C. Diabetes mellitus type 2
   D. Frequent catheterization
   E. Multiple sex partners

6. A 12-year-old male presents with swelling and tenderness of the left testicle. Two weeks ago, he had a fever, loss of appetite, and tenderness and swelling under his ears, which resolved within 3 days. What is the recommended management?
   A. Antibiotics to cover Gram-negative bacilli
   B. Fine needle aspirate of scrotal fluid
   C. Ice and analgesia
   D. Order a testicular ultrasound to rule out a mass
   E. Refer to urology for further workup

7. A 26-year-old male presents with fever and dull, achy pain in his scrotum, which radiates to the left flank. The epididymis is swollen and very tender. Urine dip reveals pyuria and bacteriuria. What is likely in this patient's history?
   A. High-sugar diet
   B. Kicked in groin yesterday
   C. New sex partner
   D. Recent diagnosis of diabetes
   E. Uncircumcised penis

8. A 54-year-old G5P5005 female describes sudden urges to urinate; often she cannot get to the bathroom quick enough and experiences incontinence. She denies fever, pain, hematuria, or pyuria. Urinalysis is normal. Postvoid analysis reveals minimal residual urine. What is the best management at this time?
   A. Encourage frequent toileting to avoid a full bladder
   B. Order urodynamic studies to assess bladder wall contractions
   C. Perform bedside ultrasonography to rule out mass or foreign body
   D. Prescribe oxybutynin and reassess in 1 month
   E. Recommend vaginal estrogen cream daily

9. A 60-year-old male presents with painless hematuria. He has smoked one pack per day for over 40 years. He takes metformin for diabetes and an ACE inhibitor for hypertension. Cystoscopy and biopsy reveal a TCC. What was this man's likely occupation?
   A. Car engine repair
   B. Coal mining
   C. Glass blowing
   D. Quarry work
   E. Rubber industry

10. A 58-year-old male underwent an abdominal CT after successful treatment of diverticulitis. A heterogeneous renal mass measuring 2 cm × 2 cm was found incidentally. Further workup confirms a Fuhrman grade 2 RCC confined to the kidney. What is the recommended treatment?
    A. Androgen ablation therapy
    B. Combination chemotherapy
    C. Radiation followed by resection
    D. Radical nephrectomy
    E. Surgical excision and chemotherapy

11. A 33-year-old female presents with acute flank pain and hematuria. She has a history of passing a kidney stone 4 months ago. No further workup was done at that time. She has had two vaginal births without complication, drinks three cups of caffeinated coffee daily, smokes three cigarettes per day, denies alcohol abuse, and uses condoms for birth control. She is 5 ft 5 in tall and weighs 160 lb. What is the most effective lifestyle change that should be recommended?

A. Avoid caffeine
B. Drink a glass of red wine daily
C. Push fluids
D. Stop smoking
E. Weight loss

12. A 61-year-old male fell off a ladder. He denies unconsciousness or trauma to the head. He has bruises on the left shoulder and lower back and several fractures in his wrist. Surgery is scheduled for tomorrow. The nursing staff is concerned about some abnormal ECG findings. At first, the T waves appeared large and thin, now the P waves are flat, the PR interval is prolonged, and the QRS is widened. What is the recommended management?

A. Calcium gluconate
B. Kayexalate
C. Hypertonic saline
D. Magnesium supplement
E. Sodium restriction

Practice Answers

1. B. *Nephrology/Urology; Basic Science; Renal Failure*

Expert consensus by the Acute Dialysis Quality Initiative Group defined risk as a reduction in GFR by 25% or more. Injury is defined as a reduction in GFR of 50% or more. Failure is defined as a reduction in GFR of 75% or more.

2. A. *Nephrology/Urology; Diagnosis; Acute Tubular Necrosis, Acute Kidney Failure*

ATN is a very common cause of postoperative kidney failure. The laboratory findings confirm an intrinsic cause of kidney failure. Bladder outlet obstruction would cause a postrenal acute kidney failure, but no casts would be seen. Cirrhosis, hypovolemia, and renal artery stenosis may cause prerenal acute kidney failure, but urine sodium excretion would not be elevated.

3. E. *Nephrology/Urology; Basic Science; Glomerulonephritis*

A recent streptococcal infection is the most common cause of GN in children. About 60% of all GN is in children. Children have a better prognosis than adults.

4. A. *Nephrology/Urology; Clinical Intervention; Nephrotic Syndrome*

Nephrotic syndrome occurs when sodium excretion exceeds 3.5 g protein per day. Patients present with widespread edema and proteinuria. The presence of oval fat bodies makes the diagnosis. First-line treatment is an ACE inhibitor to reduce protein loss and corticosteroids to induce remission. Dietary protein and potassium should not be excessive. Kayexalate is used to reduce high potassium levels.

5. D. *Nephrology/Urology; History and PE; Paraphimosis*

Entrapment of the foreskin behind the glans (paraphimosis) should be reduced urgently because prolonged obstruction may lead to tissue infarction. Frequent catheterization without returning the foreskin to its proper place is a frequent cause. Sexual intercourse may also lead to paraphimosis if the foreskin is left retracted too long; however, having multiple partners does not change the risk. Chronic balanitis and type 2 diabetes predispose uncircumcised men to phimosis.

6. C. *Nephrology/Urology; Clinical Intervention; Orchitis*

The most common cause of orchitis in prepubescent males is mumps. Treatment is ice and analgesics, such as

acetaminophen. Bacterial orchitis occurs more commonly in older men and is treated the same as epididymitis. If a testicular mass or torsion is suspect, ultrasonography and urgent referral are recommended.

7. C. *Nephrology/Urology; History and PE; Epididymitis*

Epididymitis in a patient younger than 35 years is most likely because of sexually transmitted infection (Chlamydia or Neisseria). Diabetes may predispose males to chronic balanitis. Local trauma may result in torsion. An uncircumcised penis is at risk for phimosis or paraphimosis.

8. D. *Nephrology/Urology; Pharmacology; Urge Incontinence*

A sudden urge to urinate followed by incontinence describes urge incontinence, which is a result of bladder wall contractions that are not under control of the brain. Urodynamic studies will confirm this but are not essential. A trial of oxybutynin is warranted. If the symptoms are resolved, no need for further studies. Frequent toileting is recommended for overflow incontinence, which is caused by retention and bladder distention. Estrogen cream is recommended for women with stress incontinence caused by laxity of pelvic musculature often secondary to pregnancies.

9. E. *Nephrology/Urology; History and PE; Bladder Cancer*

Risk factors for bladder cancer include cigarette smoking; exposure to chemicals from rubber, dye, printing, and chemical industries; exposure to cyclophosphamide; and schistosomiasis. Quarry work and glass blowing carry a risk of silicosis. Coal mining is a risk for black lung. Car break work exposes an individual to asbestos.

10. D. *Nephrology/Urology; Clinical Intervention; Renal Cell Carcinoma*

Early-stage localized RCC can be cured by radical nephrectomy. Adjuvant radiation or chemotherapy has not been shown to prolong survival. Chemotherapy and radiation are recommended for later-stage disease. Androgen ablation therapy has a role in prostate cancer.

11. C. *Nephrology/Urology; Health Maintenance; Nephrolithiasis*

The most important element in the prevention of recurrent kidney stones is hydration. According to the Kidney Stone Institute, an individual should be encouraged to drink enough water throughout the day that they must wake up during the night to urinate. Smoking, caffeine, and alcohol have no effect on the risk of kidney stones.

12. A. *Nephrology/Urology; Clinical Intervention; Hyperkalemia*

Hyperkalemia with ECG changes is a serious condition. Calcium gluconate should be given to antagonize the effects of hyperkalemia on the heart. Meanwhile, identification of the cause and treatment to prevent potassium retention should be initiated. Kayexalate may be used to reduce the potassium level; however, stabilization of cardiac function is necessary immediately. Sodium and magnesium should be monitored but are less likely the cause of the ECG changes.

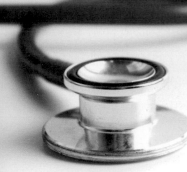

7 | Gynecology
Lori Parlin Palfreyman

Menstrual Disorders

A. Normal menstruation

   1. Understanding the hormonal timing and function in the normal menstrual cycle, including menstruation, ovulation, and proliferation of the endometrium, is important when differentiating diagnoses for a variety of gynecologic conditions, e.g., amenorrhea, abnormal uterine bleeding (AUB), endometriosis, fertility, and infertility (Fig. 7-1).

B. **Amenorrhea**

   1. General characteristics

      a. Primary amenorrhea is the absence of spontaneous menstruation by age 16 years with secondary sex characteristics or age 14 years in the absence of secondary sex characteristics.

      b. Secondary amenorrhea

         (1) In a woman who has previously menstruated, secondary amenorrhea is defined as the absence of menses for 3 months if previous cycles were normal.

         (2) In a woman with irregular menses, secondary amenorrhea is defined as the absence of menses for 6 months.

   2. **Clinical features**. The most common cause of secondary amenorrhea is pregnancy.

      a. Primary amenorrhea is divided into categories based on karyotype and clinical features (Table 7-1).

      b. Secondary amenorrhea: Pregnancy is the most common cause and secondary amenorrhea owing to a cause other than pregnancy occurs in fewer than 5% of women during their lifetime.

         (1) Common pituitary-related hormonal causes include thyroid dysfunction (consider associated symptoms and signs) and prolactinoma (often galactorrhea).

         (2) Common ovarian-related hormonal causes include polycystic ovary syndrome and premature ovarian failure (menopause before 40).

         (3) Other common causes include drug use, stress, significant weight change, or excessive exercise.

         (4) Less common structural causes include Asherman syndrome, i.e., adhesions and scarring of the endometrial lining, often caused by aggressive scraping of the uterine lining.

   3. Diagnostic studies

      a. First-line testing for amenorrhea includes β-human chorionic gonadotropin (β-hCG) for pregnancy, followed by thyroid-stimulating hormone (TSH) and prolactin.

      b. Second-line testing may include serum follicle-stimulating hormone (FSH), estrogen, luteinizing hormone (LH).

      c. Progesterone is sometimes administered; resulting menses determines that anovulatory cycles are the cause.

> 🔆 The most common cause of secondary amenorrhea is pregnancy.

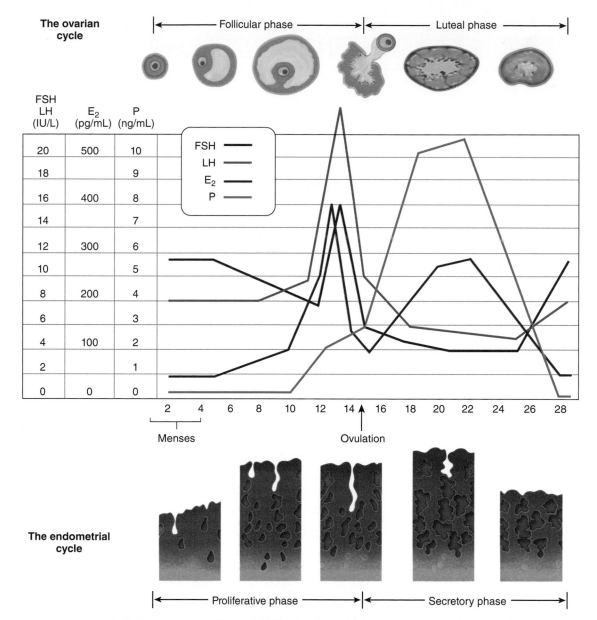

Figure 7-1 ▶ A summary of pituitary, ovarian, uterine, and vaginal changes during the reproductive cycle. E$_2$, estradiol; FSH, follicle-stimulating hormone; LH, luteinizing hormone; P, progesterone. (Reprinted with permission from Casanova R, Chuang A, Geopfert AR, et al. *Beckmann and Ling's Obstetrics and Gynecology*. 8th ed. Wolters Kluwer; 2019, Fig. 37.4.)

d. Other tests may be indicated based on the differential diagnosis, including thyroid studies; magnetic resonance imaging (MRI) or computed tomography (CT) of the hypothalamus and pituitary or pelvis; genetic testing, and pelvic and transvaginal ultrasonography.

4. Management: depends on the underlying cause

C. Abnormal uterine bleeding (AUB); formerly called dysfunctional uterine bleeding (DUB).

1. General characteristics

a. AUB is abnormal uterine bleeding in a nonpregnant woman, which represents a departure from her regular menses with regard to cycle regularity, flow, duration, and volume.

Table 7-1 | Primary Amenorrhea (Most Common Causes)[a]

Etiology #		Karyotype	Physical	Labs	Management
Negative feedback system	Hypothalamic–pituitary dysfunction/insufficiency	46, XX	Minimal to no breast development	Low FSH, LH	Surgery or cyclic estrogens and progestins
Pituitary	Pituitary microadenomas	46, XX	Normal breast development	High prolactin	Surgery
Chromosomal/ovarian	Gonadal dysgenesis (Turner's syndrome)	45, X	Short webbed neck, no breast development	High FSH	Cyclic estrogen and progestins
Structural	Mullerian dysgenesis No uterus or upper 2/3 of vagina but has ovaries	46, XX	Normal breast development	Normal hormone levels/MRI	Surgery to create vagina elongation
Structural	Anatomic imperforate hymen	46, XX	Normal breast development	Dx on PE	Surgically open
Chromosomal	Androgen insensitivity	46, XY	Normal breast development	High testosterone	Remove testes, start estrogen

[a]If all of the above is normal, do workup same as secondary amenorrhea.

FSH, follicle-stimulating hormone; LH, luteinizing hormone; Dx, diagnosis; PE, physical examination.

Adapted from Sakala E. *High-Yield Obstetrics and Gynecology.* 2nd ed. Lippincott Williams & Wilkins; 2006; DeCherney A, Nathan L, Laufer, N, Roman, A. *Current Diagnosis & Treatment: Obstetrics & Gynecology.* 12th ed. McGraw-Hill Companies; 2019.

b. AUB owing to increased anovulatory cycles is the most common cause of AUB. It can occur at any time during the reproductive years with spikes in incidence shortly after menarche and during perimenopause.

c. Terminology to describe bleeding has been refined to more accurately describe AUB (Table 7-2). The terms menorrhagia, metrorrhagia, and menometrorrhagia are no longer used.

d. Clinical features depend on the cause. Differentiating the typical patient (age and other characteristics) and the pattern of bleeding for each diagnosis in the differential is critical. Physical examination includes speculum examination and evaluation for bleeding from other sources.

Table 7-2 | Nomenclature for Normal and Abnormal Uterine Bleeding (AUB), Replacing Menorrhagia and Metrorrhagia

Terms	Definitions	Common Causes
Normal menstrual cycle	• Every 24–38 days; average 28, for 2–8 days • Predictable month to month • Volume <80 mL/cycle	
Heavy menstrual bleeding (Most common AUB)	Subjective "excessive blood loss that interferes with a woman's physical, social, or emotional quality of life"	• Von Willebrand's disease • Molar pregnancy • Malignant endometrial CA • Perimenopause • Leiomyomas • Adenomyosis
Prolonged menstrual bleeding	Exceeds 8 days	
Heavy and prolonged menstrual bleeding	Combo of the two above	
Intermenstrual bleeding	Irregular episodes of bleeding between normal periods	• Polyps • Cervical CA • Oral contraceptive pills • Vaginal trauma (sex/instrumentation)
Postmenopausal bleeding	Bleeding after 1 year of no menses	• Vaginal atrophy • HRT • Cancer

Adapted from DeCherney A, Nathan L, Laufer, N, Roman, A. *Current Diagnosis & Treatment: Obstetrics & Gynecology.* 12th ed. McGraw-Hill Companies; 2019.
CA, cancer; HRT, hormone replacement therapy.

e. Diagnostics depend on the suspected cause.

(1) Urinary β-hCG levels should be done first to rule out pregnancy prior to a workup for other causes.

(2) CBC is helpful to evaluate the extent and impact of a blood-loss hypovolemic state.

(3) Pap smear, pelvic ultrasonography, hysterosalpingography, hysteroscopy, and/ or dilation and curettage (D&C) may be indicated based on history and physical examination.

(4) An endometrial biopsy should be done on all women over 35 years with obesity, hypertension, or diabetes, and on all patients after menopause to rule out pathologic causes of the bleeding such as cancer.

f. Management depends on diagnosis and severity of bleeding; it may include observation, iron therapy, and volume replacement. Acute hemorrhage may necessitate intravenous (IV) or oral high-dose estrogens.

g. D&C may be both diagnostic and curative.

2. AUB-specific diagnoses, workups, and management: Causes of AUB can be remembered using the PALM–COEIN acronym.

a. PALM denotes structural causes: **P**olyp, **A**denomyosis, **L**eiomyoma, **M**alignancy, and hyperplasia.

b. COEIN denotes nonstructural causes: **C**oagulopathy, **O**vulatory dysfunction, **E**ndometrial, **I**atrogenic, and **N**ot otherwise classified (Table 7-3).

3. Structural causes of AUB: PALM

a. Polyps can be cervical or endometrial.

(1) Most commonly found in women older than 40 years and most likely to present with intermenstrual spotting/bleeding

(2) On examination, cervical polyps protrude from the os and appear red, purple, or flesh colored.

b. Adenomyosis is not common.

(1) Endometrial glands within the uterine musculature. Typically affects women aged 40 to 50 years and causes heavy and painful, prolonged bleeding.

(2) It is usually diagnosed by direct visualization in the uterine wall after a hysterectomy.

c. Uterine leiomyomas (fibroids)

(1) Most common in ages 40 to 50 years, resulting in heavy and prolonged menses.

(2) Fibroids are classified by their location: subserosal (deforming external serosa), intramural (within the uterine wall), and submucosal (deforming uterine cavity) (Fig. 7-2).

(3) Submucosal leiomyomas are the fibroids responsible for AUB.

> Pregnancy must be ruled out before any further workup of amenorrhea.

Table 7-3 | Causes for Abnormal Uterine Bleeding (AUB)

PALM—Structural Causes	COEIN—Nonstructural Causes
Polyp	Coagulopathy
Adenomyosis	Ovulatory dysfunction
Leiomyoma (submucosal or other)	Endometrial
Malignancy and hyperplasia	Iatrogenic
	Not classified

Adapted from Munro MG, Critchley HO, Broder MS, et al. FIGO classification system (PALM-COEIN) for causes of abnormal uterine bleeding in nongravid women of reproductive age. FIGO Working Group on Menstrual Disorders. *Int J Gynaecol Obstet*. 2011;113:3–13.

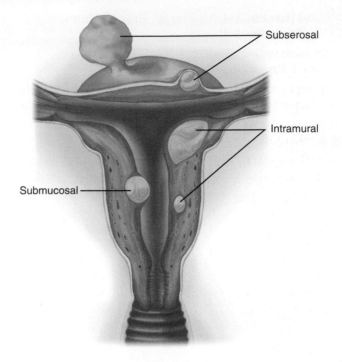

Figure 7-2 ▶ Locations of leiomyomas. (From Gilliam T. *A Text-Book of Practical Gynecology for Practitioners and Students*. FA Davis; 1913, 323. In the public domain.)

(4) Most women have no symptoms. For those who do, bleeding is the most common presenting symptom. Some will also complain of pressure or fullness in the pelvis.

(5) A firm, enlarged, irregular uterine mass indicates subserosal or intramural fibroids.

(6) Ultrasonography is most common to aid in diagnosis. Hysteroscopy and hysterosalpingography are the best methods to diagnose submucosal fibroids.

(7) Observation is recommended for asymptomatic patients.

(8) For symptomatic patients who wish to maintain their fertility, D&C or myomectomy is the best choice. Gonadotropin-releasing hormone (GnRH) agonists and mifepristone may reduce tumor size; in women with small leiomyomas (fibroids), GnRH agonists may restore fertility. Treatment is limited to 6 months.

(9) For symptomatic women who do not desire fertility, uterine artery embolization or endometrial ablation are promising treatments.

(10) Hysterectomy is the final step if symptoms cannot be resolved with other interventions.

d. Malignancy (endometrial cancer) and hyperplasia

(1) Endometrial cancer is the most common gynecologic cancer and the fourth most common malignancy in women in the United States. Median age at presentation is 58 years.

(2) Adenocarcinomas make up 75% of cancer cell types.

(3) Prognosis is influenced by histologic appearance, age (older women have poorer outcomes), and extent of spread.

(4) Risk factors include obesity, nulliparity, infertility, late menopause, diabetes mellitus, unopposed estrogen stimulation, hypertension, gallbladder disease, and chronic tamoxifen use; it is not related to sexual history. Oral contraceptives seem to have a protective effect.

(5) Clinical features: The cardinal symptom is postmenopausal uterine bleeding (90% of patients).

(6) Diagnostic testing: Women with postmenopausal bleeding should have an ultrasound, Pap smear, and endometrial biopsy.

(7) Although endocervical curettage is considered the definitive choice, endometrial biopsy is more common and has an accuracy rate of 90% to 95%.

(8) Management usually is a total hysterectomy combined with bilateral salpingo-oophorectomy; treatment and staging occur after surgery.

(9) Radiotherapy may be indicated. Chemotherapy is used at advanced stages.

(10) Recurrence is treated with high-dose progestins or antiestrogens.

> The cardinal presenting symptom for endometrial cancer is postmenopausal uterine bleeding; median age at presentation is 58 years.

4. Nonstructural causes of AUB: COEIN

   a. Coagulopathy

   (1) A history of bleeding during dental work, easy bruising, or a family history helps make the diagnosis.

   (2) Prothrombin time (PT) and partial thromboplastin time (PTT) assess the extrinsic and intrinsic clotting pathways, respectively.

   (3) Von Willebrand's disease, an inherited bleeding dyscrasia, should also be considered. Up to 13% of White adolescents have AUB owing to this disorder, which may result in heavy prolonged bleeding.

   b. Ovulatory dysfunction

   (1) Ovulatory dysfunction is the most common cause of AUB in nonpregnant women.

   (2) Common causes for anovulatory cycles include thyroid dysfunction, pituitary tumors, stress, and transition to menopause.

   (3) Polycystic ovary syndrome (PCOS) also leads to anovulatory cycles.

   (4) A menses tracking diary may be helpful. Thyroid function tests and LH are the initial workup. A serum progesterone level is helpful. A high FSH indicates the beginning of menopause.

   (5) A progestin trial should be performed. If the bleeding stops, anovulatory cycles are confirmed.

> Cessation of abnormal uterine bleeding with progestin trial confirms lack of ovulation.

   (6) For women not desiring pregnancy at this time, oral contraceptive pills are the first line of treatment.

   (7) Oral contraceptives should not be used in women over 35 years who smoke or who have hypertension, diabetes, history of vascular disease, breast cancer, liver disease, or focal headaches.

   (8) Women older than 35 years without risk factors can be prescribed oral contraceptives.

   c. Endometrial: Nonstructural causes include infection and inflammation; this is usually a diagnosis of exclusion.

   d. Iatrogenic: uterine bleeding caused by medical treatment

   (1) Oral contraception, intrauterine device (IUD), and hormone replacement therapy are common causes, resulting in spotty, intermittent bleeding.

   (2) Other causes include anticoagulants, serotonin reuptake inhibitors (SSRIs), and tricyclic antidepressants.

   e. AUB not otherwise classified: Includes rare arteriovenous malformations and hydatidiform mole (discussed in Chapter 8—Obstetrics).

D. Dysmenorrhea

   1. **Primary Dysmenorrhea**

   a. General: Painful menstruation caused by excess prostaglandin and leukotriene levels, leading to painful uterine cramping, nausea, vomiting, and diarrhea. Onset is usually within 2 years of menarche and peak incidence is late teens to early 20s, but it can occur at any age. It is important to note that there is no pathologic abnormality.

b. Clinical features

(1) Women with primary dysmenorrhea have cramping in the central lower abdomen or pelvis radiating to the back or thighs, beginning 1 to 3 days prior to menses and resolving 1 to 2 days after the onset of menses.

(2) Physical examination, labs, and radiologic tests are normal.

c. Diagnostic studies: Diagnosis is established based on history, daily charting of symptoms (menstrual diary), and physical examination.

d. Management

(1) Start nonsteroidal anti-inflammatory drugs (NSAIDs) just before the expected menses and continue for 2 to 3 days.

(2) Oral contraceptives, vitamin B (B_1, thiamine; B_6, pyridoxine), magnesium, acupuncture, application of heat, and regular exercise may reduce pain.

2. Secondary dysmenorrhea

a. General

(1) Secondary dysmenorrhea is painful menstruation caused by an identifiable clinical condition, usually of the uterus or pelvis (e.g., endometriosis, adenomyosis, uterine fibroids, pelvic inflammatory disease [PID], and use of an IUD).

(2) It usually affects women older than 25 years and increases with age.

b. Clinical features: Depending on the cause, symptoms may include heavy menstrual bleeding and dyspareunia. It is less related to the first day of flow than primary amenorrhea.

c. Diagnosis

(1) Specific tests for secondary dysmenorrhea target possible pelvic pathology.

(2) Hysteroscopy, D&C, and laparoscopy allow both diagnosis and treatment.

d. Management: Obvious underlying conditions should be treated. Symptomatic treatment may be sufficient.

E. Premenstrual syndrome (PMS) and premenstrual dysphoric disorder (PMDD)

1. General characteristics

a. PMS hypothesized causes include abnormal levels of serotonin and psychological, social, and genetic factors.

b. The prevalence is greatest between 20 and 40 years of age; 70% of women have some premenstrual symptoms.

c. PMDD is PMS symptoms severe enough to cause dysfunction in daily living. Fewer than 4% of women meet the criteria for PMDD.

d. An association exists among postpartum depression, perimenopausal depression, other affective disorders, and PMS.

2. Clinical features

a. Diagnosis is based on *Diagnostic and Statistical Manual of Mental Disorders*, Fifth edition (*DSM-5*) criteria (Table 7-4).

b. Symptoms begin 1 to 2 weeks before menses and end 1 to 2 days after the onset of menses.

c. In order to make the diagnosis, the symptoms must be absent during the first 2 weeks of the menstrual cycle.

d. The most common complaints are mood alteration and psychological effects (e.g., irritability, anxiety, depression, sleep and appetite changes, poor concentration, fatigue, insomnia).

> 💡 Regular exercise and sleep coupled with avoidance of caffeine, nicotine, and alcohol are often affective in reducing symptoms in dysmenorrhea.

> 💡 PMS and PMDD are characterized by irritability, anxiety, depression, sleep changes, and poor concentration.

Table 7-4 | Differentiation of Premenstrual Syndrome (PMS) and Premenstrual Dysphoric Disorder (PMDD)

PMS/PMDD Symptoms	PMS/PMDD Symptoms
Column 1	Column 2
• Depression or hopelessness • Anxiety/tension • Mood swings—sudden sadness, sensitivity to rejection • Anger or irritability	• Decreased interest in activities • Sleep changes • Appetite changes • Decreased concentration • Feeling overwhelmed • Bloating/breast tenderness • Lethargy, fatigue

	Premenstrual Syndrome	Premenstrual Dysphoric Disorder
Prevalence (in population)	75%	10%
Number of symptoms required	One from each column (minimum of two total)	5 of 11
Social impairment	Not required (but may be present)	Required
Prospective charting	Not required (but recommended)	Required

Adapted from the American Psychiatric Association. *Diagnostic and Statistical Manual of Mental Disorders.* 5th ed. 2013. https://doi.org/10.1176/appi.books.9780890425596

    e. Symptoms related to fluid retention include bloating, weight gain, and breast pain.

    f. Symptoms are consistent month to month within the same patient, although they vary widely from woman to woman.

  3. Diagnostic studies

    a. Menstrual diary is helpful to chart symptoms; the pattern of occurrence is more important than the specific constellation of symptoms.

    b. Thyroid studies and complete blood count (CBC) are used to rule out thyroid disease and anemia, respectively.

  4. Management

    a. Lifestyle modifications include reduction of caffeine, alcohol, tobacco, chocolate, and sodium intake; small, frequent meals of complex carbohydrates, low-fat dairy, and fruits and vegetables; increased exercise; relaxation strategies; stress reduction; and light therapy.

    b. Drug treatment

      (1) NSAIDs are useful for general pain and also seem to relieve other symptoms.

      (2) Oral contraceptives may improve, worsen, or not change symptomatology; clinical studies have not shown progesterone to be useful.

      (3) Diuretics (e.g., spironolactone) may be used for fluid retention symptoms; bromocriptine may help relieve mastalgia.

      (4) SSRIs have proven to be beneficial in some patients; anxiolytics, including buspirone and cyclic alprazolam, may relieve anxiety.

      (5) Pyridoxine (vitamin B_6) and evening primrose oil show no benefit over placebo in clinical trials but relieve breast tenderness and depression in some women; some preliminary studies show the benefits of calcium carbonate, magnesium, and vitamin E supplementation.

F. Menopause

  1. General characteristics

    a. By definition, menopause is the last menses, and perimenopause (usually lasting 3 to 5 years) is the time surrounding it. The climacteric is that portion of the aging process where a woman moves from her reproductive years to her nonreproductive years.

b. Mean age at natural menopause is 51 years; 95% of women stop menstruating between 44 and 55 years of age. Smoking is associated with early menopause.

c. The subjective experience of menopause varies by individual and is influenced by cultural expectations and life circumstances.

d. Premature menopause (spontaneous premature ovarian failure) is the cessation of menses before age 40 years.

e. The ovaries continue to produce testosterone and androstenedione; estrone is the predominant postmenopausal circulating estrogen.

2. **Clinical features** (Table 7-5)

   a. All of the symptoms associated with menopause are a result of low estrogen.

   b. Vasomotor symptoms (hot flashes/flushes) vary in intensity; when they occur frequently at night, they may cause insomnia, tiredness, and irritability. They usually resolve in 2 to 3 years.

   c. Urogenital atrophy may cause poor vaginal lubrication, dyspareunia, dysuria, urge incontinence, pelvic relaxation, atrophic cystitis, and easy bleeding.

   d. Accelerated bone loss may result in osteoporosis.

   e. Estrogen-related cardiovascular protection declines.

   f. Changes in the sleep cycle can be one of the most disabling effects.

   g. The skin thins and becomes less elastic, and facial hair may increase. Hair loss increases and nails become brittle.

   h. Confusion, loss of memory, lethargy, inability to cope, depression, and loss of interest in sex have been associated with menopause. Causes are not clear, but symptoms may be relieved with hormone administration.

3. Diagnostic studies: FSH >30 mIU per mL is diagnostic of menopause.

4. **Management**

   a. Women should be treated on the basis of individual risk factors and symptoms.

   b. Lifestyle modifications may ameliorate symptoms and decrease risks. Regular exercise has consistently been correlated with a reduction in menopausal symptoms.

   c. Combined hormone replacement therapy is effective and indicated for short-term treatment of hot flashes. Although it is also effective in reducing bone loss, vasomotor symptoms and vaginal atrophy are the only indications for its use.

   d. Contraindications to hormone replacement therapy include undiagnosed vaginal bleeding, acute vascular thrombosis, liver disease, and history of endometrial or breast cancer.

   e. Calcium and vitamin D supplementation, bisphosphonates, selective estrogen receptor modulators (SERMs), or calcitonin may be used in women at risk for osteoporosis.

> 💡 Menopausal symptoms are related to low estrogen; elevated FSH confirms the diagnosis.

Table 7-5 | Menopause Symptoms

Early Symptoms/Signs	Late Symptoms/Signs
Irregular or cessation of menses	Cystocele/rectocele/uterine prolapse
Hot flashes	Memory loss
Decreased vaginal lubrication	Osteoporosis
Loss of sexual desire	Cardiovascular disease
Depression	
Mood swings/irritability	
Thin skin	
Hair loss	
Nails brittle	
FSH >30 mIU/mL	

Adapted from DeCherney A, Nathan L, Laufer, N, Roman, A. *Current Diagnosis & Treatment: Obstetrics & Gynecology.* 12th ed. McGraw-Hill Companies; 2019.

f. Topical estrogens may improve urogenital symptoms. Systemic unopposed estrogen administration places a woman at increased risk for endometrial cancer.

g. Soy, black cohosh, and ginseng may also help alleviate symptoms.

Uterine Disorders

A. Endometriosis

1. General characteristics

a. Endometriosis is a condition in which endometrial tissue is found outside the endometrial cavity. Most sites are found in the pelvis or on the ovary (60%), but they may also be distant (e.g., lung).

b. It most commonly occurs in nulliparous women in their late 20s or early 30s.

c. Infertility is common. Endometriosis is found in 25% to 34% of infertile women.

2. Clinical features

a. Endometriosis presents with dysmenorrhea, deep-thrust dyspareunia, dyschezia (difficulty passing bowel movement), pelvic pain, and infertility.

b. Signs include tender nodularity of the cul-de-sac and uterine ligaments and a fixed uterus.

c. The degree of endometriosis does not correlate with symptomatology.

3. Diagnosis: Usually made clinically. Ultrasonography is used to rule out other conditions. Definitive diagnosis is by laparoscopy.

4. Management

a. Endometriosis treatment is based on severity of symptoms, location and severity of disease, and desire for childbearing.

b. In women with few symptoms, expectant management may suffice.

c. NSAIDs and prostaglandin synthetase inhibitors may relieve discomfort.

d. Combined oral contraceptives or progestins may relieve symptoms.

e. Surgery may be conservative or definitive; large endometriomas must be resected.

f. After surgical resection, fertility is often improved.

B. Endometrial cancer and hyperplasia (see AUB section above)

C. Leiomyomas (Uterine fibroids) (see AUB section above)

D. Uterine prolapse

1. General characteristics

a. Prolapse of the uterus typically occurs after pregnancy, labor, and vaginal delivery but may also occur in nulliparas. Risk increases to 50% after menopause for all women.

b. Any condition that increases intra-abdominal pressure may predispose a woman to prolapse, including obesity, chronic cough, constipation, or repetitive heavy lifting.

c. Systemic problems, such as obesity, asthma, and chronic obstructive pulmonary disease (COPD), as well as local factors, such as pelvic tumors and ascites, predispose to prolapse.

2. Clinical features

a. Symptoms include vaginal fullness, lower abdominal aching, or low back pain. Symptoms vary but are usually worse after prolonged standing or late in the day and are relieved by lying down.

b. Uterine prolapse is graded as 0 (no descent) to 4 (through the introitus).

> Presentation of endometriosis often includes infertility, and treatment may involve NSAIDs, COCs, or surgery.

> It is estimated that 50% of postmenopausal women have some sort of pelvic organ prolapse.

      c. With moderate prolapse, patients describe a falling-out sensation or a feeling of sitting on a ball.

      d. Most prolapses are accompanied by cystocele, rectocele, or enterocele.

   3. Diagnosis is made by visualization; no testing is indicated.

   4. Management

      a. Nonsurgical approaches include weight reduction, smoking cessation, pelvic muscle exercises, and use of a vaginal pessary.

      b. Surgical treatment includes sacrohysteropexy, which involves attaching the cervix to the sacrum with surgical mesh. Hysterectomy is also an option. Both surgeries relieve symptoms, restore normal anatomic relationships and visceral function, and allow coitus.

Ovarian Disorders

A. **Ovarian cysts**

> Most ovarian cysts are functional, are confirmed by ultrasound, and reduce within two to three cycles.

   1. General characteristics

      a. Cysts are the most common ovarian growths.

      b. Most cysts are functional; these include follicular, corpus luteum, and, much less commonly, theca lutein cysts.

   2. Clinical features: Cysts may present as asymptomatic masses or with pain and menstrual delay.

   3. Diagnostic studies: Cysts are usually confirmed by pelvic ultrasonography as mobile, simple, and fluid filled.

   4. Management

      a. Follow for one or two cycles in premenopausal women with cysts smaller than 8 cm.

      b. Large or persistent cysts require laparoscopic evaluation.

      c. Cysts in postmenopausal women are presumed to be malignant until proven otherwise.

      d. The use of oral contraceptives has not been validated in treating functional cysts.

B. **Ovarian Torsion**

> Unlike testicular torsion, ovarian torsion is more likely not to be idiopathic but owing to some structural change.

   1. In torsion, the ovary flips on the fallopian tube, occluding blood supply, leading to necrosis of the tube and ovary and ensuing peritonitis. Diagnosis must be swift to preserve the ovary.

   2. Torsion most commonly occurs as a result of a cyst or neoplasm. Sometimes the cause is idiopathic, especially when it occurs in premenarchal girls aged 10 to 15 years old.

   3. Pain and a unilateral pelvic mass are present in 85% to 95% of cases. Nausea/vomiting is also common; fever is present <20% of the time.

   4. Ultrasound is the imaging of choice.

   5. Treatment is surgical intervention.

C. **Polycystic ovary syndrome (PCOS)**

   1. General characteristics

      a. Formerly known as Stein–Leventhal syndrome, PCOS is the most common cause of androgen excess and hirsutism (male-patterned hair growth) in females.

      b. Patients with PCOS have bilaterally enlarged polycystic ovaries, amenorrhea or oligomenorrhea, and infertility.

c. Patients usually have normal menses during adolescence, followed by progressively longer episodes of amenorrhea.

d. The underlying abnormality is thought to be hypothalamic–pituitary dysfunction and insulin resistance, although the pathophysiology is not entirely clear. A genetic predisposition exists.

e. Patients are at increased risk for endometrial hyperplasia and carcinoma because of unopposed estrogen stimulation.

2. **Clinical features**

    a. Half of patients with PCOS are hirsute, and many show truncal obesity.

    b. Patients usually present for treatment of hirsutism or infertility. Others present with intractable acne or menstrual irregularities (oligomenorrhea or amenorrhea).

    c. Impaired glucose tolerance is present in 30% of patients; frank diabetes mellitus (type 2) is present in 8%.

3. Diagnostic studies

    a. Ultrasonography may demonstrate a characteristic "string of pearls" or "oyster ovaries" appearance within the ovaries (Fig. 7-3).

    b. Laboratory testing reveals mildly elevated serum androgen levels, increased LH/FSH ratio, lipid abnormalities, and insulin resistance.

4. **Management**

    a. Weight reduction improves hirsutism, lipid and glucose parameters, and fertility.

    b. Hirsutism is treated with androgen-lowering agents, including oral contraceptives, or nonpharmacological treatments such as shaving, waxing, laser, or electrolysis.

    c. Infertility is treated with letrozole or, secondarily, clomiphene citrate.

    d. Lipid abnormalities and insulin resistance should be managed medically. Adding metformin increases ovulation and pregnancy rates.

> Increased androgens account for the menstrual irregularities, hirsutism, and obesity and metabolic syndrome in PCOS.

D. **Ovarian cancer**

1. General characteristics

    a. High-risk women are older (mean age is 69 years), nulliparous, have early menses, late menopause, and have a positive family history of ovarian or endometrial cancer.

    b. Long-term oral contraceptive use may be protective because of the suppression of ovulation.

> Ovarian cancer has the highest mortality rate of any malignancy, mainly owing to delayed diagnosis.

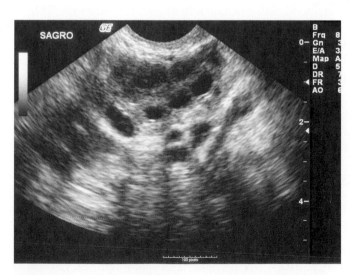

Figure 7-3 ▶ Polycystic ovarian syndrome "string of pearls." Ultrasound picture.

c. A leading cause of death, ovarian cancer is the fifth most common cancer in American women and the second most common gynecologic malignancy, with the highest mortality rate: 60% of patients die within 5 years.

d. Ten percent of patients have a genetic predisposition; 90% of cases are sporadic.

e. Hereditary ovarian cancer has two forms: breast and ovarian cancer (BOC) syndrome or hereditary nonpolyposis colorectal cancer (HNPCC) syndrome.

f. Eighty percent of ovarian cancers are epithelial tumors.

2. **Clinical features**

a. Diagnosis is often delayed because of a lack of specific symptoms. Late in the disease, women present with ascites, abdominal distention, early satiety, change in bowel habits, or a fixed mass.

b. Sister Mary Joseph nodule, a metastatic implant in the umbilicus, can be associated.

3. Diagnostic studies

a. The *BRCA1* gene is associated in 5% of cases; cancer antigen 125 (CA-125) may be used to follow treatment, particularly in postmenopausal women.

b. An association exists with mutations in the *P53* tumor suppressor gene.

c. Transvaginal or abdominal ultrasonography is useful in distinguishing benign from potentially malignant masses. Histologic examination via biopsy is the definitive diagnosis.

4. **Management** involves surgery plus chemotherapy and radiation therapy.

> Sister Mary Joseph nodule is a rare but important finding indicating advanced cancer in the abdomen or pelvis.

Cervical Dysplasia and Neoplasia

A. General characteristics

1. Human papillomavirus (HPV) infection (especially types 16, 18, 31, and 33) is the cause of over 90% of cervical cancer cases; types 6 and 11 are linked to condylomata acuminata.

2. HPV infection alone may not be sufficient for the development of cervical intraepithelial neoplasia (CIN); cofactors play a strong role. Other risk factors include early age at first intercourse, multiple sexual partners or a high-risk sex partner, history of sexually transmitted disease, low socioeconomic status, and cigarette smoking.

a. Mild dysplasia (CIN-1) may progress to moderate dysplasia (CIN-2), severe dysplasia (CIN-3), and carcinoma in situ (CIS); however, CIN-1 may remain unchanged or, most commonly, the immune system will eventually clear the virus from the body.

b. About one-third of patients with CIN-3 develop microinvasive or invasive carcinoma.

c. CIN most commonly occurs in women in their 20s, CIS in those aged 25 to 35 years, and cervical cancer after age 40 years.

B. **Clinical features**

1. Most women with abnormal Pap smears or other screening tests have no symptoms.

2. Advanced or invasive cervical cancer may cause abnormal vaginal bleeding and vaginal discharge and postcoital bleeding, and tumor may be visible on clinical examination.

3. The mean age at diagnosis of cervical cancer is 47 years overall but 39 years in lower socioeconomic status groups.

C. Diagnostic studies

1. Pap smear, liquid-based specimen, and other cytologic screening techniques are highly effective and should begin at age 21 years and continue every 3 years. HPV screening should begin at age 30, and occur every 5 years. Regular Pap smear screening reduces the incidence of invasive cervical carcinoma by 95%.

> Pap smears starting at age 21, every 3 years; HPV screening starting at age 30, every 5 years.

Table 7-6 | Comparison of Results of Bethesda Classification System, Cytology, and Corresponding Diagnoses

Cytology (from PAP) Bethesda Classification System	Histology (Biopsy from Colposcopy)	Diagnosis
ASC-US ASC-H LSIL AGC	CIN 1	Mild dysplasia
HSIL	CIN 2	Moderate dysplasia
	CIN 3	Severe dysplasia
		Carcinoma in situ

ASC-US, atypical squamous cells of undetermined significance; ASC-H, atypical squamous cells; LSIL, low-grade squamous intraepithelial lesion; HPV, human papillomavirus; HSIL, high-grade squamous intraepithelial lesion; CIN, cervical intraepithelial neoplasia; AGC, atypical glandular cells.

2. Abnormal cytologic screenings (Table 7-6) indicate terminology of PAP results and colposcopy screening.

   a. Because cervical dysplasia is considered slow growing, age at first irregular PAP dictates workup. The age 24 years is the current set point: If younger than 24 years with irregular PAP, a more conservative approach is indicated.

   b. Biopsy of suspicious lesions is mandatory if the patient is over 24 years and the PAP results are low-grade squamous intraepithelial lesion (LSIL) or more.

   c. Colposcopy with biopsies is the most appropriate technique for histologic evaluation.

3. HPV DNA testing is now common.

D. **Management** is based on the classification of disease.

   1. Mild lesions may resolve spontaneously.

   2. Preinvasive neoplasia may be treated with electrocautery or cryocautery, laser therapy, conization, large loop excision of transitional zone, or loop electrosurgical excision procedure (LEEP).

   3. Conization is used when the neoplasia is larger. Conization is more likely to lead to incompetent cervix compared to LEEP.

   4. Hysterectomy and pelvic lymphadenectomy or radiation therapy is indicated for more severe abnormalities.

   5. Vaccine against HPV is available.

      a. The Centers for Disease Control and Prevention has recommended HPV vaccine for all girls and boys; the most common dosing recommendation is at age 11 to 12 years, but it is available approved for ages 9 to 26 years. The vaccine is a two-dose regimen if the doses are given at age 14 years or before; vaccine initiated at age 15 years or later requires three doses.

      b. It prevents four types of HPV (types 6, 11, 16, and 18). In those not previously exposed, the vaccine protects against cervical cancer 90% of the time; in previously exposed, it protects 66% of the time; it is also protective for 90% of genital warts.

      c. Boosters are not recommended at this time.

> 💡 HPV vaccine against types 6, 11, 16, and 18 is recommended for boys and girls starting around age 12.

Vaginal and Vulvar Neoplasms

A. General characteristics

   1. Neoplasias of the vulva and vagina are the rarest of the gynecologic neoplasms. Primary vaginal neoplasms are far less common than cervical or vulvar neoplasms.

2. Most vulvar malignancies are squamous cell carcinomas and occur in postmenopausal women (mean age at diagnosis, 65 years).

3. Women with in utero exposure to diethylstilbestrol (DES) are at increased risk for clear cell adenocarcinoma of the vagina.

4. About 80% of vaginal cancers are metastatic; it may arise from the urethra, Bartholin's gland, rectum, bladder, endometrial cavity, endocervix, kidney, or other distant sites.

5. Vaginal melanoma also occurs.

B. **Clinical features**

1. Vulvar cancer is more often found in women who are obese and who have hypertension, diabetes mellitus, and arteriosclerosis. A history of chronic vulvar itching is common.

2. Vulvar cancer in younger women is associated with HPV infection and smoking; 25% of patients have coexisting cervical carcinoma.

3. Most vaginal intraepithelial neoplasms occur in the upper one-third of the vagina and are asymptomatic; the most common presenting problems are postmenopausal bleeding or bloody discharge.

4. DES-exposed women may have vaginal adenosis and structural changes of the cervix, vagina, and upper genital tract, leading to an increased risk of miscarriage, premature delivery, and ectopic pregnancy.

C. Diagnostic studies

1. Application of acetic acid or staining with toluidine blue may help to direct biopsies of suspicious vulvar lesions.

2. Vaginal biopsy for suspected vaginal invasive neoplasm should be directed by colposcopy or Lugol staining.

3. Clear cell adenocarcinoma is diagnosed by careful inspection and palpation of the vagina and cervix, followed by biopsies.

D. **Management**

1. Local excision, topical 5-fluorouracil, and laser therapy are used for early vulvar lesions.

2. Surgical excision is required for most vaginal neoplasms; primary vaginal cancer is treated with radiotherapy.

3. For clear cell lesions, radical hysterectomy and vaginectomy or radiation therapy is effective.

> 💡 Vaginal and vulvar neoplasms are rare; 80% are metastatic.

Breast Disorders

A. Benign breast disorders (Table 7-7)

1. Mammography, ultrasonography, and biopsy may be indicated for breast complaints. Ultrasonography differentiates between solid and cystic masses; however, the value in using mammography in young women can be problematic because of the increased density of breast tissue.

2. It is important to be able to distinguish clinically among the four most likely breast conditions: mastitis, fibrocystic breasts, breast fibroadenomas, and breast cancer.

   a. Mastodynia (mastalgia), or the symptom of breast tenderness, is common, often premenstrual.

      (1) Mastodynia increases in women taking contraceptive pills or hormone replacement therapy.

      (2) Treat mastodynia with reassurance or vitamin B_6; if severe, consider bromocriptine, tamoxifen, or danazol.

Table 7-7 | Differentiation Among Breast Disorders

Disorder	Main Points	Key Physical Findings	Treatment
Mastitis/breast abscess	Breastfeeding women Abscess forms from untreated mastitis	Fever Erythema Tender fluctuant mass in one quadrant of the breast	Antibiotics Aspiration of abscess
Fibrocystic changes	Reproductive age	Multiple bilateral painful cysts that vary in size and fluctuate in size during the menstrual cycle	Supportive bra Avoidance of caffeine
Fibroadenoma	Young women, usually aged 20–30	Single, round, rubbery mobile nontender breast mass	Monitor or excise under local anesthesia
Cancer	Women over 40 years	Fixed, irregular painless mass, most commonly in the upper outer quadrant	Surgery

b. Mastitis, or breast infection, and breast abscesses are most often caused by *Staphylococcus aureus* and occur primarily in lactating women.

(1) Mastitis and abscesses (progression of mastitis) present with unilateral tenderness, heat, significant fever, chills, and other flu-like symptoms. Usually, one quadrant or a lobule of one breast is affected.

(2) *S. aureus* is present in approximately 50% of patients with mastitis; culture of purulent material or milk is usually not performed.

(3) Treat mastitis with a penicillinase-resistant antibiotic (cloxacillin, dicloxacillin, nafcillin) or a cephalosporin and warm or cool compresses to the affected area.

(4) Breastfeeding should continue as it will hasten recovery. Renewal of breastfeeding techniques is helpful.

(5) Abscesses often cause a greater severity of symptoms, and surgical treatment may be required for abscesses or duct ectasia.

> Mastitis is almost exclusively found in lactating women; *Staphylococcus aureus* is the primary pathogen.

c. Fibrocystic changes—the most frequent benign condition of the breast—include cysts, papillomatosis, fibrosis, adenosis, and ductal epithelial hyperplasia.

(1) Fibrocystic changes are most common in women 30 to 50 years of age and may present as multiple asymptomatic masses or as painful and tender masses with bilateral breast pain. Multiple lesions that fluctuate in size during the menstrual cycle distinguish fibrocystic changes from carcinoma.

(2) In suspected cysts, fine-needle aspiration is both diagnostic and therapeutic; cysts usually contain straw-colored fluid.

(3) Many types of fibrocystic breast problems need no treatment other than a supportive bra. Heat or ice on the breast and over-the-counter analgesics may be helpful.

(4) The role of caffeine restriction in the treatment of fibrocystic changes is controversial; some patients respond to low-salt diet, vitamin E supplementation, or premenstrual hydrochlorothiazide.

> Treat fibrocystic changes with supportive care: supportive bra, local heat or ice, avoid caffeine, reduce salt intake.

d. Fibroadenomas are the second most common benign breast disorder and occur in young women; they are more common in Black women.

(1) Fibroadenomas typically are round, firm, smooth, discrete, mobile, and nontender.

(2) In a woman younger than 25 years of age, a fibroadenomatous mass should be biopsied.

(3) Fibroadenomas may be excised or managed expectantly.

B. Breast neoplasms (Refer to Table 7-7)

1. General characteristics

> The vast majority of breast cancers are infiltrating ductal carcinomas.

a. Breast cancer is the most common cancer in women (excluding skin cancer) and the second leading cause of death from cancer in women.

b. Most women with breast cancer have no identifiable risk factors other than female sex and increasing age (mean age at diagnosis, 60 to 61 years); *BRCA1* and *BRCA2* genes are associated with 5% to 10% of cases of breast cancer but appear in only 1% of the population.

c. Associated factors include nulliparity, early menarche, late menopause, long-term estrogen or radiation exposure, and delayed childbearing.

d. Women with first-degree relatives with breast cancer are at increased risk, especially if the cancer was premenopausal or bilateral or found in two of these relatives.

e. Breast cancer increases the risk of endometrial cancer and vice versa.

f. Infiltrating ductal carcinomas account for 80% to 85% of breast cancers; the remainder are lobular carcinomas. Lobular CIS and atypical ductal hyperplasia predispose to cancer.

g. Paget's disease is a ductal carcinoma presenting as an eczematous lesion of the nipple.

h. All invasive lobular carcinomas and two-thirds of ductal carcinomas are estrogen receptor–positive. Estrogen receptor–negative cancer has a poorer prognosis.

2. Clinical features

a. Breast cancer most often presents as a single, nontender, firm, immobile mass; 45% occur in the upper outer quadrant and 25% under the nipple and areola.

b. Early carcinoma may be identified through mammographic changes and no palpable masses.

c. Rarer presentations include nipple discharge or retraction, dimpling, breast enlargement or shrinkage, skin thickening or *peau d'orange* (orange peel skin), eczematous changes, breast pain, fixed mass, axillary node enlargement, ulcerations, arm edema, and palpable supraclavicular nodes.

3. Screening

a. Mammography is the best screening modality.

b. Guidelines vary among professional groups as to age to initiate screening and frequency of testing for the general population.

> Most guidelines recommend mammographic testing every 1 to 2 years between the ages of 50 and 74 years.

c. Most guidelines recommend mammographic testing every 1 to 2 years between the ages of 50 and 74 years.

d. Screening women aged 40 to 49 years is controversial because of the high rate of false positives and should be individualized.

4. Diagnostic studies

a. A combination of physical examination, mammography (the best screening tool), ultrasonography, and fine-needle or stereotactic core-needle biopsy is highly accurate in establishing the diagnosis. Open biopsy may be required.

b. Biopsy specimen should undergo estrogen and progesterone receptor analysis as well as histologic analysis.

c. Oncotype DX test is used to help determine the need for chemotherapy for women with stage I or II hormone receptor–positive cancer. The test looks at 21 genes within the tumor to determine the likelihood of the cancer recurring or spreading.

5. Management

a. TNM staging should occur before treatment begins. Metastatic workup is recommended for all breast cancers.

b. Treatment with the intent to cure most likely occurs for patients with stage I, IIA, or IIB cancer.

c. Breast conservation therapy (lumpectomy) with sentinel node biopsy is often preferred with early-stage cancer. Modified radical mastectomy and partial mastectomy have equivalent survival rates when surgery is followed by radiation therapy.

d. Adjuvant chemotherapy and/or hormonal manipulation benefit some women.

e. Tamoxifen is used to treat women with estrogen receptor–positive disease and postmenopausal women.

f. Aromatase inhibitors are first-line treatment for metastatic hormone–receptive CA.

Contraceptive Methods

A. Noninterventional methods (Table 7-8)

1. Total abstinence (no sexual intercourse) is the most effective in preventing pregnancy; however, abstinence as a recommendation for pregnancy prevention, especially in the adolescent population, has been ineffective.

2. Coitus interruptus (withdrawal) and postcoital douching are ineffective and unreliable.

3. Lactational amenorrhea may be effective in delaying conception for 6 months after birth if the woman breastfeeds exclusively and amenorrhea is maintained.

4. Periodic abstinence methods rely on abstinence from just before the time of ovulation until 2 to 3 days thereafter. Failure rate is approximately 25%.

Table 7-8 | Contraceptive Methods from Most to Least Effective

Category	Method	Key Points	Best
Sterilization	• Vasectomy • Tubal ligation	Permanent surgical procedure	Those who do not want to maintain their fertility
LARC	• Intrauterine device • Levonorgestrel • Copper Implant rod	• Surgically placed every 3–10 years, depending on the type • Quick return to fertility • Implanted subdermal in arm • Slow-release progesterone	• Desire low maintenance "get it and forget it" • Progesterone devices may help decrease heavy menses.
Injectable	Depo-Provera Progestin-only injection every 3 months	• Breakthrough bleeding; weight gain; black box warning bone loss • Injection: can take up to 18 months for ovulation to return	• Desire low maintenance "get it and forget it" • Can help with endometriosis
Estrogen and progestin combination	Oral contraceptive pills Patch Vaginal ring	• Pills: must take daily at the same time • Change weekly for 3 weeks • Contraindicated if over 200 lb • Plastic ring placed in vaginal fornix for 3 weeks	• Patient who will reliably use as directed and does not want LARC Nulliparous; wants less maintenance but does not want LARC
Mini-pill	Progesterone-only oral contraceptive	• Must take every day at the same time; no days off	Breastfeeding; cannot take estrogen
Barrier methods	Diaphragm Cervical cap Condom	• Effective immediately • Must be fitted by the provider • Made of latex • Protective against STIs • Readily available, inexpensive, low side effects	If hormones are contraindicated Anyone seeking nonpharmacologic intervention and prevention of STIs
Fertility awareness (natural family planning)	Periodic abstinence	• Abstinence from 4 to 5 days before ovulation until 2–3 days after ovulation • High level of motivation required to closely track basal body temperature and ovulation cycle	Other forms of contraception are undesired or contraindicated because of religious or medical reasons.

LARC, long-acting reversible contraception; STI, sexually transmitted infection.

a. Fertility awareness, i.e., "calendar method" predicts the day of ovulation based on average menstrual patterns, is based on the relative constancy (14 days) of the luteal phase and has a 25% to 35% failure rate.

b. The basal body temperature (BBT) method requires recording daily vaginal or rectal temperature before any activity is undertaken. Around ovulation, there is a rise of 0.3 to 0.48°C in the temperature that remains at a plateau for the rest of the cycle.

c. Although combining the calendar and BBT methods for contraception can be up to 95% effective, actual failure rates are 25% because of compliance issues.

d. The cervical mucus method requires daily evaluation of the mucus; fertile mucus is clear and stringy, resembling egg whites.

> Noninterventional birth control methods fail most often owing to noncompliance.

B. Sterilization methods are permanent, and most states require a 30-day waiting period before the procedure.

    1. Male: vasectomy entails cutting the vas deference bilaterally; blocks the transport of sperm from testicles. Must use backup method of birth control for 3 months or until semen sample shows absence of sperm.

    2. Female: salpingectomy or tubal ligation bilaterally; blocks the transport of the egg to the fallopian tube, where fertilization occurs.

C. Long-acting reversible contraception (LARC)

    1. General

        a. LARC includes the IUD and implantable rods.

        b. LARC used to be considered mainly for multiparous who desire reversible contraception; however, in recent years, they have become popular for younger, nulliparous women desiring a "get it and forget it" birth control option.

        c. Contraindications for both include current pregnancy, history of deep vein thrombosis (DVT); liver disease; breast cancer; or AUB.

    2. IUD

        a. Create changes in the endometrium that create a hostile environment for sperm.

        b. Failure rate is about 1%.

        c. IUDs are usually inserted during menses to assure the woman is not pregnant, and placement is easier because the cervical os is slightly open.

        d. Pros include immediate return to fertility upon removal.

        e. Relative contraindications include previous ectopic pregnancy, severe dysmenorrhea, and uterine abnormalities.

        f. Small risk of uterine perforation; higher incidence of spontaneous abortion if pregnancy occurs; increased risk of ectopic pregnancy

        g. Two IUDs are currently available in the United States.

            (1) Levonorgestrel-releasing IUD; usable for 3 to 5 years

                Small levels of progesterone released into bloodstream; results in light menses to amenorrhea for many women

            (2) Copper T; usable for 10 years

                May cause heavier menstrual bleeding and cramping

> IUDs have relative contraindications of previous ectopic pregnancy, dysmenorrhea, and uterine structural abnormality.

    3. Implantable rods

        a. Nexplanon relies on the implantation of rods that release levonorgestrel for 3 years.

        b. Failure rate is <1%.

        c. Pros include quick return to fertility upon removal.

        d. Side effects include menstrual irregularity, headache, and weight gain.

D. Estrogen and Progesterone Combination Contraception

    1. Estrogen and progesterone combination birth control (CBC) includes oral contraception pills, the patch, and the ring.

2. CBCs contain synthetic steroids (similar to natural estrogens and progestins) used in doses and combinations that inhibit ovulation. The estrogen component is usually ethinylestradiol or mestranol. The progestin component is one of the 19 nortestosterones such as norethindrone acetate, or others.

3. Mechanism of action includes suppressing ovulation by inhibiting FSH and LH; thickening the cervical mucus; thinning the endometrium.

4. Theoretical failure rate for combination is <1%; actual rates are 5% to 10% owing to compliance issues.

5. Advantages

  a. Lower rates of benign breast disease, iron deficiency anemia, and PID, as well as fewer ovarian cysts.

  b. Protection against ectopic pregnancy; reduced risk of ovarian and endometrial cancer; reduction of AUB (dysmenorrhea and menorrhagia); and improvements in hirsutism, acne, and symptoms of endometriosis. Oral contraceptives may also protect against rheumatoid arthritis.

> The risk of vascular complications with combined contraceptives increases with age and smoking status

6. Disadvantages

  a. Increased risk of thromboembolic disease, particularly in smokers older than 35 years of age, and abnormal lipids

  b. Possible increased risk of breast cancer and, rarely, hypertension, cholelithiasis, and benign liver tumors

7. Adverse effects

  a. Missed periods, intermenstrual bleeding, bloating, acne, nausea, headaches, and weight gain

  b. Most of these problems resolve within the first few months of use and are less common with current low-dose formulations.

  c. The warning signs for combination methods can be summarized in the acronym ACHES: Abdominal pain, Chest pain, Headaches, Eye problems, Severe leg pain.

> Warning signs for patients using combination birth control is ACHES: Abdominal pain, Chest pain, Headache, Eye problems, Severe leg pain.

8. Types of CBCs

  a. A pill taken daily, at the same time.

    (1) Most often begins with the onset of menses or the following Sunday; active pills are taken for 21 days, followed by 7 days of no pills or placebos.

    (2) A newer method allows for 84 days of active pills; this results in limiting menses to four times per year.

    (3) Withdrawal bleeding begins within 3 to 5 days of the last active pill.

  b. The transdermal patch is applied in alternating locations, once a week, for 3 weeks. In the fourth week, the last patch is removed and a woman has menses.

    (1) The patch should never be placed on the breast.

    (2) It is not effective in women who weigh more than 200 lb.

  c. The Ring: A hormone-impregnated vaginal ring is inserted for 3 weeks and then removed for 1 week; withdrawal bleeding should occur. This device is best for young, nulliparous women.

E. Progesterone-only methods

  1. Progesterone-only methods are often used for patients who have an intolerance or contraindication to estrogen-containing methods.

  2. Minipills (progestin-only) are half as effective as combination pills and may cause AUB, especially intermittent spotting. They are most useful in lactating women and for smokers over 35 years of age.

  3. Intramuscular (IM) injection (Depo-Provera): Medroxyprogesterone acetate, 150 mg every 90 days

        a. Black box warning: may lead to calcium loss, bone weakness, and osteoporosis; use should be limited to 2 years.

        b. The failure rate is 0.3% in the first year.

        c. Fertility rates return to normal within 18 months of discontinuation, so this is not a good choice for women looking for short-term birth control.

        d. Side effects include weight gain, headache, and mood fluctuations.

F. Barrier methods include male and female condoms, cervical caps, and diaphragms.

    1. Condoms provide additional protection against sexually transmitted infections.

    2. Condoms have up to a 20% failure rate because of noncompliance with best practices.

    3. The common spermicides used with barrier methods are nonoxynol-9 and octoxynol-3.

G. Emergency (postcoital) contraception

> *Emergency contraception is best within 72 hours of unprotected intercourse.*

    1. The most common formulation is high-dose progestin-only pills given within 72 hours of unprotected intercourse. It is available over the counter.

    2. One product is effective up to 120 hours post intercourse but requires a prescription.

    3. Emergency contraception is over 85% effective.

    4. Nausea and vomiting are frequent adverse effects.

H. Termination of pregnancy

    1. There is significant variation in state laws allowing elective termination of pregnancy, especially for minors.

    2. Medical abortion

        a. Recommended up to 70 days (10 weeks) from last menstrual period (LMP). Effectiveness is 98%. Patient must be reliable to return to office to be candidate.

        b. Contraindications are long-term corticosteroid use, hematologic disorders, and anticoagulation use.

        c. Step 1 is oral mifepristone. Step 2, given 24 to 48 hours later, is oral misoprostol. Step 3 is follow-up with ultrasonography 2 to 14 days later.

    3. Surgical abortion

        a. D&C or suction, up to 16 weeks from LMP.

        b. Dilation and evacuation, up to 24 weeks in some states.

Infertility

A. General characteristics

    1. Infertility is generally defined as a failure to conceive after 1 year of unprotected intercourse. Surveys estimate that up to 15% of reproductive-age couples in the United States are infertile. Prevalence ranges from 7% to 28%, increasing as a woman ages.

    2. The most common female factor is anovulatory menstrual cycles. Common causes of anovulatory cycles include polycystic ovarian syndrome, thyroid dysfunction, and stress. Other causes include infection, endometriosis, and endometrial and cervical structural abnormalities.

> *A thorough history including sexual activity is the first and most important step in the workup of infertility.*

    3. The most common male factor is abnormal sperm count or morphology. Other causes include epididymitis, varicocele, and endocrine disorders.

B. A detailed history of pregnancy with past partners and current coitus practices are the first step in determining a cause. Clinical examination is typically normal.

C. Diagnostic studies

    1. Phase I is inexpensive and noninvasive.

        a. Ovulation tracking, including menstrual diary, BBT, ovulation prediction tests, and progesterone levels on day 21 of menstrual cycle confirm ovulation (or anovulation).

b. High FSH indicates perimenopausal state. Prolactin and TSH tests may be helpful.

c. Semen analysis to confirm sperm count and motility.

d. Ultrasonography to assay pelvic structure.

2. Phase 2 is more expensive and/or more invasive

a. Hysteroscopy/endometrial biopsy to view the internal lining of the uterus and obtain tissue samples.

b. Hysterosalpingography determines tubal patency and uterine abnormalities.

c. Laparoscopy may be recommended to view internal structures and tissues.

D. Treatments currently have an overall success rate of about 85%.

1. Clomiphene citrate, 50 to 100 mg for 5 days beginning on day 3, 4, or 5 of the cycle, should be given to anovulatory women to promote ovulation.

2. Artificial insemination is an alternative for couples with abnormal postcoital tests.

3. Other treatments depend on the cause of infertility, the couple's resources, and the age of the woman.

4. Assisted reproductive technologies include in vitro fertilization, gamete intrafallopian transfer, zygote intrafallopian transfer, and surrogate options.

> Chlamydia is the most common cause of PID; always cotreat empirically for gonorrhea.

Pelvic Inflammatory Disease

A. General characteristics

1. PID includes acute salpingitis (gonococcal or nongonococcal), IUD-related pelvic cellulitis, tubo-ovarian abscess, and pelvic abscess.

2. It is usually polymicrobial (mixed aerobic and anaerobic). Most are bacterial, but viral, fungal, or parasitic causes are known.

3. Complications include infertility and ectopic pregnancy.

> The most common etiology of PID is chlamydia, a sexually transmitted infection.

B. **Clinical features**

1. Lower abdominal and pelvic pain is typically bilateral. Nausea (with or without vomiting), headache, and lower back pain are common. Fever may or may not be present.

2. Examination reveals lower abdominal and pelvic pain and cervical motion tenderness (chandelier sign). Purulent discharge and inflammation of Bartholin's or Skene glands may be present.

3. An adnexal mass may indicate a tubo-ovarian abscess.

C. Diagnostic studies

1. DNA probes for gonorrhea and chlamydia (most common cause of PID) have largely replaced Gram staining and culture of any discharge.

2. Indications for hospitalization include pregnancy; lack of response or tolerance to oral medications; nonadherence to treatment; inability to take oral medication secondary to nausea; severe illness (high fever, nausea, vomiting, severe abdominal pain); complicated PID (i.e., pelvic or tubo-ovarian abscess); and possible need for surgical intervention or diagnostic exploratory. Women with severe disease should be hospitalized for IV antibiotic therapy and possible surgery.

3. Transvaginal ultrasonography is helpful in differentiating acute and chronic inflammation or the presence of adnexal masses.

D. **Treatment**

1. Women with mild disease can be treated as outpatients with antibiotics, antipyretics, analgesics, and bed rest; if present, an IUD should be removed.

2. Treatment varies, based on local resistance to antibiotics.

3. Sex partners should be evaluated and treated.

Practice Questions

Directions: *Each of the numbered items or incomplete statements in this section is followed by a list of answers or completions of the statement. Select the ONE lettered answer or completion that is BEST in each case.*

1. A 19-year-old presents at the emergency department with acute abdominal and pelvic pain. She is febrile and nauseated. Examination reveals lower abdominal and pelvic tenderness as well as moderate cervical motion tenderness. What is the next best step?
   A. Cervical scraping for culture and sensitivity
   B. Diagnostic culdocentesis
   C. Hospitalization and IV antibiotics
   D. Oral antibiotics and analgesics, follow-up in 2 days
   E. Surgical consult

2. A 36-year-old G3P3003 is seeking information regarding contraception. She smokes ½ pack per day, is allergic to latex, weighs 212 lb, and is unsure about future pregnancies. Which of the following would be the best choice for this patient?
   A. Coitus interruptus
   B. Diaphragm
   C. IUD
   D. Oral contraception pills (OCPs)
   E. Transdermal patch

3. A new mother presents for evaluation of her right breast. She has been breastfeeding successfully for 6 weeks. The baby is growing and satisfied. She has a low-grade fever, and the lateral right breast is red and warm. What is the most likely pathogen?
   A. *Candida albicans*
   B. *Escherichia coli*
   C. *Malassezia furfur*
   D. *Staphylococcus aureus*
   E. *Streptomyces viridans*

4. A Pap smear from a 23-year-old female returns as CIN-1; HPV is positive. What is the recommended follow-up?
   A. Colposcopy with biopsy
   B. Conization
   C. Cryocautery
   D. LEEP
   E. Repeat Pap in 6 months

5. A 32-year-old G0P0 presents for infertility workup. She and her partner have been trying unsuccessfully to get pregnant for 2 years. Menses are irregular, coming every 3 to 6 weeks; she has no history of abnormal Pap or pelvic examination. She is overweight and states her weight has always been a problem despite diet and exercise. Her primary physician has warned her that she is prediabetic and has high lipid levels. What is the expected result of a pelvic ultrasound?
   A. Abnormally thick uterine wall
   B. Bicornuate uterus
   C. Scar tissue surrounding Fallopian tubes
   D. Shortened cervix
   E. String of pearls appearance in ovaries

6. Pelvic examination of a 23-year-old female reveals an ovarian mass. Ultrasonography confirms a 2 × 2 cm simple, fluid-filled cyst. What is the recommended next step?
   A. Draw blood for *BRAC1* and *BRAC2*
   B. Laparoscopic evaluation with possible biopsy
   C. Monitor over the next one to two cycles and then reassess
   D. Begin oral contraceptives
   E. Peritoneal fine-needle aspiration (FNA)

7. A 29-year-old presents for workup of extremely painful menses which often require absence from work. She denies dyspareunia, dyschezia, or intermittent bleeding. On examination, she is tender with palpation of the right cul-de-sac. What is the recommended management at this time?
   A. Exploratory laparotomy to investigate for external uterine tissue
   B. Order pelvic ultrasonography to investigate for an abnormal uterus
   C. Prescribe a tapering dose of prednisone
   D. Treat with danazol × 3 months and reassess
   E. Give a trial of OCPs for symptoms relief

8. A 33-year-old G3P2102 complains of pressure or fullness in the pelvis. Menses remain regular, although she has had a few episodes of intermenstrual spotting in the past year. LMP was 3 weeks ago. Examination reveals an enlarged, irregular uterine mass. What is the most likely diagnosis?
   A. Ectopic pregnancy
   B. Endometrial cancer
   C. Hydatidiform mole
   D. Leiomyomata
   E. Ovarian cancer

9. A 27-year-old female describes symptoms of irritability, insomnia, bloating, depression, and fatigue that begin each month about 1 week prior to menses and abate within 2 days of menses. She denies a history of mental health problems, vaginal discharge, or dyspareunia. Pelvic examination is normal. Which of the following lifestyle changes is most likely to help alleviate her symptoms?
   A. Avoid exercise the week before menses
   B. Recommend B-complex vitamin daily
   C. Recommend OCPs
   D. Reduce caffeine
   E. Reduce complex carbohydrates

10. A 17-year-old complains of painful lower pelvic cramping and breast tenderness with menses. She has one sexual partner and uses condoms for contraception. She denies vaginal discharge, abnormal bleeding, or dyspareunia. Pelvic examination is unremarkable. What is the recommended management?
    A. Assure here that symptoms will abate with time
    B. Avoid cardio exercises during menses
    C. Encourage a diet very low in sodium
    D. Increase caffeine intake prior to menses
    E. NSAID, begin 2 to 3 days before menses and continue through the cycle

11. A 32-year-old presents for evaluation of sore breasts. Examination reveals multiple tender lesions. Further questioning confirms that the breast fluctuates in size and tenderness through her menses cycles. What lifestyle intervention will most likely relieve her discomfort?
A. Avoid exercise 1 week prior to menses
B. Avoid simple carbohydrates in diet
C. Local ice packs as needed
D. Reduce alcohol intake during the second half of cycle
E. Wear a supportive bra

12. A 26-year-old is concerned because she had unprotected sex 2 days ago. She decides to take synthetic progestin pills (emergency contraception) as directed to prevent pregnancy. What is the most common side effect for which she should be warned?
A. Acne-like lesions
B. Headaches
C. Galactorrhea
D. Nausea and vomiting
E. Swollen labia

Practice Answers

1. C. *Gynecology; Clinical Intervention; PID*

Acute pain and cervical motion tenderness indicate PID. Patients with mild disease may be treated as outpatients with oral antibiotics and close follow-up. However, more severe disease, as indicated by fever and nausea, warrants hospitalization and IV antibiotics. Once stable, she can be switched to oral antibiotics and discharged. Cervical specimens are not routinely taken but may be needed if the patient does not respond to antibiotics in order to get a more definitive diagnosis.

2. C. *Gynecology; Clinical Intervention; Contraception*

This patient should avoid hormone therapies because of her increased risk of thromboembolism (age and smoking history). Latex allergy rules out use of the diaphragm. The transdermal patch is not effective in patients weighing more than 200 lb. Coitus interruptus is safe but very unreliable.

3. D. *Gynecology; Basic Science; Mastitis*

Mastitis is almost universally found in lactating women. The area is inflamed and tender. *S. aureus* is notoriously implicated. If there is suspicion of an abscess, it should be drained. Otherwise, ice to the area and mild analgesia are recommended. The mother should pump her breast to maintain mild production but discard for the first 24 to 48 hours until afebrile. *Candida* is the cause of thrush. *Malassezia furfur* is the causative agent in tinea versicolor.

4. E. *Gynecology; Clinical Intervention; Cervical Dysplasia*

CIN-1 in a young woman who is HPV-positive will likely resolve with time. A greater level of dysplasia may warrant further investigation. LEEP or cryotherapy is an option for higher grade, preinvasive neoplasia. Conization is done if the lesion is large. A colposcopy with biopsy is necessary if the specimen returns CIS or beyond.

5. E. *Gynecology; Diagnostic Studies; PCOS*

This patient likely has PCOS. Hirsutism, infertility, acne, and menses irregularity are hallmarks. Impaired glucose tolerance is present in 30%. Patients should be treated with metformin which will improve lipid and glucose levels and improve fertility.

6. C. *Gynecology; Clinical Intervention; Ovarian Cyst*

A single simple ovarian cyst in a woman under the age of 35 is likely benign. Signs of malignancy include heterogeneous mass, debris or solid filled, and nontender. For simple cysts, monitoring through the next few cycles may prove sufficient as most will resolve. Laparoscopic or percutaneous specimen finding is not recommended unless the patient progresses or symptoms are irregular. Evaluation of cancer markers is not routinely done until after a diagnosis of a malignancy. Oral contraceptives are no help with ovarian cysts.

7. E. *Gynecology; Clinical Intervention; Endometriosis*

Endometriosis is defined as functional uterine tissue outside the uterine wall. It is a common cause of infertility. A laparotomy will provide a definitive diagnosis, but this is not necessary. Patients are treated empirically. NSAIDs and prostaglandin synthetase inhibitors will provide symptomatic relief, but oral contraceptive pills may also prevent symptoms. Danazol or a GnRH may improve fertility.

8. D. *Gynecology; Diagnosis; Leiomyomata*

Leiomyomata (fibroids) most commonly develop in women in their 30s. Asymptomatic fibroids can be watched; once symptomatic, surgical options should be considered. Menses would be late with an ectopic pregnancy. Endometrial cancer presents with abnormal bleeding, most commonly post menopause. Hydatidiform moles are usually diagnosed in the first trimester of an assumed pregnancy. Ovarian cancer is often missed until late in disease; early symptoms are vague and nonspecific; however, the uterine mass is unlikely.

9. D. *Gynecology; Health Maintenance; Premenstrual Syndrome*

PMS manifests symptoms 1 week prior to 2 days after onset of menses; patients are symptom-free for the first 2 weeks of each cycle. There is no consensus regarding pathology or treatment. Evidence supports the following recommendations to reduce symptoms: reduce caffeine, restrict salt, low-dairy and low-fat diet, increased high complex carbohydrates, increased exercise, and stress reduction.

10. E. *Gynecology; Clinical Intervention; Dysmenorrhea*

Primary dysmenorrhea is thought to be because of excess prostaglandins and leukotrienes. A trial of NSAIDs is recommended. Dietary and physical interventions have not proven helpful.

11. E. *Gynecology; Health Maintenance; Fibrocystic Changes*

Fibrocystic breasts can be asymptomatic or painful and tender masses. The key to diagnosis is fluctuation during the cycles.

Avoidance of caffeine and a supportive bra are the best recommendations. Ice packs may reduce tenderness but are impractical on an ongoing basis.

12. D. *Gynecology; Pharmacology; Emergency Contraception*

The most common side effect of emergency contraception is nausea and vomiting. Breast tenderness may occur, but not galactorrhea. Headache, acne, and swollen labia are not seen.

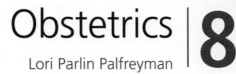

Obstetrics | 8

Lori Parlin Palfreyman

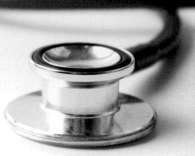

Routine Prenatal Care and Prenatal Diagnostic Testing

A. Routine prenatal care

  1. General characteristics

    a. An initial obstetric history includes subjective symptoms and signs (Table 8-1) of pregnancy as well as the patient's general medical, obstetric, and family history (Table 8-2).

    b. The due date or expected date of confinement (EDC) can be calculated using Nägele or McDonald's rule: Start at the first day of the last menstrual period (LMP), go back 3 months, and add 7 days. For example, if the LMP is January 15, go back 3 months to October 15 and add 7 days, making the EDC October 22. This is based on a 28-day menstrual cycle and must be adjusted for shorter or longer cycles.

    c. The patient's obstetric history can be expressed as gravida (G; number of total pregnancies) and parity (P; number of deliveries). The parity is denoted as a sequence of four digits P####. The full expression is written $G_\#P_{TPAL}$, signifying the

Table 8-1 | **Manifestations of Pregnancy**

Symptoms
Amenorrhea
Nausea/vomiting
Breast tenderness
Quickening (fetal movement)
Nullipara: 18–20 weeks
Multipara: 14–16 weeks
Easy fatigability
Urinary frequency, nocturia, infection

Signs
Chadwick's sign (bluish discoloration of vagina and cervix)
Increased basal body temperature
Skin changes
Melasma/chloasma (dark patches on face)
Linea nigra (dark vertical line through the midline of abdomen)
Positive pregnancy test
Hegar's sign (softening between fundus and cervix)
Uterine growth
12 weeks: at symphysis pubis
16 weeks: midway between pubis and umbilicus
20 weeks: at umbilicus
After 20 weeks: 1 cm for every week of gestation
Fetal heart tones: 9 weeks by Doppler
Palpation of fetus
Ultrasonography of fetus: heartbeat at 5–6 weeks

Table 8-2 | Patient History on Initial Prenatal Office Visit

Menstrual history
    Last menstrual period
Present pregnancy
    See Table 8-1
Previous pregnancies
    Vaginal vs. cesarean section and reason for cesarean section
    Complications
    Size of baby, Apgar scores
Medical history
    Gynecologic history: Pap smears, ovarian cysts, fibroids, STIs
    Cardiovascular
    Asthma
    Autoimmune disorders
    Bleeding disorders
    Seizure disorders
Surgical history
    Abdominal surgery
    Pelvic surgery
Family history
    Chromosomal abnormalities
    Mental retardation
    Diabetes
Social history
    Alcohol
    Drugs
    Diet

STIs, sexually transmitted infections.

number of **T**erm infants (37 to 42 weeks of gestation), **P**remature deliveries (20 to 36 weeks of gestation), **A**bortions (therapeutic and/or spontaneous, occurring before 20 weeks of gestation), and **L**iving children.

d. The initial visit should take place 6 to 8 weeks after the LMP. Generally, a woman is examined every 4 weeks until 32nd week of gestation, every 2 weeks up to 36 weeks of gestation, and then weekly until delivery.

e. See Table 8-3. After the initial visit, each subsequent prenatal visit includes a focused history and physical examination, including assessment of general health, diet, activity, compliance with vitamins, maternal weight gain, edema, fetal movement, and blood pressure (BP); check of fundal height starting at 20 weeks' gestation and fetal heart tones starting at 10 weeks' gestation; and urinalysis for glucosuria, ketonuria, and proteinuria. Vaginal examination to assess cervical dilation is added after 36 weeks or as indicated.

2. Clinical features

    a. Uterine growth throughout pregnancy (Fig. 8-1)

        (1) At 20 weeks, the fundus is at the umbilicus.

> Nägele's rule:
> LMP − 3 months
> + 7 days.
> Parity = TPAL (**t**erm, **p**remature, **a**bortion, **l**iving)

Table 8-3 | Components of Routine Prenatal Visit

- Focused history and physical examination
- General health, diet, activity
- Compliance with vitamins
- Maternal weight gain
- Edema
- Fetal movement
- Blood pressure
- Fundal height (starting at 20 weeks)
- Fetal heart tones (starting at 10 weeks)
- Urinalysis (glucose, ketones, protein)
- Vaginal examination (after 36 weeks or as indicated)

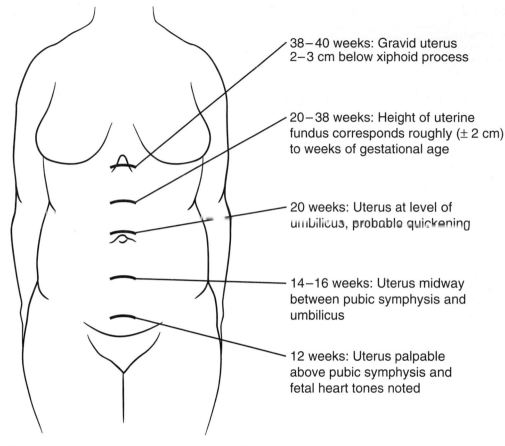

38–40 weeks: Gravid uterus
2–3 cm below xiphoid process

20–38 weeks: Height of uterine
fundus corresponds roughly (± 2 cm)
to weeks of gestational age

20 weeks: Uterus at level of
umbilicus, probable quickening

14–16 weeks: Uterus midway
between pubic symphysis and
umbilicus

12 weeks: Uterus palpable
above pubic symphysis and
fetal heart tones noted

Figure 8-1 ▶ Uterine size and position throughout gestation.

(2) From 21 weeks on, the height of the uterine fundus from pubic bone should correlate roughly with the number of weeks of gestation.

b. Fetal heart tones can be appreciated beginning at 9 to 12 weeks using a handheld transabdominal Doppler; normal fetal heart rate (HR) is 110 to 160 bpm.

c. Quickening, or the first awareness of fetal movement, usually occurs at 18 to 20 weeks in a primigravida and as early as 14 to 18 weeks in a multigravida.

d. Common complaints such as backache, increasing varicosities, heartburn, hemorrhoids, bleeding gums, profuse salivation, and fatigue need to be evaluated but can be associated with an otherwise healthy pregnancy.

e. Normal physiologic changes include an increase in blood volume up to 45%; pulse rate increase up to 20 bpm; elevated plasma cholesterol levels, white blood cell count, total T3 and T4, and insulin levels. There may also be a normal physiologic decrease in hemoglobin, hematocrit, thyroid-stimulating hormone (TSH), fasting glucose, blood urea nitrogen (BUN), creatinine, and uric acid.

B. Prenatal screening and diagnostic testing

1. Table 8-4 lists the most common laboratory and prenatal testing by gestational age. All women should be offered screening tests, regardless of maternal age.

2. First-trimester screening and diagnostic testing

a. Maternal blood levels of pregnancy-associated plasma protein A (PAPP-A) and free β-human chorionic gonadotropin (free β-hCG): Abnormally low PAPP-A and abnormally high free β-hCG indicate increased risk of trisomy 21 and other genetic disorders.

Table 8-4 | Prenatal Laboratories and Screening/Diagnostic Tests

First Prenatal Visit	First Trimester	Second Trimester	Third Trimester
• CBC • Blood type and Rh • Rubella titer • Urinalysis • Hepatitis B serum antigen • Hepatitis C • VDRL or RPR (syphilis screen) • HIV testing offered • Chlamydia and gonorrhea, as indicated • PPD, as indicated • Random glucose (risk for diabetes or past gestational diabetes • Cystic fibrosis, sickle cell, other conditions per maternal and paternal history • Coombs' test (irregular antibody screen) • Pap smear, as indicated	• PAPP-A • Free β-hCG • Nuchal translucency (10–13 weeks) • Ultrasound (confirm EDC) • CVS (10–13 weeks)	• Unconjugated estriol • Maternal serum AFP • Inhibin A • Ultrasound (anatomy scan) • Amniocentesis (15–18 weeks)	• Screen for gestational diabetes (24–28 weeks) • In unsensitized Rh patients, repeat antibody titers (followed by Rh immunoglobulin) (28 weeks) • Vaginal culture for group B streptococci (35 weeks) • Ultrasound, as needed • Hemoglobin and hematocrit (35 weeks) • NST, as needed • Biophysical profile, as needed

AFP, α-fetoprotein; CBC, complete blood count; CVS, chorionic villi sampling; NST, nonstress test; PAPP-A, pregnancy-associated plasma protein A; β-hCG, β-human chorionic gonadotropin; RPR, rapid plasma regain test; VDRL, venereal disease research laboratory.

Recommended from American College of Obstetricians and Gynecologists. ACOG Practice Bulletin. Clinical management guidelines for obstetrician gynecologists. *Obstet Gynecol*. June, 2020. https://www.acog.org/womens-health/faqs/routine-tests-during-pregnancy

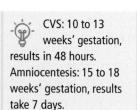

CVS: 10 to 13 weeks' gestation, results in 48 hours. Amniocentesis: 15 to 18 weeks' gestation, results take 7 days.

  b. Ultrasonography for establishing or confirming EDC and detecting multiple gestations is usually done at 6 to 8 weeks at the first prenatal visit: Transvaginal ultrasound can detect fetal heart activity as early as 5 to 6 weeks after the LMP.

  c. Nuchal translucency screening test (also known as a *nuchal fold scan*)

   (1) Ultrasound measurement of the nuchal space is performed at 10 to 13 weeks. It screens for trisomies 13, 18, and 21 as well as for Turner's syndrome (45,X0).

   (2) If an abnormally wide measurement for gestational age is detected, genetic counseling is recommended. Chorionic villus sampling (CVS) or amniocentesis is offered as part of the genetic counseling.

   (3) The combination of the first-trimester nuchal translucency measurement and PAPP-A and β-hCG screening can detect 82% to 87% of trisomy 21 disorders.

  d. Chorionic villus sampling

   (1) CVS is performed between 10 and 13 weeks; a catheter or needle is inserted through the cervix or the abdomen, based on the location of the placenta, under ultrasound guidance to biopsy placental tissue.

   (2) Indications for CVS are listed in Table 8-5.

   (3) The advantage of CVS is its ability to be performed during the first trimester, allowing the option of a first-trimester termination if a major malformation is detected. Also, preliminary results are available within 48 hours after the procedure. CVS is considered a diagnostic, and not screening, test.

   (4) The disadvantage of CVS is that, unlike amniocentesis, CVS specimens cannot detect neural tube defects. The risk of spontaneous abortion after CVS is the same as amniocentesis when adjusted for the earlier gestational age for the CVS procedure.

Table 8-5 | Indications for Genetic Counseling, Including Chorionic Villus Sampling or Amniocentesis

- Maternal age of 35 years or older
- Previous child with chromosomal abnormality
- Patient or father of baby with chromosomal anomaly
- Family history of chromosomal anomaly
- Neural tube defect risk (amniocentesis only)
- Abnormal first-trimester or second-trimester maternal serum screening tests
- Two previous pregnancy losses
- Known exposure to teratogens
- Abnormal ultrasound

3. Second-trimester screening and diagnostic testing

   a. Screening tests include serum levels of unconjugated estriol, maternal α-fetoprotein (AFP), and inhibin A.

     (1) Abnormally low unconjugated estriol and AFP and abnormally high inhibin A indicate increased risk of trisomy 21 and other genetic disorders.

     (2) Abnormally high levels of AFP indicate increased risk for neural tube defects. AFP can detect up to 75% to 85% of open neural tube defects such as spina bifida and anencephaly.

     (3) Combining the first-trimester maternal serum blood tests with second-trimester maternal serum blood tests can detect 94% to 96% of trisomy 21 disorders.

   b. Ultrasound is an accurate modality to check for fetal viability, correlate appropriate growth in relation to gestational age, check for placental status and location, and evaluate amniotic fluid level. It can also be used to help detect lethal malformations and as a follow-up to abnormal prenatal serum screening tests.

   c. Amniocentesis involves the withdrawal of amniotic fluid via needle through the maternal abdomen under ultrasound guidance for prenatal diagnosis.

     (1) It is usually performed between 15 and 18 weeks of gestation.

     (2) Indications for amniocentesis are listed in Table 8-5.

     (3) The advantage of amniocentesis is its availability after the second-trimester screening tests and routine sonographic fetal anatomy scan at 16 to 20 weeks. The disadvantage of amniocentesis is that it is performed during the second trimester; therefore, if termination of the pregnancy is chosen, a more complicated procedure is involved. Also, results from the test are not available for a minimum of 7 days.

> In third trimester, nonstress test (NST) and sonographic biophysical profile (BPP) are fetal well-being assessments.

4. Third-trimester screening for fetal well-being

   a. The nonstress test (NST), conducted with an external Doppler monitor to assess the fetal HR and an external monitor for uterine contractions, is used near term to monitor fetal well-being. The NST is the first-line antepartum test to assess fetal well-being. When a pregnancy is impacted by preexisting maternal conditions or pregnancy-related complications that warrant increased surveillance, the NST will be routinely performed.

     (1) Baseline fetal HR is 110 to 160 bpm.

     (2) The NST is conducted for 20 minutes. A normal (reactive) NST requires a minimum of two accelerations of fetal HR in 20 minutes; the accelerations must increase at least 15 bpm from the baseline HR for a duration of 15 seconds; there must also be an absence of HR decelerations.

     (3) A nonreactive NST may be caused by a variety of factors including benign fetal sleep cycles or maternal dehydration or insufficient eating; or more worrisome fetal conditions. Routine antepartum tests to evaluate a nonreactive NST include vibroacoustic stimulation and the sonographic biophysical profile (BPP).

(4) Contractions usually decrease the flow of blood to the placenta. This may be poorly tolerated by the stressed fetus, which can lead to a variety of fetal HR decelerations. The pattern of the deceleration, in relation to maternal contractions, identifies different conditions.

   (a) Early decelerations, defined as a mirror of the contraction, usually indicate that the cervix is fully dilated and the mother may begin to push.

   (b) Late decelerations, defined as a decrease in the fetal HR *after* the peak of the contraction, indicate fetal hypoxia and warrant intervention.

b. Ultrasonography is used late in pregnancy to monitor fetal well-being. It can be used either alone or in the form of a scored examination (BPP).

   (1) The BPP examines five parameters: NST, amniotic fluid level, gross fetal movements, fetal tone, and fetal breathing.

   (2) Each parameter has a maximum of two points; a total of 10 points is possible. The risk of asphyxia increases with lower scores.

> Biophysical profile (BPP):
> nonstress test
> amniotic fluid level
> gross fetal movement
> fetal tone fetal breathing

High-Risk Pregnancy

A. Teenage pregnancy has an increased risk of premature delivery and low fetal birth weight.

B. Multiple gestation

   1. General characteristics

   a. The overall incidence of multiple births in the United States is 3% and has been increasing during the past 30 years, in part as a result of the use of assisted reproductive techniques and ovulation induction.

   b. With multiple gestation, all the same symptoms of pregnancy generally occur, but they are often more severe. Prenatal visits should occur more frequently than with single gestations.

   c. Prenatal screening tests are less reliable in multiple pregnancies compared to singleton pregnancies.

   d. Twins are the most common form of multiple gestation.

> Twinning occurs in approximately 1 in 250 pregnancies.

   (1) Two-thirds of twins are dizygotic or fraternal (i.e., formed by the fertilization of two ova). The incidence of dizygotic twins is increased in those with a family history of twins and those undergoing fertility treatment.

   (2) Monozygotic twins (i.e., those formed from the fertilization of one ovum) occur randomly and may be associated with fetal transfusion syndrome and discordant fetal growth.

   e. Maternal complications

   (1) The most common complications of multiple gestation are spontaneous abortion and preterm birth.

   (2) There is also an increased maternal risk for preeclampsia and anemia.

   f. Fetal complications include intrauterine growth restriction, cord complications, death of one fetus, congenital anomalies, abnormal or breech presentation, and placental abruption or placenta previa.

Complications of Pregnancy

A. Ectopic pregnancy

   1. General characteristics

   a. Ectopic pregnancy is the implantation of a pregnancy anywhere but the endometrium.

   b. More than 95% of ectopic pregnancies occur in the fallopian tube, and 70% of tubal pregnancies occur in the ampulla of the tube.

   c. The most common cause of ectopic pregnancy is occlusion of the tube secondary to adhesions.

   d. The most common risk factors for ectopic pregnancy include conditions that lead to adhesions including history of a previous ectopic pregnancy, previous salpingitis (caused by pelvic inflammatory disease), previous abdominal, or tubal surgery. The use of an intrauterine device and assisted reproduction also lead to higher risk.

> The #1 location of ectopic pregnancy is the ampulla of the fallopian tube.

2. Clinical features

   a. Ectopic pregnancy universally results in pelvic or abdominal pain. The classic presentation includes unilateral adnexal pain, amenorrhea or spotting, and tenderness or mass on pelvic examination (Table 8-6). Other symptoms may include dizziness or syncope as well as gastrointestinal (GI) distress.

   b. Signs and symptoms associated with a ruptured ectopic pregnancy are severe abdominal or shoulder pain associated with peritonitis, tachycardia, syncope, and orthostatic hypotension.

3. Diagnostic studies

   a. Serum levels of hCG normally double every 48 hours. If serial increases of hCG are less than expected, ectopic gestation should be suspected until the diagnosis has been definitively excluded.

   b. Transvaginal ultrasonography is diagnostic in 90% of cases of ectopic gestation.

   c. Women with an hCG titer of 1,000 to 2,000 mU per mL (some references say as high as 3,500 mU/mL) should show evidence of a developing intrauterine gestation on transvaginal ultrasound. If no such evidence is found, ectopic pregnancy is the clinical diagnosis.

4. Management

   a. Medical treatment with methotrexate, a folic acid analog, can be used to treat up to one-third of ectopic gestations when diagnosed early and the patient is hemodynamically stable. Criteria for methotrexate treatment are listed in Table 8-7.

   b. Surgical treatment usually involves removal of the ectopic gestation, most commonly via laparoscopy.

   c. Follow-up testing using serial quantitative serum hCG levels is crucial to exclude any remaining evidence of pregnancy.

> Medical management is contraindicated if ectopic pregnancy is >3.5 cm.

B. Spontaneous abortion

   1. General characteristics

     a. Abortion is the ending of a pregnancy, by any means, before 20 weeks of gestation.

     b. Spontaneous abortion is the spontaneous, premature expulsion of the products of conception; it occurs in up to 15% to 20% of clinically recognized pregnancies.

Table 8-6 | Signs and Symptoms Associated with Ectopic Pregnancy

Signs/Symptoms	Percent of Cases
Pain	90
Abnormal menstruation	75
Tachycardia, hypotension	75
Pelvic mass	30–50
Dizziness or syncope	30–50
Shock	10
Gastrointestinal symptoms	Often

Adapted from DeCherney A, Nathan L, Laurfer, N, Roman, A. *Current Diagnosis & Treatment: Obstetrics & Gynecology*. 12th ed. McGraw-Hill Companies; 2019.

Table 8-7 | Indications for Medical Treatment for Ectopic Pregnancy

Criteria for Methotrexate	Surgical Intervention
• Ectopic measures <3.5 cm • β-hCG <5,000 mIU/mL • Thrombocytes >100,000 • Hemodynamically stable • No blood disorders • No pulmonary disease • No peptic ulcer • Normal renal function • Normal hepatic function • Compliant patient and able to return for follow-up	• Emergency situations • Anyone who does not meet the criteria for methotrexate management

β-hCG, β-human chorionic gonadotropin.

    c. Eighty percent of spontaneous abortions occur during the first trimester of pregnancy; of these, up to 50% are associated with chromosomal abnormalities.

    d. The biggest single risk factor is advanced maternal age (over 35 years) and secondarily a prior spontaneous abortion. Other factors that increase the risk of spontaneous abortion include smoking, infection, maternal systemic disease, immunologic parameters, and drug use.

2. Clinical features

    a. Table 8-8 indicates the various classifications of spontaneous abortion.

    b. Bleeding is variable on examination.

    c. Uterine size often does not correlate appropriately with the LMP, and the fundus of the uterus may be boggy or tender.

3. Diagnostic studies

    a. Serial hCG titers, serum progesterone, or serial ultrasonography may be required to confirm a viable pregnancy.

    b. Ultrasound findings in a nonviable pregnancy may include inappropriate development or interval growth, poorly formed or unformed fetal pole, and fetal demise.

    c. Blood type and Rh status are necessary tests to prevent possible Rh sensitization in the mother.

4. Management

    a. If the pregnancy has been definitively determined to be no longer viable, the uterus must be emptied.

    b. If the patient desires, she may be permitted to go home and allow the products of conception to pass naturally, provided the pregnancy is early and the patient is committed to return for follow-up. Careful monitoring with pelvic examinations, serial hCG titers, and transvaginal ultrasonography can be used to determine whether the abortion is complete.

    c. Dilation and curettage also may be necessary to ensure complete emptying of the uterus or as one form of induced abortion. Possible complications of the procedure include uterine perforation or cervical laceration.

Table 8-8 | Classification of Spontaneous Abortions[a]

Type	Vaginal Bleeding	Cervix Open	Products of Conception Passed
Threatened	Yes	No	No
Inevitable	Yes	Yes	Not yet, but no way to maintain pregnancy
Incomplete	Yes	Yes	Partial
Complete	Yes	No	Yes
Missed	No	No	No (fetal demise has occurred without symptoms)

[a]Three or more consecutive abortions are classified as recurrent, and any abortion with associated sepsis is classified as septic.

   d. Immunoglobulin should be administered to Rh-negative women in the event of either an elective or a spontaneous abortion.

   e. Septic or infected abortion requires hospital admission for complete evacuation of the uterine contents, medical support, and antibiotics.

C. Gestational trophoblastic disease (GTD)

   1. General characteristics

   a. GTD is a spectrum of diseases arising from the placenta and includes complete and partial hydatidiform moles, placental site–invasive moles, trophoblastic tumors, and choriocarcinomas.

   b. GTD is divided into benign and malignant forms. A hydatidiform mole (also called a *molar pregnancy*) is the benign form of GTD.

   2. Hydatidiform moles are divided into complete and incomplete molar pregnancies.

   a. Complete hydatidiform moles occur when the egg is fertilized by two sperm and the maternal genetic material disappears or is inactivated. Incomplete hydatidiform moles occur when the egg is fertilized by two sperm and the maternal genetic material persists, resulting in 69 chromosomes. Complete molar pregnancies are the most common form of GTD. See Table 8-9.

   > GTD includes complete and incomplete hydatidiform moles, and <5% of incomplete moles progress to malignancy.

   b. Complete hydatidiform moles are characterized by an empty egg and the appearance of "grapelike vesicles" or a "snowstorm pattern" on ultrasound. Approximately 20% progress to malignancy.

   c. Incomplete hydatidiform moles have a fetus present, but the fetus is nonviable. Less than 5% progress to malignancy.

   3. Clinical features: A complete or partial molar pregnancy most commonly presents with abnormal vaginal bleeding, uterine size greater than dates, hyperemesis gravidarum (excessive vomiting), or preeclampsia-like symptoms before 20 weeks of gestation.

   4. Diagnostic studies

   a. With complete molar pregnancy, the hCG level is often >100,000 mU per mL. Persistently elevated levels of hCG may indicate a gestational trophoblastic tumor.

   > hCG level is abnormally high in GTD and should be monitored until it returns to normal after evacuation.

   b. Ultrasonography of a complete hydatidiform mole shows characteristic grapelike vesicles or snowstorm appearance consistent with the swelling of the chorionic villi. Ultrasonography may aid in establishing the diagnosis of a partial molar pregnancy.

   5. Management

   a. Treatment depends on tumor classification. Benign tumors and metastatic low-risk tumors can be treated without chemotherapy. Metastatic high-risk tumors require a combination of chemotherapy with or without adjuvant radiation and surgery.

   b. Surgical treatment includes suction curettage (for those desiring to preserve fertility) or hysterectomy. These treatments all carry high cure rates of 80% to 100%.

   c. After evacuation, patients must be monitored with serial hCG to assure return to baseline and to diagnose and manage sequelae properly. Contraception is recommended for 12 months after remission.

Table 8-9 | **Key Features of a Complete Hydatidiform Mole (i.e., Molar Pregnancy)**

- Empty egg, no viable fetus
- Abnormal vaginal bleeding
- Uterine size greater than gestational age (based on LMP)
- Hyperemesis gravidarum (excessive vomiting)
- High blood pressure during the first 20 weeks of pregnancy
- "Snowstorm pattern" or "grapelike vesicles" on ultrasound

LMP, last menstrual period.

D. Gestational diabetes mellitus

1. General characteristics

a. Gestational diabetes mellitus is carbohydrate intolerance of variable severity that is only present during pregnancy.

b. The lifetime risk of developing diabetes after pregnancy in women who have had gestational diabetes is increased to >50% (vs. 5% in the general population). If insulin is required during the pregnancy, there is a 50% risk of developing diabetes within 5 years from the pregnancy.

c. Recurrence of gestational diabetes is common, occurring in 60% to 90% of subsequent pregnancies.

d. Maternal complications associated with gestational diabetes mellitus include pre-eclampsia, hyperacceleration of general diabetic complications, and traumatic birth, including shoulder dystocia.

e. Fetal complications associated with gestational diabetes mellitus include macrosomia, prematurity, delayed fetal lung maturity, and fetal demise.

2. Clinical features

a. Patients with gestational diabetes are usually asymptomatic.

b. Risk factors for the development of gestational diabetes include a history of a previous large-for-gestational-age infant, obesity, age older than 25 years, glucosuria, a family history of diabetes, or having the following ethnic or racial heritage: African American, Asian, Hispanic, or Native American.

3. Diagnostic studies

a. Screening recommendations; typical screening occurs at 24 to 28 weeks' gestation.

b. Obtain a random glucose on all pregnant women.

c. Glycosylated hemoglobin (HgbA$_{1c}$), which measures average glycemic control across the prior 3 months, is not recommended as a screening method in gestational diabetes because gestational glycemic intolerance does not occur before 24 weeks' gestation.

d. In recent years, recommendations for screening protocols from medical organizations have diverged.

e. The American College of Obstetrics and Gynecology (ACOG) recommends the traditional two-step approach. Step 1 consists of an oral administration of a non-fasting 50-g glucose challenge test, followed by a serum glucose level 1 hour later. If the 1-hour serum glucose value is >140 mg per dL, a 3-hour glucose tolerance test is performed.

f. The 3-hour glucose tolerance test consists of a 100-g glucose load in the morning after an overnight fast. Serum glucose levels are taken at fasting and then at 1, 2, and 3 hours after the glucose load. If two or more of the values are abnormal, the patient is diagnosed with gestational diabetes (Table 8-10).

(1) Antepartum testing, including regular NSTs and BPPs, is often used in gestational diabetes beginning at 34 weeks of gestation.

(2) Women who have had gestational diabetes should be screened at 6 weeks postpartum for diabetes and at yearly intervals thereafter.

4. Management

a. Careful management of gestational diabetes with diet and exercise is essential.

b. Patients with gestational diabetes are recommended to check their blood glucose levels four times daily: after fasting overnight and after each meal. At each office visit, the patient's home glucose levels should be reviewed, and if necessary, a fasting or a 2-hour postprandial blood glucose measurement should be done during the office visit.

 Screening for GDM of all pregnant women is recommended at 24 to 28 weeks with random glucose and HA1c.

The management of gestational diabetes begins with diet and exercise; if control is not achieved, insulin is recommended.

Table 8-10 | Diagnosis of Gestational Diabetes Mellitus with a 100-g Oral Glucose Load[a]

Test	Results (mg/dL)
Fasting	95
1-hour	180
2-hour	155
3-hour	140

[a]Two or more of the venous plasma concentrations must be met or exceeded for a positive diagnosis. The test should be done in the morning after an overnight fast of between 8 and 14 hours and after at least 3 days of unrestricted diet and unlimited physical activity.

Adapted from DeCherney A, Nathan L, Laurfer, N, Roman, A. *Current Diagnosis & Treatment: Obstetrics & Gynecology.* 12th ed. McGraw-Hill Companies; 2019.

   c. Patients who have fasting blood glucose measurements of >105 mg per dL or 2-hour postprandial blood sugar measurements of >120 mg per dL may need medical management.

   d. The current mainstay of treatment in the United States is insulin and is recommended by the ACOG because it does not cross the placental barrier and it is easier to maintain tighter control. However, for patients resistant to insulin management, some medical providers may consider oral hypoglycemic agents. Metformin is most commonly recommended.

   e. If a patient is well controlled and there are no signs of macrosomia, induction of labor should occur at 40 weeks' gestation. If glucose is poorly controlled or there are signs of macrosomia, induction occurs at 38 weeks' gestation.

   f. To help avoid the development of type 2 diabetes later in life, the patient should be advised to obtain and maintain an ideal body weight. Annual evaluations of fasting glucose concentrations are recommended.

E. **Preterm labor and delivery**

   1. General characteristics

   a. Preterm delivery is the delivery of an infant after 20 weeks' but before 37 weeks' gestation and occurs in 8% to 10% of births.

   b. Preterm delivery is the most common cause of neonatal deaths not resulting from congenital malformations.

   c. Low birth weight infants born prematurely often have significant developmental delays, cerebral palsy, and lung disease.

   d. The cause of preterm labor is poorly understood. The most common cause is maternal infection (vaginal group B streptococci or urinary tract infection). Other risk factors include smoking, cocaine use, uterine malformations, cervical incompetence, and low prepregnancy weight.

   e. Complications of maternal or fetal health, such as hypertension, diabetes mellitus, premature rupture of membranes (PROM), and abruptio placentae, are associated with preterm delivery.

> 💡 Preterm delivery is the birth of an infant between 20 and 37 weeks' gestation.

   2. **Clinical features**

   a. Preterm labor is defined as regular uterine contractions (>4/hour) between 20 and 36 weeks of gestation and the presence of one or more of the following signs:

   (1) Cervical dilation ≥2 cm at presentation

   (2) Cervical dilation ≥1 cm on serial examinations

   (3) Cervical effacement >80%

   b. Late symptoms of preterm labor include painful or painless contractions, pressure, menstrual-like cramps, watery or bloody discharge, and low back pain.

3. Diagnostic studies

a. Ultrasonography can be used to examine the length of the cervix. Normal length is 4 cm. A length of 2 cm at 24 weeks' gestation increases the risk to deliver prematurely.

b. Examination of the cervicovaginal secretions for fetal fibronectin, a glycoprotein, has been used as a marker for preterm labor. Its absence means a low risk of delivery within 2 weeks.

c. When cervical length and fetal fibronectin are used together, if both are abnormal, there is a 50% chance of delivery before 34 weeks' gestation. If both are normal, there is only an 11% chance of delivery before 34 weeks' gestation.

d. Vaginal cultures and urinalysis with culture and sensitivity should also be obtained.

4. Management

a. Management techniques include bed rest; oral or intravenous (IV) hydration; steroids administered to the mother to enhance fetal lung maturity; antibiotics if there is known infection, including group B streptococci; and tocolytics, if indicated.

b. Tocolytics are used in an attempt to stop contractions. They are recommended for up to 48 hours if the cervix is dilated <5 cm. Currently, no one agent is recommended over others.

(1) Prostaglandin inhibitors (e.g., indomethacin) block naturally occurring prostaglandins that cause uterine contractions. It is only used before 32 weeks because it may cause premature closing of the fetus' ductus arteriosus.

(2) β-Mimetic adrenergic agents, including ritodrine and terbutaline, are infrequently used because of potentially fatal maternal heart complications.

(3) Calcium channel blockers inhibit smooth muscle contractility by decreasing intracellular Ca^{2+} ions, which, in return, relax uterine muscle. Side effects include maternal hypotension and tachycardia.

(4) Magnesium sulfate ($MgSO_4$) inhibits myometrial contractility mediated by calcium. It is sometimes preferred because maternal serum levels can be easily monitored. Side effects include nausea, fatigue, and muscle weakness.

(a) Magnesium sulfate can lead to decreased reflexes, respiratory depression, and cardiac collapse.

(b) In the case of magnesium sulfate toxicity, calcium gluconate can be given.

c. The goal in treatment is to identify patients at risk and to diagnose the condition before labor is irreversibly established.

5. Prevention

a. Cervical cerclage (i.e., closure of cervix by suturing the cervix closed) is an option for women with known cervical incompetence or a history of preterm birth. For these patients, the cerclage is placed between 12 and 14 weeks and removed at 37 weeks or earlier if the patient goes into preterm labor despite the cerclage.

b. For women with a history of preterm delivery, weekly injections of 17α-hydroxyprogesterone caproate from 16 to 36 weeks' gestation can sometimes reduce the rate of recurrent preterm birth.

F. Premature rupture of membranes (PROM)

1. General characteristics

a. PROM is rupture of the amniotic membranes before the onset of labor. It occurs in ~8% of pregnancies at 37 weeks' gestation or beyond. Most women (up to 90%) will go into spontaneous labor within 24 hours after PROM.

b. Preterm premature rupture of membranes (PPROM) occurs before 37 weeks' gestation and precedes 30% to 40% of all preterm deliveries.

c. The major risk associated with both PROM and PPROM is infection (chorioamnionitis and endometritis). This risk increases with time and hastens delivery.

d. The risk of cord prolapse, when the cord slips out of the open cervix before the baby is delivered, is increased because of the force of the gush of fluids when the fetal head is not well engaged. Cord prolapse is identified as a ropelike, soft, elongated mass on speculum or bimanual examination. This is considered an obstetric emergency necessitating immediate delivery.

2. Clinical features

    a. Symptoms of ruptured membranes are a gush or persistent leakage of fluid from the vagina. Some women have difficulty distinguishing PROM from urine incontinence.

    b. Ruptured membrane is suspected with direct visualization of pooling using a sterile speculum and the use of nitrazine paper; PROM is confirmed with the fern test. Ultrasonography can be used to check the amniotic fluid index.

    c. Vaginal digital examination should be avoided unless delivery is imminent.

3. Management

    a. Gestational age is the primary factor when considering management.

    b. Antibiotic treatment for any woman with known group B streptococci is indicated.

    c. PROM (after 37 weeks)

        (1) Deliver: The baby should be delivered within 24 hours of ruptured membranes to decrease the risk of maternal and fetal infection. The patient should be hospitalized, and the fetus carefully monitored. Labor is induced with most patients if labor does not occur spontaneously within 6 hours of rupture. Women should be allowed a trial of labor for 12 to 18 hours before considering cesarean section, provided that maternal and fetal vital signs are normal and labor is progressing.

        (2) Active management of PROM involves induction of labor with prostaglandin cervical gel or oxytocin, depending on the cervical examination and the presence of contractions.

    d. PPROM (34 0/7 to 36 6/7 weeks)

        (1) Management during this period is controversial. Traditionally, recommended management was the same as for a term gestation (see earlier). However, recent data show there may be benefit from the administration of steroids (betamethasone) to enhance fetal lung maturity and continue expectant management. In each case, the risks and benefits must be weighed to determine the appropriate management.

    e. PPROM (24 0/7 to 33 6/7 weeks)

        (1) Expectant management: If there is no sign of maternal or fetal infection or distress, waiting to induce labor is preferred. The patient is admitted to the hospital and put on strict bed rest.

        (2) Steroids (betamethasone) should be administered to enhance fetal lung maturity. Depending on gestational age, steroids can be administered up to two times, 2 weeks apart.

        (3) Antibiotics are administered to prevent infection and help prolong the pregnancy in order to decrease infant mortality.

        (4) Magnesium sulfate for maternal neuroprotection is given between 24 0/7 and 32 0/7 weeks' gestation.

        (5) NST and BPP should be performed daily to assess fetal well-being.

        (6) Amniocentesis can be performed to check for lung maturity.

        (7) If there is any indication of maternal or fetal infection or distress, delivery of the fetus is warranted.

> Ferning of the fluid confirms premature rupture of membranes.

> 💡 Elevated BP before 20 weeks is chronic hypertension. Elevated BP that develops after 20 weeks is pregnancy-induced hypertension (PIH).

   f. PPROM (20 to 23 6/7 weeks)

     (1) Previable pregnancy: Patient counseling and maternal–fetal medicine consultation required.

     (2) Expectant management or induction of labor is indicated.

G. Hypertension in pregnancy

   1. Chronic hypertension is hypertension that presents before 20 weeks' gestation.

   2. PIH is hypertension that presents after 20 weeks' gestation but has no other associated symptoms.

     a. Chronic hypertension and PIH are treated in the same manner: monthly ultrasonography to check for intrauterine growth retardation, serial BP and urine protein, and weekly NST and BPP during the third trimester.

     b. The basic underlying pathophysiology of PIH is thought to be vasospasm or arteriolar constriction.

     c. Medication for chronic hypertension and PIH is only given in severe cases. Methyldopa is the treatment of choice, with labetalol being an alternative.

   3. **Preeclampsia/eclampsia**

     a. General characteristics

       (1) To be diagnosed as preeclampsia/eclampsia, the symptoms must occur after 20 weeks' gestation. It most often occurs near term but can occur up to 6 weeks postpartum.

       (2) Classic criteria of preeclampsia include new-onset hypertension and proteinuria. Terms used to define preeclampsia have recently changed from mild and severe to preeclampsia and preeclampsia with severe features (Table 8-11).

       (3) HELLP syndrome is the presence of severe preeclampsia with the addition of **H**emolysis, **E**levated **L**iver enzymes, and **L**ow **P**latelets.

       (4) Eclampsia is severe preeclampsia with the addition of new-onset seizures.

Table 8-11 | Classification Preeclampsia and Preeclampsia with Severe Features

	Preeclampsia	Preeclampsia with Severe Features
Blood pressure	>140/90 mm Hg but <160/110 mm Hg, *or* increase in 30 mm Hg systolic and 15 mm Hg diastolic from prepregnancy blood pressure on at least two occasions at least 4 hours apart	>160–180 mm Hg systolic or >110 mm Hg diastolic on two occasions at least 4 hours apart
Proteinuria	>300 mg/24 hour *or* protein/creatinine ratio of 0.3 *or* protein dipstick reading of 2+	>300 mg/24 hour *or* protein/creatinine ratio of 0.3 *or* protein dipstick reading of 2+ BUT diagnosis can be made without proteinuria if there is presence of thrombocytopenia, renal insufficiency, impaired liver function pulmonary edema, or headache (see details below)
Platelet count		Thrombocytopenia (platelet count <100 × 10⁹/L)
Liver function		• LDH elevated to 600 IU/L • AST twice normal limit • ALT twice normal limit • Severe persistent right upper quadrant or epigastric pain
Renal function		Creatinine >1.1 mg/dL
Respiratory function		Pulmonary edema
Symptoms/signs		• Visual disturbances • New-onset headache unresponsive to medication

ALT, alanine aminotransferase; AST, aspartate aminotransferase; LDH, lactate dehydrogenase.

Adapted from DeCherney A, Nathan L, Laurfer, N, Roman, A. *Current Diagnosis & Treatment: Obstetrics & Gynecology.* 12th ed. McGraw-Hill Companies; 2019; Gestational hypertension and preeclampsia: ACOG practice bulletin, number 222. *Obstetr Gynecol (New York 1953).* 2020;135(6):e237-e260. doi:10.1097/AOG.0000000000003891

(5) The most common risk factor for preeclampsia is nulliparity. Other risk factors include multiple gestation, preeclampsia in a previous pregnancy, chronic hypertension, diabetes, autoimmune disease, body mass index (BMI) >30, and maternal age over 35.

(6) Women at high risk (see earlier) should receive low-dose aspirin for prophylaxis, starting at 12 weeks' gestation through delivery.

(7) Maternal complications of preeclampsia include progression to eclampsia or HELLP syndrome, abruptio placentae, renal failure, cerebral hemorrhage, pulmonary edema, and disseminated intravascular coagulation.

(8) Fetal complications include hypoxia, low birth weight, preterm delivery, and perinatal death.

b. Clinical features: Symptoms include new-onset headache, visual disturbances, nausea, vomiting, right upper quadrant (RUQ) pain, and decreased urine output.

c. Diagnostic studies

(1) Sterile urine protein, 24-hour urine protein level, complete blood count (CBC), fibrinogen, and prothrombin time/partial thromboplastin time are followed.

(2) Chemistry panel, including liver enzymes and creatinine, aids in identifying risk for complications.

d. Management

(1) Delivery of the infant is the ultimate treatment for hypertensive disorders of pregnancy.

(2) Preeclampsia without severe features

(a) After a full evaluation of the fetus, including NST and sonogram for estimated fetal weight and amniotic fluid levels, the patient may be followed as an outpatient if she is reliable.

(b) Regular BP monitoring and weekly evaluation including sonogram for fetal growth and NST are necessary.

(c) Delivery through induction is indicated at 37 weeks of gestation.

(3) Preeclampsia with severe features

(a) The patient is always hospitalized for close monitoring.

(b) The presence of any of the following requires delivery of the fetus, regardless of gestational age: uncontrolled BP >160/110, persistent headache or visual disturbance, RUQ pain, HELLP, pulmonary edema, stroke, or suspected placental abruption.

(c) Magnesium sulfate, administered by IV drip, is the first-line medication for inpatient management to decrease chance of seizures. $MgSO_4$ should be continued for 24 hours after delivery.

(d) Urine output must be closely monitored as $MgSO_4$ is cleared through the kidney, leading to an increased risk of $MgSO_4$ toxicity when urine output is low.

(e) Hydralazine or labetalol may be given for acute management of high BP.

(f) Betamethasone is given before 34 weeks of gestation to enhance fetal lung maturity.

4. Delivery through induction of labor or cesarean section is guided by evaluation of the gestational age, maternal symptoms, and control of BP.

H. Rh incompatibility

1. General characteristics

a. The most common problem of mismatched blood typing between mother and father involves the rhesus D factor (Rh factor). Approximately 15% of the population is Rh negative. Although 98% of isoimmunizations are secondary to the Rh factor,

43 other antigens exist. Rh incompatibility is only a problem if mother is Rh negative and father is Rh positive.

b. If mother is Rh negative and father is Rh positive, and the baby is subsequently Rh positive, the mother may develop antibodies against fetal blood, and as a result, hemolysis can occur, leading to fetal anemia. The anemia may be mild or severe, leading to fetal death.

c. The key to management is not allowing the Rh-negative mother to become sensitized and make antibodies against the Rh-positive blood.

d. Rh immunoglobulin (RhoGam) is administered routinely at 28 to 29 weeks of gestation to all Rh-negative mothers for prophylactic protection. After delivery, if the baby is found to be Rh positive, the mother receives RhoGam again to protect subsequent pregnancies. RhoGam prevents the development of these antibodies to fetal blood in 99% of cases.

e. The most common time of maternal–fetal blood mixing is at delivery. However, RhoGam should be administered after any event that may allow fetal cells to enter maternal circulation, such as ectopic pregnancy, spontaneous or therapeutic abortion, CVS, amniocentesis, or trauma. The Kleihauer–Betke (KB) test measures the occurrence and degree of fetomaternal hemorrhage.

f. If antibodies develop, the mother's immune system will attack Rh-incompatible fetus in a subsequent pregnancy, which can lead to severe fetal anemia and death (fetal hydrops).

2. Diagnostic studies

a. Routine prenatal blood work should include blood type, Rh factor, and Coombs' test for antibodies.

b. Antibody titers of <1:16 probably will not adversely affect the pregnancy.

c. In a sensitized pregnancy, a combination of Coombs' test, amniocentesis, and ultrasonography is used to follow up the developing fetus for evidence of distress or fetal hydrops.

3. Management

a. Routinely give RhoGam 300 mg to Rh-negative, nonimmunized women at 28 weeks of gestation and within 72 hours of delivering an Rh-positive infant.

b. RhoGam is also to be administered at amniocentesis and other instances when there is a risk of fetal blood entering the maternal bloodstream, as previously noted.

c. Massive fetal–maternal hemorrhage may require larger doses of immunoglobulin.

d. Maternal sensitization is rare; management varies based on a variety of factors.

I. Abruptio placentae (Table 8-12)

1. General characteristics

a. Abruptio placentae is the premature separation of a normally implanted placenta after 20th week of gestation but before birth.

b. Abruptio placentae is the cause of one-third of third-trimester bleeding. Bleeding may freely flow through the cervix and vagina or may be concealed between a partially detached placenta and uterus (Fig. 8-2).

c. Several risk factors are known for the development of abruptio placentae: trauma, smoking, hypertension, decreased folic acid, cocaine use, alcohol (>14 drinks/week), uterine anomalies, high parity, previous abruption (recurrence rate is 10%–17%), and advanced maternal age.

d. Abruption is classified into three categories based on clinical and laboratory findings. Category 1 is mild vaginal bleeding, and both the mother and the fetus are hemodynamically normal; category 2 is moderate bleeding, contractions, and maternal hypotensive, and fetus shows signs of distress such as decreased variability or deceleration of heartbeat; category 3 is severe bleeding, mom is hemodynamically unstable, and there is high risk of fetal death.

💡 Administer RhoGam to Rh-negative mothers at 28 weeks, within 72 hours of delivery, and in any other invasive procedure during pregnancy.

Table 8-12 | Abruptio Placentae Versus Placenta Previa

	Abruptio Placentae	**Placenta Previa**
Definition	Premature separation of a normally implanted placenta after 20th week of gestation	Placenta is partially or completely covering the cervical os
Key feature	**_Painful_** vaginal bleeding with associated uterine camps or searing back pain	**_Painless_** bright red bleeding
Main risk factors	Trauma Smoking Hypertension Cocaine use Alcohol Uterine anomalies	Advanced maternal age Smoking Multiple gestation Previous scarring on endometrium
Diagnosis	Usually clinical	Ultrasound
Management	Depends on the degree of separation, viability of fetus, and status of mother Vaginal delivery is possible	Delivery always via cesarean section

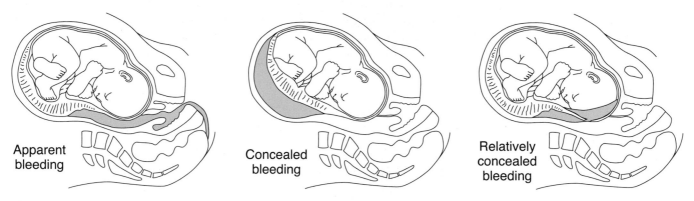

Apparent bleeding   Concealed bleeding   Relatively concealed bleeding

Figure 8-2 ▶ Types of abruptio placentae: external (apparent) and concealed.

    e. Abruption can lead to liberation of tissue thromboplastin or consumption of fibrinogen, thereby activating the extrinsic clotting mechanism. This could eventually lead to disseminated intravascular coagulation.

2. Clinical features

    a. Painful vaginal bleeding is the hallmark to diagnosis and occurs in the majority of cases (85%).

    b. Uterine, abdominal, or back pain is a frequent symptom of abruptio placentae and, if bleeding is concealed, may be the only symptom.

    c. The uterus becomes hypertonic, irritable, or tender when the placenta has abrupted.

    d. Evidence of fetal distress may or may not be present, depending on the degree of separation.

    e. Complications of abruptio placentae, in addition to the obvious compromise of placental blood flow to the fetus and hemorrhage, are renal failure, coagulation failure, and death.

3. Diagnostic studies

    a. Diagnosis is almost always clinical.

    b. Ultrasonography is not routinely reliable in establishing the diagnosis of abruption.

4. Management

    a. Delivery of the fetus and placenta is the definitive treatment of abruptio placentae. However, ultimate management depends on the degree of separation and the age and viability of the fetus.

    b. Blood type, crossmatch, and coagulation studies are indicated in a stable patient, as is placement of a large-bore IV line.

    c. Cesarean section most often is the preferred route for delivering the infant in cases of abruptio placentae.

J. Placenta previa

    1. General characteristics

        a. Placenta previa occurs when the placenta partially or completely covers the cervical os.

        b. Placenta previa is rare, occurring in 0.3% to 0.5% of pregnancies, and is associated with advanced age, smoking, high parity, and any process that could cause scarring of the lower uterine segment (e.g., cesarean delivery).

        c. Performing a digital examination in a patient with placenta previa is contraindicated because it can incite severe bleeding.

    2. Clinical features

        a. Painless vaginal bleeding is the hallmark of placenta previa. Bleeding may be mild spotting to severe hemorrhage.

        b. Bleeding may continue from the placenta's implantation site after delivery because the lower uterus contracts poorly.

        c. Placenta previa usually diagnosed during the routine 16- to 20-week sonographic anatomy scan. Up to 50% of affected placentas will spontaneously "migrate off" the os owing to the expansion of the uterine wall because of growth during pregnancy; and as a result, these placentas are not ultimately covering the cervical os at term.

    3. Diagnosis

        a. Ultrasonography is the test of choice for establishing the diagnosis of placenta previa.

        b. When the patient is hemodynamically unstable, studies for blood type, crossmatch, and coagulation should be ordered; a large-bore IV line should be placed.

        c. Differentiating placenta previa from placental abruption is of utmost importance (Table 8-12).

    4. Management

        a. Intervention depends on the amount of bleeding and gestational age. Some women with placenta previa never experience bleeding and have uncomplicated term births.

        b. Before term, observation is warranted if the patient is stable.

            (1) Blood transfusion may be necessary while waiting for fetal maturity.

            (2) Patients with previa should abstain from vaginal penetration.

            (3) Vaginal delivery is an absolute contraindication; cesarean section is always indicated.

            (4) The patient should be scheduled for cesarean section at 38 weeks' gestation. She should not be allowed to go into labor.

> A placenta previa may migrate over weeks; careful monitoring is required. If it does not migrate, vaginal delivery is contraindicated.

> Painful third-trimester bleeding: think abruption. Painless third-trimester bleeding: think previa.

Labor and Delivery

A. Routine vaginal labor and delivery

    1. General characteristics

        a. Approximately 20% of perinatal morbidity and mortality occurs during the intrapartum period in otherwise healthy pregnancies.

        b. Most infants present with a vertex (head-down) presentation. However, other possibilities include breech, face, transverse, and compound (arm or leg).

2. Clinical features

a. Cervical examination to assess labor

(1) Dilatation: opening of the cervical os, expressed in centimeters (fully dilated is 10 cm)

(2) Effacement: cervical softening and thinning out, expressed as a percentage (up to 100%)

(3) Station

(a) Location of the presenting part (usually the head) in relation to the maternal ischial spines

(b) The level at the spines is denoted as "0" station. Stations above the spines are expressed in negative numbers (e.g., −1 cm, −2 cm), and stations below the spine in positive numbers (e.g., +1 cm, +2 cm).

> "0" station indicates the presenting part is at the level of the ischial spines.

b. Stages of labor (Table 8-13)

(1) The first stage of labor begins at the onset of true, regular contractions and ends at full dilation. The length of the first stage of labor is generally 6 to 20 hours for primiparous women and 2 to 14 hours for multiparous women (or 1 to 1.5 cm/hour).

(2) The second stage of labor begins at full dilation and ends with the delivery of the infant. The length of the second stage of labor is generally 30 minutes to 3 hours (average 50 minutes) for primiparous women and 5 to 60 minutes (average 20 minutes) for multiparous women.

(3) The third stage of labor begins after the delivery and entails separation and expulsion of the placenta. The length of the third stage of labor is 0 to 30 minutes but usually is about 5 minutes.

(4) The hour after delivery sometimes is called the fourth stage and is critical in assessing and treating tears, lacerations, and hemorrhage.

c. Bloody show, which is the passage of a small amount of blood-tinged mucus that has been plugging the cervical os, often precedes true labor.

d. Amniotic fluid rupture can occur before or during the first stage of labor.

3. Diagnostic studies

a. On admission, urinalysis for protein, glucose, and hematocrit may be obtained.

b. Fetal monitoring is used in labor to assess the fetus' response to labor.

(1) An external fetal monitor is attached to the maternal abdomen and assesses an estimated fetal HR via transmitted sound waves.

(2) An internal fetal monitor is an electrode attached to the infant's head and gives the most accurate fetal HR pattern because it transmits the true R wave (as with an electrocardiogram) of electroactivity. The cervix must be dilated at least 2 cm and membranes ruptured to attach an internal fetal monitor.

(3) Specific patterns visible on monitoring include:

Table 8-13 | Stages of Normal Labor

Stage of Labor	Definition	Average Length
1	Onset of true contractions until fully dilated	Primiparous: 6–20 hours Multiparous: 2–14 hours
2	Fully dilated to delivery of fetus	Primiparous: 30 minutes to 3 hours, average 50 minutes Multiparous: 5–60 minutes, average 20 minutes
3	Delivery of fetus to delivery of the placenta	0–30 minutes, average 5 minutes
4	The hour after delivery of the placenta when patient is monitored for lacerations and hemorrhage	

> Accelerations of an increase in 15 bpm for 15 seconds above the normal baseline HR (110 to 160 bpm) are reassuring and denote fetal well-being.

(a) Accelerations of an increase in 15 bpm for 15 seconds above the normal baseline HR (110 to 160 bpm) are reassuring and denote fetal well-being.

(b) Early decelerations mirror the images of the contractions and denote fetal head compression. They are often present as a woman approaches the second stage of labor and are considered to be benign.

(c) Variable decelerations are rapid drops in fetal HR with a return to baseline with variable shape and no identifiable pattern. They often occur with cord compression and, if mild or infrequent, are benign.

(d) Late decelerations are fetal HR drops during the second half of the contractions. They denote uteroplacental insufficiency and always are worrisome.

(e) When a nonreassuring fetal HR is present, the following management is appropriate: stop oxytocin (if applicable), change maternal position, administer oxygen via face mask, and measure fetal scalp pH.

4. **Management**

a. Regular cervical examinations for dilation, station, and effacement are necessary to check the progress of labor.

b. Continued monitoring of maternal BP, temperature, and pulse are critical to exclude late preeclampsia and infection.

c. Analgesia such as epidural is offered to provide comfort and prevent fatigue. Delaying administration of the epidural until the cervix is 5 cm dilated decreases the chances of arrest of labor and increases the chance of a successful vaginal delivery.

d. After crowning of the presenting part, pressure applied from the coccygeal region upward will extend the head at the proper time and help to protect the perineal musculature.

e. When the head has been delivered, the baby's mouth can be suctioned with a rubber suction bulb.

f. When the rest of the body passes, the cord is clamped and cut.

g. Episiotomy (surgical incision of the perineum to prevent traumatic tearing) is sometimes performed to protect the perineum as the head crowns for such indications as a large baby or a short perineum.

h. Signs of placental separation include umbilical cord lengthening, a fresh show of blood flow, fundus rising, and the uterus becoming firm and globular.

i. The infant is suctioned, kept warm, and assessed for Apgar score at 1 and 5 minutes after delivery (Table 8-14).

j. The placenta and umbilical cord should be examined to ensure that the entire placenta and membranes are passed and that the cord contains three vessels (two arteries and one vein).

k. Oxytocin may be administered in the third and fourth stages of labor to reduce blood loss by stimulating the contractions.

Table 8-14 | Apgar Scoring[a]

		Points		
Letter	**Sign**	**0**	**1**	**2**
A	Activity (muscle tone)	Absent	Arms and legs flexed	Active movement
P	Pulse	Absent	<100 bpm	>100 bpm
G	Grimace (reflex irritability)	No response	Grimace	Sneezes, coughs, pulls away
A	Appearance (skin color)	Blue gray, pale all over	Pink, except extremities	Pink all over
R	Respiration	Absent	Slow, irregular	Good, crying

[a]A score is determined for each sign at 1 and 5 minutes after birth; if there are problems with the neonate, a score is determined at 10 minutes as well. Scores are classified as follows: 7–10 = normal; 4–7 = may require some resuscitative measures; ≤3 = immediate resuscitation required.

B. Abnormal labor and delivery

1. General characteristics

   a. Dystocia, or abnormal labor, occurs when the cervix fails to dilate progressively over time or the fetus fails to descend.

   b. Dystocia is a leading indication for cesarean section.

   c. Common causes include abnormalities with the pelvis, power, or passenger.

   (1) Pelvis refers to cephalopelvic disproportion. Sometimes, the maternal pelvis is not large enough to allow the infant to pass through, which denotes cephalopelvic disproportion.

   (2) Power refers to the contractions, which are needed to dilate the cervix and expel the infant. If the contractions are inadequate, IV oxytocin (Pitocin) can be given to enhance labor.

   (3) Passenger refers to the baby. The head is usually the biggest part. The bigger the baby is in relation to the pelvis, the greater the likelihood of cephalopelvic disproportion.

2. **Clinical features**

   a. Inability to deliver vaginally after full cervical dilation is a good marker of true dystocia.

   b. Macrosomia, nonvertex presentation, and the adequacy of the pelvis can be evaluated by clinical examination and ultrasound before the onset of labor.

   c. Shoulder dystocia occurs when the fetus' anterior shoulder gets lodged under the symphysis pubis.

   d. Risk factors include fetal macrosomia and normal weight fetus with large shoulder-to-head ratio.

   e. Diagnosis is made during delivery when the head retracts back into the perineum.

   f. Risks to the fetus include brachial plexus injury, fetal asphyxia, and death.

3. **Management**

   a. Inadequate uterine contractions can be augmented with oxytocin after the maternal pelvis and fetus are assessed.

   b. If maternal pushing does not result in decent and delivery of the baby, rest or assisted delivery with vacuum extraction or forceps may be used to shorten the second stage of labor. Forceps or vacuum extractors may be indicated for fetal distress or for maternal indications only if the head is engaged and the cervix is fully dilated.

   c. If the baby is in a nonvertex presentation, external version with ultrasound guidance can be attempted after 37 weeks of gestation.

   d. Shoulder dystocia is an emergency. Management includes episiotomy, manually rotating the fetal trunk and fracturing the clavicle to dislodge the shoulder; if these maneuvers fail, the fetus is pushed back into the uterus and an emergency cesarean is performed.

C. Cesarean delivery and vaginal birth after cesarean delivery (VBAC)

1. General characteristics

   a. Cesarean section is defined as the birth of the fetus through an incision in the abdominal and uterine walls and constitutes about 32% of deliveries in the United States.

   b. The most frequent indications for cesarean section are repeat cesarean (one-third of cesareans), dystocia or failure to progress, breech presentation, and fetal distress.

   c. The success rate of VBAC depends on the indications for and the number of the previous cesarean sections.

   (1) When dystocia was the indicator for a previous cesarean delivery, the rate of successful VBAC is the lowest. Conversely, women who have a cesarean delivery for malpresentation (e.g., breech) have a higher rate of success with VBAC.

> Common causes for issues during labor and delivery include *pelvis* (cephalopelvic disproportion), *power* (inadequate contractions), and *passenger* (big infant head).

(2) Although the incidence of uterine rupture in a VBAC after use of a low transverse incision is relatively low (0.2% to 1.5%), it can lead to death of the fetus and significantly increased morbidity and mortality of the mother.

    d. Risks of cesarean section include a greater likelihood of thromboembolic events, increased bleeding, and development of infection.

    e. With each subsequent cesarean section, the risk of complications is higher.

2. Management

    a. Prophylactic antibiotics are often used after a cesarean section to prevent infection.

    b. A low transverse uterine incision is usually made because of the decreased blood loss associated with its use, the ease of repair, and the lower likelihood of rupture compared with that of a classical incision. A classical incision is vertical through the entire length of the uterus.

    c. Recovery time is longer following a cesarean. Breastfeeding may be difficult secondary to abdominal pain.

D. Induction of labor

1. General characteristics

    a. Induction of labor can be done by medical or surgical means.

    b. Induction of labor is considered when prolongation of pregnancy might expose the mother or fetus to complications and when vaginal delivery is not contraindicated (Table 8-15).

2. Methods

    a. Early induction of labor (when minimal dilation or effacement has occurred) is initiated with prostaglandin gel or tablet applied directly on the cervix, which may be repeated once in 12 hours. This helps to soften or "ripen" the cervix. A balloon catheter or laminaria can also be used.

    b. Later induction (when the cervix is dilated >1 cm and some effacement has occurred) is initiated with oxytocin (Pitocin) given IV, with systematic increases in the oxytocin level until strong contractions are occurring approximately every 3 minutes.

    c. Amniotomy, or artificially rupturing the membranes with a small hook, can also induce labor.

E. Postpartum hemorrhage

1. General characteristics (Table 8-15)

    a. Postpartum hemorrhage is defined as blood loss requiring transfusion or a 10% decrease in hematocrit between admission and the postpartum period. It is the third leading cause of maternal mortality in advanced gestation.

    b. Early postpartum hemorrhage occurs <24 hours after delivery and is associated with abnormal involution of the placental site, cervical or vaginal lacerations, and retained portions of placenta.

Table 8-15 | Induction of Labor

Indications	Relative Contraindications	Absolute Contraindications
• Prolonged pregnancy • Diabetes mellitus • Rh isoimmunization • Preeclampsia • Premature rupture of membranes • Chronic hypertension • Placental insufficiency • Suspected intrauterine growth retardation	• Breech presentation • Oligohydramnios • Multiple gestation • Prematurity • Grand multiparity • Previous cesarean section with transverse scar • Fetal macrosomia	• Cephalopelvic disproportion • Placenta previa • Uterine scar from previous classical cesarean section • Transverse lie • Myomectomy

Adapted from DeCherney A, Nathan L, Laurfer, N, Roman, A. *Current Diagnosis & Treatment: Obstetrics & Gynecology.* 12th ed. McGraw-Hill Companies; 2019.

Table 8-16 | Postpartum Hemorrhage

Condition	Uterine atony *most common* (50%)	Genital laceration (20%)	Retained placenta (10%)
Risk factors	Excessively short or long labor Infected uterus	Uncontrolled vaginal delivery	Noncontracted uterus
Findings	Soft uterus	Visual laceration	Missing cotyledon on placenta
Management	Uterine massage Oxytocin	Suture	Manual exploration

    c. Late postpartum hemorrhage occurs >24 hours after delivery to 6 weeks postpartum and is most commonly caused by subinvolution of the uterus, retained products of conception, or endometritis.

2. Clinical features

    a. Complaints of increased bleeding after delivery signal a need to evaluate for hemorrhage.

    b. A subinvoluted uterus will feel enlarged and soft on examination, and the patient may present with complaints of increased bleeding, pain, fever, and foul-smelling lochia.

3. Diagnostic studies

    a. Hemoglobin and hematocrit tests are necessary to quantify complaints of bleeding and evaluate for acute anemia.

    b. Ultrasonography can sometimes detect obvious retained placental fragments.

4. Management

    a. Initially, uterine massage and compression can be used.

    b. Establish IV access and prepare blood components.

    c. The use of IV oxytocin, ergonovine, methylergonovine, or prostaglandins is often the first line of treatment for early postpartum hemorrhage.

    d. Subinvolution of the uterus often responds to oral agents that increase uterine contraction (e.g., methylergonovine maleate, ergonovine maleate). Antibiotic treatment may also be necessary.

    e. Postpartum hemorrhage may require surgical intervention, depending on the cause and severity.

F. Endometritis

1. General characteristics

    a. Endometritis most commonly occurs after cesarean section or when membranes are ruptured >24 hours before delivery.

    b. Findings most commonly present 2 to 3 days postpartum. Fever >38.3°C (101°F) and uterine tenderness are highly suspicious for endometritis.

    c. Adnexal tenderness, peritoneal irritation, and decreased bowel sounds may occur.

2. Diagnostic studies

    a. White blood cell count is commonly >20,000/μL.

    b. Causative bacteria vary widely from hospital to hospital, but anaerobic streptococci are most common.

    c. Urinalysis should also be performed.

3. Management

    a. Antibiotics are administered until afebrile for 24 hours.

      (1) Clindamycin plus gentamicin is the first line of treatment.

> Endometritis is pelvic inflammatory disease in a pregnant patient.

(2) Ampicillin is added if there is no response in 24 to 48 hours.

(3) Metronidazole is added if sepsis is present.

b. A single dose of antibiotic at the time of cord clamping reduces the incidence of endometritis.

Puerperium

A. Definition: The 6-week period after delivery is known as the puerperium or the postpartum period.

B. **Normal puerperium**

   1. General characteristics

     a. Immediately after delivery, the uterus is at the level of the umbilicus.

      (1) After 2 days, the uterus shrinks or involutes.

      (2) After 2 weeks, it descends into the pelvic cavity.

      (3) By 6 weeks, it is back to its antenatal size.

     b. Lochia, or bleeding that occurs after delivery, represents the sloughing off of decidual tissue. It can last for 4 to 5 weeks postpartum.

     c. In a nonbreastfeeding mother, menses resume 6 to 8 weeks postpartum. In contrast, breastfeeding mothers typically are anovulatory and may remain amenorrheic for the duration of lactation.

   2. **Clinical features**

     a. The first postpartum visit should be ~6 weeks after delivery. This should include a thorough history with attention to bleeding, breastfeeding or bottle-feeding, pelvic pain, sexual and contraceptive history, bowel and bladder function, and emotional well-being. Postpartum blues are common and relatively benign. Postpartum depression and postpartum psychosis can be debilitating.

     b. On pelvic examination at 6 weeks, the perineum should be well healed, and the uterus back to its pregravid size.

     c. Occasionally, a lactating mother will have atrophic vaginitis.

   3. Diagnostic studies

     a. During the first postpartum visit, hemoglobin and hematocrit may be recommended as indicated by history.

     b. If the patient had developed gestational diabetes, a fasting blood glucose should be ordered.

     c. The Edinburgh Postnatal Depression Scale screens for depressive symptoms. Patients scoring 10 or more should receive further assessment and treatment.

   4. **Management**

     a. It is important to emphasize contraceptive counseling at the postpartum examination.

     b. Vitamin supplementation should be continued for the nursing mother.

     c. Atrophic vaginitis can be treated with vaginal estrogen as needed.

> 💡 Crucial follow-up postpartum concerns beyond Ob-Gyn include glucose if GDM; hemoglobin if indicated; and depression screening in all women.

Practice Questions

Directions: *Each of the numbered items or incomplete statements in this section is followed by a list of answers or completions of the statement. Select the ONE lettered answer or completion that is BEST in each case.*

1. A 26-year-old who is 8 weeks pregnant presents with vaginal bleeding. Speculum examination reveals an open cervix without any visible products of conception. What is the most likely diagnosis?
   A. Complete abortion
   B. Inevitable abortion
   C. Missed abortion
   D. Threatened abortion
   E. Inevitable abortion

2. A 27-year-old at 9 weeks' gestation presents with vaginal bleeding. Examination reveals a 20-week–sized uterus. β-hCG levels are exceptionally high. Ultrasonography reveals a mass with a snowstorm appearance. What is the recommended treatment?
   A. Combination chemotherapy
   B. Methotrexate
   C. Suction curettage
   D. Targeted radiation
   E. Watchful waiting

3. A 29-year-old at 24 weeks' gestations has an elevated glucose (152) after a 50-g challenge. The 3-hour glucose tolerance test reveals fasting 92 g; 1-hour 201 g; 2-hour 180 g; 3-hour 138 g. What is the best diagnosis?
   A. Normal results
   B. Type 2 diabetes
   C. Gestational diabetes
   D. Unable to diagnose without further testing

4. A 23-year-old at 33 weeks' gestation presents with painful contractions and watery discharge. Cervix is 3 cm dilated and 80% effaced. Fetal HR is 160 and regular. BP is 140/88; urine is positive for blood. What is the diagnosis?
   A. Incomplete abortion
   B. Incompetent cervix
   C. Placenta abruption
   D. Preeclampsia
   E. Preterm labor

5. A 26-year-old pregnant female with normal BMI presents for prenatal care. She is unsure of her last menses. The top of her uterus is felt about 2 cm below the umbilicus. What is the best estimate of gestational age?
   A. 8 weeks
   B. 12 weeks
   C. 16 weeks
   D. 20 weeks
   E. 26 weeks

6. A 25-year-old female presents with right side lower abdominal pain and spotting. LMP was 6 weeks ago. What diagnostic study is warranted at this time?
   A. Abdominopelvic computed tomography (CT) scan
   B. β-hCG level
   C. CBC with differential
   D. PAPP-A
   E. Transvaginal ultrasonography

7. A 33-year-old G1P0 at 37 weeks presents with headache and blurred vision. She has a BP of 166/112; urine is positive for protein 4+. She is admitted and started on magnesium sulfate and labetalol. Two hours later, she complains of difficulty breathing; BP is 148/98, HR 100; RR 26; deep tendon reflexes are slow. What is the recommended management at this time?
   A. Add potassium to IV fluids
   B. Calcium gluconate
   C. Betamethasone
   D. Increase labetalol
   E. Terbutaline

8. A 24-year-old G1P0 undergoes NST at 36 weeks. Tracing shows accelerations of fetal heart of 10 to 12 bpm from baseline lasting 15 seconds; there are no decelerations. What is the recommended management?
   A. Have mother lie on the left side and repeat the test.
   B. Order an acoustic stimulation test.
   C. Prepare for induction of labor.
   D. Reassure mother that the results are normal.
   E. Send mother for a high-risk ultrasound.

9. A 29-year-old G1P0 presents for initial prenatal care. LMP was 8 weeks ago. Mother is B (−ve); father is A (+ve). Which of the following is recommended to include in her prenatal care?
   A. Administer RhoGam at 28 to 29 weeks and again after delivery.
   B. Administer RhoGam at this visit and again after delivery.
   C. Draw blood for further antibody testing.
   D. Prepare for cesarean section to reduce maternal–fetal blood mixing.
   E. Prepare for transfusion for the fetus after delivery.

10. A 41-year-old overweight female is 9 weeks pregnant. BP is 160/114; repeat after 5 minutes of rest results in a BP of 162/110. What is the treatment of choice?
    A. Bed rest and low-salt diet
    B. Magnesium sulfate
    C. Methyldopa
    D. Labetalol
    E. Plasma exchange

11. A 32-year-old G3P2 is in labor. Baby is moving and has a HR of 170. Monitor shows decelerations of fetal HR that begin at the peak of contractions. There are no accelerations. What is the best interpretation?
    A. Check fluid for ferning.
    B. Order a KB test.
    C. Perform a digital vaginal examination.
    D. Place mother on her left side.
    E. Perform ultrasonography to assess placenta.

12. A 31-year-old at 34 weeks presents with painless vaginal bleeding. Vital signs are stable. Baby is moving, and HR is 166. What is the next best step?
    A. Fetal head compression
    B. Oligohydramnios
    C. Placental abruption
    D. Uterine irritability
    E. Uteroplacental insufficiency

Practice Answers

1. C. *Obstetrics; Diagnosis; Abortion*

An open cervix indicates an inevitable abortion. An open cervix with partial products of conception visible is termed an *incomplete abortion*, whereas with full products of conception is termed a *complete abortion*. A missed abortion is defined as no bleeding with closed cervix but no products of conception in the uterus. The cervix is closed in a threatened abortion.

2. C. *Obstetrics; Clinical Intervention; Molar Pregnancy*

A complete molar pregnancy (hydatidiform mole) is the most common form of GTD. A marked high hCG and "snowstorm" or "grapelike vesicles" is characteristic. The cure rate following suction curettage of a molar pregnancy is 80% to 100%. The hCG level should be followed to assure resolution. Benign tumors can be treated with chemotherapy; high-risk tumors require combination chemotherapy.

3. C. *Obstetrics; Diagnosis; Gestational Diabetes*

A 50-g glucose challenge is the standard screening for gestational diabetes. If abnormal, a 3-hour 100-g glucose tolerance test is recommended. If two or more of the values are abnormal, a diagnosis of gestational diabetes is made.

4. E. *Obstetrics; Diagnosis; Preterm Labor*

Preterm labor is diagnosed before 37 weeks' gestation and is the most common cause of neonatal deaths. It is defined as regular uterine contractions and the presence of one or more of the following: cervical dilation 2 cm or more at presentation; cervical dilation of 1 cm or greater on serial examination; cervical effacement ≥80%. Watery or bloody discharge may occur. Placenta abruption causes painful contraction and a tense irritable uterus. Preeclampsia is characterized by hypertension, edema, and proteinuria. Inevitable abortion is defined as an open cervix without visible products of conception before 20 weeks' gestation. An incompetent cervix places a woman at risk for spontaneous abortion.

5. C. *Obstetrics; History and physical examination; Normal Pregnancy*

At 8 weeks, the uterus is in the pelvis. At 12 weeks, the uterus is at the pelvic rim. At 16 weeks, it is about 2 cm below umbilicus. At 20 weeks, it is at the umbilicus. At 26 weeks, it is far above the umbilicus.

6. E. *Obstetrics; Diagnostic Studies; Ectopic Pregnancy*

A transvaginal ultrasonography is warranted to identify placement of the fetus. β-hCG will confirm the pregnancy, but not diagnose an ectopic pregnancy. A CT scan will expose the fetus to unnecessary radiation. PAPP-A evaluates risk of trisomy. A CBC is nonspecific.

7. B. *Obstetrics; Pharmacology; Preeclampsia*

This patient presented with preeclampsia but has developed magnesium toxicity. Calcium gluconate is needed to reduce the cardiac effects of the toxicity. Betamethasone is recommended at this stage if the gestational age is <34 weeks.

Tocolytics, such as terbutaline, are given to reduce contractions, which is not needed in this patient. Ultimate treatment for preeclampsia is delivery.

8. D. *Obstetrics; Diagnostic Studies; NST*

An NST is considered reactive (normal) if there are at least two accelerations of fetal HR in 20 minutes for up to 15 bpm from baseline for a duration of 15 seconds and in the absence of decelerations. Mother can be reassured and continue routine care.

9. A. *Obstetrics; Clinical Intervention; Rh Incompatibility*

Mothers who are Rh negative should receive RhoGam at 28 to 29 weeks; if the baby is found to be Rh positive, mother should receive another injection of RhoGam after delivery to protect subsequent pregnancies. Although there are 43 other antigens in the blood, 98% of all isoimmunizations are secondary to the Rh factor. There is no need to recommend C-section.

10. C. *Obstetrics; Pharmacology; Chronic Hypertension in Pregnancy*

Elevated BP before 20 weeks' gestation is considered chronic hypertension. PIH is elevated BP after 20 weeks' gestation. Medication is recommended for severe hypertension in pregnancy; methyldopa is the drug of choice; labetalol is an alternative. Hypertension, edema, and proteinuria after 20 weeks indicate preeclampsia; magnesium sulfate is given to lower the risk of seizure. Bed rest and low-salt diet will not be adequate for this level of hypertension. Plasma exchange is the separation of the blood components leaving a filtered plasma product; it is indicated in cases where immunoglobulins have become pathologic, such as thrombotic thrombocytopenia.

11. E. *Obstetrics; Scientific Concepts; Fetal Heart Monitoring*

Late decelerations (starting at the peak of contraction and into the second half of the contraction) are worrisome; the most likely cause is uteroplacental insufficiency. Urgent delivery is recommended. Early decelerations (mirroring the contraction) or variable decelerations (rapid drops of fetal HR with variable return to baseline) indicate fetal head compression and are typically benign. Uterine irritability affects the shape of the contractions. Placental abruption is the most common cause of third-trimester bleeding; it presents with painful bleeding.

12. E. *Obstetrics; Diagnostic Studies; Placenta Previa*

The most common cause of painless bleeding in the second half of pregnancy is placenta previa (placenta covering the cervical os). An ultrasound is a noninvasive method to identify placental placement. A digital examination should be avoided because it can cause more severe bleeding. Ferning of vaginal fluid confirms rupture of membranes. Placing mother on the left side reduces pressure on the vena cava, thus allowing improved blood return to the heart. KB test evaluates for fetomaternal hemorrhage; it is indicated after trauma.

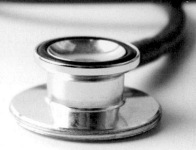

Rheumatology and Orthopedics (Musculoskeletal System) | 9

Jennifer Joseph

Arthritis/Rheumatologic Conditions

A. Osteoarthritis (OA)

  1. General characteristics

    a. OA is characterized as progressive loss of articular cartilage with reactive changes in the bone, resulting in pain and destruction of the joint.

    b. Among persons aged 40 years or older, 90% display radiographic signs of the disease.

    c. See Table 9-1 for a comparison of OA versus rheumatoid arthritis (RA).

  2. Clinical features

    a. Decreased range of motion (ROM), joint crepitus, morning stiffness, and pain gradually worsening throughout the day are features of OA.

    b. Common sites of involvement are the distal interphalangeal joint (DIP, Heberden's nodes), proximal interphalangeal joint (PIP, Bouchard's nodules), wrist, hip, knee, and spine. The metacarpophalangeal (MCP) joints (except the thumb), ankle, and elbow are usually spared.

    c. Joints can become unstable during the late stages of OA.

  3. Diagnostic studies

    a. Laboratory tests are nonspecific.

    b. Radiographs show asymmetric narrowing, subchondral sclerosis, bony cysts, and marginal osteophytes.

  4. Treatment

    a. Nonpharmacologic management: Weight reduction, moderate physical activity, bracing, canes, and muscle strengthening may be useful in managing OA.

    b. Topical nonsteroidal anti-inflammatory drugs (NSAIDs) are considered first-line treatment by the American College of Rheumatology when pain is mild to moderate and there is no evidence of inflammation. If topical NSAIDs fail, oral NSAIDs can be prescribed along with gastrointestinal (GI) protection in patients who are at risk.

    c. Intra-articular treatment with steroids or viscosupplementation injections (e.g., hyaluronic acid) are appropriate second-line treatments,

    d. Total joint replacement may be indicated in advanced cases. Osteotomy and surgical arthrodesis generally do not have long-term benefits.

B. Rheumatoid arthritis (RA)

  1. General characteristics

    a. RA is a chronic inflammatory disease with synovitis affecting multiple joints as well as other systemic extra-articular manifestations.

> 💡 OA is the most common arthropathy among adults, particularly the elderly.

> 💡 Bony cysts and osteophytes are seen in OA but not in RA.

255

Table 9-1 | Osteoarthritis Versus Rheumatoid Arthritis

	Osteoarthritis (Noninflammatory)	**Rheumatoid Arthritis (Inflammatory)**
Age	>60 years	30–50 years
Sex	F > M	F > M
Symmetry	Asymmetric	Symmetric
Joints	Hip, knee, DIPs	Hands, wrists, ankles
Physical examination	↓ ROM, crepitus, stiffness lasting <1 hour, no systemic symptoms, Heberden and Bouchard's nodes	Ulnar deviations, swan neck and Boutonniere deformities, sub Q nodules, stiffness lasting >1 hour plus systemic symptoms
Treatment	Weight loss, exercise, topical NSAIDs, oral NSAIDs, joint injections, joint replacement	NSAIDs, DMARDs, physical therapy, splinting

DMARDs, disease-modifying antirheumatic drugs; DIP, distal interphalangeal joint; NSAID, nonsteroidal anti-inflammatory drugs; ROM, range of motion.

    b. Females are affected more often than males (3:1 ratio), with onset typically occurring between 30 and 50 years of age. The juvenile form occurs in patients younger than 16 years of age.

    c. A cascade of events leads to joint destruction. Hyperplastic synovial tissue (pannus) may erode cartilage, subchondral bone, articular capsule, tendons, and ligaments.

2. Clinical features

    a. See Table 9-2 for diagnostic criteria of RA. To make the diagnosis, a score of 6/10 should be attained.

    b. The DIP joints are usually spared.

    c. RA causes joint pain and deformity as well as muscle weakness, myositis, myopathy, osteopenia, and osteoporosis.

    d. Extra-articular manifestations of RA include changes in the skin, lungs, kidneys, eyes, liver, blood system, and heart (Table 9-3). Osteoporosis is frequently diagnosed.

3. Diagnostic studies

    a. Aspiration and joint fluid analysis (Table 9-4) are useful laboratory tests to quantify inflammation and exclude the presence of gout or septic arthritis.

Table 9-2 | Diagnostic Criteria for Rheumatoid Arthritis[a]

1. Joint involvement (0–5 points)
   - 1 medium or large joint (0 point)
   - 2–10 medium or large joints (1 point)
   - 1–3 small joints (2 points)
   - 4–10 small joints (3 points)
   - >10 joints (at least one small) (5 points)

2. Serology (0–3 points)
   - RF and ACPA negative (0 point)
   - RF or ACPA low positive (2 points)
   - RF or ACPA high positive (3 points)

3. Duration of symptoms (0–1 point)
   - <6 weeks (0 point)
   - >6 weeks (1 point)

4. Acute phase reactants (0–1 point)
   - CRP and ESR not elevated (0 point)
   - Increased CRP or ESR (1 point)

[a]Score of 6/10 is required for a definite diagnosis of RA.

RF, rheumatoid factor; ACPA, anticitrullinated protein antibody; CRP, C-reactive protein; ESR, erythrocyte sedimentation rate.

Adapted from the American College of Rheumatology (ACR) and the European League Against Rheumatism (EULAR) diagnostic criteria for rheumatoid arthritis from 2010.

Table 9-3 | Extra-articular Manifestations of Rheumatoid Arthritis

System	Typical Manifestation
Constitutional	General achiness, stiffness Fever Weight loss Fatigue Sleep disturbance Cognitive and emotional dysfunction Depressive symptoms
Dermatologic	Rheumatoid nodules Skin ulcers Neutrophilic dermatoses
Eye	Episcleritis, scleritis Uveitis, iritis Ulcerative keratitis Keratoconjunctivitis sicca Sjögren's syndrome
Pulmonary	Pleuritis, pleural effusion Interstitial fibrosis Pulmonary nodules Bronchiolitis obliterans Organizing pneumonia Pulmonary embolus
Hematologic	Anemia Neutropenia Felty syndrome Lymphoproliferative disease
Cardiovascular	Myocarditis Pericarditis Coronary artery disease Heart failure Atrial fibrillation Vasculitis Peripheral vascular disease Venous thromboembolus
Renal	Glomerulonephritis Chronic kidney disease Amyloidosis
Neurologic	Carpal tunnel, tarsal tunnel Cervical subluxation Cervical myelopathy CNS vasculitis Stroke Meningitis

CNS, central nervous system.

    b. Erythrocyte sedimentation rate (ESR) and C-reactive protein (CRP) are elevated.

    c. Rheumatoid factor (RF), although nonspecific, is positive in 80% of patients. Anti-cyclic citrullinated peptide (ACPA or anti-CCP) antibodies are more specific and are positive in 95% of patients with RA; levels may be low in early disease.

    d. Soft-tissue swelling and juxta-articular demineralization are seen on radiography.

  4. Treatment

    a. Consultation with a rheumatologist is recommended for initiation of treatment and development of a long-term plan.

    b. Physical and occupational therapy should be implemented.

    c. Pharmacologic management (Table 9-5) should be early and aggressive to reduce pain, preserve function, and prevent deformity.

Table 9-4 | Differentiation of Joint Fluid Analysis

	Color	WBCs (/IL)	PMNs (%)	Culture
Osteoarthritis	Yellow	200–300	25	Negative
Rheumatoid arthritis (or other inflammatory conditions)	Yellow to opalescent	3,000–50,000	25–50	Negative
Septic	Yellow to green	>50,000	75	Positive

WBCs, white blood cells; PMNs, polymorphonucleocytes.

(1) NSAIDs may be used in conjunction with disease-modifying antirheumatic drugs (DMARDs).

(2) DMARDs are begun as soon as the diagnosis is made.

(a) Methotrexate is frequently the initial DMARD.

(b) Other DMARDs include corticosteroids, sulfasalazine, antimalarials, and leflunomide.

(c) Newer biologic DMARDs include etanercept, abatacept, rituximab, infliximab, and adalimumab.

(d) Combination therapy is typically required, although there is concern about safety and cost. Methotrexate plus a biologic DMARD is a common choice.

(e) Reconstructive surgery is indicated for severe cases.

Table 9-5 | Antirheumatoid Arthritis Drugs

Class/Type	Examples	Notes
NSAIDs	Ibuprofen Naproxen	Available without prescription
Traditional DMARDs	Methotrexate Sulfasalazine Leflunomide	GI and liver side effects
Biologic DMARDs	Etanercept Infliximab Adalimumab Certolizumab Golimumab Anakinra Abatacept Rituximab Tocilizumab	Costly Increased risk of infection
Nonbiologic DMARDs	Azathioprine Tofacitinib Auranofin Iguratimod Tacrolimus Temsirolimus Hydroxychloroquine	
Immunologics	Cyclosporine Prednisone	Negative long-term side effects

DMARDs, disease-modifying antirheumatic drugs; NSAIDs, nonsteroidal anti-inflammatory drugs.

C. Juvenile idiopathic arthritis (JIA); juvenile rheumatoid arthritis (JRA)

1. General characteristics

a. JIA is characterized by chronic synovitis and a number of extra-articular manifestations (fever, rash, weight loss, other organ involvement).

b. Females are affected more often than males (2:1 ratio) and have an earlier age of onset (females, 1 to 3 years of age; males, 8 to 12 years of age).

2. Clinical features: The American College of Rheumatology defines JIA by age (younger than 16 years old) and duration of the disease (>6 weeks) and divides JIA into three subtypes listed as follows:

a. Systemic, 15% of cases (Still disease)

(1) This type is characterized by spiking fevers (39°C to 40°C; 102.2°F to 104°F), myalgias, polyarthralgias, and a typical salmon-pink maculopapular rash appearing in the evening and with the fever.

(2) The rash may be elicited by scratching the skin in susceptible areas (Koebner phenomenon).

(3) There are minimal articular findings, but hepatosplenomegaly, lymphadenopathy, leukocytosis, pericarditis, or myocarditis may occur.

b. Oligoarticular, 50% of cases

(1) This type is characterized by involvement of four or fewer medium to large joints.

(2) Patients are also at risk for the development of asymptomatic uveitis, which may lead to blindness if they have a positive antinuclear antibody (ANA) test.

c. Polyarticular, 35% of cases

(1) This type resembles adult RA with its symmetric involvement and involves five or more small and large joints.

(2) Systemic symptoms include low-grade fever, fatigue, rheumatoid nodules, and anemia.

3. Diagnostic studies

a. There are no specific diagnostic tests for JIA, but 10% to 15% of patients have a positive RF; ACPA antibody test may be positive as well.

(1) ESR and CRP are increased or normal with the systemic type.

(2) The ANA test may be increased in the oligoarticular type and indicates a tendency for uveitis.

b. Imaging studies may be similar to those for adults with soft-tissue swelling and synovitis. Periarticular osteoporosis and joint space narrowing may occur. Joint destruction is less frequent.

4. Treatment (may differ based on subtype of diagnosis)

a. NSAIDs and physical and occupational therapy are most beneficial. Methotrexate, leflunomide, or anakinra may be used as second-line agents, early on, if there is no improvement with NSAIDs alone.

b. Monitor children with JIA for any growth abnormalities, nutritional deficiencies, and school/social impairment.

c. Seventy-five percent to 80% remit without serious disability. Patients who are RF positive are at the greatest risk of progressing to disabling arthritis into adulthood.

D. Other types of arthritis

1. Infectious (septic) arthritis

a. General characteristics and clinical features

(1) The hematogenous spread of bacteria from periarticular osteomyelitis, infection caused by diagnostic or therapeutic procedure (e.g., intra-articular injection), or infection elsewhere (e.g., cellulitis, bursitis) may lead to infectious arthritis. Bacterial septic arthritis involves a single joint in 90% of cases (most commonly the knee, followed by hip, shoulder, ankle, and wrist).

> The most common type of JIA is oligoarticular: ≤4 med to large joint involvement.

> Septic arthritis stems from hematogenous spread of infection (often *Staphylococcus aureus*) into a joint space, resulting in swelling, fever, and effusion.

> Gonococcal arthritis occurs twice as often in males compared to females.

(2) *S. aureus* is the most common pathogen in joint infections followed by methicillin-resistant *S. aureus* (MRSA) and group B streptococcus.

(3) Sexually active young adults are at risk for septic arthritis caused by infection with *Neisseria gonorrhoeae*. Gonococcal arthritis is typically monoarticular.

(4) Patients usually present with acute swelling, fever, joint warmth and effusion, tenderness to palpation, and increased pain with minimal ROM in the involved joint(s). Cutaneous lesions may also be present.

b. Diagnostic studies

(1) Synovial fluid should be collected. The fluid is typically yellow to green with elevated white blood cell (WBC) and polymorphonucleocytes (PMNs). Forty percent of patients will have a positive blood culture. See Table 9-4.

(2) Radiographs usually only show soft-tissue swelling.

c. Treatment

(1) Aggressive treatment with intravenous (IV) antibiotics for 2 weeks is required. Vancomycin and ceftriaxone are recommended for empiric treatment; adjustment post culture and sensitivity is based on identified organism.

(2) Arthrotomy (surgical opening into a joint to drain and debride the infection) or joint drainage by arthrocentesis (puncture of joint space with a needle for synovial fluid analysis and culture) is required early in the presentation.

(3) Oral antibiotics should follow the IV antibiotics for generally up to an additional 4 weeks.

2. Psoriatic arthritis

a. General characteristics: This is an inflammatory arthritis with skin involvement usually preceding joint disease by months to years.

b. Clinical features

(1) The course usually is mild and intermittent, affecting a few joints.

(2) Symmetric arthritis resembles RA and may involve the hands and feet. Pitting of the nails and onycholysis are seen.

(3) Sausage-finger appearance (caused by arthritis and tenosynovitis of the flexor tendon) is a common feature.

> In psoriatic arthritis, more severe skin involvement is often associated with increased uric acid.

c. Diagnostic studies

(1) ESR and CRP may be elevated; normocytic normochromic anemia is common.

(2) Hyperuricemia may occur when skin involvement is severe.

(3) RF is generally normal.

(4) "Pencil in cup" deformities of the proximal phalanx are demonstrated on radiography.

d. Treatment

(1) Lifestyle management: Weight loss, physical and occupational therapy should be recommended.

(2) NSAIDs are sufficient for mild cases.

(3) Methotrexate is beneficial for both skin inflammation and arthritis. Biologic DMARDs are recommended for severe cases. Corticosteroids and antimalarials should be avoided as they may exacerbate skin problems.

(4) Reconstructive surgery (arthrodesis or joint replacement) is indicated if movement is limited or patients have decreased mobility.

3. Reactive arthritis (Reiter syndrome)

a. General characteristics

(1) Reactive arthritis is a seronegative arthritis that presents with a tetrad of urethritis, conjunctivitis, oligoarthritis, and mucosal ulcers.

(2) It is often seen as a sequelae to sexually transmitted infections (chlamydial urethritis or *Ureaplasma*) or gastroenteritis (*Shigella, Salmonella, Yersinia,* or *Campylobacter, Clostridium difficile*).

b. Clinical features

(1) Patients typically have asymmetric arthritis that involves large joints usually below the waist (i.e., knee and ankle); mucocutaneous lesions (balanitis, stomatitis), urethritis, and conjunctivitis are common.

(2) The gender ratio is 1:1 after enteric infections and 9:1 after sexually transmitted infections, with a male predominance. It is the leading cause of nontraumatic monoarthritis.

c. Diagnostic studies

(1) Up to 80% of patients are human leukocyte antigen (HLA)-B27 positive.

(2) Synovial fluid culture is usually negative.

(3) Evidence of permanent and progressive joint disease may be present on radiography.

d. Treatment

(1) Physical therapy and NSAIDs are the mainstay of treatment.

(2) Antibiotics given at the time of infection will reduce the chance of developing the disorder but do not alleviate the symptoms of reactive arthritis.

> Post-STI reactive arthritis has a 9:1 male predominance.

E. Gout

1. General characteristics

a. Gout is a systemic disease of altered purine metabolism and subsequent sodium urate crystal precipitation into the synovial fluid.

b. It is more common in men than in women (9:1) until menopause, after which the ratio approaches parity.

2. Clinical features

a. The most common feature is an initial attack of the metatarsophalangeal (MTP) joint of the great toe (podagra). It is the presenting manifestation in 70% of cases.

b. Other joints of the feet, ankles, and knees are commonly affected.

c. Pain, swelling, redness, and exquisite tenderness develop suddenly at and surrounding the joint.

d. In chronic gout, tophi (chalky deposits of urate crystals) may form adjacent to the joint and are considered diagnostic.

e. Table 9-6 provides a comparison of gout and calcium pyrophosphate dihydrate (CPPD; pseudogout).

> Seventy percent of gout presents with a red, swollen, supremely tender MTP joint of the great toe.

Table 9-6 | Gout Versus CPPD (Pseudogout)

	Gout (Inflammatory)	CPPD—Pseudogout (Inflammatory)
Age	Young, >30 years	Old, >60 years
Sex	M > F	M = F
Symmetry	Asymmetric	Asymmetric
Joints	Great toe, lower extremity	Large joints, knee, lower extremity
Physical examination	Painful, red, swollen, tophi	Painful, red, swollen, no tophi
Synovial fluid crystals	Sodium urate, needle-like crystals that are *negatively* birefringent	Rhomboid-shaped crystals that are *positively* birefringent

CPPD, calcium pyrophosphate dihydrate.

> Foods high in purine include meats, beer, and certain seafoods.

3. Diagnostic studies

   a. Joint fluid analysis is diagnostic if rod-shaped, negatively birefringent urate crystals are seen. The diagnosis of gout may also be inferred by clinical examination.

   b. Serum uric acid level of >8 mg/dL is suspicious but not diagnostic.

4. Imaging: Characteristic erosions (small, punched-out lesions and interosseous tophi) on plain radiographs make the diagnosis of gout highly suspect.

5. **Treatment**

   a. Treatment includes both lifestyle modification and pharmacologic treatment.

   b. Elevation and rest may alleviate symptoms.

   c. Dietary modifications such as decreased ingestion of purines (found in foods such as certain meats, beer, and certain seafood) and decreasing alcohol intake can reduce elevated urate levels.

   d. Weight loss is important if the patient is overweight.

   e. Protein should be increased; plant sources are recommended.

   f. Alcohol intake should be limited.

   g. Pharmacotherapy

      (1) NSAIDs are generally the initial drug of choice (i.e., indomethacin, 25 to 50 mg po three times daily, until symptoms resolve).

      (2) Colchicine is also very effective. Use is limited because of the pervasive GI side effects.

      (3) Corticosteroid injections are recommended for accessible joints if the patient cannot take NSAIDs or colchicine; oral prednisone (or adrenocorticotropic hormone [ACTH]) may be used if other medicines (oral or injected) are not tolerated and septic arthritis has been ruled out.

      (4) Patients should avoid thiazide diuretics and aspirin prophylaxis.

      (5) Patients with severe or recurrent attacks may benefit from lowering the uric acid level.

      (6) Management between acute attacks can be achieved with colchicine, probenecid, sulfapyrazine, xanthine oxidase inhibitors (allopurinol or febuxostat), or uricase medications (pegloticase, rasburicase).

      (7) Allopurinol should not be started during an acute attack, although it should not be discontinued in a patient already on allopurinol maintenance.

> Gout: negatively birefringent urate crystals
>
> Pseudogout: positively birefringent calcium pyrophosphate crystals

F. **Calcium pyrophosphate dihydrate disease (CPDD or pseudogout)** can present with similar symptoms to gout (see Table 9-6).

   1. General characteristics

      a. Pseudogout affects peripheral joints, usually in the lower extremity, and results from intra-articular deposition of calcium pyrophosphate.

      b. Acute presentations may mimic gout; recurrent and abrupt onset of attacks is characteristic.

   2. **Clinical features**

      a. Painful inflammation results when crystals are shed into the joint.

      b. The joints most involved are the knee, wrist, and elbow.

   3. Diagnostic studies

      a. Rhomboid-shaped calcium pyrophosphate crystals that are positively birefringent are found in joint aspiration.

      b. Radiographs show fine, linear calcifications in cartilage (chondrocalcinosis).

   4. **Treatment**: NSAIDs, colchicine, and intra-articular steroid injections may be beneficial. Colchicine is most often used as prophylaxis; NSAIDs for treatment of acute attacks.

G. Systemic lupus erythematosus (SLE)

1. General characteristics

    a. SLE is an autoimmune disorder characterized by inflammation, a positive ANA, and involvement of multiple organs.

    b. SLE commonly affects women of childbearing age. Prevalence also is found among certain familial and ethnic groups (most common in African American women).

2. **Clinical features**

    a. The diagnosis of SLE is based on the presence of certain criteria (Table 9-7).

    b. Diagnosis requires at least four criteria to be met, including a significantly high-titer ANA.

    c. Drug-induced lupus must be ruled out. Some drugs may cause a lupus-like syndrome, including procainamide, hydralazine, isoniazid, methyldopa, quinidine, and chlorpromazine. If the offending agent is stopped, the symptoms typically resolve. These patients have positive antihistone antibodies.

    d. A relapsing and remitting pattern of symptoms is characteristic.

3. Diagnostic studies

    a. Routine laboratory studies at diagnosis should include complete blood count (CBC), blood urea nitrogen (BUN), creatinine, urinalysis, ESR, and serum complement (C3 or C4).

    b. Antibodies to Smith antigen, double-stranded DNA, or depressed levels of serum complement may be used as markers for the progression of the disease.

    c. ANA is present (99%), but low titers have a low predictive value.

4. **Treatment**

    a. Lifestyle modifications: Regular exercise, smoking cessation, and sun protection are important for all patients.

    b. NSAIDs are often used for musculoskeletal complaints.

    c. Antimalarials (hydroxychloroquine or chloroquine) may be used for musculoskeletal complaints and cutaneous manifestations.

    d. Corticosteroids

        (1) Topical or intralesional preparations are often used for cutaneous manifestations.

> Goals when treating chronic autoimmune disorders:
> - prevent flares
> - treat flares early and actively
> - reduce organ damage

Table 9-7 | Diagnostic Criteria for Systemic Lupus Erythematosus[a]

Malar rash
Discoid rash
Photosensitivity
Oral ulcers
Arthritis
Serositis (heart, lungs, or peritoneal)
Renal disease (proteinuria, cellular casts)
ANA
Hematologic disorders (hemolytic anemia, leukopenia, leukocytosis, thrombocytopenia)
Immunologic disorders (LE cell, anti-DNA, anti-Sm, false-positive serologic test for syphilis)
Neurologic disorders (seizures or psychosis in absence of any other cause)

[a]Presence of 4 of the 11 criteria required for diagnosis.

ANA, antinuclear antibody; LE, lupus erythematosus.

Adapted from Tan EM, Cohen AS, Fries JF, et al. The 1982 revised criteria for the classification of systemic lupus erythematosus. *Arthritis Rheum.* 1982;25:1271–1277.

(2) Low- or high-dose oral corticosteroids are used for disease flares and tapered as symptoms resolve.

e. Methotrexate is used at low doses for arthritis, rashes, serositis, and constitutional symptoms.

H. **Polymyositis/Dermatomyositis**

1. General characteristics

a. Polymyositis is an inflammatory disease of striated muscle affecting the proximal limbs, neck, and pharynx. The skin also can be affected (dermatomyositis).

b. Other organ systems affected include joints, lungs, heart, and GI tract.

c. Cause is unknown, but there is a strong association with an occult malignancy.

d. Women are more commonly affected than men (3:1).

2. **Clinical features** may include insidious, painless, proximal muscle weakness; dysphagia; skin rash (malar or heliotrope rash around the eyes); Gottron papules develop on the extensor surfaces of the hands; polyarthralgias; and muscle atrophy.

3. Diagnostic studies

a. The muscle enzymes creatine phosphokinase (CPK) and aldolase will be elevated.

b. Muscle biopsy should be performed and will show myopathic inflammatory changes.

4. **Treatment**: Polymyositis is treated with high-dose steroids, methotrexate, or azathioprine until symptoms resolve.

I. **Polymyalgia rheumatica**

1. General characteristics

a. Polymyalgia rheumatica is characterized by pain and stiffness in the neck, shoulder, and pelvic girdles and is accompanied by constitutional symptoms (e.g., fever, fatigue, weight loss, depression).

b. It affects women twice as often as men and usually presents in patients older than 50 years of age.

c. Cause is unknown. It is associated with giant cell (temporal) arteritis in up to 30% of cases.

2. **Clinical features**

a. Pain and stiffness is usually the predominant feature, being most severe after rest and in the morning.

b. Musculoskeletal symptoms are usually bilateral, proximal, and symmetrical.

c. Giant cell (temporal) arteritis must be ruled out. It characteristically presents with scalp tenderness, jaw claudication, headache, and temporal artery tenderness and may lead to vision loss.

3. Diagnostic studies: ESR is markedly elevated (>50 mm/hour). Temporal arteritis is confirmed by biopsy (minimum length 1 to 2 cm).

4. **Treatment**: Patients respond quickly to low-dose corticosteroid therapy, which may be required for up to 2 years and slowly tapered. Higher doses are required if giant cell arteritis is present; treatment should not be delayed while awaiting biopsy.

J. **Polyarteritis nodosa**

1. General characteristics

a. Small and medium artery inflammation and necrosis involving the skin, kidney, peripheral nerves, muscle, and gut occurs.

b. The male to female ratio is 3:1.

c. Onset is generally between 40 and 60 years of age, although it may occur in every age group.

d. Cause is unknown, but association with hepatitis B is seen in up to 10% of patients.

A heliotrope rash around the eyes is characteristic of dermatomyositis.

Polymyalgia rheumatica is associated with giant cell/temporal arteritis 30% of the time.

Polyarteritis nodosa is a chronic inflammation and necrosis of arterial walls.

2. Clinical features

a. Fever, anorexia, weight loss, abdominal pain, peripheral neuropathy, arthralgias, and arthritis are commonly seen.

b. Skin lesions, including palpable purpura and livedo reticularis, occur in some patients.

c. Renal involvement leads to hypertension, edema, oliguria, and uremia.

3. Diagnostic studies

a. The diagnosis requires confirmation by vessel biopsy or angiography.

b. Elevated ESR and CRP and proteinuria may be present as well as a positive hepatitis B surface antigen (HBsAg).

c. Presence of antineutrophil cytoplasmic antibody (ANCA) is usually not found.

4. Treatment

a. Initial management is with high doses of corticosteroids.

b. Cytotoxic drugs and immunotherapy may also be used. Concomitant treatment of hepatitis B may be required.

c. Hypertension should be treated with angiotensin-converting enzyme inhibitor (ACEI) or angiotensin receptor blockers (ARBs) when diagnosed.

K. Systemic sclerosis (SS; scleroderma)

1. General characteristics

a. Scleroderma is of unknown cause and is characterized by deposition of collagen in the skin and, less commonly, in the kidney, heart, lungs, and stomach.

b. The female to male ratio is 4:1.

c. The peak age of onset is between 30 and 50 years.

2. Clinical features

a. There are two types of scleroderma: *diffuse* (35%), which affects the skin as well as the heart, lungs, GI tract, and kidneys; and *limited* (65%), which mostly affects the skin of the face, neck, and distal to the elbows and knees and late in the disease causes isolated pulmonary hypertension.

b. Skin involvement occurs in 95% of patients. Changes most often begin with swelling in the fingers and hands and may spread to involve the trunk and the face.

c. Raynaud's phenomenon, vasospasm of the digital arteries causing a characteristic white–blue–red pattern, is seen in more than 75% of patients.

d. The following conditions, Calcinosis cutis, Raynaud's phenomenon, Esophageal dysfunction, Sclerodactyly, and Telangiectasias comprise "CREST" syndrome, which is associated with limited scleroderma.

e. Patients usually present with skin changes, polyarthralgias, esophageal dysfunction, and a history of Raynaud's phenomenon.

3. Diagnostic studies

a. ANA is present in 90% of patients with diffuse scleroderma.

b. Anticentromere antibody is associated with CREST syndrome. Anti-SCL-70 antibody and anti-RNA polymerase III are associated with diffuse disease and portend a poor prognosis.

c. Patients should be monitored for development of lung disease and renal involvement that can present as hypertensive renal crisis.

4. Treatment

a. There is no cure for scleroderma.

b. Treatment is aimed at organ-specific disease processes (i.e., proton pump inhibitors for reflux disease, ACEIs for renal disease, avoidance of triggers and treatment with calcium channel blockers for Raynaud's, and immunosuppressive drugs for pulmonary hypertension).

The mottled discoloration seen in livedo reticularis is owing to blood vessel spasms in circulation near the surface of the skin.

Scleroderma is from the Greek for "hard skin."

The most common cause of death in patients with systemic sclerosis is pulmonary disease.

L. Sjögren's syndrome

    1. General characteristics

        a. Sjögren's syndrome is an autoimmune disorder that destroys the salivary and lacrimal glands (exocrine glands).

        b. It may also be a secondary complication to a preexisting connective tissue disorder such as RA, SLE, polymyositis, or scleroderma.

        c. It is most often diagnosed in middle-aged females.

    2. **Clinical features**

        a. Mucous membranes are most affected. Dry mouth (xerostomia) and dry eyes (xerophthalmia or keratoconjunctivitis sicca) are characteristic features of primary Sjögren's syndrome.

        b. The parotid glands may also be enlarged.

    3. Diagnostic studies

        a. RF is present in 70% of cases, ANA in 60%, anti-Ro antibodies in 60%, and anti-La antibodies in 40% of cases.

        b. A Schirmer test evaluates tear secretions by the lacrimal glands. Wetting of <5 mm of filter paper placed in the lower eyelid for 5 minutes is positive for decreased secretions.

        c. Biopsy of the lower lip mucosa confirms lymphocytic infiltrate and gland fibrosis.

    4. **Treatment**

        a. Management is mainly symptomatic, with the goal of keeping mucosal surfaces moist. This can be achieved by using artificial tears and saliva, increased oral fluid intake, and ocular and vaginal lubricants.

        b. Pilocarpine or cevimeline improves symptoms by stimulating the exocrine glands.

        c. Topical cyclosporine or lifitegrast may improve ocular symptoms. Punctal plugging is also helpful.

> Sjögren's syndrome:
> - dry eyes
> - dry mouth
> - parotid gland disease

M. **Fibromyalgia syndrome**

    1. General characteristics

        a. The fibromyalgia syndrome is a central pain disorder whose cause and pathogenesis are poorly understood.

        b. Fibromyalgia may occur spontaneously or may occur with RA, SLE, and Sjögren's syndrome, hypothyroidism, and sleep apnea in men.

    2. **Clinical features**

        a. Patients have nonarticular musculoskeletal aches, pains, and multiple tender "trigger" points on examination. Fibromyalgia is characterized by pain above and below the waist that is bilateral and axial for a duration of at least 3 months.

        b. Nonspecific complaints include fatigue, sleep disruption, mood changes, and cognitive disturbances. Anxiety, depression, headaches, irritable bowel syndrome, dysmenorrhea, and paresthesias are also associated with this condition.

    3. Diagnostic studies

        a. Fibromyalgia is recognized by the typical pattern of pain and other symptoms as well as by exclusion of contributory or underlying diseases such as hypothyroidism, hepatitis C, and vitamin D deficiency.

        b. There are no routine laboratory markers; it is often a diagnosis of exclusion.

        c. Abnormality of the T-cell subsets has been described.

    4. **Treatment**

        a. Pharmaceutical: Antidepressants: Selective serotonin reuptake inhibitors (SSRIs), selective serotonin and norepinephrine reuptake inhibitors (SSNRIs), and tricyclic

> The widespread pain and resulting fatigue of fibromyalgia is caused by hypersensitive abnormal pain processing in the central nervous system; this is why NSAIDs are not effective.

antidepressants (TCAs) have all been shown to be helpful in subsets of patients with fibromyalgia. NSAIDs are not effective.

b. Pregabalin or gabapentin can be effective in reducing pain and improving sleep. Side effects, however, include fatigue, trouble concentrating, sleepiness, and edema.

c. Lifestyle: Aerobic exercise improves conditioning and has been shown to improve functioning as long as overtraining is avoided.

d. Cognitive-behavioral therapy and mindfulness training are often helpful. Patient education, stress reduction, sleep assistance, and treatment of psychological problems may alleviate some symptoms.

N. Table 9-8 is a summary of typical seroconversions in common autoimmune disorders.

> Musculoskeletal pain is a complex interplay of sensory, psychological, and motor factors.

Bone and Joint Disorders

A. **Tendinopathy and tenosynovitis**

1. General characteristics

a. Tendinopathy refers to inflammation of the tendon.

b. Tenosynovitis is inflammation of the enclosed tendon sheath.

c. Common causes include overuse injuries and systemic disease (e.g., arthritides).

2. **Clinical features**

a. Tendinopathy and tenosynovitis commonly appear in the following sites: rotator cuff, supraspinatus, biceps, flexor carpi ulnaris, flexor carpi radialis, flexor digitorum, patella, hip adductor, and Achilles.

b. Tendinopathy and tenosynovitis generally occur together, causing pain with movement, swelling, and impaired function.

c. The conditions may resolve over several weeks, but recurrence is common.

3. **Treatment**

a. Nonpharmaceutical: Ice, relative rest, and active stretching and rehabilitation to allow recovery.

b. NSAIDs may alleviate pain but do not penetrate the tendon circulation adequately. An injection with corticosteroids combined with anesthesia and administered alongside the tendon may be beneficial. Intratendon injection should be avoided because of the risk of rupture.

c. Surgery for excision of scar tissue and necrotic debris may be performed if conservative measures are unsuccessful. The scar tissue is caused by repetitive microtrauma to the tissue.

> Relative rest, not full rest, is recommended in tendinopathies.

Table 9-8 | Summary of Typical Seroconversions in Common Autoimmune Disorders

Autoimmune Disease	% with Specific Positive Seroconversions
Ankylosing spondylitis	90% HLA-B27
Juvenile rheumatoid arthritis	50% ANA, 15% RF, anti-CCP (95% spec.)
Polymyositis	May have positive ANA and anti-JO 1 antibodies
Reactive arthritis (Reiter)	80% HLA-B27
Rheumatoid arthritis	80% RF, 30%–60% ANA, anti-CCP (95% spec.)
Systemic sclerosis (scleroderma)	90% ANA, 25% anti-topoisomerase antibody (diffuse) and 75% anti-centromere antibodies (limited), anti-RNA polymerase III
Sjögren's syndrome	90% ANA, 65% anti-SS-A (Ro) and anti-SS-B (La) antibodies, 70% RF
Systemic lupus erythematosus	95% ANA, 60% anti-ds-DNA, 20% RF, anti-Smith antibody

ANA, antinuclear antibody; CCP, cyclic citrullinated peptide; HLA, human leukocyte antigen; RF, rheumatoid factor; SS, systemic sclerosis.

B. Bursitis

1. General characteristics

   a. Bursitis is an inflammatory disorder of the bursa (a thin-walled sac lined with synovial tissue).

   b. The inflammation is caused by trauma or overuse.

2. Clinical features

   a. Common sites of presentation include subacromial, subdeltoid, trochanteric, ischial, iliopsoas, olecranon, and prepatellar and suprapatellar (housemaid's knee).

   b. Pain, swelling, and tenderness may persist for weeks.

3. Treatment

   a. Prevention of the precipitating factors is essential to avoid relapse.

   b. Rest, brace/support as needed, NSAIDs, and steroid injections may be helpful.

C. Osteomyelitis

1. General characteristics

   a. Osteomyelitis is an infection of the bone caused by a pyogenic organism (most commonly *S. aureus*) and is described by duration (acute, chronic), cause (hematogenous, exogenous, surgical, true contiguous spread), site (spine, hip, other), extent (size of defect), and type of patient (infant, child, adult, immunocompromised host).

   b. Types

      (1) Acute hematogenous osteomyelitis most commonly affects the long bones of children and the spine in adults.

      (2) Patients with sickle cell anemia are at risk for *Salmonella* osteomyelitis.

      (3) Osteomyelitis is termed chronic hematogenous osteomyelitis when, after the original acute infection has completed appropriate treatment (antibiotics, surgery), viable colonies of bacteria harbored in necrotic and ischemic tissue cause a recurrence of infection.

      (4) Exogenous osteomyelitis results from open fracture or surgery.

2. Clinical features

   a. Acute hematogenous osteomyelitis

      (1) Pain, loss of motion, and soft-tissue swelling occur.

      (2) Drainage is rare.

   b. Chronic hematogenous osteomyelitis

      (1) Recurrent acute flare-ups of tender, warm, sometimes swollen areas occur, and patients often complain of malaise, anorexia, fever, weight loss, and night sweats as well as pain and drainage from a sinus tract (an abnormal channel permitting escape of exudate to the surface).

      (2) Bone necrosis, soft-tissue damage, and bone instability can occur.

3. Diagnostic studies

   a. WBC count, CRP, and ESR may be mildly elevated in acute and chronic osteomyelitis, although normal results are possible.

   b. Identification of the infectious organism by blood culture or bone biopsy is best.

   c. Radiographic evidence of osteomyelitis lags behind symptoms and pathologic changes by 7 to 10 days. Ultrasonography can be useful for the early detection of acute osteomyelitis.

   d. Late sequestra (i.e., dead bone surrounding granulation tissue) and involucrum (i.e., periosteal new bone) take several weeks to months to appear.

   e. Magnetic resonance imaging (MRI) shows the changes before plain-film radiography or bone scan.

Bursitis risk factors:
- increasing age
- repetitive motion
- chronic pressure
- overweight and obesity

Acute osteomyelitis presents with pain and swelling near the infected bone. Most commonly caused by *S. aureus*, it requires prolonged antibiotic treatment.

4. Treatment

   a. Acute osteomyelitis is treated with a 6- to 8-week course of bacteria-specific antibiotics (typically IV; however, some bacteria respond as well to oral antibiotics).

   b. Chronic osteomyelitis is treated with a minimum of 4 weeks to 24 months of IV and oral antibiotics depending on the organism involved and the comorbidities of the patient.

   c. Immobilization and surgical drainage may be indicated. Attention to open wounds must be part of the treatment as well as the removal of any hardware present.

   d. Surgical debridement may be required to remove sequestra, sinus tract, infected bone, and scar tissue.

D. Neoplasms

   1. General characteristics

   a. Metastasis to the bone is more commonly caused by primary cancers of the prostate, breast, lung, kidney, and thyroid.

   b. Primary bone neoplasm

   (1) Benign tumors of the bone and soft tissue are more common than primary malignant tumors.

   (2) Enchondroma (cartilaginous tumor) is the most common primary benign bone neoplasm of the hand and is asymptomatic unless complicated by pathologic fracture.

   (3) Lipomas (soft, nontender, movable mass) and ganglions (soft, nontender, transilluminant mass, usually on the dorsum of the hand or wrist) are common benign soft-tissue masses.

   (4) Mucous cysts are ganglia originating from the DIP joint and are often associated with Heberden's nodules.

   (5) Soft-tissue sarcomas occur three times more often than primary bone malignancies. The most common types of primary sarcomas of bone are chondrosarcoma, Ewing's sarcoma, and osteosarcoma.

   (6) Multiple myeloma is the most common primary malignant bone tumor.

   c. Age groups

   (1) Ewing's sarcoma is found in patients between 5 and 25 years of age, usually in the diaphyses of long bones, ribs, and flat bones. Osteosarcomas are most common in individuals 10 to 20 years of age, arising in the metaphyseal area of the long bones.

   (2) In adults 60 years of age or older, metastatic carcinoma is the most common source of bone lesion. Chondrosarcomas also increase in incidence in adults older than 60 years of age and can present within the central metaphyseal area.

2. Clinical features

   a. Night pain is often associated with malignancy.

   b. A painful mass attached to bone is likely to be malignant; however, some malignant tumors are nonpainful.

   c. Severe pain preceded by dull, aching pain may indicate pathologic fracture.

   d. Systemic symptoms, such as fever, weight loss, anorexia, or fatigue, should be noted.

   e. Rule out areas of metastases, such as the lungs, breasts, prostate, thyroid, and kidneys.

3. Diagnostic studies

   a. Routine laboratory studies are noncontributory, but with suspected malignancy, routine labs can provide a baseline for patients who will need chemotherapy.

> The spine is the most common site of bony metastases, often from prostate, breast, and lung cancers.

> Most common benign bone tumor is enchondroma.
> Most common primary malignant bone tumor is multiple myeloma.

> Bony night pain is a red flag for malignancy.

> **b.** Alkaline phosphatase and lactate dehydrogenase are elevated when the bone is broken down and remodeled.
>
> **c.** Serum and urine protein electrophoresis studies can detect the specific abnormal globulin of multiple myeloma.
>
> **d.** Biopsy is essential to diagnose whether benign or malignant, the cell type, and the grade of lesion.
>
> > **(1)** Open incisional biopsy is best and should be done by a specialist.
> >
> > **(2)** The capsule is then closed tightly to prevent bleeding and local spread.

4. Imaging studies

a. Radiology

> **(1)** Radiographic signs may help to distinguish benign from malignant tumors because certain tumors have a characteristic appearance.
>
> **(2)** Radiography may also help to determine a tumor's location and may narrow the diagnostic possibilities.
>
> **(3)** If multiple myeloma is suspected, a bone scan is best to document lytic lesions.

> Lytic lesions, such as in multiple myeloma, are documented best by bone scan, not radiographs.

b. Computed tomography (CT) is used to determine if pulmonary metastasis is present.

c. MRI is used to determine the local extent of a tumor.

d. Bone scans can evaluate distant osseous metastasis and noncontiguous tumor or skip lesions. They are not diagnostic in multiple myeloma.

5. Treatment

a. The goals of treatment are to relieve pain and maintain function.

b. For benign tumors, simple excision is the treatment.

c. Malignant neoplasms

> **(1)** Wide surgical resection is used when feasible.
>
> **(2)** The success of chemotherapy, either alone or in conjunction with radiation therapy, depends on the type of tumor, its location, and whether metastasis has been found.
>
> **(3)** Limb salvage (using cadaver allograft or endoprosthetic devices) is part of definitive treatment.
>
> **(4)** Radiation therapy followed by local resection is the common treatment for soft-tissue sarcomas.

E. Osteoporosis

1. General characteristics

a. Osteoporosis is a disease of abnormal bone remodeling.

> **(1)** It is characterized by a decrease in total bone volume. Although the bone that is present is normal, it is less dense.
>
> **(2)** This decrease in mass leads to an increased susceptibility to fractures.

b. Osteoporosis is divided into two categories, primary and secondary:

> **(1)** Primary osteoporosis is further divided.
>
> > **(a)** Type I (postmenopausal) occurs primarily in women but can occur in men. It is the most prevalent form of primary osteoporosis.
> >
> > **(b)** Type II (senile) occurs in both men and women.
>
> **(2)** Secondary osteoporosis is recognized by conditions in which bone is lost owing to the presence of other diseases or medications (malignancies, corticosteroid use, GI disorders, or hormonal imbalances).

> Most common fracture sites of Type I/postmenopausal osteoporosis are vertebrae, hip, and distal radius.

c. Risk factors include those that are modifiable and nonmodifiable (Table 9-9).

```

**Table 9-9 | Risk Factors—Osteoporosis**

| Modifiable | Nonmodifiable |
| --- | --- |
| Alcohol abuse | Advanced age |
| Smoking cigarettes | Caucasian race |
| Low body weight | Asian race |
| Sedentary lifestyle | Female gender |
| Low calcium and vitamin D intake | |
| Corticosteroid use | |
| Recurrent falls | |

2. **Clinical features**

   a. Type I commonly is associated with loss of estrogen in postmenopausal women and with testosterone deficiency in men

      **(1)** The trabecular bone is primarily affected.

      **(2)** The vertebrae, hip, and distal radius are the most common fracture sites.

   b. Type II is seen in patients older than 75 years with poor calcium absorption.

      **(1)** Both trabecular and cortical bone are affected.

      **(2)** The hip and pelvis are the most common fracture sites.

3. Diagnostic studies

   a. Calcium, phosphate, alkaline phosphatase, and serum protein electrophoresis should be measured and serum markers should be considered as well to rule out other secondary causes of osteoporosis (i.e., hyperthyroidism, hyperparathyroidism, Cushing's syndrome, hematologic disorders, malignancy, and vitamin D deficiency).

   b. Dual-energy x-ray absorptiometry (DEXA scan) is the most helpful way to measure bone density with the least amount of radiation. Screening bone density is recommended in the following groups:

      **(1)** Postmenopausal women younger than 65 years of age who have one or more additional risk factors

      **(2)** All postmenopausal women older than 65 years and men older than 70

      **(3)** Postmenopausal women who present with fractures

      **(4)** All women considering therapy for other conditions in which the bone mineral density will affect that decision

      **(5)** Women who have been on hormone replacement therapy (HRT) for prolonged periods

      **(6)** Patients who experience fractures after minimal trauma

      **(7)** Patients with evidence of osteopenia on radiography or a disease known to increase the risk for osteoporosis

      **(8)** Patients with RA

   c. Radiographs show features of decreased bone density when 30% bone loss is present.

   d. A diagnosis of osteoporosis is made if the T score is 2.5 standard deviations or more below the normal young adult reference.

4. **Treatment**

   a. Preventive measures include weight-bearing exercises; adequate calcium, vitamin D, and phosphorus intake; smoking cessation; and limited alcohol intake.

   b. The bisphosphonate class of drugs is the first-line treatment for osteoporosis. These drugs must be taken on an empty stomach, and the patient must be able to sit upright for 30 to 60 minutes after ingestion. Long-term use may be associated with weakened bones or complications such as jaw necrosis; close monitoring is recommended.

> World Health Organization (WHO) bone density t-scores: −1 to −2.5 = osteopenia; <−2.5 = osteoporosis
```

c. Teriparatide (a parathyroid hormone [PTH] analog) can be used if patients are unable to use bisphosphonates, but it is not recommended to be used longer than 2 years because of risk of osteosarcoma.

d. Selective estrogen receptor modulators (SERMs) may also be used in the treatment of osteoporosis; however, the risk for deep venous thrombosis is increased.

e. HRT and calcitonin are no longer recommended for the treatment of osteoporosis.

Fractures, Dislocations, Sprains, and Strains

> 💡 Fractures are described by location, direction, alignment, and associated features.

A. Classification of fractures. Fractures are classified by location, direction, and alignment.

    1. Examples of location are proximal, middle, and distal third.

    2. Examples of direction are transverse (at a right angle to the axis of the bone), spiral (bone has a twisted appearance; also called torsion), oblique (fracture line between horizontal and vertical direction), comminuted (splintered or crushed in multiple pieces), and segmental (double).

    3. Examples of alignment are angulation (deviation from straight line) and displacement (abnormal position of fracture fragments), such as dorsal displacement of the bone fragment in a Colles' fracture of the wrist and volar displacement of the bone fragment in a Smith fracture of the wrist; both may be complicated by injury to the median nerve or radial artery.

    4. Examples of associated factors are open fracture (disruption of the skin), closed fracture (skin is intact), and dislocation (displacement of bone from a joint).

B. Imaging studies

> 💡 Imaging in fractures: plain x-rays are first line; CT for pelvic or intra-articular fractures; MRI for occult or spinal column fractures.

    1. Plain-film radiographs are sufficient to visualize most fractures.

        a. Both anteroposterior (AP) and lateral films should be taken to ensure visualization of the bony structures 90 degrees away from each other.

        b. Concurrent fractures may also be seen at the joints proximal and distal to the fracture (e.g., distal tibia, proximal fibula, dome of the talus, lateral malleolus).

        c. Comparative films of the contralateral joints may be helpful, especially in patients with open growth plates.

    2. Radionucleotide bone scanning shows increased uptake at the site of an occult fracture or stress fracture (common in athletes and associated with disuse osteopenia when weight-bearing resumes after long periods of immobilization).

    3. CT is a better diagnostic method than plain-film radiography or bone scans. It allows visualization of the bone's articular surface otherwise obscured by overlying structures (e.g., carpal bones, elbow, tibial plateau). CT is helpful in establishing the diagnosis of pelvic, facial, or intra-articular fractures.

    4. MRI is the study of choice to diagnose an occult hip fracture.

C. Treatment

    1. Fractures are initially treated with analgesics, immobilization, and emergent referral to an orthopedist after adequate stabilization of the patient.

    2. Open fractures

        a. Any bleeding fracture should be considered an open fracture until proven otherwise.

        b. Ideally, open fractures must be debrided and irrigated (in the operating room) within 4 to 8 hours of injury.

        c. IV antibiotics (first- and second-generation cephalosporins and aminoglycosides) should be administered for 48 hours after fracture and for 48 hours after surgical procedures. Confirm patient's tetanus status.

        d. Immobilization and fixation should be performed to preserve function.

3. Intra-articular fractures (the fracture line enters a joint cavity)

   a. Open treatment may be indicated to restore and maintain articular congruity.

   b. When stable, consider active ROM.

4. Femur fractures

   a. Surgical approach: Treat femoral neck fractures with percutaneous screws or hemiarthroplasty, femoral shaft fractures with intramedullary rods or plates, and intertrochanteric fractures with sliding hip screw fixation or a long gamma nail.

   b. There is significant potential for hemorrhage with fractures of the femur.

5. Fractures of the tibia and fibula in adults

   a. Fractures of the tibia and fibula are associated with ligamental, meniscal, and vascular injuries.

   b. For simple fractures, closed reduction with cast placement is appropriate; for more complicated or unstable fractures, open reduction combined with internal fixation (ORIF) is required.

D. **Fractures in children**

1. The physis, or growth plate, is more susceptible to fracture than to injury of attached ligaments.

   a. Swelling and tenderness over the physis are the common findings when fractured.

   b. Growth plate fractures are classified with the Salter–Harris classification system (Fig. 9-1).

   c. Comparison films may be helpful and should be obtained as part of any pediatric fracture workup.

2. Incomplete fractures occur when the line of fracture does not continue through to the other side of the bone.

   a. Torus fractures (buckle fractures) occur when one side of the cortex buckles as a result of a compression injury (e.g., falling on an outstretched hand). It differs from a greenstick fracture by the mechanism of injury and sometimes buckles on both sides of the bone. Treatment is 4 to 6 weeks in a cast.

   b. Greenstick fractures

      (1) These fractures occur in long bones when bowing causes a break in one side of the cortex.

> The physis is the translucent cartilage disc between epiphysis and metaphysis responsible for longitudinal bone growth.

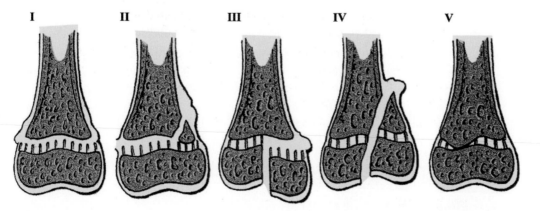

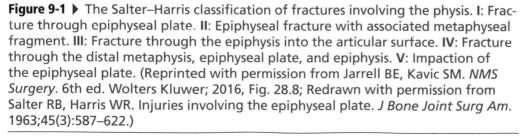

Figure 9-1 ▶ The Salter–Harris classification of fractures involving the physis. **I:** Fracture through epiphyseal plate. **II:** Epiphyseal fracture with associated metaphyseal fragment. **III:** Fracture through the epiphysis into the articular surface. **IV:** Fracture through the distal metaphysis, epiphyseal plate, and epiphysis. **V:** Impaction of the epiphyseal plate. (Reprinted with permission from Jarrell BE, Kavic SM. *NMS Surgery.* 6th ed. Wolters Kluwer; 2016, Fig. 28.8; Redrawn with permission from Salter RB, Harris WR. Injuries involving the epiphyseal plate. *J Bone Joint Surg Am.* 1963;45(3):587–622.)

(2) When the angulation of the fracture is <15 degrees, a long-arm or leg cast can be applied for 4 to 6 weeks.

(3) Fractures with angulation of >15 degrees need referral to an orthopedic surgeon.

3. When radiographs of a young child show multiple fractures at various stages of healing, abuse should be suspected and the child referred to a protective agency.

E. Dislocations and subluxations

1. General characteristics

a. Dislocation is a total loss of congruity that occurs between the articular surfaces of the joint.

b. Subluxation is any less serious loss of congruity or a less than complete dislocation.

2. Sites of dislocation

> ⚡ Axillary nerve damage is present in up to 40% of shoulder dislocations.

a. Common sites of dislocation are the anterior shoulder, posterior hip (a common complication of a posterior dislocation is osteonecrosis of the femoral head), and dislocations of the posterior elbow.

b. Less common sites of dislocation are the navicular and subtalar joints, as part of a combination of Lisfranc fracture (a dislocation of the tarsometatarsal joint complex), and the second metatarsal joint (often, one metatarsal is fractured at the base and the others are dislocated).

3. Treatment

a. After assessment of the neurovascular status, most dislocations are treated with closed reduction.

b. Dislocations that reduce spontaneously require immobilization for 2 to 4 weeks, followed by ROM activity and return to normal activity.

c. If associated fractures or interposed soft tissues are present, the patient needs to undergo open reduction and internal fixation.

d. It is imperative to assess the neurovascular status pre- and postreduction as well as get postreduction radiographs to ensure adequate reduction.

F. Strains and sprains

1. A strain is an injury to the bone–tendon unit at the myotendinous junction or the muscle itself.

2. A sprain involves collagenous tissue such as ligaments or tendons.

3. A strain or sprain injury often follows a sudden stretch.

a. It can lead to avulsion of tendon (e.g., mallet finger avulsion or stretch of the terminal extensor tendon, which is treated with extensor splinting for 6 weeks).

b. It can also lead to ligamentous sprain (e.g., stretch of the anterior talofibular ligament [ATL], which causes the common ankle sprain).

4. Treatment: Both strains and sprains require supportive therapy: rest, ice, compression, elevation, and support/bracing (RICES).

Disorders of the Head and Neck

A. Temporomandibular joint (TMJ) disorder

1. General characteristics

a. TMJ disorder, which is the most common cause of facial pain, involves pain that affects the TMJ and muscles of mastication.

b. Causes

(1) Neuropsychologic components, such as psychologic stress, may play a role.

(2) Joint capsulitis from bruxism, such as grinding of teeth, clenching of teeth, and posturing of the jaw, may cause TMJ disorder.

(3) Hypermobility syndrome and malocclusion may lead to pain in the jaw area.

2. Clinical features

    a. Pain is aggravated by movement of the jaw.

    b. There may be restricted ROM; a click or pop may be felt or heard.

3. Imaging studies

    a. Initial radiographic studies are normal.

    b. Arthritis is a late finding.

    c. Other systemic causes need to be ruled out, such as OA, RA, growth abnormalities, and tumor.

4. Treatment

    a. Most cases resolve without identification of the cause.

    b. Suggestion of conservative lifestyle changes and behavior modification can be helpful.

    c. Referral to a specialist, such as an odontologist or oral and maxillofacial surgeon, is required if the symptoms warrant.

> TMJ occurs in females 4× as often as in males.

B. Neck pain

    1. General characteristics

        a. Spondylosis is the most common condition affecting the cervical spine.

            (1) Degenerative changes occur in the disk, most frequently in C5–C6, with the formation of osteophytes and disk narrowing.

            (2) Later, facet joints and the joints of Luschka are affected.

            (3) Paresthesias and numbness occur in the fingers.

            (4) Pain increases with extension and decreases with flexion of the neck.

        b. Compression by central disk protrusion or osteophytes may cause long-tract signs (e.g., clonus, Babinski sign) and gait disturbance.

    2. Treatment

        a. Conservative treatment involves the use of a cervical collar, traction, physical therapy, and analgesics.

        b. In advanced disease, cervical fusion or diskectomy may be necessary.

C. Other conditions of the neck

    1. Whiplash and extension injury are common causes of pain and can last 18 months or longer.

        a. Injury occurs as a result of a rear impact, with rapid extension followed by flexion of the cervical spine.

        b. Treatment includes a soft cervical collar (2 to 3 days), application of ice or heat, analgesics, and gentle active ROM very soon after injury.

    2. Rheumatoid spondylitis of the neck is found in most of the patients with adult RA.

        a. Ligamentous stretching causes progressive atlantoaxial and midcervical subluxation. Posterior subluxation at C1–C2 can lead to cord compression.

        b. Surgical stabilization is often necessary.

> Whiplash is caused by rapid extension followed by flexion of the cervical spine; treatment is supportive.

Disorders of the Shoulder and Upper Extremity

A. Shoulder pain

    1. Shoulder pain can be referred pain caused by cervical spondylosis.

    2. Pain, if localized to a particular area of the shoulder, may be the site of pathology; referred pain is diffuse and cannot be well localized.

B. Rotator cuff syndrome

1. General characteristics

   a. This syndrome occurs with eccentric overload (e.g., a throwing athlete), underlying glenohumeral instability, poor muscle strength, and training errors.

   b. A common cause in adults is impingement of the supraspinatus tendon as it passes beneath the subacromial arch.

2. **Clinical features**

   a. Dull aching in the shoulder is the main clinical feature.

   b. The pain is caused by inflammation, fibrosis, and tears.

   c. The pain may interfere with sleep and is exacerbated by abduction of the arm.

3. Diagnostic studies

   a. Radiographs are helpful in ruling out calcific tendinitis, glenohumeral or acromio-clavicular arthrosis, and bone tumors.

   b. MRI is most often used to diagnose rotator cuff tears.

4. **Treatment**

   a. Lifestyle: Aggravating factors, such as repetitive throwing, other overhead activities, and improper mechanics, must be avoided.

   b. NSAIDs and local steroid injections may help to alleviate inflammation and pain.

   c. Physical therapy may provide relief. Begin nonoperative management of cuff tears with a ROM and strengthening program.

   d. Arthroscopic subacromial decompression should be considered for adults with persistent impingement.

   e. If the patient is still symptomatic after conservative treatment, surgical repair should be considered.

> 💡 MRI is the study of choice in rotator cuff disease. Treatment centers on conservative treatment; surgery is reserved for refractory cases.

C. Shoulder dislocations

1. General characteristics

   a. Fall on outstretched arm in abduction and extension is the most common cause of shoulder dislocation.

   b. Anterior shoulder dislocations are more common than posterior shoulder dislocations.

2. **Clinical features**

   a. Patient usually presents supporting the affected extremity with the other arm.

   b. Loss of shoulder contour is observed, with the elbow pointing outward (anterior dislocation).

   c. Careful neurovascular assessment must be performed to rule out axillary artery or nerve, musculocutaneous nerve, or brachial plexus injury before reduction attempts.

3. Diagnostic imaging should include an AP view of the shoulder as well as a transthoracic "Y" view. Humeral head deformities (Hill–Sachs lesions) may be noted in recurrent dislocations. Bankart lesion, a tear of the glenoid labrum, may be picked up on MRI.

4. **Treatment** includes reduction and immobilization.

   a. As with all orthopedic reductions, postreduction films should be obtained and neurovascular status should be assessed.

   b. Immobilization by sling and swath (Velpeau sling) is recommended for all. For patients younger than 40 years, therapy should begin after 3 weeks, and for those older than 40 years, therapy should begin after 1 week.

> 💡 Recurrent dislocation is an indication for surgical referral.

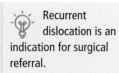

D. Other conditions of the shoulder

1. Adhesive capsulitis (frozen shoulder) is an inflammatory process that may follow injury to the shoulder or arise on its own (with an increased risk in patients with diabetes).

   a. It is characterized by pain and restricted glenohumeral movement.

   b. Arthrography may show a decreased volume of the joint capsule and capsular contraction.

   c. Treatment includes NSAIDs, physical therapy for passive ROM, and, occasionally, manipulation under anesthesia.

2. OA of the humeral head can be secondary to osteonecrosis, trauma, septic arthritis, and endocrine disorders or neuropathic disorders.

   a. Pain, stiffness, and limited ROM are features of the condition.

   b. Radiographs show osteophytes and joint space narrowing.

   c. Treatment includes NSAIDs, cortisone injections, activity modification, and debridement or total joint replacement in severe cases.

3. Rupture of the long head of the biceps tendon

   a. This rupture can occur as a result of spontaneous or forced overload.

   b. In the elderly, this rupture may be caused by degenerative or attritional changes.

   c. Treatment: Rupture is managed by surgical repair.

> Adhesive capsulitis occurs at higher frequency in patients with diabetes.

E. Fractured clavicle

1. General characteristics

   a. This is the most common fracture in children and adolescents.

   b. It is usually caused by a fall on an outstretched hand (FOOSH).

   c. It can be found in up to 3% of live births as a result of trauma.

2. Clinical features

   a. Visible deformity is usually present.

   b. The arm is supported by the contralateral extremity.

   c. Look for brachial plexus injuries (pain, weakness, reflex, and sensory abnormalities).

   d. The proximal portion may be displaced superiorly because of the attachment of the sternocleidomastoid muscle.

3. Imaging studies: An AP view generally will visualize the fracture.

4. Treatment

   a. In children, a figure-of-eight splint or arm sling is used for 4 to 6 weeks.

   b. In adults, a sling for 6 weeks is generally enough to treat the fracture.

   c. Early ROM is recommended.

> Most clavicle fractures occur in the middle portion (shaft) of the bone.

F. Acromioclavicular separations

1. General characteristics

   a. Acromioclavicular separation is also referred to as a "separated shoulder."

   b. It involves a "tearing" of the acromioclavicular and/or coracoclavicular ligaments.

   c. It is usually caused by a fall on or impact to the tip of the shoulder.

2. Clinical features: Patients may have a clinically apparent step-off at the acromioclavicular joint.

3. Imaging studies

   a. An AP view of both shoulders is usually necessary.

   b. Mild separations may require stress films that are obtained while the patient holds a weighted object to reveal the separation.

4. **Treatment**

   a. Conservative management is possible for mild to moderate injuries because they can be managed with a sling and analgesia.

   b. More severe injuries will usually require operative repair.

G. **Humeral head fractures**

   1. General characteristics

      a. Most fractures of the proximal humerus occur in older patients with osteoporosis.

      b. The female to male ratio is 2:1.

   2. **Clinical features**

      a. Pain, swelling, and tenderness, especially in the region of the greater tuberosity, are the most common findings.

      b. Ecchymosis typically does not appear for 24 to 48 hours.

      c. The patient will hold the affected extremity against the chest wall.

      d. Look for injuries to the brachial plexus and/or axillary artery.

   3. Imaging studies

      a. AP, lateral, and "Y" views typically are diagnostic.

      b. Humeral fractures are assessed most commonly by the Neer classification. Displaced fractures are two-part, three-part, or four-part based on whether or not the fracture parts (e.g., head, greater tuberosity, lesser tuberosity, shaft) are involved.

   4. **Treatment**

      a. Closed reduction with the application of a sling and swath (Velpeau sling) can treat most nondisplaced fractures. Early mobilization with pendulum exercises is indicated to prevent frozen shoulder.

      b. ORIF is reserved for the management of displaced fractures.

H. **Humeral shaft fractures**

   1. General characteristics

      a. The mechanism of injury includes motor vehicle accidents, FOOSH, and penetrating injuries, such as gunshot wounds.

      b. The degree of comminution and amount of soft-tissue injury relate directly to the amount of energy causing the fracture.

   2. **Clinical features**

      a. Pain, arm swelling, deformity, and shortening are all possible initial complaints.

      b. Radial nerve injury is common and should be looked for carefully.

   3. Imaging studies: AP and lateral views that include the elbow and shoulder should be performed.

   4. **Treatment**

      a. Initial treatment is usually the application of a coaptation splint.

      b. The coaptation splint can be followed by a hanging cast, Sarmiento brace, or operative repair.

   5. Complications: Fractures of the humeral shaft may be associated with radial nerve injury at the time of fracture or during reduction.

I. **Supracondylar humerus fractures**

   1. General characteristics: The usual mechanism of fracture is a FOOSH with hyperextension of the elbow.

   2. **Clinical features**

      a. Initially, patients may have pain with minimal swelling. Extension of swelling around the elbow is a delayed finding.

> 💡 Humeral head fractures: often with osteoporosis history, painful swelling of greater tuberosity, and treatment with sling and swath.

> 💡 When a FOOSH is described, think of fractures in the humeral shaft, supracondylar humerus, distal radius, and radial head.

b. Full neurovascular examination must be performed. Special attention to brachial artery injuries should be given. The brachial artery is the most spastic artery in the body and can lead to Volkmann ischemic contractures.

3. Imaging studies

   a. AP and lateral views generally are sufficient to make the diagnosis. Evidence of an effusion is indicated by the presence of a posterior fat pad on x-ray.

   b. In children, always obtain comparative views.

4. Treatment

   a. For children with displaced fracture, treatment involves closed reduction in the operating room with pin placement and posterior splint application.

   b. Adults should undergo ORIF.

5. Complications

   a. Besides Volkmann ischemic contractures (permanent shortening), injuries to the radial, ulnar, and median nerves have been described.

   b. Varus (gunstock) or valgus deformities of the elbow also may result from arrest of the medial or the lateral growth plate, respectively.

> Radiologic fat pads indicate effusion.

J. **Elbow, Hand, and wrist pain**

1. OA and RA are the most common painful conditions of the hand and wrist.

   a. OA commonly affects the carpometacarpal joint of the thumb and DIP joints.

   b. OA of the wrist can be posttraumatic or follow osteonecrosis of the lunate (Kienböck's disease).

2. Clinical features

   a. OA presents with Heberden's nodes and mucous cysts in DIP joints and Bouchard's nodes in PIP joints.

   b. RA causes soft-tissue swelling that is symmetrical and primarily affects the MCP and PIP joints, usually sparing the DIP joints.

   c. Dupuytren's disease affects the palmar aponeurosis, ring, and little and middle fingers, causing painful nodules, pitting, and contractures.

3. Treatment

   a. Nonsurgical treatment includes heat, stretching, ultrasound therapy, and steroid injections.

   b. Surgical release is indicated for contractures of the metacarpal phalangeal joint that are >30 degrees and for proximal phalangeal contractures of any degree, pain (rare), or nerve compression (digital).

K. **Carpal tunnel syndrome**

1. General characteristics

   a. Carpal tunnel syndrome, the most common mononeuropathy, involves compression of the median nerve under the transverse carpal ligament.

   b. It can be precipitated by premenstrual fluid retention, early RA with thickening of the synovial tendon sheath, acromegaly, pregnancy, repetitive flexion or extension of the wrist (e.g., production line work, keyboard work), and alcohol abuse.

> The most common mononeuropathy in the United States is carpal tunnel syndrome.

2. Clinical features

   a. Classic findings of night pain, numbness, paresthesias (sparing the little finger), clumsiness, and weakness are seen.

   b. Thenar atrophy may occur late in the disease.

   c. Tinel's sign (tingling with percussion over the volar aspect of the wrist) may be noted.

   d. Phalen's test (symptoms with full flexion of the wrist for >1 minute) may be positive.

3. Diagnostic studies: Electromyography (EMG) and nerve conduction velocity (NCV) studies may help confirm the diagnosis when considered with the clinical presentation.

4. **Treatment**

   a. Activity modification, volar wrist splint worn at night, and NSAIDs (except in pregnancy) make up the initial recommended treatment.

   b. Steroid injections may be used.

   c. Surgical intervention may be needed to decompress the nerve if symptoms don't resolve with conservative treatment.

L. **Fractures and dislocations of the hand**

   1. A boxer's fracture is a fracture of the metacarpal neck of the fourth or fifth finger.

      a. Examination reveals loss of prominence of the knuckle with tenderness and pain.

      b. Inspect for a puncture wound over the metacarpal phalangeal joint. If the fracture was caused by a punch to another's mouth, it may also be necessary to treat with antibiotics (*Eikenella corrodens* is an organism specific to the human mouth).

      c. Fractures with 25 to 30 degrees of angulation should be reduced with the application of an ulnar gutter splint with follow-up in 1 to 2 weeks.

   2. A Colles' fracture is a distal radius fracture with dorsal angulation.

      a. It is the most common injury of the wrist and results from a fall onto the dorsiflexed hand, described as a silver fork deformity.

      b. Cast immobilization is adequate after reduction in most cases.

   3. Gamekeeper's thumb is a sprain or tear of the ulnar collateral ligament of the thumb.

      a. There usually is a history of a sprained thumb or a fall on the hand.

      b. Examination reveals ligamentous laxity of the ulnar collateral ligament, with instability and weakness of pinch.

      c. Surgical repair is indicated for a complete rupture; a partial rupture may be treated by immobilization with a thumb spica cast.

> Colles fracture is most common in elderly women, especially in those with osteoporosis.

M. **Lateral epicondylosis ("tennis elbow")**

   1. General characteristics

      a. This is the most common overuse injury of the elbow.

      b. It is most common during the fourth decade of life.

      c. It involves the tendinous insertion of the extensor carpi radialis brevis on the lateral aspect of the elbow.

   2. **Clinical features**

      a. Pain on lifting objects, primarily when the arm is pronated, is characteristic.

      b. The pain can be duplicated by having the patient extend the elbow, hold the forearm in the pronated position, and then extend the fingers and wrist against resistance.

   3. Imaging studies

      a. AP and lateral views of the elbow may demonstrate osteophytes overlying the lateral epicondyle.

      b. MRI is useful in demonstrating tendon disruption.

   4. **Treatment**

      a. Activity modification for at least 6 weeks is probably the most important component in the treatment.

      b. Counterbalance braces (tennis elbow braces) are beneficial.

      c. Instruct the patient to pick up objects with the extremity in supination.

      d. Physical and occupational therapy are important adjuncts to care.

    e. Steroid injections may give short-term relief but do not offer long-term treatment.

    f. NSAIDs are frequently used for their analgesic effect; their role as an anti-inflammatory is controversial.

    g. Surgery is reserved for patients who fail at least 6 months of conservative management.

N. Medial epicondylitis ("golfer's elbow" or "baseball elbow")

  1. General characteristics: This affects the flexor–pronator muscles at their origin, anterior to the medial epicondyle.

  2. Clinical features

    a. A history of repetitive stress is obtained in most patients.

    b. Pain is reproduced by resisted pronation or flexion of the wrist.

    c. Patients may complain of paresthesias in the distribution of the ulnar nerve.

  3. Imaging studies: MRI is typically not indicated but is useful for assessing the ulnar nerve.

  4. Treatment

    a. Conservative management, including activity modification, NSAIDs, and physical and occupational therapy, is commonly sufficient.

    b. A medial counterforce brace is frequently applied.

    c. Surgical intervention to debride the epicondyle is usually not necessary but is an option.

> Lateral epicondylitis pain is with resisted wrist extension of a pronated arm; medial epicondylitis pain is with resisted pronation or flexion of wrist.

O. Olecranon bursitis

  1. General characteristics

    a. It is caused either by an acute injury or by repetitive trauma to the olecranon bursa.

    b. Less frequently, it can result from breaks in the skin, leading to a septic cause. The most common organism is *S. aureus*.

  2. Clinical features

    a. Swelling overlying the olecranon process is the most common finding. This swelling may be mildly painful, but in chronic cases, it is usually painless.

    b. ROM is usually preserved.

  3. Imaging studies are generally not indicated unless there is a significant history of trauma or a fracture is suspected.

  4. Treatment

    a. Avoid continued trauma to elbow and use an ace wrap for compression. Aspiration of the bursa is not recommended unless infection is suspected.

    b. NSAIDs and warm compresses are used for their analgesic properties.

    c. Surgical removal of the bursa is reserved for septic bursal sacs that are nonresponsive to conservative management.

> Students often develop olecranon bursitis owing to prolonged pressure from leaning on tabletops.

P. Radial head injuries

  1. General characteristics

    a. Fractures of the radial head result from a FOOSH.

    b. Subluxation of the radial head in children, or nursemaid's elbow, is caused by excessive longitudinal traction. It is most common before the age of 4 years. The radial head slips anteriorly out of the annular ligament.

  2. Clinical features

    a. Fractures of the radial head present with pain over the lateral aspect of the elbow that worsens with forearm rotation. They are the most common fracture of the elbow in adults.

       b. Children who have sustained a subluxation of the radial head usually present with the extremity fully pronated, partially flexed, and held tightly to the side.

   3. Imaging studies

       a. AP and lateral films of the elbow are usually sufficient to establish the diagnosis. Displacement of the anterior fat pad and presence of a posterior fat pad imply the presence of a hemarthrosis. CT is useful in determining the degree of comminution.

       b. AP and lateral films are usually performed to rule out fracture in children who are suspected of having a subluxed radial head.

   4. Treatment

       a. Treatment of radial head fractures depends on the type of fracture. If the fracture is nondisplaced, it can be treated with a sling for 2 to 4 weeks. Displaced fractures may require ORIF.

       b. Radial head subluxations can be reduced by holding the affected arm just above the wrist and just below the elbow. The practitioner then places the thumb of the proximal hand over the radial head while fully supinating and flexing the forearm and applying posteriorly directed pressure. The objective is to effect a "screwing" action and place the radial head back within the annular ligament.

Q. Scaphoid (navicular) fracture

   1. General characteristics

       a. The scaphoid bone is the most commonly fractured carpal bone.

       b. Blood supply is from the radial artery by way of lateral and distal branches. The proximal pole of the scaphoid has a poor blood supply that is further compromised with fractures through the waist of the bone; this poor blood supply can lead to avascular necrosis or nonunion of the scaphoid.

   2. Clinical features

       a. Cardinal finding is pain over the anatomic snuffbox.

       b. Swelling over the region in association with ecchymosis implies a fracture–dislocation.

       c. It is often confused with a "sprain" of the wrist, so clinical suspicion is key.

   3. Imaging studies

       a. AP, lateral, and scaphoid views should be ordered. If negative initially, films may be repeated after 2 to 3 weeks, at which time the fracture may become apparent.

       b. Bone scan or MRI can be used to make diagnosis at the time of injury.

   4. Treatment

       a. A delay in diagnosis should be avoided. Suspicion of scaphoid fracture without radiologic evidence should be treated as a fracture in a long-arm thumb spica cast until bone scan or MRI can be performed.

       b. The initial treatment for a displaced scaphoid fracture is long-arm thumb spica cast and then referral to an orthopedic surgeon. A short-arm thumb spica cast is used for nondisplaced fractures with referral to an orthopedic specialist.

       c. Displacement of ≥1 mm requires ORIF.

   5. Complications include nonunion of the fracture or development of avascular necrosis. In avascular necrosis, radiography may reveal a ground-glass appearance of the proximal pole or an increased bone density.

R. de Quervain's disease

   1. Clinical characteristics

       a. deQuervain's disease is a stenosing tenosynovitis involving the abductor pollicis longus and extensor pollicis brevis.

       b. It is more common in females older than 30 years and in patients with diabetes.

> 💡 Keys to diagnosing scaphoid fracture are clinical suspicion and repeat hand x-rays 2 weeks after injury. Failure to diagnose risks nonunion and avascular necrosis.

2. Clinical features

   a. Pain and tenderness occur at the wrist and base of the thumb. Radiation of pain up the forearm is common.

   b. Swelling and thickening of the tendon sheath may be appreciated during examination.

   c. The patient places the thumb within his or her fist, and the wrist is then ulnarly deviated, reproducing the pain (Finkelstein test).

3. Imaging studies: not usually required

4. Treatment

   a. Conservative treatment for at least a month using a thumb spica splint, NSAIDs, and physical/occupational therapy is required.

   b. Injection of a steroid into the tendon sheath can be employed if conservative measures fail. No more than three injections should be given before referral to an orthopedist.

   c. Surgical decompression of the first dorsal compartment may be required in cases that are resistant to all conservative measures.

> The pain of deQuervain's disease is at the base of the thumb; proximal radiation is common.

Disorders of the Back

A. **Low back pain and sciatica**

1. General characteristics

   a. The most common causes of low back pain are prolapsed intervertebral disk and low back strain.

   b. When back pain is unrelated to the mechanical use of the back, it can be referred from the intra-abdominal, pelvic, or retroperitoneal areas.

   c. Table 9-10 shows a comparison of important disorders of the spine and back.

2. Clinical features

   a. Pain originating in the back and radiating down the leg suggests nerve root irritation.

   b. Pain from musculoskeletal causes may be localized to an area of point tenderness.

   c. Sciatica (pain in the distribution of the sciatic nerve) is pain felt in the buttock, posterior thigh, and posterolateral aspect of the leg around the lateral malleolus to the lateral dorsum of the foot and the entire sole.

Table 9-10 | Disorders of the Spine and Back

	Cauda Equina Syndrome	Herniated Disk	Low Back Pain	Spinal Stenosis
Pain	LE radicular pain and numbness	Radicular pattern	No radicular pattern	Low back and buttock
Onset	Sudden	Sudden or insidious	Usually within 24 hours of injury or overuse	Insidious
Physical examination	Bowel/bladder dysfunction, ↓ sphincter tone, saddle anesthesia	May have diminished DTR and abnormal motor and sensory examination, +SLR	Neuro examination normal, paraspinal muscle tenderness/spasm	25% diminished DTRs, 65% LE weakness
Imaging study	MRI	MRI	x-ray if symptoms persist	MRI, CT, or CT myelogram
Treatment	Find the cause and fix it	Conservative, surgery if not better in 6–12 weeks	Conservative	Conservative, ESI, surgery

LE, lower extremity; DTR, deep tendon reflex; SLR, straight leg raise; ESI, epidural steroid injection; MRI, magnetic resonance imaging; CT, computed tomography.

d. Unilateral low back and buttock pain that gets worse with standing in one position may have sacroiliac joint involvement.

e. Pain in the elderly that is increased by walking and is relieved by leaning forward suggests spinal stenosis.

3. Diagnostic studies

a. Radiography of the spine in nontraumatic low back pain is often not required when pertinent directed history and physical examination reveal no sign of a serious condition.

b. Red flags that indicate a need for urgent radiography include fever, weight loss, morning stiffness, history of IV drug or steroid use, trauma, history of cancer, saddle anesthesia, loss of anal sphincter tone, or major motor weakness.

c. CT is helpful in demonstrating bony stenosis and identifying lateral nerve root entrapment.

d. MRI can be useful in identifying cord pathology, neural tumors, stenosis, herniated disks, and infections.

4. Treatment

a. Short-term relative rest (maximum of 2 days) with support under the knees and neck and administration of NSAIDs or analgesics are the first components of treatment.

b. Progressive ambulation to normal activities may follow if pain has subsided.

c. A fitness program, including postural exercises (e.g., McKenzie exercises for disk derangement), should be implemented for back rehabilitation.

d. If no improvement occurs in 6 weeks, perform further evaluation with bone scan, CT, MRI, or EMG and a medical workup to rule out spinal tumor or infection.

e. If studies are normal, continue back rehabilitation.

f. When conservative treatment fails, consider surgical intervention (~5% of those who present with low back pain).

B. Scoliosis and kyphosis

1. Scoliosis

a. General characteristics

(1) Scoliosis is defined as lateral curvature of the spine.

(2) Some curves are secondary to underlying causes (i.e., upper or lower motor neuron disease, myopathies); some are idiopathic.

(3) Girls between onset of the puberty growth spurt and cessation of spinal growth are at the greatest risk for idiopathic scoliosis.

(4) The vertebrae at the apex of the curve are used for its description. Right thoracic curves (T7 or T8) are the most common, followed by the double major (right thoracic, left lumbar), left lumbar, and right lumbar.

(5) A thoracic curve to the left is rare; other spinal cord pathology needs to be ruled out before making a diagnosis of scoliosis.

2. Clinical features

(1) Physical examination reveals asymmetry in the shoulder and iliac height; asymmetric scapular prominence; and a flank crease with forward bending, showing right thoracic and left lumbar prominence.

(2) Gait and neurologic examinations are normal.

(3) Curves of <20 degrees, diagnosed <2 years postmenarche, and Risser stage 2 to 4 are less likely to progress than are other curves.

a. Imaging

(1) Single, standing AP radiographs should be obtained when a patient has scoliometer (a device used for measuring curves) readings of >5 degrees.

Low back pain red flags for urgent imaging (TUNAFISH):
Trauma
Unexplained weight loss
Neurologic symptoms
Age>50
Fever
IVDU
Steroid use
History of cancer

Idiopathic adolescent scoliosis is the most common spinal deformity evaluated by a clinician.

(2) Vertebral levels are identified on radiography.

(a) The greatest anterior tilt is measured by the Cobb method (measurement is perpendicular to the end plate of the most tilted [end] vertebra).

(b) Curves of >15% are significant.

(3) Accurate measurement is best performed by an orthopedic specialist.

3. Treatment

(1) Curves of 10 to 15 degrees are treated by 6- to 12-month follow-up with clinical evaluation and possibly x-rays.

(2) Curves of 15 to 20 degrees need serial AP radiographic follow-up every 3 to 4 months for larger curves and every 6 to 8 months for smaller curves or for patients near the end of growth.

(3) Curves of 20 degrees or greater need referral to an orthopedist for continuous monitoring and management (bracing, electrical stimulation, or surgery).

> In scoliosis, orthopedic intervention is recommended with >20° curvature.

4. Kyphosis

a. General characteristics

(1) Kyphosis is defined as increased convex curvature of the thoracic spine.

(2) Scoliosis is also present in one-third of patients with kyphosis.

(3) Juvenile kyphosis (Scheuermann disease) is idiopathic osteochondrosis of the thoracic spine.

(4) Tuberculosis of the spine (the most common extrapulmonary location of tuberculosis after the lymph nodes) causes progressive kyphosis (Pott disease).

b. Clinical features

(1) When several vertebrae are involved, there is a round back appearance; when only one vertebra is involved, there is an angular curve.

(2) If the curve is a result of faulty posture, it will disappear with spinal flexion.

(3) Excessive lumbar lordosis is common.

c. Imaging: Standing lateral films are definitive.

d. Treatment

(1) Curves of 45 to 60 degrees should be observed every 3 to 4 months and exercises prescribed for lumbar lordosis and the thoracic spine.

(2) Curves of >60 degrees or with persistent pain can be treated using a Milwaukee brace.

(3) Surgery is indicated when curvature is unresponsive to conservative treatment.

C. Spinal stenosis

1. General characteristics

a. Spinal stenosis is nerve compression caused by narrowing of the spinal canal or neural foramina.

b. Types

(1) Central stenosis (compression of the thecal sac) can be idiopathic or developmental.

(2) Lateral stenosis (impingement of the nerve root lateral to the thecal sac) often accompanies central stenosis or is an isolated entity in young adults and the middle-aged.

c. Spinal stenosis is usually symptomatic in late middle age and is more common in men than in women.

2. Clinical features

a. Neural claudication and exacerbation of pain with walking is typical. The pain is relieved by leaning forward.

b. Variable back and leg pain may occur.

> Spinal stenosis features: a later middle-aged patient with low back pain relieved by leaning forward (shopping cart sign), progressively treated with conservative management or epidural steroids or surgical fusion.

3. Imaging

    a. Radiographs show soft-tissue and thecal narrowing.

    b. Plain CT, postmyelographic CT, and MRI are standard imaging modalities.

4. Treatment

    a. Conservative management includes rest, isometric abdominal exercises, pelvic tilt, flexion exercises, NSAIDs, and weight reduction.

    b. Lumbar epidural corticosteroid injections provide symptomatic relief; 25% of patients will gain sustained relief of symptoms following steroid injection.

    c. Decompression and fusion are indicated when studies are positive for neural compressive pathology and quality of life is unacceptable to the patient.

D. Ankylosing spondylitis (AS)

1. General characteristics

    a. AS is a seronegative spondyloarthropathy that progresses to fusion of the vertebrae.

    b. This condition involves onset of back pain, stiffness, and hip pain during the third and fourth decades of life and is seen more often in men than in women.

    c. This disorder affects the sacroiliac joint symmetrically and the spine in a progressively ascending manner.

> In AS, chronic inflammation of the axial spine leads to pain, stiffness, and immobility.

2. Clinical features

    a. Lumbar motion is restricted.

    b. Limited motion in the shoulders and hips, synovitis of the knees, plantar fasciitis, and Achilles tendinitis are seen.

    c. Patients also have hip contractures and fixed cervical, thoracic, and lumbar hyperkyphosis.

    d. Fracture of the fused osteopenic spine may occur (commonly cervical), as may sciatica.

    e. Extra-articular manifestations may occur, including uveitis, cardiac abnormalities, and interstitial lung disease, and inflammatory bowel disease.

    f. Noninvasive tests for spine and thoracic mobility include the Schober test, thoracolumbar rotation and flexion, finger-to-floor distance, cervical rotation, occiput–wall distance, and chest expansion.

3. Diagnostic studies

    a. Elevated levels of ESR and CRP are seen. Ninety percent of white and 50% of black patients with AS are HLA-B27 positive.

    b. Sacroiliitis is an early radiographic finding. The "bamboo spine appearance" on radiography occurs because of radiographic obliteration and marginal syndesmophyte ossification of the paraspinal ligaments.

    c. Generalized osteopenia of the spine may be seen.

> A (+) HLA-B27 antigen is found in up to 90% of whites and 50% of blacks with AS.

4. Treatment

    a. The mainstay of treatment is physical therapy with emphasis on posture, extension exercises, and breathing exercises. Swimming is considered the best overall exercise.

    b. NSAIDs are the first-line treatment and may slow the radiographic progression of spinal disease. For those who are resistant to NSAIDs, TNF inhibitors have been used with great success to prevent pain and disease progression.

    c. Spine fractures need intervention and stabilization.

E. Cauda equina syndrome

1. General characteristics: This is a rare condition that can be caused by a large midline disk, epidural abscess, tumor, or hematoma that compresses several nerve roots, usually at L4–L5 level.

2. Clinical features

    a. Bowel and bladder function is severely impaired.

    b. Leg pain, numbness, saddle anesthesia, and/or paralysis are noted.

3. Treatment: This is a surgical emergency requiring immediate referral.

Disorders of the Hip and Lower Extremity

A. Aseptic necrosis of the hip

> Aseptic necrosis of hip presents as dull aching or throbbing pain in groin/hip/buttock. MRI is imaging of choice. Hip replacement is often indicated.

  1. General characteristics

    a. Aseptic necrosis (also known as osteonecrosis or avascular necrosis) of the hip results from loss of blood supply to the trabecular bone, which causes a collapse of the femoral head.

    b. It can occur at any age but is seen with greater frequency during the third to fifth decades of life and is often bilateral.

    c. In children, it is known as Legg–Calvé–Perthes (LCP) disease; it typically develops in children aged 2 to 11 years, with a peak incidence between 4 and 8 years of age.

    d. The cause is generally unknown but is associated with obesity in children and is often seen in adults with a history of trauma, steroid use, alcohol abuse, RA, radiation therapy, and SLE.

  2. Clinical features

    a. Patients present with a dull ache or throbbing pain localized to the groin, lateral hip, or buttocks.

    b. Pain with weight-bearing and activity that is relieved with rest may also occur.

    c. Loss of rotation (internal and external) or abduction and an antalgic limp are observed.

    d. Children with LCP usually present with persistent pain, a limp, and loss of motion, particularly internal rotation and abduction.

    e. Adverse outcomes include secondary OA, femoral head collapse, and disability.

  3. Imaging

    a. MRI is the study of choice for early detection.

    b. Radiography may be normal early in the course of adult disease; later, progression of necrosis may reveal a crescent sign in lateral films.

    c. Bone scans are useful but are less sensitive than MRI.

    d. Radiography should be done early in children and may show soft-tissue swelling, joint distension, increased bone density, fragmentation, or a deformed femoral head, all various stages of the disease.

  4. Treatment

    a. Protected weight-bearing for early-stage disease is considered to be a temporary treatment. Alendronate has been used to prevent early collapse.

    b. Surgical options range from core decompression to total hip replacement.

    c. In children, the treatment is protected weight-bearing. Little benefit has been shown from bracing.

B. Slipped capital femoral epiphysis (SCFE)

  1. General characteristics

    a. SCFE is a weakening of the epiphyseal plate of the femur, resulting in a displacement of the femoral head. It may be bilateral.

    b. It typically presents in children between 10 and 16 years of age.

> Insidious pain with a painful limp in young adolescents indicates SCFE.

    c. Boys are affected more often than girls, and there is a higher incidence in black and Hispanic children, the athletically inclined, and obese children.

    d. Most cases of SCFE are idiopathic, but in the younger child, consider a metabolic cause (hypothyroidism or hypopituitarism).

  2. Clinical features include a history of insidious hip, thigh, or knee pain associated with a painful limp.

  3. Imaging: Lateral radiographs show posterior and medial displacement of the epiphysis. SCFE is best assessed with the patient in the frog-leg lateral pelvis or lateral hip view.

  4. Treatment

    a. Definitive treatment for chronic SCFE is pinning in situ.

    b. The child should be placed on crutches and should avoid weight-bearing before and after surgery.

C. Meniscal injuries of the knee (see Table 9-11 for comparison of common knee disorders)

  1. General characteristics

    a. Meniscal injury occurs with excessive rotational force of the femur on the tibia.

    b. The medial meniscus is injured most often.

    c. Injuries may be isolated or may occur with other ligamentous ruptures.

  2. Clinical features

    a. Patients report joint line pain on the side of the injury, which may be palpable during examination.

    b. Inability to fully extend the knee is described as locking.

    c. The patient may describe a feeling of the knee giving way.

    d. Swelling occurs gradually, over hours to days.

    e. Walking up and down stairs or squatting is difficult and may be painful.

    f. The McMurray and Apley tests may be helpful in detecting a meniscal tear.

  3. Imaging

    a. Radiography usually is negative.

    b. MRI often makes the diagnosis of a meniscal tear, but occasionally, arthroscopy is required for diagnosis.

  4. Treatment

    a. Initial treatment is conservative: activity modification, NSAIDs, quadriceps strengthening exercises, and time.

    b. Indications for arthroscopy include persistent symptoms unresponsive to conservative treatment or irreducible locking.

> Osgood-Schlatter is pain and swelling localized to the tibial tubercle, just below the kneecap.

D. Osgood–Schlatter's disease (see Table 9-11 for comparison of common knee disorders)

  1. General characteristics

    a. Osgood–Schlatter's disease is apophysitis of the tibial tubercle caused by trauma or overuse.

    b. The age of onset is between 8 and 15 years. Males are affected two to three times more often than females.

    c. A self-limited disease, symptoms resolve when the epiphysis closes.

  2. Clinical features

    a. Patients complain of anterior knee pain, with localized pain and swelling over the tibial tubercle.

    b. Pain is typically related to activity and is relieved with rest.

3. Imaging: Lateral radiography is usually normal but may show fragmentation at the tibial tubercle.

4. Treatment

    a. Activity modification for as long as several months

    b. Stretching, ice, and NSAIDs after exercise are indicated.

E. Cruciate ligament injuries (see Table 9-11 for comparison of common knee disorders)

    1. General characteristics

        a. The anterior cruciate ligament (ACL) is more commonly injured than the posterior cruciate ligament (PCL).

        b. ACL injury is commonly associated with a pivoting motion during running, jumping, or cutting activities like skiing, basketball, or soccer.

        c. Women are affected more often than men.

    2. Clinical features

        a. Patients usually report hearing a pop and complain of knee instability.

        b. Hemarthrosis develops quickly within 3 to 4 hours.

        c. Lachman test is the most sensitive for diagnosing an ACL tear.

    3. Imaging

        a. Radiographs are done to rule out associated avulsion fracture of the knee.

        b. MRI is useful as an adjunct to physical examination to diagnose an ACL tear.

    4. Treatment

        a. Nonoperative treatment with physical therapy and bracing is appropriate in patients who do not participate in competitive activities or who do not report instability with desired activities.

        b. Surgical reconstruction with autograft or allograft is appropriate in patients who are younger than 40 years, those who participate in competitive activities, or those who report instability with desired activities.

        c. Complications from surgery may include limited or loss of full ROM or anterior knee pain.

F. Ankle sprain/strain (see Table 9-12 for comparison of common foot and ankle injuries)

    1. General characteristics

        a. Ankle sprains are one of the most common sports-related injuries; 85% result from an inversion injury.

        b. Ankle sprains most often involve the lateral ligaments, particularly the ATL.

    2. Clinical features

        a. Patients will often report hearing a pop and will present with ecchymosis and tenderness of the lateral ankle.

        b. Stability of the ankle can be assessed using the anterior drawer test.

Table 9-11 | Comparing Common Knee Disorders

Osgood–Schlatter's (Apophysitis)	Meniscal Disorder	Cruciate Ligament Disorder
8–15 years old	Rotation injury	Typically from a pivoting force
Male > female	Force from femur	Knee instability
Anterior knee pain	Joint line pain	Pop is heard or felt
Swelling at tibial tubercle	Locking, giving way	Lachman test positive
Treatment with rest, stretching	Swells over hours to days	Hemarthrosis possible 3–4 hours later
Ice, NSAIDs for acute pain	Stairs increase pain	
	McMurray's or Apley's maneuvers +	

Table 9-12 | Comparing Common Foot and Ankle Problems

Ankle Strain/Sprain	Achilles Tendinitis	Hallux Valgus (Bunions)	Morton Neuroma	Plantar Fasciitis
- Inversion injury most common - Anterior talofibular ligament most often injured - Pop, then pain - Ecchymosis - Tenderness	- Runners, overuse injury - Improper stretching - Gradually increasing pain, posterior calf - Pain increases with passive dorsiflexion and with resisted plantar flexion - Thompson test to rule out rupture	- Affects metatarsophalangeal joint - Medial eminence and metatarsal head pain - Females > males - Requires wide toe box shoe for comfort	- Third web space pain - Females > males - Growing mass - Squeeze test positive - Wide toe box shoe - Good support shoes	- Pain with first steps of the day - Heel pain at night - Calcaneal origin, inflexible Achilles tendon - Stretching, heel pads, arch supports - Massage

> Ottawa Rules indicate x-ray of the ankle if the injury is acutely painful plus point tender at posterior medial malleolus; *or* point tender at posterior lateral malleolus; *or* unable to bear weight upon injury.

3. Imaging: Radiography should be done to rule out a fracture, especially if the patient is unable to bear weight or has tenderness to palpation over a bone.

4. **Treatment**

   a. Treatment should be tailored to the severity of the sprain but should always include "RICE" (rest, ice, compression, elevation).

   b. Patients should use crutches for the first 48 to 72 hours, and a brace should be used for support.

   c. Referral to physical therapy may speed recovery. Length of recovery could be 3 to 4 months.

G. **Achilles tendinitis** (see Table 9-12 for comparison of common foot and ankle injuries)

   1. General characteristics

      a. Pain is attributed to inflammation and degeneration of the Achilles tendon and its attachment to the calcaneus.

      b. It is common in runners and in patients who suddenly increase their activity level.

      c. It is considered an overuse injury and is usually the result of improper stretching and training.

      d. If untreated, it may result in rupture of the Achilles tendon.

   2. **Clinical features**

      a. Patients usually report a gradual onset of pain during activity or after an activity is completed.

      b. The pain is located on the posterior calf, 2 to 6 cm above the insertion of the Achilles tendon.

      c. Patients will be tender over the posterior calf above the calcaneus and will report pain on passive dorsiflexion and resisted plantar flexion.

      d. Ankle ROM and strength should be normal.

      e. Thompson test should be done to rule out Achilles tendon rupture.

   3. Imaging

      a. Radiographs may show a soft-tissue shadow and calcifications along the tendon and its insertion.

      b. MRI may show hypertrophy of the Achilles tendon or help rule out a rupture.

   4. **Treatment**: The patient should be started on a regimen of NSAIDs and physical therapy for stretching and strengthening exercises. Corticosteroid injections are contraindicated in Achilles tendinitis.

H. **Bunions (hallux valgus)** (see Table 9-12 for comparison of common foot and ankle injuries)

   1. General characteristics

> Common presentation of Achilles tendinitis is the aging athlete returning to a sport. MRI is indicated to evaluate rupture if Thompson test is positive.

    a. The most common deformity of the MTP joint is hallux valgus; it is the result of a lateral deviation of the proximal phalanx.

    b. Bunions are more common in women than in men (10:1). They are often caused by wearing tight, pointed shoes.

    c. Other causes include congenital deformity and systemic diseases such as RA.

2. Clinical features

    a. Patients will often complain of medial eminence pain, metatarsal head pain, deformities of the toes, and the inability to find shoes that fit.

    b. Examination may show a hallux valgus deformity, MTP enlargement, and pain and crepitation on movement of the MTP joint.

    c. Patients may also have limited ROM and pain on extreme ROM of the MTP joint.

3. Imaging: Weight-bearing radiography of the foot will show the valgus deformity of the proximal phalanx; an angle of >15 degrees is considered abnormal.

4. Treatment

    a. Encourage patients to buy shoes with a wide toe box and to use pads on the medial eminence of the bunion deformity or between the first and second toes if they are rubbing together.

    b. Surgical treatment is for severe deformity or pain that is not relieved with conservative measures.

I. **Morton neuroma** (see Table 9-12 for comparison of common foot and ankle injuries)

    1. General characteristics

        a. Morton neuroma is a result of traction of the interdigital nerve against the transverse metatarsal ligament causing degeneration of the nerve and chronic inflammation.

        b. It usually affects the third web space and is more common in women than in men (10:1).

    2. Clinical features

        a. Patients complain of pain and localized numbness when walking and standing, and may say they feel like they are walking on a marble, which is relieved with rest.

        b. Pain is usually localized to the web space, and a mass is often palpable.

        c. Squeezing the forefoot will often reproduce the symptoms.

    3. Imaging

        a. Plain radiography is normal.

        b. MRI is sensitive but not usually needed, as the diagnosis is made clinically.

    4. Treatment

        a. Conservative treatment using a soft metatarsal pad and shoes with a wide toe box are helpful.

        b. Steroid injections into the web space can be helpful.

        c. Surgical removal of the neuroma is possible in cases that are not resolved with conservative treatment, but the patient should be aware that the affected toes will be chronically numb.

J. **Plantar fasciitis** (see Table 9-12 for comparison of common foot and ankle injuries)

    1. General characteristics

        a. Plantar fasciitis is very common in runners and patients who are overweight.

        b. It is caused by microscopic tears in the plantar fascia at the calcaneal origin.

    2. Clinical features

        a. Patients will complain of pain with the first few steps in the morning and possibly heel pain at night.

        b. Examination will show pain at the calcaneal origin and an inflexible Achilles tendon.

> Avoiding tight shoes and high heels will reduce the frequency of painful flare-ups of Morton neuroma.

3. Imaging

    a. Plain radiography is typically normal but may reveal a calcaneal fracture or bone spur.

    b. MRI may reveal calcifications of the plantar fascia.

4. Treatment

    a. Conservative treatment is recommended for 6 to 12 months, including physical therapy for stretching of the plantar fascia and the Achilles tendon, heel pads, arch supports, and massage of the area with a tennis ball.

    b. Steroid injections should be used with caution because of the risk of rupture of the plantar fascia.

    c. Surgery is reserved for extreme cases.

Practice Questions

Directions: *Each of the numbered items or incomplete statements in this section is followed by a list of answers or completions of the statement. Select the ONE lettered answer or completion that is BEST in each case.*

1. A 62-year-old obese female complains of pain in her left knee that has been getting worse for the past year. The pain is better in the morning after her shower and worse in the evening after normal daily activities. On examination, there is crepitus noted and decreased, painful ROM. What is the initial recommended treatment for the most likely diagnosis?

A. Topical NSAIDs

B. NSAIDs

C. Opioids

D. Topical capsaicin

2. A 56-year-old male presents with pain in his first toe that awakened him from sleep last night. He states it is so painful that he is unable to move his toe or touch it. History reveals he drinks four beers each night after dinner. On examination, his toe is erythematous with a dusky appearance, swollen, and tender to touch. Uric acid level is 8.4 mg per dL. Which of the following would most likely be found on examination of the synovial fluid?

A. Gram-negative diplococci

B. Normal synovial fluid

C. Rhomboid-shaped, positively birefringent crystals

D. Rod-shaped, negatively birefringent crystals

3. A 27-year-old female presents with a history of 3 months of joint pain and stiffness. On examination, you note a rash over her nose and cheeks and small ulcers on her buccal mucosa. Which of the following positive lab tests will best support the most likely diagnosis?

A. Anti-double-stranded DNA antibody

B. RF

C. Anti-SS-A (ro) antibody

D. ESR

4. A 68-year-old female presents complaining of weakness in her shoulders and hips. She states it is difficult for her to comb her hair and get up from a chair. Examination confirms weakness of the proximal muscles of the arms and legs and a purplish rash over the eyelids. Which of the following will confirm the most likely diagnosis?

A. Elevated aldolase

B. Elevated ESR

C. Muscle biopsy showing inflammation

D. Presence of anti-native DNA antibody

5. A 50-year-old female presents with complaints about her skin looking strange lately. She also complains of Raynaud-like symptoms and achiness of her muscles and joints over the past few months. The skin on the hands and face appears edematous and thickened and seems to have lost its normal folds. Laboratory data reveal mild anemia, a positive ANA, and anti-SCL-70 antibody. What is the most likely diagnosis?

A. Primary Raynaud's phenomenon

B. RA

C. SLE

D. Scleroderma syndrome

6. A 32-year-old female presents with complaints of headaches, insomnia, all-over body pain, and difficulty concentrating for the past 3 months. Physical examination reveals multiple trigger points on the body; no other physical signs are present. Which of the following would be most effective for treating the most likely diagnosis?

A. Diphenhydramine

B. Cognitive and behavioral therapy

C. Massage therapy

D. NSAIDs

7. A 62-year-old healthy female returns to the office to discuss her DEXA scan results. Her T score is –2.6. She is diagnosed with osteoporosis. What is the first-line treatment for this patient?

A. Bisphosphonates

B. Teriparatide

C. Nasal calcitonin

D. Watchful waiting

8. A 7-year-old male presents after falling off a slide at school. He complains of pain in his left wrist. x-ray shows an epiphyseal fracture with associated metaphyseal fragment. What type of fracture is this according to the Salter–Harris classification?

A. Type I

B. Type II
C. Type III
D. Type IV

9. A 56-year-old female presents complaining of a dull pain in her right shoulder. She states it is painful when she reaches over her head and the pain wakes her up at night. On examination, the patient has pain and difficulty abducting her arm but has normal ROM. Radiographs are negative. What is the most likely diagnosis?
   A. Adhesive capsulitis
   B. Cervical spondylosis
   C. Rotator cuff syndrome
   D. Shoulder dislocation

10. A 32-year-old female presents complaining of pain in her wrist and forearm and numbness and tingling in her thumb, index, and middle fingers. The symptoms are worse at night. On examination, there is no thenar atrophy noted, but she does have a positive Tinel's sign and Phalen's test. What is the recommended treatment for the most likely diagnosis?
    A. Nighttime volar splinting
    B. NSAIDs

C. Steroid injection
D. Surgical decompression

11. A 68-year-old female presents complaining of a swelling on her left elbow. She states she bumped her elbow on a railing 2 days ago and now it looks like there is a golf ball on her elbow. She denies pain and has full ROM. What is the recommended treatment for the most likely diagnosis?
    A. Angiotensin-converting enzyme wrap and rest
    B. Aspiration of the bursa
    C. NSAIDs
    D. Surgical removal

12. A 38-year-old female presents with pain and numbness near the ball of the foot. She states the pain is worse when wearing shoes and is relieved when she removes the shoes and rests. On examination, there is no palpable mass, but her pain is reproduced when you squeeze the forefoot. What is the most likely diagnosis?
    A. Bunion
    B. Lumbar disk disease
    C. Morton neuroma
    D. Plantar fasciitis

Practice Answers

1. **A.** *MSS; Pharmacology; OA*

   Topical NSAIDs are the first-line medical therapy in patients with mild OA. Patients should also be counseled to lose weight and start or continue a regular exercise program. Oral NSAIDs can be used if topical NSAIDs are not effective, but because of the side-effect profile they are not used until a patient has tried the topicals. Opioid medications are not generally used for OA because they have a dangerous side-effect profile and can be addictive. Topical capsaicin can be used in patients with OA affecting the hands but is not recommended in patients with OA of the knee or hip.

2. **D.** *MSS; Diagnostic Studies; Gout*

   Acute gout is typically characterized by sudden onset pain in a single joint (usually the first MTP joint). Uric acid is elevated in 95% of patients. Synovial fluid will show an elevated WBC, a negative culture, and rod-shaped, negatively birefringent crystals. Pseudogout (CPPD) presents like gout but does not have an elevated uric acid level and shows rhomboid-shaped, positively birefringent crystals in the synovial fluid. Gram-negative diplococci is indicative of *N. gonorrhoeae*, a common cause of septic arthritis.

3. **A.** *MSS; Diagnostic Studies; SLE*

   Anti-ds DNA antibody is seen in patients with SLE 60% of the time. RF is seen in patients with SLE about 20% of the time but is more likely (70% to 75%) seen in patients with RA and Sjögren's syndrome. Anti-SS-A (ro) antibody is occasionally (20%) seen in patients with SLE but is also more likely (65%) seen in patients with Sjögren's syndrome. Elevated ESR is seen in SLE but is not specific for this diagnosis.

4. **C.** *MSS; Diagnostic Studies; Dermatomyositis*

   Muscle biopsy showing inflammation in the muscles is the only way to confirm the diagnosis of polymyositis. Elevated aldolase

may be seen in polymyositis/dermatomyositis but does not confirm the diagnosis. The ESR is typically normal in a patient with polymyositis but will be very high in a patient with polymyalgia rheumatica which can sometimes be confused with polymyositis. Anti-native DNA antibody is seen in patients with SLE, which can sometimes be confused with polymyositis, especially when the skin is involved (dermatomyositis).

5. **D.** *MSS; Diagnosis; Systemic Sclerosis*

   Patients with SS typically present with skin changes, arthralgias, and Raynaud's disease. A positive ANA and anti-SCL-70 antibody are found in patients with SS >95% and 20% to 30% of the time, respectively. Primary Raynaud's phenomenon presents with the typical symptoms of color changes in the hands (white, blue, red) and is not usually associated with other symptoms. Patients with RA often present with arthralgias but typically do not have skin symptoms; although an ANA is often positive in a patient with RA, a positive anti-SCL-70 antibody is rare. SLE usually presents with arthralgias and skin rashes; laboratory data usually include a positive ANA and anti-native DNA antibody.

6. **B.** *MSS; Clinical Intervention; Fibromyalgia*

   This patient has fibromyalgia which is treated with a multimodal approach of pain control, cognitive and behavioral therapy, and moderate exercise. Benadryl (diphenhydramine) can be used for occasional insomnia but should not be prescribed in patients who have a chronic disease that may be contributing to their insomnia. Massage therapy is not part of the multimodal approach to treating fibromyalgia and may cause the patient pain. NSAIDs do not effectively treat fibromyalgia.

7. **A.** *MSS; Pharmacology; Osteoporosis*

   This patient has osteoporosis and is at risk for developing a fracture; medical treatment should not be delayed.

Bisphosphonates are the first-line treatment for patients with osteoporosis if they can sit up for 30 minutes after ingestion. Teriparatide can be used if a patient cannot tolerate bisphosphonates. Nasal calcitonin is not considered first-line therapy for osteoporosis, and watchful waiting is not appropriate with this T score.

8. B. *MSS; Diagnosis; Salter–Harris Fracture*

Type I only involves a fracture through the epiphyseal plate. Type II involves the epiphyseal plate with a metaphyseal fragment. Type III involves a fracture through the epiphysis into the articular surface. Type IV involves the metaphysis, epiphyseal plate, and epiphysis.

9. C. *MSS; Diagnosis; Rotator Cuff Syndrome*

Rotator cuff syndrome is usually caused by either inflammation/impingement of the rotator cuff tendons or a rotator cuff tear. It typically presents with a dull aching pain in the shoulder that is exacerbated by abduction of the arm. The pain often wakes patients up at night; pathology would not be seen on x-ray. Adhesive capsulitis presents with severe pain and diminished ROM. Cervical spondylosis usually presents with neck pain and numbness and tingling down the arms and below the elbow. Shoulder dislocation is usually caused by a traumatic injury, and the patient presents unable to move the arm; a dislocation would be seen on x-ray of the shoulder.

10. A. *MSS; Clinical Intervention; Carpal Tunnel Syndrome*

The initial treatment for a patient with carpal tunnel syndrome is nighttime volar splinting and activity modification. NSAIDs may help alleviate the pain but should not be used exclusively. Steroid injections may be used in patients whose symptoms do not resolve with splinting and activity modification. Surgical decompression is used as a last resort in patients who do not respond to conservative management.

11. A. *MSS; Clinical Intervention; Bursitis*

This patient has olecranon bursitis which can be caused by acute injury or repetitive trauma. Initial treatment, if there is no concern for infection, is conservative with an ACE wrap, rest, and heat. Aspiration of the bursa is only recommended in patients who have redness and tenderness over the bursa and there is a possibility of infection. NSAIDs can be used in olecranon bursitis if the patient is experiencing pain, but this patient denies pain. Surgical removal is only indicated in cases where infection is a concern and the patient has not responded to more conservative treatment.

12. C. *MSS; Diagnosis; Morton Neuroma*

A Morton neuroma is caused by the traction of the interdigital nerve against the ligaments in the foot. Patients often complain of localized pain and numbness that is worse with tight-fitting shoes and relieved with loose shoes or barefoot. Patients may say it feels like they are walking on a marble. A bunion is a deformity of the MTP joint that causes lateral deviation of the proximal phalanx; patients may complain of pain where their shoes are rubbing on the bone, but not numbness. Lumbar disk disease can cause foot pain and numbness, but because the problem is in the back the symptoms would not worsen with compression of the forefoot. Plantar fasciitis presents as pain that is worse in the morning when the patients get out of bed and is located on the bottom of the foot near the arch; pain is not exacerbated by squeezing the forefoot.

Endocrinology | 10

Michael Cirone

Parathyroid Disorders

A. Hyperparathyroidism

1. General characteristics

a. There are four pea-sized parathyroid glands on the posterior aspect of the thyroid gland. These glands secrete parathyroid hormone (PTH), which causes serum calcium levels to rise. The parathyroid gland responds to low or falling calcium levels and thus mobilizes calcium from bones by osteoclast stimulation. It also stimulates the kidneys to resorb calcium and increases gastrointestinal (GI) absorption of calcium.

b. Benign parathyroid gland adenomas cause 85% of primary hyperparathyroidism. Parathyroid gland hyperplasia is the cause in 15%. Carcinoma is rare and accounts for <1% of cases.

c. Hyperparathyroidism is more common in women than men at a 2:1 ratio, and the incidence increases after age 50 years.

d. Primary hyperparathyroidism is the most common cause of hypercalcemia in ambulatory patients, and there are 100,000 new cases each year in the United States. Malignancy is the most common cause in hospitalized patients. Hypercalcemia is also common with renal failure, milk–alkali syndrome, multiple myeloma, head–neck–lung cancers, sarcoidosis, tuberculosis (TB), medications (thiazides, calcium or vitamin D, lithium), Hodgkin's lymphoma, adrenal insufficiency, prolonged bed rest, and hyperthyroidism (secondary hyperparathyroidism).

e. In patients with chronic kidney disease, secondary hyperparathyroidism occurs because of hyperphosphatemia, causing increased ionized calcium levels and decreased renal production of active vitamin D.

2. **Clinical features**

a. Mild hypercalcemia is likely to be asymptomatic.

b. More severe hypercalcemia causes thirst, anorexia, nausea, vomiting, abdominal pain, constipation, fatigue, anemia, weight loss, peptic ulcer disease, pancreatitis, hypertension (HTN), and depressed deep tendon reflexes. Symptoms are summarized as follows:

(1) Renal loss of calcium and phosphate = kidney *stones*

(2) Enhanced release of calcium from bones = pain in *bones*

(3) Increased GI absorption and abdominal cramps = *groans*

(4) Irritability, psychosis, and depression = *moans*

c. Patients may develop polydipsia and polyuria caused by hypercalcemia-induced nephrogenic diabetes insipidus (DI).

d. Other findings include arrhythmias, HTN, renal failure, pancreatitis, gastric ulcers, weakness, fatigue, anorexia, polydipsia, and polyuria.

> Carcinoma accounts for <1% of all cases of hyperparathyroid disease.

> The leading cause of hypercalcemia in the United States is hyperparathyroidism. The most common complaints are summarized as stones, bones, groans, and moans.

Calcium levels should be adjusted for serum albumin level.

3. Diagnostic studies

   a. Hypercalcemia of hyperparathyroidism is often identified on routine chemistry panels in asymptomatic patients; abnormal screening studies should be repeated.

   b. Adjusted serum calcium level >10.5 mg per dL and phosphate <2.5 mg per dL with PTH >55 pg per mL indicates a primary disorder. Adjusted total calcium = measured serum calcium (mg/dL) + [0.8 × (4.0 − serum albumin [g/dL])].

   c. Urine calcium excretion is usually low for the degree of hypercalcemia.

   d. Elevated serum levels of intact PTH confirm primary hyperparathyroidism.

   e. Elevated calcium with low PTH indicates secondary disorder such as a malignancy.

   f. Extreme elevations of both calcium and PTH indicate parathyroid cancer.

   g. Imaging studies, including ultrasonography, computed tomography (CT), magnetic resonance imaging (MRI), and sestamibi scan, are less useful in the diagnosis of hyperparathyroidism but more helpful if surgery for parathyroid adenoma is anticipated.

   h. All patients should be screened for familial benign hypocalciuric hypercalcemia with a 24-hour urine for calcium and creatinine before treating for hyperparathyroidism.

   i. Patients with low bone mineral density, normal serum calcium, and elevated PTH level should be assessed for secondary hyperparathyroidism from vitamin D or calcium deficiency, hyperphosphatemia, or renal failure.

   j. Electrocardiographic (ECG) findings may include prolonged PR interval, shortened QT interval, bradyarrhythmias, heart block, and asystole.

4. **Treatment**

   a. Patients with mild asymptomatic primary hyperparathyroidism may only need to keep active, avoid immobilization, and drink adequate fluids.

   b. Patients should avoid thiazide diuretics, lithium carbonate, large doses of vitamins A and D, and calcium-containing antacids and supplements.

   c. Monitoring includes a schedule of serum calcium and albumin levels, kidney function and urinary calcium excretion, and bone density studies. Bisphosphonates may be a temporizing measure to decrease serum calcium levels. Cautious administration of vitamin D may be indicated.

   d. Intravenous (IV) hydration and bisphosphonates are recommended for acute hypercalcemic crisis. Furosemide may promote urinary calcium excretion.

   e. Parathyroidectomy is indicated for symptomatic primary disorder. Hypocalcemia and transient hyperthyroidism may occur postoperatively. Surgery is indicated in the presence of the following:

      (1) Symptomatic hypercalcemia (proximal muscle weakness, gait disturbance, atrophy, hyperreflexia, syncope from arrhythmias)

      (2) History of an episode of life-threatening hypercalcemia

      (3) Adjusted calcium level >1 mg per dL above upper limit

      (4) Urinary calcium excretion >400 mg in 24 hours (differentiate familial benign hypocalciuric hypercalcemia)

      (5) Creatinine clearance <60 mL per min, or reduced by over 30%

      (6) Bone density consistent with osteoporosis (≥2.5 standard deviation below normal) or previous fragility bone fracture

      (7) Age younger than 50 years

      (8) Osteitis fibrosa cystica

      (9) Nephrolithiasis

      (10) Pregnancy

      (11) Parathyroid carcinoma

Fluids are the foundation of treatment for hypercalcemia regardless of cause.

B. Hypoparathyroidism

1. General characteristics

a. Acquired hypoparathyroidism is most commonly encountered following parathyroidectomy or thyroidectomy.

b. It may also be caused by autoimmune disease, heavy metal toxicity (e.g., Wilson's disease, hemochromatosis), thyroiditis, or hypomagnesemia (chronic alcoholism).

c. DiGeorge syndrome is a congenital cause of hypocalcemia arising from parathyroid hypoplasia, thymic hypoplasia, and outflow tract defects of the heart.

d. Congenital pseudohypoparathyroidism results from a group of disorders characterized by alterations in serum calcium related to resistance to PTH.

2. Clinical features

a. Hypocalcemia may cause tetany resulting in carpopedal spasms, muscle or abdominal cramps, paresthesias, and hyperreflexia, as well as teeth, nail, and hair defects.

b. Chvostek sign is contraction of eye, mouth, or nose muscles elicited by tapping along the course of the facial nerve anterior to the ear. Trousseau sign produces spasm in the hand and wrist with compression to the forearm.

c. Findings in patients with chronic disease include lethargy, anxiety, parkinsonism, mental retardation, personality changes, and blurred vision caused by cataracts.

3. Diagnostic studies

a. The hallmark is decreased PTH, decreased adjusted serum calcium, and increased phosphate levels. Serum magnesium may be low. Alkaline phosphatase will be normal. Hypomagnesemia may worsen symptoms.

b. ECG changes may include prolonged QT intervals and T-wave abnormalities.

c. Radiography may demonstrate chronic increased bone mineral density, especially in the lumbar spine and skull.

4. Treatment

a. PTH, as a drug (Natpara), has been available for use in the treatment of osteoporosis. It is approved as an adjunct to calcium and vitamin D to control hypocalcemia in patients with hypoparathyroidism. This medication has been linked to osteosarcoma. It is reserved for those who do not respond to vitamin D and calcium treatment.

b. Treatment should be directed at correcting the hypocalcemia with calcium and vitamin D. Maintenance therapy includes oral calcium (1 to 2 g/day) and vitamin D preparations to keep serum calcium at 8 to 8.6 mg per dL. Calcitriol (activated vitamin D) is also used. Magnesium supplementation may be required.

c. Monitoring of treatment includes measurement of adjusted serum and urine calcium levels.

d. Phenothiazines and furosemide should be avoided because of the risk of further calcium loss.

e. Emergency treatment for tetany includes airway maintenance and slow administration of IV calcium gluconate.

> Hypocalcemia is associated with muscle abnormalities including spasms, hyperreflexia, and the Chvostek and Trousseau signs.

> The approach to treatment of hypothyroid disease begins with calcium and vitamin D.

Thyroid Disorders

A. Hyperthyroidism

1. General characteristics

a. Thyrotoxicosis is the clinical syndrome caused by excess circulating thyroid hormone (thyroxine [T_4] or triiodothyronine [T_3]). Serum thyroid-stimulating hormone (TSH) is suppressed in primary hyperthyroidism.

   b. The condition is more common in women than in men (8:1) and occurs in 2% of the U.S. society. Typical age of onset is between 20 and 40 years.

   c. Graves' disease is the most common cause of hyperthyroidism (80% of cases). Other causes include toxic multinodular goiter (second most common cause), Hashimoto thyroiditis, pituitary tumor, pregnancy, exogenous thyroid hormone, excessive dietary iodine intake, radiographic contrast, and amiodarone use.

   d. Graves' disease is an autoimmune disease affecting TSH receptors. Some antibodies act like TSH to cause secretion of thyroid hormone, whereas others stimulate glandular growth only. Diffuse, symmetric enlargement and goiter may be seen.

   e. Graves' disease is associated with specific human leukocyte antigen (HLA) markers and other autoimmune diseases.

   f. Thyroid cancer can coincide with Graves' disease.

2. **Clinical features** (Table 10-1)

   a. Weight loss despite good intake may be seen.

   b. Anxiety, warm, moist skin, onycholysis, and insomnia are common, as are a fine tremor, fatigue, muscle cramps, and weakness. Women report menstrual irregularity; amenorrhea occurs with severe disease. Three percent of patients with hyperthyroidism experience pretibial myxedema (a characteristic more common in hypothyroid disease).

   c. Cardiac presentations may include tachycardia, palpitations, forceful heartbeat, systolic HTN, widened pulse pressure, and premature ventricular contractions (PVCs). Atrial fibrillation occurs in 10% to 15% of patients, with greater frequency in elderly men with ischemic or valvular heart disease.

   d. There may be a change in bowel pattern, oligomenorrhea, brittle hair, or heat intolerance. Diffuse, symmetric thyroid enlargement and goiter may be seen.

   e. A brisk hyperreflexia may be seen on examination of deep tendon reflexes.

   f. Graves' disease is the only type of hyperthyroidism that is associated with ophthalmopathy, which manifest as inflammation of the eyes, upper eyelid retraction, lid lag with downward gaze, swelling of the tissue around the eyes, and protrusion or bulging of the eyes. Infiltrative ophthalmopathy is seen in 20% to 40% of patients, but true exophthalmos is seen in only 5%. The risk is higher in smokers.

> 💡 Thyroid ophthalmopathy is only seen in Graves' disease; true exophthalmos is seen in only 5%, but the rate is higher in smokers.

Table 10-1 | Comparison of Common Clinical Features of Hyper- and Hypothyroidism

Hypothyroidism	Hyperthyroidism
Dry, coarse hair	Hair loss
Dry skin	Clammy skin
Brittle nails	Soft nails
Puffy face	Exophthalmos
Bradycardia	Tachycardia, palpitations
Weight gain	Weight loss
Constipation	Diarrhea
Cold intolerance	Heat intolerance
Fatigue, lethargy	Muscle weakness, cramps
Muscle aches	Sleep difficulties
Hyporeflexia	Hyperreflexia
Memory loss, forgetfulness	Fine tremor
Depression	Anxiety, nervousness
Heavy menstrual periods	Oligomenorrhea or amenorrhea

g. Only 50% of older patients have thyroid enlargement compared with 94% of younger patients. Symptoms that occur more frequently in older patients than in younger patients include anorexia (32% vs. 4%) and atrial fibrillation (35% vs. 2%). Older patients, therefore, need routine screening.

h. Complications include atrial fibrillation, hypercalcemia, osteoporosis, impotence, nephrocalcinosis, decreased libido, gynecomastia, and decreased sperm count.

i. Chronic thyrotoxicosis may cause osteoporosis, clubbing, and finger swelling.

j. About 15% of Asian or Native American men with thyrotoxicosis may develop hypokalemic periodic paralysis lasting 7 to 72 hours, often after IV dextrose, oral carbohydrate, or vigorous exercise.

3. Diagnostic studies

a. Laboratory data reveal elevated T_3 and free T_4 levels. Elevation of T_3 is more pronounced than T_4.

b. T_4 can be normal, which indicates T_3 toxicosis that has a more favorable treatment prognosis to antithyroid medication. T_3 toxicosis is seen more commonly in early disease or relapse.

c. TSH levels are extremely low or undetectable in primary hyperthyroidism.

d. Peroxidase antibodies and thyroglobulin antibodies are positive in Graves' disease but not in toxic multinodular goiter.

e. Radioactive iodine uptake (RAIU) study (which should never be done in pregnant women or in those with laboratory-confirmed disease) shows increased uptake in Graves' disease and toxic multinodular goiter; uptake is more diffuse and symmetric in Graves' disease.

f. MRI and CT scanning of the orbits is performed for severe or unilateral ocular signs or when causation may be other than Graves.

> TSH is the most sensitive study in primary thyroid disease: It is elevated in hypothyroidism and reduced in hyperthyroidism.

4. Treatment

a. β-Blockers (primarily propranolol) control symptoms (tachycardia, tremor, diaphoresis, anxiety, palpitations) in any hyperthyroid episode and are the initial treatment of choice for thyroid storm and periodic paralysis. Rapid drug metabolism may initially occur, effecting dose titration.

b. The thiourea class of drugs includes propylthiouracil (PTU) and methimazole (MM). PTU is the drug of choice during pregnancy or breastfeeding. PTU is associated with arthritis, lupus, aplastic anemia, thrombocytopenia, and hepatic necrosis. MM is generally preferred over PTU because of dosing convenience and less risk of fulminant hepatic necrosis. It is associated with serum sickness, cholestatic jaundice, alopecia, nephrotic syndrome, and hypoglycemia. Fetal anomalies include aplasia cutis and esophageal or choanal atresia. Both PTU and MM cross the placenta and affect fetal thyroid function but PTU to a lesser effect. TSH levels should be checked 4 to 6 weeks after treatment is started.

> β-Blockers provide first-line symptomatic treatment until definitive treatment based on cause is decided: medication, ablation, or surgical resection.

c. Radioactive iodine ablation is used in older patients, those with prior PTU/MM reaction or failure, or poor compliance. Stop antithyroid medications 3 to 5 days prior to the procedure. RAIU is used to determine dosing. Improvement may be seen after 4 to 6 weeks. Almost 80% are cured with one dose. At least 50% of patients treated will become hypothyroid in a year. Ablation is contraindicated in pregnancy/nursing as iodine is concentrated in fetal thyroid tissue. It can also induce thyroiditis and swelling (life threatening).

d. Thyroidectomy is indicated for large obstructing glands, malignant nodules, or in pregnancy. Patients should be euthyroid before surgery. Potassium iodide may be given prior. Complications include laryngeal nerve damage, bleeding, and hypoparathyroidism.

e. Iodinated contrast agents provide temporary treatment and may be helpful in highly symptomatic patients. T_3 levels may drop by >50% in 24 hours.

f. Ophthalmopathy responds best to IV methylprednisolone but may respond to high-dose, tapered prednisone treatment, particularly in nonsmokers. Retrobulbar radiation treatment or optic nerve decompression surgery may be indicated.

g. Atrial fibrillation is not likely to convert electrically while the patient is hyperthyroid and should be promptly treated.

(1) Digoxin may be used, but may require larger doses, and β-blockers with caution (especially in the presence of cardiomyopathy or heart failure).

(2) Anticoagulation with warfarin is recommended to prevent thromboembolism.

(3) Congestive heart failure must be treated as usual, along with aggressive treatment for hyperthyroidism.

5. Thyroid storm

a. Thyroid storm (thyroid crisis) is a rare but life-threatening condition of extreme hyperthyroidism. Illness, sepsis, trauma, surgery, RAI administration, and pregnancy may precipitate this condition.

b. It may not be identified by lab testing but may reveal findings of elevated T_3 and free T_4 as well as decreased TSH.

c. Clinical presentation includes high fever, tachycardia, agitation, sweating, tremor, instability, delirium, vomiting, and diarrhea. Mortality is high, and these patients should be admitted to the intensive care unit (ICU).

d. PTU may be given orally, but the patient should be monitored for liver dysfunction. IV sodium iodide may be considered as well as IV hydrocortisone 50 to 100 mg every 6 hours. Iodide may be administered as Lugol solution.

e. Propranolol or similar medications may alleviate signs and symptoms of sympathetic discharge; use with caution in heart failure.

f. Hypokalemic periodic paralysis responds to propranolol, which normalizes the serum potassium and phosphate levels and reverses the paralysis within 3 hours. Avoid IV dextrose or oral carbohydrates. Therapy is continued with propranolol along with PTU or MM.

B. **Hypothyroidism**

1. General characteristics

a. Hypothyroidism is common; it affects >3% of the U.S. population and >5% of the U.S. elderly. Incidence is 5% to 15% in iodine-deficient countries. It is second only to diabetes as the most common endocrine disorder in the United States.

b. Pathology most commonly starts in adulthood. It is usually autoimmune in nature, which causes antibodies against TSH receptors, antiperoxidase, and thyroglobulin.

c. It is associated with other autoimmune disorders such as pernicious anemia, rheumatoid arthritis, systemic lupus erythematosus, Sjögren's syndrome, and myasthenia gravis. The antiperoxidase and antithyroglobulin antibodies serve as disease markers, but the anti-TSH antibodies actually cause disease.

d. Primary hypothyroidism accounts for 95% of cases of hypothyroidism. Causes include autoimmune thyroid destruction such as in Hashimoto thyroiditis and end-stage Graves' disease. Hashimoto thyroiditis is the most common cause.

e. Other primary causes include iodine therapy causing gland shrinkage, surgical thyroidectomy, iodine-deficient diet, amyloidosis, lymphoma, scleroderma, lithium, amiodarone, interferon, and birth enzyme/hormone defects (rare).

f. Secondary causes of hypothyroidism (causes not involving the gland itself) include pituitary or hypothalamic neoplasms, congenital hypopituitarism, pituitary necrosis such as Sheehan's syndrome, and TSH or thyrotropin-releasing hormone (TRH) deficiency (rare).

g. Up to 30% of Down's syndrome patients will have hypothyroidism.

High fever with acute severe symptoms of thyroid disease indicates a thyroid storm. Propranolol reduces symptoms and helps normalizer serum potassium.

Hypothyroidism is almost always autoimmune.

2. **Clinical features** (see Table 10-1)
   a. Mild hypothyroidism is often missed without TSH screening.
   b. Signs and symptoms may include weakness (99%), dry or coarse skin (97%), lethargy (91%), slow speech (91%), cold intolerance (89%), eyelid edema (90%), forgetfulness, facial edema, constipation, coarse hair, weight gain, facial dullness, depression, anemia, bradycardia, and hyporeflexia.
   c. A palpable, diffusely enlarged thyroid with fine nodules is often present.
   d. Myxedema is a nonpitting fluid retention state caused by mucopolysaccharide buildup. It most commonly occurs in the pretibial area.
   e. Hyponatremia may occur secondary to alteration in renal tubular sodium reabsorption.
   f. There is an increased risk of hypercholesterolemia and coronary artery disease (CAD).
   g. Anemia can result from iron deficiency or from chronic disease. There is decreased absorption of iron and folate as well as decreased GI motility.

   > Pretibial edema (myxedema) is characteristic of moderate hypothyroidism.

3. Diagnostic studies
   a. The single best screening test is the TSH.
   b. Normal or low-normal free T_4 and TSH indicate a euthyroid state.
   c. Low free T_4 and elevated TSH indicate a primary hypothyroid disorder.
   d. Low free T_4 and low or normal TSH indicate secondary hypothyroidism.
   e. Normal free T_4 and elevated TSH without symptoms indicate subclinical hypothyroidism; 18% will develop overt hypothyroidism.
   f. Presence of antithyroid peroxidase and antithyroglobulin antibodies in the serum confirms autoimmune disease.
   g. Imaging is not routinely required unless there is concern for malignancy (i.e., nodularity).

4. **Treatment**
   a. Levothyroxine is a replacement T_4 and doses range from 25 to 200 μg daily. The T_4 is converted into T_3. Adjust dose every 4 to 6 weeks based on TSH value.
   b. Assess patients for adrenal insufficiency and angina prior to initiating treatment. Start at a lower dose in the elderly or in those with coronary disease and titrate up as needed.
   c. T_4 needs increase in the third trimester of pregnancy and with some medications; lab monitoring should be interpreted with this in mind.
   d. In the newly diagnosed patient, levels of thyroid hormone should be checked frequently. Once stable, levels can be checked twice yearly.

   > Myxedema coma signifies profound hypothyroidism and must be treated with bolus doses of thyroxine.

5. Myxedema coma
   a. Myxedema coma is a life-threatening crisis of severe hypothyroidism characterized by obtundation, CO_2 retention, and coma; however, coma does not need to be present. Altered mental status is the hallmark. Even with optimal treatment, mortality is between 20% and 50%. The patient should be admitted to the ICU.
   b. Patients may exhibit severe hypothermia, hypoventilation, hyponatremia, hypoglycemia, hypotension, rhabdomyolysis, and acute kidney injury.
   c. Crisis can be precipitated by sepsis, cardiac disease, respiratory distress, central nervous system (CNS) disease, cold exposure, drug use, or noncompliance with treatment.
   d. Treatment may include thyroxine IV bolus 300 to 400 μg, then 50 to 100 μg daily. Also consider hydrocortisone if adrenal insufficiency is suspected.
   e. Patients are overly sensitive to morphine, which can lead to death.

C. Thyroiditis

1. Suppurative or infectious thyroiditis

    a. This is a rare, nonviral condition caused by Gram-positive bacteria (most commonly *Staphylococcus aureus*).

    b. Findings include pain and a tender thyroid gland, fever, pharyngitis, and overlying erythema along with leukocytosis and elevated erythrocyte sedimentation rate (ESR).

    c. Fine-needle aspiration (FNA) with Gram stain and culture is required.

    d. Treatment includes medications for the underlying cause and surgical drainage when fluctuation occurs.

2. Subacute painful (de Quervain's, granulomatous, or giant cell)

    a. First described in 1825, the disorder was pathologically identified in 1904 by de Quervain.

    b. It is the most common cause of a painful thyroid gland, peaks in the summer, and most commonly affects young and middle-aged women.

    c. It is believed to be the result of a preceding viral illness such as coxsackievirus infection, Epstein–Barr virus infection, mumps, measles, adenovirus infection, echovirus infection, or influenza.

    d. The thyroid gland is often tender. Fever, fatigue, dysphagia, and otalgia may be present and may persist for months.

    e. Thyrotoxicosis initially presents, followed by a period of hypothyroidism with resumption of euthyroid within 12 months.

    f. The ESR is markedly elevated and antithyroid antibody titers are low.

    g. Treatment of choice is aspirin; steroids provide no additional benefit. Symptoms may be lessened with β-blockers and iodinated contrast products. Antithyroid medication is usually of no benefit.

3. Drug induced (amiodarone)

    a. Amiodarone has a 100-day half-life, contains 37% iodine by weight, and each 200 mg tablet contains 75 mg of iodide. It causes thyroid dysregulation in up to 20% of patients.

    b. It may cause a serum increase of T_4 by 20% to 40% during the first month of therapy but causes cellular resistance to T_4. A resultant hypothyroid picture ensues with elevated TSH and symptoms typical of hypothyroidism.

4. Chronic lymphocytic (Hashimoto)

    a. Hashimoto thyroiditis (aka chronic lymphocytic thyroiditis) is the most common thyroid disease in the United States, with rising incidence. This is also the most common cause of sporadic goiter in children. It is six times more common in females and may be familial.

    b. The thyroid is diffusely enlarged with firm, small nodules. It is painless and often progresses to hypothyroidism with detectable thyrotropin receptor–blocking antibodies and antithyroid peroxidase.

5. Fibrous thyroiditis (Riedel)

    a. First described in 1898, this is the rarest form of thyroiditis. There is development of dense fibrous tissue in the thyroid gland.

    b. There may be extraglandular fibrous involvement such as sclerosing cholangitis, retroperitoneal fibrosis, and orbital pseudotumor.

    c. Over 80% of cases are in females.

    d. An asymmetric, hard, "woody" thyroid may be palpated.

    e. RAIU is decreased in the involved areas of the thyroid gland, and thyroid antibodies may be present in 45% of patients.

   f. Diagnosis is made by biopsy because the differentiation with carcinoma can be difficult.

   g. It may respond to long-term tamoxifen treatment.

D. Nontoxic goiter

   1. This is a slowly enlarging thyroid gland progressing over years.

   2. It affects about 5% of the U.S. population and women more often than men.

   3. It is usually asymptomatic unless impinging or causing an obstruction. Multiple painless nodules are palpable. Labs may show a euthyroid, hyperthyroid, or hypothyroid state.

   4. Endemic goiter is when 10% of the population has goiter, usually found in iodine-deficient areas.

   5. Certain foods (sorghum, millet, maize, and cassava) and mineral deficiencies (selenium and iron) may cause or enhance risk in iodine-deficient states.

E. Solitary thyroid nodule

   1. General characteristics

   a. A solitary thyroid nodule is common in the general population and affects women more often than men. One in 12 to 15 young women has a thyroid nodule.

   b. Nodules must generally be over 1 cm in diameter to be palpated. Most are asymptomatic and are discovered incidentally via physical examination or through imaging. The presence of one palpable nodule increases the risk of additional nodules.

   c. Thyroid adenoma is the most common benign nodule. Only 5% of palpable nodules are malignant.

   d. The nodule of adenoma is encapsulated, but the nodules of multinodular goiter are not encapsulated.

   e. Bleeding into the nodule may cause pain and enlargement.

   2. Types

   a. Follicular adenoma is the most common type.

   b. Papillary adenomas are very rare.

   c. Hurtle cell has eosinophilic staining and has a malignant potential.

   3. Workup (Fig. 10-1)

   a. Differentiation of a thyroid adenoma and thyroid cancer can be very difficult. True adenomas are not cancer precursors.

   b. If the TSH is low, the patient should be assessed for hyperthyroidism and undergo radionuclide thyroid scan. Cold nodules (no uptake) are hypofunctioning and require surgery. Hot nodules (increased uptake) are functional and, therefore, carry a lower risk of malignancy.

   c. High-resolution ultrasonography is the most sensitive test to detect thyroid lesions, determine size and structure, and assess diffuse changes in the gland. Ultrasonography is preferred over CT scan because of higher accuracy, lower cost, and lack of radiation.

   d. Malignancy is suspected in the presence of irregular or indistinct margins, heterogeneous echogenicity, intranodular vascular margins, microcalcifications, complex cyst patterns, or size >1 cm.

   e. Lesions suspicious for malignancy should undergo ultrasound-guided FNA. Approximately 75% of FNA of solitary nodules show benign lesions.

   f. All thyroid nodules need periodic monitoring. In benign lesions, T_4 replacement is shown to decrease nodule size by 20%. If no response to T_4 therapy and the patient is euthyroid, the T_4 therapy can be discontinued.

> Suspicious ultrasound findings include irregular, indistinct margins; heterogeneous echogeneity; intranodular vascular margins; microcalcifications; and complete cyst pattern.

> Cold nodules are hypofunctioning; they require surgery. Hot nodules are functional; they have a lower malignant risk.

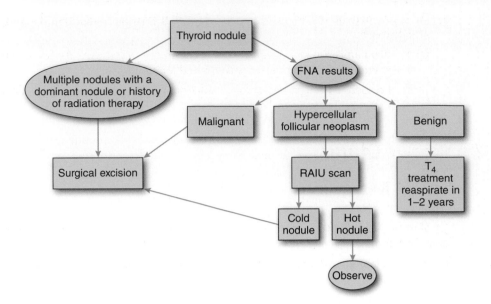

Figure 10-1 ▶ Approach to the patient with a thyroid nodule. FNA, fine-needle aspiration; RAIU, radioactive iodine uptake; T₄, thyroxine.

F.   Thyroid cancer

1. General characteristics

a. Thyroid cancer is more common in women (3:1), but the prognosis is worse in men. The incidence has increased threefold over the last 50 years.

b. About 9% of thyroid cancers are fatal. Most thyroid cancers remain microscopic and indolent.

c. Prognosis depends on staging, with a 99% 5-year survival with locally confined, <1.0 cm diameter papillary carcinoma.

2. Types

a. Papillary type is most common (76%) but least aggressive and spreads by local extension. They are caused by genetic mutation or translocation.

b. Follicular type (16%) often metastasizes to lung, bone, brain, and liver.

c. Anaplastic type (1%) is seen in the elderly and is the most aggressive, often causing dysphagia or vocal cord paralysis.

d. Medullary type (4%) is distributed as one-third sporadic, one-third familial, and one-third associated with multiple endocrine neoplasia (MEN) syndrome. These tumors may cause symptoms from their possible secretion of calcitonin, prostaglandins, serotonin, adrenocorticotropic hormone (ACTH), and other peptides.

e. Thyroid lymphoma and other malignancies represent 3%.

3. Risk factors

a. Childhood irradiation to head and neck confers a 25-fold increase in thyroid cancer and may emerge 10 to 40 years postexposure.

b. Other risks include family history, Gardner's syndrome, and MEN type II syndrome.

4. Presentation and treatment

a. Painless neck swelling and a palpable, single firm nodule is the most common presentation of thyroid cancer.

b. Imaging

(1) Ultrasonography is routinely performed. It is noninvasive and can differentiate cystic from solid and provide evidence of architectural distortion.

> **Thyroid cancer types:**
> - most common = papillary
> - most aggressive = anaplastic
> - associated with MEN = medullary
> - most likely to metastasize = follicular

(2) RAIU may be helpful to assess risk of malignancy and help plan the surgical approach.

(3) Positron emission tomography (PET) scanning is particularly useful in detecting thyroid cancer metastases with limited iodine uptake.

   c. Surgical resection is indicated and RAI ablation may be useful for residual disease. Patients require T_4 replacement for life.

Pituitary Gland

A. Anatomy and physiology

   1. Anatomy

     a. The pituitary gland lies below the hypothalamus attached by a stalk called the infundibulum.

     b. It lies in close proximity to the optic chiasm, which accounts for the frequent visual involvement.

   2. Physiology

     a. The anterior lobe (adenohypophysis) secretes hormones within negative feedback loops to adrenals, thyroid, and gonads. The anterior pituitary produces six major hormones (ACTH, TSH, luteinizing hormone [LH], growth hormone [GH], follicle-stimulating hormone [FSH], and prolactin [PRL]) (Fig. 10-2).

     b. The posterior pituitary (neurohypophysis) does not produce its own hormones but stores antidiuretic hormone (ADH or vasopressin) and oxytocin, which are made in the hypothalamus.

     c. There is also an intermediate lobe that secretes melanocyte-stimulating hormone to control skin pigmentation.

     d. The pituitary gland is called the master gland because it controls the functions of the other endocrine glands.

> Anterior pituitary: secretes six major hormones
> Posterior pituitary: stores ADH and oxytocin

B. **GH excess**

   1. Etiology

     a. Most often caused by a benign pituitary adenoma, often >1 cm in diameter, which stimulates GH release. The excess GH stimulates release of insulin-like growth factor 1 (IGF-1) from the liver. Somatotroph-producing tumors account for 10% to 15% of pituitary tumors.

     b. Usually mixed cell tumors, pituitary adenomas are often associated with PRL secretion (40%).

     c. Ectopic tumors (islet cell type) and MEN type I are uncommon causes of excess growth hormone–releasing hormone (GHRH). Other causes are neurofibromatosis, McCune–Albright syndrome (affects bones and skin pigmentation), and Carney complex (causes benign tumors of skin, heart, and endocrine system).

   2. Presentation

     a. GH excess causing excess IGF-1 in childhood prior to closure of the epiphyses leads to gigantism, which causes excess growth of long bones. It is extremely rare compared to acromegaly.

     b. GH excess causing excess IGF-1 in adulthood results in acromegaly, which causes enlargement and elongation of the hands, feet, and jaw as well as internal organ involvement. Onset is in the 30s so it does not affect long bones.

       (1) Affected individuals have an increased risk of diabetes mellitus (DM) (30%), HTN, and CAD.

       (2) Other features include doughy, moist handshake; macroglossia; carpal tunnel syndrome; deep, coarse voice; obstructive sleep apnea; goiter; HTN and

> Excessive GH in childhood = giantism; in adulthood = acromegaly

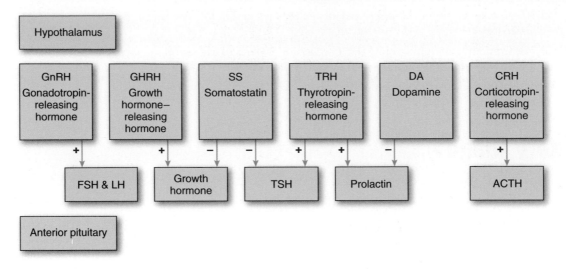

Figure 10-2 ▶ Hormonal effects of hypothalamus on the pituitary gland. ACTH, adrenocorticotropic hormone; FSH, follicle-stimulating hormone; LH, luteinizing hormone; TSH, thyroid-stimulating hormone.

cardiomegaly; weight gain and insulin resistance; arthralgias and arthritis; colon polyps; hyperhidrosis; cystic acne; acanthosis nigricans; headaches; spinal stenosis; bitemporal hemianopia; decreased libido; erectile dysfunction; and menstrual abnormalities.

> **(3)** At diagnosis, 10% have overt heart failure with dilated left ventricle and reduced ejection fraction.

3. Diagnostic studies

   a. Screening with random serum IGF-1 may be done and, if normal for age, rules out acromegaly. If elevated fivefold, it is highly suggestive of an adenoma. PRL levels should also be measured because GH-secreting tumors often cosecrete PRL.

   b. A 75-g loading dose 1-hour oral glucose tolerance test (OGTT) will show failure of GH to decrease to <2 µg per L.

   c. Random measurement of GH is not accurate as levels may fluctuate.

   d. MRI is the imaging modality of choice; a negative scan virtually rules out a GH pituitary adenoma. MRI will reveal a pituitary tumor in 90% of patients. Skull radiography often shows enlarged sella and thickened skull. Radiography of hands or feet may reveal tufting of the terminal phalanges.

4. **Treatment**

   a. Somatostatin analogs (octreotide/lanreotide) are inhibitory and may decrease tumor size.

   b. Dopamine agonists like cabergoline or bromocriptine suppress GH levels in some patients with acromegaly who fail surgery but are not considered first-line therapy.

   c. Transsphenoidal microsurgery is most successful in patients with preoperative blood GH levels below 50 ng per mL (normal is 0.4 to 10 ng/mL) and with pituitary tumors no larger than 2 cm in diameter. The best measure of surgical success is normalization of GH and IGF-1 levels.

   d. Pegvisomant, a GH receptor antagonist, blocks hepatic IGF-1 production, thereby providing symptomatic relief and normalization of IGF-I in about 90% of patients. It may be added when somatostatin therapy has not been successful.

   e. Acromegalic patients have increased morbidity and mortality from cardiovascular disorders and progression of acromegalic symptoms.

   f. Regardless of treatment modality, IGF-1 should be measured every 3 to 4 months, then every 6 months once well controlled.

C. Dwarfism

1. There are over 400 types of dwarfism, which is divided into disproportionate types (average size torso with shorter arms and legs or shorter trunk with longer limbs) or proportionate.

2. Achondroplasia accounts for 70% of dwarfism; this is a genetic mutation of cartilage and bone growth. Other forms are less common; many times a cause cannot be identified.

3. **Clinical features**

   a. Achondroplastic dwarfs are the most common type of short-limbed dwarfism. This syndrome affects 1 in 15,000 to 40,000 newborns and results from a failure to ossify cartilage.

   b. The average height of an adult male with achondroplasia is 4 feet 4 inches; the average height for an adult female is 4 feet 1 inch.

   c. Dwarfs have short limbs, long and narrow trunks, large heads with midface hypoplasia, and prominent brows. They have delayed motor milestones and fall below normal height standards. Intelligence is normal. Neurologic complications, bowing of the legs, obesity, dental problems, and frequent otitis media are common.

   d. Although not usually apparent at birth, pituitary dwarfism may present in male infants with hypoglycemia and micropenis.

4. Laboratory studies: The achondroplasia group of disorders are all caused by mutations in the *FGFR3* gene.

5. **Treatment**

   a. The cornerstone of management is maximizing function, monitoring growth, and preventing complications.

   b. Limb-lengthening procedures and surgical correction of orthopedic problems may be indicated in achondroplasia.

   c. Use of human GH is controversial. Investigational drugs using recombinant peptides is underway.

> Achondroplasias (mutations in *FGFR3* genes) account for 70% of dwarfism.

D. Diabetes insipidus

1. General characteristics

   a. Insipid means tasteless, as opposed to sweet (mellitus).

   b. DI is caused by a deficiency of, or resistance to, vasopressin (ADH).

   c. Serum osmolality is 285 to 295 mOsm per kg. At 295 mOsm per kg, maximum antidiuresis occurs; at 290 mOsm per kg, thirst kicks in. Normal urine specific gravity is between 1.010 and 1.030. In DI, urine specific gravity may be closer to 1.00.

   d. Primary DI may be familial (genetic) or sporadic.

   e. Secondary DI is a result of hypothalamic or pituitary pathology; it may be caused by tumor, anoxic encephalopathy, surgery, accidental head trauma, infection, sarcoidosis, multifocal Langerhans cell granulomatosis, or metastatic disease.

2. Types

   a. There are four types of DI: central, nephrogenic, gestational, and primary polydipsia. All manifest with polydipsia, polyuria, and a dilute urine. Hypothalamic (central) and nephrogenic are more common; see Table 10-2 for comparison.

   b. Hypothalamic DI: inability to produce and secrete vasopressin (levels will be low)

   c. Nephrogenic DI: kidney unable to respond to vasopressin (levels are high)

   d. Transient DI of pregnancy and the puerperium: rapid destruction/breakdown of vasopressin

   e. Primary polydipsia: disorder of thirst mechanism (ADH levels low)

> Deficiency or lack of ADH leads to diabetes insipidus.

Table 10-2 | Comparison of Central and Nephrogenic Diabetes Insipidus

Central	Nephrogenic
Commonly occurs after head trauma or brain surgery	Associated with chronic renal failure, lithium toxicity, hypercalcemia, and hypokalemia
May be inherited	May be inherited
May lack "osmostat"	Abnormal receptors in the kidneys
Responds to desmopressin	No response to desmopressin

> Diabetes insipidus manifests with polydipsia with polyuria and excessively dilute urine.

3. **Clinical features**
   a. Intense thirst with fluid intake of 2 to 20 L per day, craving for ice water, and large-volume polyuria are most common; other possible presentations are hypernatremia and dehydration.
   b. Unremitting enuresis may be present in partial disease.
4. **Diagnostic studies**
   a. There is no single diagnostic test, and clinical judgment is needed.
   b. Serum osmolality is high; urine osmolality is low.
   c. Serum sodium can be normal or high depending on compensatory fluid intake. Blood urea nitrogen (BUN) may be elevated. Uric acid may be elevated.
   d. A supervised vasopressin challenge test may distinguish central from nephrogenic DI.
   e. MRI of the pituitary, hypothalamus, and the skull may reveal mass lesions.
5. **Treatment**
   a. Desmopressin acetate is the treatment of choice for central DI and DI associated with pregnancy and the puerperium.
   b. Mild cases may require no treatment except adequate hydration.
   c. Central and nephrogenic DI respond partially to hydrochlorothiazide with potassium or amiloride supplementation.
   d. Nephrogenic DI may respond to indomethacin, either alone or in combination with hydrochlorothiazide, desmopressin, or amiloride.
   e. With treatment, prognosis is good with no reduction in life expectancy.

Diabetes Mellitus

A. General characteristics
   1. DM describes a group of disorders characterized by disordered metabolism and inappropriate hyperglycemia. This may be because of deficiencies in insulin secretion, inadequate response to insulin, or both. It affects 30.3 million (9.4%) of the U.S. population and is the seventh leading cause of death in the United States. Many individuals remain undiagnosed.
   2. Most patients with diabetes have type 1 (<10%) or type 2 (>90%).
   3. Rare types of diabetes include maturity-onset diabetes of the young (MODY), diabetes caused by mutant insulins or insulin receptors, diseases affecting the exocrine pancreas (e.g., cystic fibrosis), endocrinopathies, drug- and chemical-induced diabetes, and other genetic syndromes.
   4. Type 1 DM is characterized by early-onset, autoimmune phenomena, insulinopenia or absence of insulin, and a risk of diabetic ketoacidosis (DKA). It has an association with HLA *DR3-DQ2* and *DR4* genes.

5. Type 2 DM typically has a later onset and is associated with excess weight or obesity, positive family history, and associated hyperinsulinemia. However, it is presenting in youth with increasing incidence because of the obesity epidemic.

6. Prediabetes is defined as blood glucose levels above normal but without meeting the criteria for a diagnosis. Based on fasting glucose or hemoglobin A_{1c} (HbA_{1c}) levels, 35% of the U.S. population older than age 20 years and 50% of those older than age 65 years have prediabetes. Most individuals eventually diagnosed with DM type 2 had signs of prediabetes prior to diagnosis. Screening and identification at this stage should prompt aggressive lifestyle changes to delay or prevent the onset of diabetes.

7. Criteria for a diagnosis of DM and prediabetes are listed in Table 10-3.

8. Gestational diabetes mellitus (GDM) is defined as glucose intolerance hyperglycemia with onset or first diagnosis during pregnancy and is discussed in Chapter 8.

B. Metabolic syndrome

1. Metabolic syndrome is also known as "syndrome X" and "insulin resistance syndrome." It is a constellation of findings that predisposes to DM, CAD, and cerebrovascular accidents (CVAs, strokes).

2. Criteria include the following:

   a. High-density lipoprotein (HDL) <40 mg per dL in males or <50 mg per dL in females

   b. Elevated blood pressure (BP) (>130/85 mm Hg)

   c. Elevated triglycerides (>150 mg/dL)

   d. Fasting blood sugar 100 to 125 mg per dL (impaired fasting glucose)

   e. Two-hour OGTT of 140 to 199 mg per dL (impaired glucose tolerance)

   f. Waist circumference above 35 inches for females or 40 inches for males

3. Individuals should be counseled regarding diet and exercise to reduce their risk of disease progression. Metformin may be recommended for many.

C. Acute complications of diabetes

1. Diabetic ketoacidosis

   a. DKA is complex metabolic dysfunction because of insulin deficiency and occurs predominantly in type 1 DM, but may also occur in type 2 DM.

   b. Patients often present in times of physiologic stress: infection, trauma, sepsis, or other acute pathologic process. Patients may present with symptoms of polyuria, nocturia, polydipsia (before presenting); nausea/vomiting; and fatigue. Physical findings may include hypotension, tachycardia, tachypnea (Kussmaul breathing), abdominal pain, and fruity acetone breath.

   c. Key typical lab findings include elevated plasma glucose (typically >250 mg/dL); low serum bicarbonate (<15 mEq/L); low (acidotic) serum pH (<7.3), with ketonemia and ketonuria. The anion gap is elevated. Other abnormal labs may include hyperkalemia, hyponatremia, elevated BUN and creatinine, abnormal phosphorus, elevated urine and plasma acetone.

> Prediabetes is often a precursor to diabetes. Strict adherence to diet and exercise recommendations can prevent progression of the disease.

> DKA: the presence of ketonemia and ketonuria signifies the body's inability to utilize the excessive glucose. Management: fluids, insulin, potassium as needed.

Table 10-3 | Diagnosis of Diabetes and Prediabetes

	HbA$_{1c}$ (%)	Fasting Glucose (mg/dL)	Oral Glucose Tolerance Test (mg/dL)
Diabetes	6.5 or higher	126 or higher	200 or higher
Prediabetes	5.7–6.4	100–125	140–199
Normal	5.0 or lower	≤99	≤139

HbA$_{1c}$, hemoglobin A$_{1c}$.

    d. DKA patients are managed in the inpatient setting, often in the ICU initially. Management is focused on correcting the metabolic abnormalities, restoring the acid–base imbalance, aggressive IV hydration, and treatment of related conditions or causative factors.

    e. Normal saline is the preferred initial IV fluid; change to D5NS when the glucose approaches <250 mg per dL.

    f. Potassium must be closely monitored. If <3.3 mEq per L, replace potassium and hold insulin. If >5.5 mEq per dL, hold the potassium, give insulin. If potassium is between 3.3 and 5.5 mEq per dL, start both and adjust according to lab returns.

    g. Insulin is given as 0.1 units per kg per hr; begin with IV administration and switch to subcutaneous as the patient stabilizes.

2. Hyperosmolar hyperglycemic state (HHS; formerly hyperosmolar hyperglycemic nonketotic coma [HHNC])

> *Ketonemia and ketonuria are* **absent** *in HHS.*

    a. HHS most commonly occurs in type 2 DM patients, often with a comorbid condition, usually during an infection, myocardial infarction, or surgery; it is also because of (relative or partial) insulin deficiency often in the setting of dehydration. HHS typically has a slower onset compared with DKA.

    b. Patients commonly present in a time of acute illness with symptoms of polyuria, polydipsia, fatigue. Change in mental status or lethargy can occur. Physical findings may include tachycardia, hypotension, and possible neurologic findings of aphasia, muscle tone abnormalities, and nystagmus.

    c. Key lab findings include elevated serum glucose (>600 mg/dL); elevated serum osmolality (>310 mOsm/kg); high bicarbonate (>15 mEq/L), with a normal blood pH (>7.3) and normal anion gap.

    d. Management is focused on careful yet assertive intervention: rehydration with IV fluids is paramount; begin with NS. Monitor electrolyte balance; correct hyperglycemia and other electrolyte disturbances; and treat the related conditions or causative factors.

D. Long-term complications of diabetes

1. Diabetic retinopathy leads to blindness, premature cataracts, and glaucoma. It is the leading cause of blindness in people older than age 60 years in the United States. About 28% of diabetic individuals have retinopathy.

2. Diabetic nephropathy accounts for almost half of the cases of end-stage renal disease (ESRD) in the United States.

3. Diabetes is associated with accelerated large vessel atherosclerosis, which increases CAD and CVA risk. Two-thirds of diabetes-related death certificates note cardiovascular disease (CVD). Risk of stroke is two to four times greater in diabetics. Diabetes is also associated with cardiomyopathy.

4. Diabetic peripheral vascular disease is caused by poor perfusion and inadequate delivery of nutrients. It accounts for half of all lower leg amputations in the United States.

5. Neuropathy is the most common complication of DM; it may be peripheral or autonomic.

    a. It commonly causes a characteristic peripheral symmetric polyneuropathy (stocking and glove) but may cause a peripheral mononeuropathy or mononeuropathy multiplex.

    b. Painful foot neuropathy may be physically and emotionally disabling.

    c. Nerve damage also causes autonomic dysfunction, leading to exercise intolerance, erectile dysfunction, atonic bladder, delayed gastric emptying, and urinary or fecal incontinence.

> *Prevent diabetic complications through tight glycemic control and monitoring for eye disease, kidney disease, vascular disease, heart disease, and neuropathy.*

6. Skin changes associated with DM include candidal infections, slow wound healing, necrobiosis lipoidica diabeticorum, and acanthosis nigricans.

7. Periodontal disease is more common in diabetic patients and is more severe with poor glucose control and tobacco use.

E. **Type 1 diabetes mellitus**

1. General characteristics

   a. Type 1 occurs most often in young people (before school age or near puberty) but rarely presents in adults in their 30s or 40s. Nonautoimmune type 1 disease occurs primarily in those of Asian or African origin.

   b. There is little or no endogenous insulin secretion.

      (1) Plasma glucagon is elevated.

      (2) Pancreatic β-cells fail to respond to stimuli and undergo autoimmune destruction. If untreated, this is a catabolic state with ketosis.

   c. Most type 1 DM is an autoimmune disease (90%), with antibodies to insulin, islet cells, and glutamic acid decarboxylase (GAD). Most Caucasians with type 1 diabetes carry alleles 3 and/or 4 of the *HLA-DR* gene. The *HLA-DR7* allele plays a role in diabetes in blacks, whereas *HLA-DR9* allele is important in diabetes among Japanese. About 85% of individuals with *HLA-DQ* genes have islet cell antibodies.

   d. It is estimated that genetic factors account for one-third of the susceptibility and environmental factors one-third. Theories related to viruses, toxic chemicals, cow milk exposure, and other environmental factors are under investigation.

2. **Clinical features**

   a. The most common presentation includes polydipsia, polyuria, nocturia, and rapid weight loss despite normal or increased appetite associated with a random plasma glucose of 200 mg per dL or greater.

   b. Blurred vision is common; pruritus, weakness, postural hypotension, paresthesias, and balanitis or vulvovaginitis may occur.

   c. Untreated type 1 DM results in DKA, leading to anorexia, nausea, vomiting, dehydration, stupor, and, ultimately, coma. Fruity breath suggests ketoacidosis.

3. Diagnostic studies

   a. A random plasma glucose of >200 mg per dL with classic symptoms or fasting levels of 126 mg per dL or greater on more than one occasion is diagnostic.

   b. Most patients with new-onset type 1 DM will have a severely elevated glucose, warranting no further diagnostic study; suspected cases may be confirmed by glucose tolerance testing.

   c. Patients are likely to have glucosuria; they may also have ketonemia and/or ketonuria.

   d. HbA_{1c} reflects glycemic control over the preceding 8 to 12 weeks; 6.5% or higher is diagnostic of DM.

   e. Serum fructosamine reflects control over the preceding 1 to 2 weeks, resulting in more rapid change than HbA_{1c}. This test should be complementary to HbA_{1c} and not substitutive.

   f. Self-monitoring of blood glucose is encouraged to assess glucose control, guide insulin administration, and teach patients the relationship between dietary intake and blood glucose excursions.

   g. Well-controlled type 1 DM results in normal lipid values.

   h. Patients with DM should also be closely monitored for risk of CVD, nephropathy, neuropathy, and retinopathy.

4. **Treatment**

   a. Diet is central to management.

      (1) Diet must be individualized according to the patient's activity level, food preferences, and need to attain and maintain ideal weight.

      (2) Patients with type 1 DM should follow a well-balanced diet and may apply the principles of carbohydrate counting, often administering 1 unit of short- or

90% of type 1 diabetes mellitus is autoimmune.

Diagnostic criteria for diabetes mellitus include random glucose >220 with symptoms; fasting glucose >126 on two or more occasions; HbA1c >6.5%.

rapidly acting insulin for each 10 to 15 g of ingested carbohydrate in addition to basal insulin needs.

(3) There is no longer a specific American Diabetes Association (ADA) diet. Patients may choose among the Mediterranean diet and other complex carbohydrate distribution schemes, emphasizing low-fat, high-fiber intake.

(4) A diet high in soluble fiber improves glucose through slowed absorption and improves cholesterol levels; insoluble fiber improves colonic transit.

(5) Patients should coordinate meals and snacks with exercise and insulin administration.

(6) Artificial sweeteners appropriate for patients with diabetes include aspartame, neotame, saccharin, sucralose, plant-derived stevia, and acesulfame potassium.

b. Insulin may be delivered by subcutaneous injection, injector pens, or insulin pump. See Table 10-4 for comparison of insulins.

(1) Glycemic response depends on amount and type of insulin, depth of injection, injection site, proximity of site to muscles being exercised, and ambient temperature.

(2) Regular insulin is absorbed most rapidly from the abdomen, but any site with ample subcutaneous tissue may be used. Analog insulins are less affected by site of injection.

(3) Human insulin causes markedly less antibody response than animal insulin and is available in regular or neutral protamine Hagedorn (NPH) formulations.

(4) Analog insulins include rapid-acting (lispro, aspart, glulisine) and long-acting (glargine, detemir) forms. The rapid-acting insulins have a more rapid onset and a shorter duration of action than regular insulin.

(5) Rapid-acting insulins (lispro, aspart, glulisine) reach peak serum values in 60 to 90 minutes and have a 4- to 5-hour duration of action; they may be taken 20 minutes before a meal.

(6) Regular insulin is short acting and is used 30 to 60 minutes before meals; the effect appears in 30 minutes, peaks in 2 to 4 hours, and lasts for 5 to 8 hours. IV administration is useful in DKA and in perioperative management of patients with diabetes.

(7) NPH insulin is an intermediate-acting form with onset of action in 1 to 3 hours, peak effect in 5 to 8 hours, and duration of action of <24 hours (range 12 to 24 hours), often requiring two injections per day. NPH is often used in combination with regular or analog insulin for improved control.

(8) Basal insulins include glargine and detemir. Basal coverage is the "background" insulin required for "housekeeping" functions and suppression of glucagon.

(a) Glargine is generally given once a day and cannot be mixed with other insulins because of its acidity. It lasts for about 24 hours without peaks.

> 💡 Regular insulin is most rapidly absorbed through abdominal subcutaneous tissue.

Table 10-4 | Insulins

		Onset	Peak	Duration	Notes
Rapid-acting analog insulin	Lispro (Humalog) Aspart (NovoRapid) Glulisine (Apidra)	10–30 minutes	60–90 minutes	4–5 hours	Take 15–20 minutes before a meal
Long-acting analog insulin	Glargine (Lantus) Detemir (Levemir)	1–2 hours	No peak	Glargine: 24 hours Detemir: 12–24 hours	"Basal insulins"
Regular insulin (short acting)	Regular	10–30 minutes	2–4 hours	5–8, up to 12 hours	Take 15–20 minutes before meals
NPH (neutral protamine Hagedorn)	NPH (Humulin-N, Novolin)	1–3 hours	5–8 hours	12–24 hours	

(b) Detemir lasts from 12 to 24 hours and is relatively peakless, often given daily or twice daily for basal coverage.

c. Daily aspirin (75 to 325 mg/day) is used in primary prevention in those with an increased 10-year cardiovascular risk (>10%). This includes men older than 50 years and women older than 60 years, with at least one additional CVD risk factor such as HTN, dyslipidemia, smoking, or albuminuria.

d. Careful foot care, regular ophthalmology examinations, moderate exercise, meticulous personal hygiene, and prompt treatment of infection are imperative.

e. Annual ophthalmologic examination and kidney function evaluation is recommended.

f. Research is ongoing in the areas of consistently successful pancreas transplantation and closed-loop insulin pump.

F. **Type 2 diabetes mellitus**

1. General characteristics

a. Type 2 DM, a heterogeneous group of diseases, occurs most often in middle-aged or older people; however, it is increasingly found in younger persons who are overweight or obese.

b. Distribution of fat to the upper body (central obesity) is associated with the highest risk; exercise and weight loss decrease the risk.

c. Type 2 DM has a strong multifactorial genetic component.

> The number one risk factor for type 2 diabetes is obesity.

d. In the United States, type 2 DM accounts for >90% of diabetes cases. Increased prevalence is found in African Americans, Hispanics, Pima Indians, and Pacific Islanders.

e. In type 2 DM, insulin levels are generally high enough to suppress ketoacidosis. The basic physiology is twofold: insulin resistance to β-cell–produced insulin and relative insulin deficiency, especially with disease progression. Resistance is increased with aging, sedentary lifestyle, and abdominovisceral obesity.

f. Untreated type 2 DM can lead to hyperosmolar nonketotic states.

2. Clinical features

a. Many patients have polyuria and polydipsia; ketonuria and weight loss are rare.

b. Patients may also present with fatigue, pruritus, recurrent balanitis or candida vaginitis, chronic skin infections, blurred vision, or poor wound healing.

c. Many patients have few symptoms; DM may be discovered during routine laboratory testing. Distribution of fat to the upper body is associated with increased risk; measuring waist-to-hip ratio is useful in monitoring treatment.

d. Women who have delivered large-for-gestational age babies or were diagnosed with gestational diabetes, polyhydramnios, preeclampsia, or unexplained fetal loss are at increased risk for type 2 DM.

3. Diagnostic studies

a. The diagnostic criteria for type 2 DM are the same as those for type 1 DM: random glucose >200 mg per dL (with symptoms), fasting glucose ≥126 mg per dL on more than one occasion, or HbA_{1c} ≥ 6.5%. The diagnostic use of HbA_{1c} is limited in the presence of severe anemia, hemoglobinopathies, and other conditions with higher than normal red blood cell (RBC) turnover.

b. An OGTT may be used with patients who have fasting glucose levels between 100 and 125 mg per dL (impaired fasting glucose) and are suspected of having overt diabetes.

> HbA_{1c} is used to diagnose and monitor chronic control.

c. Diabetic dyslipidemia includes high triglycerides, low HDL, and alteration of low-density lipoprotein (LDL) to smaller, denser particles. It is very common in type 2 DM.

d. Impaired fasting glucose (prediabetes; glucose of 100 to 125 mg/dL in fasting state) and impaired glucose tolerance (glucose of 140 to 199 mg/dL 2 hours after 75 g oral glucose) are considered strong risk factors for the development of type 2 DM. These individuals benefit most from primary prevention efforts (diet, weight loss, and exercise).

4. **Treatment**

> The initial approach to type 2 diabetes is diet, exercise, and weight loss.

a. In obese patients, weight loss should be initiated, which may improve insulin responsiveness. An initial goal of 5% to 7% weight loss is desirable. This should not delay pharmacotherapy and can be started simultaneously.

b. Cholesterol, protein, fat, fiber, and artificial sweetener recommendations are the same as in type 1 DM.

c. Regular exercise (150 min/week) is correlated with better glucose control.

d. Oral hypoglycemic agents potentiate insulin secretion (Table 10-5).

(1) The oldest oral hypoglycemic agents are the sulfonylureas; of these, glyburide, glipizide, and glimepiride are second-generation agents with few drug interactions. They are associated with weight gain and increased risk of hypoglycemia.

(2) Other newer insulin secretagogues are repaglinide and nateglinide, which are associated with lower rates of hypoglycemia.

(3) Metformin (Glucophage), which reduces hepatic glucose production, is the most common first-line agent, unless contraindicated. It decreases glucose

Table 10-5 | Selected Pharmacotherapy for Type 2 Diabetes

Drug Class	Drug Names	Mechanism	Drug Notes
Thiazolidinediones	Pioglitazone (Actos), rosiglitazone (Avandia)	Sensitize peripheral tissues to insulin. Reduce glucose without increasing risk for hypoglycemia	Not for patients with congestive heart failure (New York Heart Association class III or IV in particular) or liver disease. Rosiglitazone may cause heart failure or infarction. Use with great caution. Pioglitazone is associated with bladder cancer. Both increase fracture risk.
α-Glucosidase inhibitors	Acarbose (Precose), miglitol (Glyset)	Delays absorption of dietary carbohydrates by blocking the intestinal α-glucosidase enzyme, thereby decreasing postprandial glucose levels	The major side effects are gastrointestinal (GI) symptoms. Duration of action is short, 4 hours.
Glucagon-like peptide-1 (GLP-1) receptor agonists	Exenatide (Byetta), liraglutide (Victoza, Saxenda)	Lower blood glucose via slowing of gastric emptying, stimulating the pancreatic insulin response to glucose, and reducing glucagon release after meals	Must be injected. Adverse effects include nausea and acute pancreatitis; contraindicated in patients with gastroparesis. This class of agents is associated with weight loss. Liraglutide is associated with C-cell tumors in animals and may not be used in patients with a history of thyroid cancer.
Dipeptidyl peptidase 4 (DPP-4) inhibitors	Saxagliptin (Onglyza), sitagliptin (Januvia), linagliptin (Tradjenta)	Inhibit DPP-4 activity, prolonging the endogenous action of GLP-1, stimulating insulin secretion, and suppressing glucagon release	Dosed once daily, orally. They are weight neutral and have no associated hypoglycemia. There have been limited cases of pancreatitis and reports of urticaria/angioedema.
Selective sodium-glucose transporter–2 (SGLT-2) inhibitors	Canagliflozin (Invokana), dapagliflozin (Farxiga), empagliflozin (Jardiance)	Lower renal glucose threshold by selectively inhibiting SGLT-2, which results in increased urinary glucose excretion	Daily oral medication taken in combination with metformin or sulfonylureas. This class is contraindicated in patients with severely impaired kidney function; monitoring is critical.

levels by suppressing hepatic glucose production without the risk of hypoglycemia. It may promote weight loss and decrease triglycerides. It is contraindicated in patients at risk for lactic acidosis, those with serum creatinine >1.5 mg per dL (males) or >1.4 mg per dL (females), or abnormal creatinine clearance. It is associated with GI side effects which abate with time and are limited with medication titration. A vitamin B_{12} deficiency may occur with longer term use; this may be confused with diabetic peripheral neuropathy.

(4) Table 10-5 lists other agents that are commonly added to metformin in patients unable to meet glycemic control.

e. Approximately one-third of patients with type 2 DM require insulin, either alone or in combination with other agents. Basal insulin is recommended in patients who cannot be adequately controlled on other medications or if the HbA_{1c} is higher than desirable despite maximum treatment.

f. Acceptable glucose levels are 70 to 130 mg per dL before meals and after an overnight fast and 180 mg per dL or less at 1 hour and <150 mg per dL at 2 hours postprandially. Patients should monitor glucose levels as often as necessary to achieve desired control.

g. Careful foot care, moderate exercise, meticulous personal hygiene, and prompt treatment of infection are imperative.

h. Careful monitoring and treatment of BP to a goal of <130 mm Hg systolic and <80 mm Hg diastolic is essential to reduce the risk of CVD, retinopathy, and nephropathy. Hyperlipidemia should be treated with a goal of <100 mg per dL LDL (or <70 with cardiovascular risk factors) and >50 mg per dL HDL.

i. A joint statement between the ADA, the American Heart Association, and the American College of Cardiology Foundation suggests that low-dose aspirin is reasonable for diabetic adults who are at increased risk of CVD (with no previous history of vascular disease) and not at an increased risk for bleeding. This includes men over age 50 years and most women over the age of 60. Aspirin is not recommended for those diabetic patients with a low risk of CVD, such as men under the age of 50 and women over 60 years with no major risk factors. The suggested aspirin dose range is 75 to 162 mg daily.

j. Annual ophthalmologic examinations are recommended to monitor for diabetic retinopathy. Diabetics also have increased incidence of macular degeneration, glaucoma, and cataracts. A complete dilated retinal examination is required. Screening is recommended at the time of diagnosis of type 2 and annually or more frequently as needed.

k. Annual urine albumin and serum creatinine are also recommended; early identification and treatment will reduce risk or slow progression of diabetic nephropathy. Screening is recommended at the time of diagnosis and annually or more frequently as needed. Care must be taken as many behaviors increase renal protein excretion (fever, exercise); testing guidelines to avoid false positives should be followed.

l. Table 10-6 provides a suggested type 2 DM management algorithm, presented in 2015 by the American Association of Clinical Endocrinologists.

> Diabetic foot care:
> • manage blood sugar levels
> • inspect feet daily
> • keep feet dry
> • never go barefoot
> • wear good socks

Table 10-6 | Approach to Management of Type 2 Diabetes Mellitus

Start with education about lifestyle modifications and weight loss	Metformin (Glucophage) should almost always be your first-line choice. Then follow below guidelines:
A_{1c} < 7.5% initially start with glucophage	Add second agent if goal not achieved in 3 months
A_{1c} 7.5%–9% initially add second agent at onset	Add third agent if goal not met in 3 months
A_{1c} > 9% with symptoms initially	Add long-acting basal insulin
A_{1c} > 9% with no symptoms initially	May try triple oral therapy to start

G. **Hypoglycemia**

   1. General characteristics

      a. Fasting hypoglycemia occurs secondary to some endocrine disorders (Addison's disease, myxedema), liver malfunction, acute alcoholism, and ESRD; primary hypoglycemia is caused by either hyperinsulinism (e.g., exogenous administration), extrapancreatic tumors (insulinoma), or β-cell tumors.

      b. Postprandial or reactive hypoglycemia is classified as early (2 to 3 hours after eating) or late (3 to 5 hours after eating). It occurs after GI surgery, especially postgastrectomy with dumping syndrome, and Roux-en-Y gastric bypass surgery. It may also be alcohol-related, factitious, immunopathologic, or drug induced.

   2. **Clinical features**

      a. Symptoms begin at plasma glucose levels of 60 mg per dL; cognitive impairment begins at 50 mg per dL.

      b. Fasting hypoglycemia is often subacute or chronic and presents with neuroglycopenia.

      c. Postprandial hypoglycemia is usually acute and presents with diaphoresis, palpitations, anxiety, and tremulousness.

      d. The Whipple triad consists of a history of hypoglycemic symptoms, a fasting blood glucose of 45 mg per dL or less, and immediate recovery on administration of glucose.

   3. Diagnostic studies depend on the suspected cause.

   4. **Treatment** is directed at the underlying cause.

> 💡 Small, frequent meals help reduce the frequency of hypoglycemia.

Hyperlipidemia

A. General characteristics

   1. Elevated LDL levels increase the risk of CAD; higher HDL levels are thought to be protective. Elevated triglycerides are also a risk factor for atherosclerosis; severe elevations can cause pancreatitis.

   2. Causes of hyperlipidemia may be genetic (primary hyperlipidemia, familial hypercholesterolemia) or, more commonly, secondary to DM, alcohol use, hypothyroidism, obesity, sedentary lifestyle, renal or liver disease, or drugs (estrogen, thiazides, β-blockers).

B. **Clinical features**

   1. Most patients have no symptoms or signs.

   2. Eruptive and tendinous xanthomas are common with hyperlipidemia and usually indicate a genetic cause.

   3. Nearly two-thirds of all people with xanthelasmas (the most common form of xanthomas, affecting the eyelids) have normal lipid profiles.

   4. Patients with severe hypercholesterolemia may develop premature arcus senilis; lipemia retinalis (cream-colored retinal vessels) is seen with triglyceride levels of >2,000 mg per dL.

C. Diagnostic studies (Table 10-7)

   1. Patients with any evidence of CVD or who have a coronary heart disease (CHD) risk equivalent should be screened with a fasting complete lipid profile; those without cardiac risk factors should be screened with at least a measurement of total cholesterol.

   2. The U.S. Preventive Services Task Force (USPSTF) recommends screening for patients with no evidence of CVD and no other risk factors should begin at 35 years of age. The National Cholesterol Education Program (NCEP) recommends screening all adults at age 20 years regardless of risk factors.

> 💡 CAD is associated with elevated LDL cholesterol and triglycerides.

Table 10-7 | Lipid Levels

LDL (mg/dL)		Total Cholesterol (mg/dL)		HDL (mg/dL)	
Optimal	<100	Desirable	<200	Protective	>60
Near optimal	100–129	Borderline high	200–239	Borderline	41–59
Borderline high	130–159	High	>239	At risk	<40
High	160–189				
Very high	>189				

HDL, high-density lipoprotein; LDL, low-density lipoprotein.

3. Screening may include total cholesterol alone, total and HDL cholesterol, or LDL and HDL cholesterol levels.

D. Treatment

1. Lifestyle changes are first line and should be stressed for life regardless of pharmacologic treatment.

   a. Reduce total fat intake to 25% to 30% of diet, saturated fat to 7% or less, and dietary cholesterol to <200 mg per day. The Mediterranean diet reduces LDL cholesterol without reducing HDLs.

   b. Encourage 30 minutes of aerobic exercise daily.

   c. Increase antioxidants from fruits and vegetables. Soluble fiber may reduce LDL levels.

   d. CAD prophylaxis with aspirin 81 mg daily is recommended unless otherwise contraindicated.

   e. Smoking cessation should be encouraged at every visit.

2. Pharmacologic treatment

   a. Statins (3-hydroxy-3-methylglutaryl-coenzyme A [HMG-CoA] inhibitors)

      (1) They reduce cholesterol production in the liver and increase the ability of the liver to remove LDL cholesterol from the blood.

      (2) Statins can lower LDL by 20% to 60% and triglycerides by 15% to 30%.

      (3) Side effects include myalgias and mild GI complaints. More severe cases of myositis, liver toxicity, and rhabdomyolysis have been reported. Monitor liver enzymes; measure creatine phosphokinase if myalgias develop.

      (4) Monitor lipid levels every 6 weeks until goals are met.

   b. Niacin reduces long-term risk of CAD by reducing production of very-low-density lipoprotein, lowering LDL, and increasing HDL levels. It may also reduce triglycerides. Prostaglandin-induced niacin flushing can be reduced by taking aspirin 30 minutes prior or a daily nonsteroidal anti-inflammatory drug. Extended-release niacin is often better tolerated.

   c. Bile acid sequestrants (cholestyramine, colesevelam, and colestipol) bind bile acids in the intestine. These resins reduce the incidence of coronary events in middle-aged men, but they have no effect on total mortality. They are associated with constipation and gas and may interfere with absorption of fat-soluble vitamins, potentially effecting warfarin management.

   d. Fibric acid derivatives (gemfibrozil and clofibrate) are peroxisome proliferator–activated receptor α agonists and are the most potent medications for lowering triglyceride levels and raising HDL. Treatment may induce gallstones, hepatitis, and myositis.

   e. Ezetimibe blocks intestinal absorption of dietary and biliary cholesterol by blocking a cholesterol transporter and may be used as monotherapy or in combination with a statin.

Lifestyle changes are key to managing lipid disorders: limiting fat intake (avoid trans fats and saturated fats) and choosing better fats; increasing aerobic activity, antioxidant foods, fiber; and smoking cessation.

Adrenal Gland Disorders

A. Cushing's syndrome

1. General characteristics

   a. Cushing's syndrome (hypercortisolism, cortisol excess) is the effect of excess cortisol on the body. One-third of cases arise from excessive autonomous adrenal cortical secretion and are ACTH independent.

   b. Cushing's disease (ACTH excess) is usually caused by ACTH-secreting pituitary microadenoma, which is typically very small (<5 mm) and most often located in the anterior pituitary. Women are affected three times more often than men.

   c. Exogenous Cushing's syndrome is caused by corticosteroid drug use.

   d. Adrenocortical tumors and nonpituitary ACTH-producing tumors (most often small cell lung carcinoma) may also cause Cushing's syndrome.

2. **Clinical features** (Table 10-8)

   a. Hypercortisolism may present as obesity, HTN, and thirst and polyuria with or without glycosuria.

   b. The most specific signs are proximal muscle weakness and pigmented striae >1 cm wide; patients may present with backache and headache.

   c. Oligomenorrhea or amenorrhea and erectile dysfunction are common.

   d. Disorders of calcium metabolism may cause osteoporosis, vertebral fractures, hypercalciuria, and kidney stones. Avascular necrosis may occur.

   e. Impaired wound healing, acne, easy bruising, and superficial skin infections occur. Patients are susceptible to opportunistic infections.

   f. Psychiatric symptoms range from emotional lability to psychosis.

3. Diagnostic studies

   a. First, determine cortisol excess using overnight dexamethasone suppression test (suppression to <5 μg/dL excludes Cushing with some certainty). Additional testing includes a 24-hour urine collection for free cortisol and creatinine. Late night salivary cortisol assays may also be useful.

   b. Plasma or serum ACTH of <20 pg per mL suggests adrenal tumor; higher levels suggest pituitary or ectopic production.

   c. MRI is preferred to identify pituitary tumors. CT may show adrenocortical or other tumors. Somatostatin receptor scintigraphy is useful in detecting occult tumors.

   d. Hyperglycemia, impaired glucose tolerance, and hypokalemia (without hypernatremia) are not unusual.

   e. Consider workup for ectopic ACTH producers: small cell lung cancer, thymomas, and thyroid or pancreatic islet cell tumors.

4. **Treatment**

   a. Transsphenoidal selective resection of the pituitary tumor cures 75% to 90%.

   b. Irradiation provides remission in 50% to 60% of nonresectable tumors.

   c. Gamma knife radiosurgery is useful if the pituitary tumor is well seen on MRI and not near the optic pathway.

   d. Bilateral adrenalectomy in selected cases may be considered.

   e. Adrenal cortisol–secreting neoplasms <6 cm in diameter are resected. Ectopic ACTH-secreting tumors should be located and surgically removed if possible.

   f. Medical therapy before surgery can inhibit glucocorticoid synthesis. Mitotane, metyrapone, or ketoconazole may suppress hypercortisolism. Parenteral octreotide suppresses ACTH in one-third of cases.

Hypercortisolism presents with centripetal obesity and the extremities may appear wasted; fat deposition may cause the characteristic buffalo hump, moon facies, and supraclavicular pads.

Transsphenoidal selective resection of the pituitary tumor cures 75% to 90% of Cushing's disease.

Table 10-8 | Common Clinical Features of Cushing's Syndrome Versus Addison's Disease

Cushing's Syndrome (Hypercortisolism)	Addison's Disease (Adrenal Insufficiency)
Obesity (centripetal, with wasted extremities)	Insidious onset and often nonspecific symptoms
Hypertension	Weight loss
Thirst and polyuria with or without glycosuria	Orthostatic hypotension
Buffalo hump of upper back	Fatigue and weakness
Moon facies	Anorexia
Supraclavicular pads	Irritability
Proximal muscle weakness	Anxiety
Pigmented striae	Myalgias
Backache	Arthralgias
Headache	Nausea or diarrhea
Oligomenorrhea or amenorrhea; erectile dysfunction	Amenorrhea
	Delayed deep tendon reflexes
Osteoporosis, hypercalciuria, and kidney stones (secondary to disorders of calcium metabolism)	Hyperpigmentation (in primary disease, i.e., with elevated ACTH)
Impaired wound healing	Hyperpigmentation of hands and pressure areas
Acne	Small heart
Easy bruising	Hyperplasia of lymphoid tissues
	Scant axillary and pubic hair
	Hypogonadism

ACTH, adrenocorticotropic hormone.

g. Prognosis of Cushing's syndrome with successful excision of a benign adrenal adenoma offers a 95% 5-year survival. A similar prognosis occurs with Cushing's disease if postoperative nonsuppressed cortisol levels are <2 μg per dL. However, there is a 15% to 20% chance of recurrence over 10 years. Continued ectopic ACTH production has a 5-year survival of 65%.

B. Adrenal insufficiency (Addison's disease)

1. General characteristics

   a. The most common cause of primary adrenal insufficiency is autoimmune destruction of the adrenal cortex (80% of cases). Secondary causes are pituitary based.

   b. It may occur alone or as part of polyglandular autoimmune syndrome or genetic disorders such as adrenoleukodystrophy.

   c. TB is a leading cause of Addison's disease in areas of TB prevalence. Calcification of adrenal glands in a setting of symptoms is diagnostic.

   d. Adrenal crises may be precipitated by infection, trauma, surgery, stress, lymphoma, metastatic cancer, amyloidosis, scleroderma, hemochromatosis, or cessation of corticosteroid medication.

2. **Clinical features**

   a. Addison's disease begins insidiously with nonspecific problems, such as fatigue and weakness. Anorexia and weight loss are usually present, as is irritability/anxiety. It may coexist with other autoimmune disorders such as vitiligo.

   b. Most patients have emotional changes, myalgias, and arthralgias; many have GI symptoms. Amenorrhea is common in females.

   c. Many patients develop sensory hypersensitivities; some patients crave salt.

   d. Orthostatic hypotension is common. Systolic BP <110 mm Hg is found in 90% of patients.

   e. Delayed deep tendon reflexes are common.

   f. Hyperpigmentation is found only in primary disease (i.e., when ACTH is elevated). This may produce diffuse tanning over non–sun-exposed skin; multiple freckles; and hyperpigmentation of knuckles, elbows, knees, palmar creases, pressure areas such as bra or belt lines, and nipple areas.

> 🔆 Signs of hypercortisolism with hyperpigmentation signify primary disease of the adrenal gland.

g. Other findings include small heart, hyperplasia of lymphoid tissues, scant axillary and pubic hair, and hypogonadism.

h. Addisonian crisis is heralded by hypotension, acute pain (abdomen, low back), vomiting, diarrhea, dehydration, hypotension, and altered mental status. If untreated, it can be fatal.

3. Diagnostic studies

> A rise of >20 µg/dL is a normal response to cosyntropin stimulation and rules out primary adrenal insufficiency.

    a. Laboratory findings include hyperkalemia (only in primary disease), hyponatremia, hypoglycemia, hypercalcemia, and low BUN.

    b. Neutropenia, mild anemia, relative lymphocytosis, and eosinophilia may occur.

    c. Low (<3 µg/dL) 8:00 AM plasma cortisol accompanied by elevation of the plasma ACTH (>200 pg/mL) is diagnostic. Low levels of ACTH indicate secondary disease.

    d. The simplified cosyntropin stimulation test is also diagnostic. A serum cortisol rise of >20 µg per dL after administration of cosyntropin is normal; anything less is suspicious.

    e. Antiadrenal antibodies will be present in 50% of patients; antithyroid antibodies are found in 45% of patients.

    f. Serum dehydroepiandrosterone (DHEA) levels are <1,000 ng per mL; a level higher than this excludes Addison's disease.

    g. Chest radiography and abdominal CT scanning may be indicated for suspected secondary disease.

4. **Treatment**

    a. Primary disease is treated with a combination of corticosteroids and mineralocorticoids. These include oral hydrocortisone or prednisone (corticosteroids) and fludrocortisone acetate (mineralocorticoid) for its sodium-retaining effect.

    b. DHEA may be given; studies show improved well-being, increased muscle mass, and reversal of femoral neck bone loss. Monitoring is needed for androgenic effects.

    c. Patients must be fully informed about their condition as infections must be treated immediately and aggressively along with treatment of the underlying disease with increased hydrocortisone dosing. A medical alert bracelet or medal may be lifesaving.

    d. Prognosis for treated disease is close to normal, although patients often have chronic low-grade fatigue.

    e. Addisonian crisis requires aggressive IV saline, glucose, and glucocorticoids as well as treatment of the underlying cause.

Practice Questions

Directions: Each of the numbered items or incomplete statements in this section is followed by a list of answers or completions of the statement. Select the ONE lettered answer or completion that is BEST in each case.

1. A 43-year-old female presents complaining of palpitations and jitteriness. She quickly tires doing routine tasks. Examination is noncontributory. Labs reveal a mildly low hemoglobin and hematocrit with normal RBC indices. TSH is low and T_4 is markedly elevated. What is the most likely diagnosis?
  A. Graves' disease
  B. Toxic multinodular goiter
  C. MEN I
  D. Thyroid storm
  E. Thyroiditis

2. A 38-year-old asymptomatic female has a 1 cm rounded, nontender thyroid nodule. T_3, T_4, and TSH are within normal range. Ultrasonography confirms a single, heterogeneous lesion. What is the best next step?
  A. FNA
  B. RAIU study
  C. Open biopsy
  D. Trial of T_4 treatment
  E. Reassess in 3 months

3. A 33-year-old patient presents with weight gain, easy bruising, and proximal muscle weakness. Examination reveals excess adipose tissue in the face and upper back, violaceous striae, and purpura. What is the expected result of an overnight dexamethasone suppression test?

A. Morning cortisol level normal
B. Morning cortisol level elevated
C. Morning cortisol level decreased
D. Morning ACTH level decreased
E. Morning ACTH normal

4. A 48-year-old male presents with flank pain radiating to the groin. Urine is positive for blood. He is admitted and started on IV fluids and given analgesics. Admission labs reveal an elevated calcium and low phosphorus. Upon further questioning, he admits to fatigue, weakness, anorexia, and constipation. What is the best next step to secure the underlying diagnosis?

A. Amylase and lipase levels
B. Bone density scan
C. Glomerular filtration rate
D. PTH level
E. Renal biopsy

5. A 61-year-old male has an elevated adjusted calcium of 12.8 mg per dL and an elevated PTH at 200 mg per mL. An ECG shows a shortened QT interval. What other finding is likely in this patient?

A. Contraction of the eye, mouth, or nose muscles with tapping along the facial nerve area
B. Increased phosphate and decreased magnesium levels
C. Increased thirst, abdominal pain, and depressed deep tendon reflexes
D. Osteoporosis and hyperactive deep tendon reflexes
E. Spasms in the hand or wrist with compression of the forearm

6. A patient described coarsening of his voice and enlargement of his hands and feet. He refuses any imaging studies until laboratory testing is done. Which of the following is the best laboratory approach?

A. Administer a glucose tolerance test
B. Administer cortisol
C. Measure a random GH level
D. Measure a random IGF-1 level
E. Measure PRL level

7. A 56-year-old male complains of anxiety and insomnia. Examination reveals a fine tremor, enlarged thyroid, and an irregularly irregular heartbeat, rate of 112 bpm. BP is 162/78. Skin is moist; nails and hair are brittle. ECG shows fine atrial fibrillation with irregular ventricular beats. What is the recommended treatment?

A. Amiodarone
B. β-Blocker
C. Hydrocortisol
D. MM
E. Levothyroxine

8. A 72-year-old female with a history of rheumatoid arthritis is brought to the emergency department after almost passing out at a bridge game. She describes a week of progressive weakness, lethargy, and forgetfulness. She states she is depressed and feels cold all the time; she is experiencing worsening constipation despite use of a psyllium-based supplement. What is the most sensitive lab test to order at this time?

A. Free triiodothyronine (T_3)
B. Antithyroid peroxidase
C. Antithyroglobulin antibodies
D. Potassium level
E. TSH level

9. A 43-year-old obese female has a fasting glucose of 166 mg per dL. Repeat labs confirm elevated glucose; HbA_{1c} is 8.1%. What is the mechanism of action of the first-line treatment of the most likely diagnosis?

A. Delay absorption of dietary carbohydrates
B. Inhibit dipeptidyl peptidase 4 (DPP-4) activity and prolong the endogenous action of glucagon-like peptide-1 (GLP-1)
C. Sensitize peripheral tissue to insulin
D. Reduce hepatic glucose production
E. Stimulate insulin release from pancreatic cells

10. A 45-year-old overweight male undergoes routine screening. He is 6 feet tall and weighs 262 lb; waist circumference is 44 inches; BP is 144/88. Lab results include the following: fasting glucose 124 mg per dL; LDL 240 mg per dL; HDL 31 mg per dL; triglycerides 244 mg per dL. What is the best recommendation for this patient at this time?

A. Counsel patient on diet and exercise and begin metformin.
B. Refer to cardiologist for further workup of hyperlipidemia.
C. Obtain HbA_{1c} before deciding further plan.
D. Screen patient for HLA *DR3-DQ2* and *DR4* genes.
E. Start the patient on metformin and a thiazide diuretic.

11. A 40-year-old female presents for workup of amenorrhea. She describes insidious worsening of fatigue and irritability along with loss of appetite, irregular bowel habits, and a 12-lb unintentional weight loss. BP is 100/78, pulse is 66 and regular. Hyperpigmentation is seen on the knuckles, elbows, and knees. What is the most likely underlying pathology?

A. Autoimmune destruction of the adrenal cortex
B. Benign pituitary adenoma
C. Abnormal release of ACTH from pituitary
D. Genetic mutations affecting adrenal and thyroid glands
E. Exposure to radiation affecting multiple glands

12. A 25-year-old female has a solitary thyroid nodule. Radionuclide scan shows increased uptake in the area. Ultrasonography confirms a solitary, well-defined, homogeneous area measuring 1.2 cm. What is the recommended management?

A. FNA
B. Follow quarterly T_3, T_4, and TSH levels
C. Periodic ultrasonographic monitoring
D. 6 weeks of T_3 replacement and reevaluate
E. Surgical excision and histologic workup

Practice Answers

1. A. *Endocrinology; Diagnosis; Hyperthyroidism*

Graves' disease accounts for 80% of hyperthyroid cases. It is more common in women and affects 2% of the U.S. population. Toxic multinodular goiter is the second most common cause of hyperthyroidism; T_4 levels are not as elevated as in Graves' disease. Thyroid storm is a rare but serious complication of hyperthyroidism; it is often brought on by sepsis, trauma, major surgery, or pregnancy. Thyroiditis encompasses several disease entities that may cause inflammation or infection of the thyroid gland. MEN I is an autosomal dominant familial tumor affecting the parathyroids and possibly the skin, pancreas, and pituitary.

2. A. *Endocrinology; Diagnostic Studies; Thyroid Nodule*

In a patient with a solitary nodule and no history of radiation therapy, an FNA should be performed to guide care. RAIU studies are performed if an FNA shows a nonmalignant, hypercellular follicular neoplasm. An open biopsy and/or excision is performed when FNA shows a malignancy, there is a cold nodule on RAIU, there are multiple nodules with a dominant nodule, or there is a history of radiation therapy to the head or neck.

3. B. *Endocrinology; Diagnostic Studies; Cushing*

A patient with Cushing's disease would show a failure of dexamethasone to suppress the morning cortisol level, therefore morning cortisol is elevated. An unaffected patient (without Cushing) would have a decreased (suppressed) morning cortisol after overnight testing. A normal cortisol level after an overnight suppression test would be inconclusive. Cushing's disease displays elevated ACTH levels, if measured. An ACTH-producing pituitary tumor, as in Cushing's disease, will not turn off when challenged with dexamethasone.

4. D. *Endocrinology; Diagnostic Studies; Hyperparathyroidism*

Primary hyperparathyroidism is most commonly discovered through an elevated calcium on routine screening. Symptomatic hyperparathyroidism is manifest most commonly with renal stones, bone pain, abdominal cramping, or mild cognitive or psychologic dysfunction. An elevated calcium and low phosphorus along with an elevated PTH level confirms primary hyperparathyroidism. A benign adenoma accounts for 85% of cases of primary hyperparathyroidism.

5. C. *Endocrinology; History and PE; Hyperparathyroidism*

This is a picture of hyperparathyroidism. Although increased thirst and anorexia are nondescript findings, depressed deep tendon reflexes are more often seen with symptomatic hypercalcemia. Contraction of the eye, mouth, or nose muscles (Chvostek sign) and spasm in the hand or wrist with compression of the forearm (Trousseau sign) are seen in hypoparathyroidism. Increased phosphate and decreased magnesium levels are more commonly seen in hypocalcemic conditions. Hypercalcemia will more commonly cause a decrease in serum phosphate. Magnesium levels in hypercalcemia are variable but more often slightly elevated. Osteoporosis can be seen in both hypercalcemia (because of sequestration of calcium from bones) and hypocalcemia (because of lack of available calcium). Hypocalcemia is associated with hyperactive deep tendon reflexes.

6. D. *Endocrinology; Diagnostic Studies; Acromegaly*

IGF-1 is produced in the liver in response to GH. It is a useful test as it gives an accurate indicator of GH levels and remains stable during the day. Levels may be falsely low in liver disease and chronic illness. Because of the pulsatile nature of release, GH levels are not helpful unless used in conjunction with suppression testing or IGF-a levels. A glucose tolerance test may be useful; it is less specific than IGF-1. GH-secreting tumors are often mixed and may also secrete PRL or cortisol; they are not diagnostic of acromegaly.

7. B. *Endocrinology; Pharmacology; Hyperthyroidism*

This patient is experiencing atrial fibrillation secondary to hyperthyroidism. Although the thyroid disease should be treated long term with either MM or PTU or radioactive iodine ablation, it is more important at this time to treat the symptoms with β-blockade. Levothyroxine is appropriate for treatment of hypothyroidism.

8. E. *Endocrinology; Diagnostic Studies; Hypothyroidism*

TSH is the single best screening test for hypothyroidism, which is found in >5% of the geriatric population. TSH will be elevated; concomitant low levels of free T_4 confirm primary hypothyroid disease. Antithyroid peroxidase and antithyroglobulin antibodies confirm autoimmune disease as the cause of the hypothyroidism.

9. D. *Endocrinology; Pharmacology; Diabetes Mellitus*

Metformin is the first-line treatment for new-onset DM. It suppresses hepatic glucose production without the risk of hypoglycemia. It also aids in weight loss and will help reduce elevated triglycerides. Thiazolidinediones (pioglitazone, rosiglitazone) sensitize peripheral tissue to insulin. α-Glucosidase inhibitors (acarbose, miglitol) delay absorption of dietary carbohydrates. DPP-4 inhibitors (saxagliptin, sitagliptin, linagliptin) inhibit DDP-4 activity and prolong the endogenous action of GLP-1 receptor agonists. GLP-1 receptor agonists (exenatide, liraglutide) stimulate pancreatic release of insulin.

10. A. *Endocrinology; Clinical Intervention; Diabetes Mellitus*

This patient meets the criteria for metabolic syndrome or insulin resistance syndrome, a condition with a high likelihood of progressing to DM. Intervention is needed to reduce the patient's risk of cardiac disease. A strong commitment to diet and exercise is needed. Patient should be started on metformin and closely monitored. If the lipids remain high or worsen, referral may be warranted. If the BP remains high, intervention may be required; a thiazide diuretic is a good choice but an angiotensin-converting enzyme (ACE) inhibitor would be better as it is renal protective. HLA *DR3-DQ2* and *DR4* genes are associated with type 1 DM.

11. A. *Endocrinology; Scientific Concepts; Addison's Disease*

Primary adrenal insufficiency (Addison's disease) is caused by autoimmune destruction of the adrenal cortex and presents with fatigue, irritability, weight loss, and amenorrhea in women. Secondary adrenal insufficiency is pituitary based. Hyperpigmentation is seen only in primary adrenal insufficiency.

12. C. *Endocrinology; Clinical Intervention; Thyroid Nodule*

This lesion does not show any signs of malignancy (i.e., functioning ["hot"] nodule on radioactive scan; irregular or indistinct margins, heterogeneous echogenicity, microcalcifications, complex cyst patterns) and therefore can be monitored periodically. If the nodule had signs of malignancy, an FNA is recommended. Benign lesions may be treated with T4 replacement, which may decrease the size by 20%.

11 | Neurology

Michael A. Johnson

Diagnosis of Neurologic Disorders

A. Background

1. The accurate diagnosis of neurologic disorders requires a fundamental knowledge of neuroanatomy, a detailed patient history, a neurologic physical examination, and, when indicated, specialized neurologic testing.

2. The nervous system is composed of the central nervous system (CNS) and the peripheral nervous system (PNS).

   a. The CNS consists of the brain and the spinal cord. Gray matter in the CNS is composed primarily of neurons and dendrites, and white matter in the CNS is composed primarily of axons coated with myelin sheaths.

   b. The PNS includes 12 pairs of cranial nerves (CNs), 31 pairs of spinal nerves, peripheral nerves, and the junctions between the nerves and the muscles.

   c. The autonomic nervous system (ANS) is within the CNS and PNS and controls involuntary functions of the body, such as heart rate, digestion, and pupillary responses. The ANS can be divided into the sympathetic (fight or flight) and parasympathetic (rest and digest) systems.

B. History

1. Neurologic history should ask about symptoms such as pain, numbness, weakness, paresthesias, dizziness, poor balance, involuntary movements, and vision changes. Family history of neurologic problems is important to elicit.

2. The history should cover the onset, severity, and timing of symptoms; whether the symptoms have worsened or improved; and if any traumatic event was involved.

C. Physical examination

1. The neurologic physical examination may be brief if a single peripheral nerve is involved, such as the median nerve in carpal tunnel syndrome. The examination may need to be more comprehensive if the patient has complex symptoms or a variety of neurologic symptoms (Table 11-1).

2. Hyperreflexia, positive Babinski's (upgoing toe), and spastic weakness are consistent with upper motor neuron lesions. Cerebral palsy, multiple sclerosis (MS), and stroke are examples of pathologic conditions that may have these findings.

3. Hyporeflexia and weakness with muscle atrophy are consistent with lower motor neuron lesions. Guillain–Barré syndrome (GBS) and lumbar or cervical radiculopathy are pathologic conditions that may have these physical examination findings.

D. Special testing

1. Brain and/or spinal cord structure is imaged with computed tomography (CT) or magnetic resonance imaging (MRI).

2. The cerebrovascular system is imaged with computed tomography angiography (CTA), magnetic resonance angiography (MRA), or conventional angiography.

> A complete neurologic examination consists of seven components: CN testing, motor function, sensory function, reflexes, coordination, station and gait, and mental status.

Table 11-1 | Complete Neurologic Physical Examination

Mental status examination	Appearance, mood, cognition, speech, thought process, perception, insight, judgment
CN examination	Test motor and sensory functions of CN I–CN XII
Motor examination	Inspection (atrophy, fasciculations), tone/rigidity, strength, posture (decerebrate, decorticate, hemiparetic)
Sensory examination	Evaluate light touch, pinprick (pain), vibratory, proprioception, stereognosis
Reflexes	Check strength and speed of deep tendon reflexes; test for Babinski's, primitive reflexes
Cerebellar function testing	Test coordination and balance, Romberg, observe gait

CN, cranial nerve.

3. Electromyography (EMG) and nerve conduction tests may be indicated to help make the diagnosis or better evaluate peripheral nerve disorders.

4. Lumbar puncture (LP) and evaluation of the cerebrospinal fluid (CSF) are important diagnostic tools. LP is indicated when a patient is suspected to have meningitis, encephalitis, subarachnoid hemorrhage (SAH), or CNS disease, such as GBS.

Cerebrovascular Disease

A. Stroke

   1. General characteristics

      a. Stroke is the fifth most common cause of death in the United States, and it is the most common cause of chronic severe disability. Stroke is characterized by ischemia or hemorrhage in the CNS, resulting in infarction.

      b. The incidence of stroke increases with age and is higher in blacks, Native Americans, and Hispanics as compared to whites.

      c. The major modifiable risk factors for stroke are hypertension, hypercholesterolemia, diabetes, atrial fibrillation, carotid artery disease (with symptoms), physical inactivity, and cigarette smoking. Other, unmodifiable risk factors are increasing age and family history.

      d. Hypertension is the most significant and treatable risk factor for stroke. Hypertension is a risk factor for ischemic and hemorrhagic strokes.

      e. A previous stroke increases the susceptibility to additional strokes.

      f. Ischemic strokes account for about 85% of all strokes in the United States. Two-thirds of ischemic strokes are thrombotic, and one-third are embolic. Emboli commonly arise from the heart, aortic arch, or large cerebral arteries.

      g. Hemorrhagic strokes, which are usually secondary to hypertension, account for about 15% of strokes. A hemorrhagic stroke can be intracerebral or subarachnoid. Most hemorrhagic strokes are intracerebral. Approximately one in four hemorrhagic strokes is subarachnoid.

      h. Arteriovenous malformations (AVMs) can cause intracerebral hemorrhagic stroke and less commonly SAH. These congenital vascular malformations or tangles of vessels are areas of direct connections between arteries and veins without the usual intervening capillary vessels. This results in high flow with increased potential for bleeding. These vascular malformations are the cause of about 1% to 2% of all strokes, and about 10% of subarachnoid and intracerebral hemorrhages. These areas are usually discovered in the second to fourth decades of life, and most present with hemorrhage or seizure.

> Control of hypertension can significantly decrease the risk of ischemic stroke.

2. Clinical features

a. Signs and symptoms of stroke begin abruptly or upon awakening, and they correlate with the area of the brain that is supplied by the affected vessel, especially with ischemic events.

b. History and physical examination usually reveal hemiparesis or hemisensory deficit. One can localize the lesion to one side, contralateral to these deficits (Table 11-2).

(1) Strokes involving the anterior circulation (anterior choroidal, anterior cerebral, middle cerebral arteries), which supplies the cortex, subcortical white matter, basal ganglia, and the internal capsule, are commonly associated with hemispheric signs and symptoms (aphasia, apraxia, hemiparesis, hemisensory losses, and/or visual field defects).

(2) Strokes involving the posterior circulation (vertebral and basilar arteries), which supplies the brain stem, cerebellum, thalamus, and portions of the temporal and occipital lobes, are commonly associated with evidence of brainstem dysfunction (coma, drop attacks, vertigo, nausea, vomiting, limb ataxia, and/or gait ataxia).

c. Thrombotic strokes are often preceded by transient ischemic attacks (TIAs). Embolic strokes occur abruptly and without warning.

d. Hemorrhagic strokes are less predictable; presentation is variable because of complications of blood dispersion, cerebral edema, and increased intracranial pressure. Headache, nausea, vomiting, and change in mental status (to include coma) are some possible symptoms.

3. Diagnostic studies

a. Initial tests should include finger stick glucose, pulse oximetry, noncontrast CT or MRI of the brain, and 12-lead electrocardiogram (ECG).

b. Blood tests should include complete blood count (CBC), platelet count, prothrombin time (PT), international normalization ratio (INR), partial thromboplastin time (PTT), and troponin.

c. Additional blood tests may be indicated: comprehensive metabolic panel (CMP) to check liver function, electrolytes, and kidney function. Blood cultures should be considered if endocarditis or sepsis is suspected.

d. Noncontrast CT scan of the brain is recommended during the acute phase and is currently the preferred modality for differentiating ischemic from hemorrhagic stroke at most hospitals. It is also used to rule out an intracranial mass. MRI of the brain is also acceptable as the initial imaging, but it is frequently not available, takes longer to perform, and may be contraindicated in many patients.

e. Additional test to evaluate stroke patients is usually warranted. Neurovascular imaging can be accomplished with CTA, MRA, or, rarely, conventional

> Anterior stroke leads to unilateral functional deficits; posterior strokes more likely lead to systemic symptoms, often bilateral, and often include loss of consciousness.

> A CT scan should be done STAT in any patient with stroke symptoms to rule out a bleed.

Table 11-2 | Common Stroke Symptoms

Common Anterior Circulation Stroke Symptoms	Common Posterior Circulation Stroke Symptoms
Unilateral arm/leg weakness	Dizziness/vertigo
Aphasias (MCA dominant side, usually left hemisphere CVA)	Gait abnormality/ataxia
	Limb ataxia
Hemineglect (MCA nondominant side, usually right hemisphere CVA)	Nausea and vomiting
	Visual loss, hemianopia
Unilateral arm/leg paresthesias or anesthesias	Headache, confusion, impaired consciousness
Visual changes	Dysarthria, dysphagia
	Drop attacks

CVA, cerebrovascular accident; MCA, middle cerebral artery.

angiography. Patients who are the candidates for mechanical thrombectomy may have diffusion-weighted MRI or CT perfusion to assess for irreversible brain injury. Further diagnostic testing may include carotid ultrasonography to evaluate for carotid stenosis, and echocardiography to look for emboli.

f. Cardiac monitoring with ECG and Holter monitor may reveal an arrhythmia (e.g., atrial fibrillation) or a recent myocardial infarction (MI) as the possible source of emboli.

g. LP should be reserved for patients with suspected hemorrhage. Patients with symptoms of SAH but with a normal CT should have an LP. Findings in SAH may include increased opening pressure, increased CSF red blood cell count in all tubes, and/or xanthochromia (a yellow color of the CSF caused by breakdown of blood). LP should not be performed until an intracranial mass has been ruled out.

4. Treatment

a. Acute treatment is aimed at reversing the ischemia and salvaging tissue in the core and surrounding penumbra.

> Goal of stroke therapy—save the penumbra!

(1) Thrombolytic therapy (intravenous [IV] alteplase) for acute ischemic stroke is given to reduce the extent of deficit; it is most effective if given within 3 hours of symptoms but can be attempted up to 4.5 hours after the onset of symptoms. If alteplase is unsuccessful, mechanical thrombectomy may be considered.

(2) The major complication of thrombolytic therapy is bleeding. Most contraindications to thrombolytic therapy are related to bleeding risk (Table 11-3).

(3) If blood pressure (BP) is elevated to >185/110 and thrombolytic therapy is indicated, the BP must be controlled to <185/110 before infusion of thrombolytic and controlled to <180/105 for 24 hours thereafter. Labetalol is commonly used for BP control.

(4) If thrombolytics are not indicated, elevated BP for acute ischemic stroke is usually left untreated, unless significantly elevated over 220 mm Hg systolic or over 120 mm Hg diastolic.

(5) Patients presenting with stroke symptoms between 4.5 and 24 hours may be the candidates for mechanical thrombectomy.

(6) Antiplatelet therapy with aspirin is initiated early for acute ischemic stroke; however, if thrombolytic therapy with alteplase is given, aspirin should not be given until 24 hours after the time of thrombolytic therapy. Chronic anticoagulant therapy is indicated in the setting of cardiac emboli.

Table 11-3 | Contraindications to Thrombolytic Therapy

Absolute Contraindications	Relative Contraindications
History or evidence of hemorrhage	Pregnancy
Clinical suggestion of subarachnoid hemorrhage	Rapidly improving stroke symptoms
Known arteriovenous malformation	MI in the previous 3 months
Systolic BP >185 mm Hg or diastolic BP >110 mm Hg despite repeated measurements and treatment	Glucose <50 mg/dL or >400 mg/dL
	Recent major surgery within 3 months
Seizure with postictal residua	Heparin use within 48 hours
Platelet count <100,000 μL	
PT >15 or INR >1.7	
Active internal bleeding or acute trauma (fracture)	
Head trauma or stroke in previous 3 months	
Arterial puncture at a noncompressible site within 1 week	

BP, blood pressure; INR, international normalization ratio; MI, myocardial infarction; PT, prothrombin time.

> In any suspected hemorrhagic stroke, all anticoagulant and antiplatelet therapy must be stopped or reversed to prevent further injury.

(7) Endarterectomy may be indicated if >70% stenosis of the common or internal carotid artery is present.

(8) Hemorrhagic stroke has a high mortality. Patients with hemorrhagic stroke should have antiplatelet and anticoagulants stopped immediately. Anticoagulants should be reversed without delay. Heparin is reversed with protamine sulfate, warfarin is reversed with IV vitamin K and four-factor prothrombin complex concentrate. Dabigatran is reversed with idarucizumab.

(9) Patients with hemorrhagic stroke should have hypertension controlled acutely. Treat to bring SAH patients to <160 mm Hg and intracerebral hemorrhage patients to a systolic of 140 mm Hg. Elevated intracranial pressure can be managed with elevating the head of the bed, sedation, mannitol, or other interventions if needed. Microsurgical excision or radiosurgery is frequently the best option for patients with AVMs. Endovascular repair with surgical clipping or coil embolization is the preferred option for patients with specific anatomic foci, such as berry aneurysms causing SAH.

b. Long-term supportive therapy, follow-up physical therapy, and social supports are important.

B. Transient ischemic attack (TIA)

> TIA = acute neurologic deficit that completely resolves within 24 hours; it is often a harbinger of stroke.

1. General characteristics

a. A TIA is a sudden transient neurologic deficit secondary to disturbance of cerebral circulation that does not result in acute infarction.

b. TIAs typically relate directly to either the carotid or the vertebral vascular distribution and may be caused by atherosclerotic plaque, inflammation, or other process that leads to decreased flow of blood to an area of the brain.

c. Most TIAs only last a few minutes and typically completely resolve within 1 hour. By definition, symptoms resolve completely within 24 hours and result in no infarction of tissue.

d. Although TIAs are brief and transient, one-third of these patients will have a stroke within 5 years, making assessment and treatment important in prevention. TIAs are noted most frequently in older patients and those at risk for vascular disease.

e. TIAs may be caused by emboli from the heart, aorta, or arteries.

2. Clinical features

a. If the TIA is related to a disturbance in carotid circulation, patients may demonstrate contralateral hand–arm weakness with sensory loss, ipsilateral visual symptoms or aphasia, and/or amaurosis fugax. Carotid bruit may be present, but with a high-grade stenosis (95% or greater), it may be absent.

b. Those experiencing vertebrobasilar TIA may demonstrate diplopia, ataxia, vertigo, dysarthria, CN palsies, lower extremity weakness, dimness or blurring of vision, perioral numbness, and/or drop attacks.

c. The differential diagnosis of TIA includes focal seizure, generalized seizure, migraine, syncope, hypoglycemia in patients using insulin or oral hypoglycemic agents, and mass lesions.

3. Diagnostic studies

> Workup after a TIA is similar to stroke; aimed at finding the cause and preventing stroke.

a. The workup of a patient with TIA is similar to the workup of a patient with stroke. In some cases, the workup may be performed urgently within days instead of within minutes or hours.

b. The patient with TIA may require an inpatient environment, or in milder cases, it may be completed in an outpatient environment. Patients with TIA who are older, have elevated BP, have weakness and speech impairment, have longer symptom duration, and those with diabetes have a higher risk of stroke and may need hospitalization.

   c. If outpatient workup is chosen, the evaluation should be completed within 2 days.

   d. Head CT or MRI will exclude a possible small cerebral hemorrhage or infarct.

   e. Head CTA and MRA are minimally invasive options to evaluate the cerebrovascular system; conventional angiography remains the definitive study; as it is invasive and associated with small risk of stroke, it is rarely done.

   f. Cardiac workup should be done to exclude arrhythmia and new murmurs. The heart is a common source of emboli.

   g. A hematologic workup must be done to identify coagulopathies.

      (1) A normal erythrocyte sedimentation rate (ESR) will effectively rule out temporal arteritis.

      (2) Other studies include CBC, cholesterol, PT, PTT, antiphospholipid, serum glucose, electrolytes, blood urea nitrogen (BUN), and creatinine.

   h. Other studies to evaluate possible cardiogenic or carotid emboli are echocardiography, ECG, Holter monitor, and carotid Doppler imaging.

> TIA workup must include ruling out infarct/hemorrhage, arrhythmia, murmur, and coagulopathies.

  4. Treatment

   a. Because a TIA may indicate an impending stroke, prophylactic antiplatelet therapy is initiated when the TIA is not cardiogenic. This therapy might include aspirin, clopidogrel, ticlopidine, or aspirin/extended-release dipyridamole.

   b. Cardiogenic TIA requires anticoagulation with warfarin or a direct-acting anticoagulant (DOAC), such as apixaban, for long-term therapy.

   c. Carotid endarterectomy may be indicated in patients with anterior circulation TIAs and moderate- to high-grade carotid stenosis on the side appropriate to account for the symptoms.

   d. Adjunctive therapies include control of BP, serum cholesterol, blood glucose, and atrial fibrillation. Patients also must be urged to discontinue cigarette smoking.

C. Cerebral aneurysm/SAH

  1. General characteristics

   a. Ruptured saccular (berry) aneurysms account for the majority of cases of SAH and are associated with a high mortality rate. These aneurysms typically occur on the surface of the brain. These catastrophic events most often occur during the fifth and sixth decades of life, with slightly higher incidence in females.

   b. A ruptured cerebral arterial aneurysm or, less commonly, an AVM causes bleeding into CSF in the subarachnoid space.

   c. Risk factors for developing aneurysms include smoking, hypertension, family history, and heavy alcohol use. Cerebral aneurysms are also associated with polycystic kidney disease and coarctation of the aorta.

   d. Methamphetamine and cocaine use is associated with triggering SAH, presumably by causing elevation of the BP.

   e. Intracranial AVM accounts for <10% of SAHs. Most AVMs are congenital. AVM is typically diagnosed during the second to fourth decades.

  2. Clinical features

   a. The classic SAH presents as sudden onset of an unusually severe generalized headache of maximum intensity—a "thunderclap headache." The headache may be accompanied by nausea and vomiting, seizure activity, or altered state of consciousness.

   b. Frequently, BP rises precipitously as a result of the hemorrhage.

   c. Patients with SAH may display confusion, stupor, coma, and nuchal rigidity or other signs of meningeal irritation, or they may be alert and have a normal neurologic examination.

   d. A herald bleed, or aneurysmal leak, occurs in up to 40% of patients, producing a less severe but atypical headache and is accompanied by focal neurologic signs

> SAH is characterized as the worst headache of one's life followed by acute symptoms including nausea/vomiting, seizure activity, and loss of consciousness.

> Delayed diagnosis of SAH = poor outcomes including permanent neurologic sequelae.

resulting from pressure on the brain or CNs. The herald bleed and corresponding sentinel headache usually occur 1 to 3 weeks before severe SAH.

3. Diagnostic studies

   a. The diagnosis of SAH is frequently missed or delayed, resulting in poor outcomes.

   b. Noncontrast head CT is the initial investigational modality for suspected SAH; >90% of patients with aneurysmal rupture will be identified in this way.

   c. If the CT of the head is normal, but a high suspicion of SAH exists, an LP must be accomplished. LP with evaluation of CSF in a patient with SAH reveals markedly elevated opening pressures and grossly bloody fluid in all four tubes. Xanthochromia may also be present if the blood has been in the CSF over 2 hours.

   d. Cerebral angiography or CTA should be done to evaluate the entire intracranial vasculature because as many as 20% of individuals will have multiple aneurysms.

4. **Treatment**

   a. Supportive medical treatment involves prevention of elevated arterial or intracranial pressures that might lead to re-rupture of the affected vessel. It may also include strict bed rest, mild sedation, or administration of stool softeners to prevent straining.

   b. Management of hypertension is important, but care must be taken to prevent hypotension and inadequate cerebral perfusion. The BP should be controlled to a systolic of <160 mm Hg.

   c. Surgical management includes coil embolization or clipping of aneurysms and, depending on the clinical state of the patient, microsurgical excision of an AVM.

Seizure Disorders

> Seizure classification features include onset, etiology, and impairment of awareness.

A. General characteristics

1. Seizures are transient disturbances of cerebral function caused by abnormal paroxysmal neuronal discharges in the brain. These abnormal neuronal discharges produce transient neurologic signs and symptoms. Seizures can be clinical (full expression), subtle (minimal clinical expression), or subclinical (no clinical or outward manifestation of the electrical abnormality).

2. Seizures are categorized as generalized or focal depending on onset: bilateral or unilateral. Seizures can be further categorized as genetic, structural, or metabolic, or, in some cases, as unknown etiology, with intact awareness or without, motor onset or nonmotor onset (Table 11-4).

3. Focal seizures can be with or without cognitive impairment.

Table 11-4 | Seizure Classification

Focal onset (one hemisphere origin)	Focal without impairment of awareness	Motor onset Sensory onset Autonomic
	Focal with impairment of awareness	Motor onset Sensory onset Autonomic
Generalized onset (originating somewhere within and/or rapidly engaging both hemispheres)	Generalized with impaired awareness	Motor (tonic–clonic) Nonmotor (absence)
	Generalized without impaired awareness	Motor Nonmotor
	Focal seizures evolving into generalized/bilateral	
Unknown onset or origin	Motor	
	Nonmotor	

4. Structural or metabolic seizures may result from congenital abnormalities or perinatal injury, head trauma, withdrawal from alcohol or drugs, metabolic disorders, tumors, vascular disease, infectious diseases, or degenerative diseases, such as Alzheimer's disease (AD). Seizures in the elderly are frequently caused by strokes and/or tumors.

5. Status epilepticus, either convulsive or nonconvulsive, is diagnosed when seizures fail to cease spontaneously or recur so frequently that full consciousness is not restored between successive episodes (≥5 minutes). The length of time seizure activity must persist to diagnose status epilepticus is generally >5 minutes.

B. **Clinical features**

1. Generalized seizures are characterized as either motor (generalized tonic–clonic, myoclonic, tonic, or atonic) or nonmotor (absence).

   a. Symptoms of generalized tonic–clonic convulsive seizures often include an ictal moan or cry, a sudden stiffness of the body, a brief loss of consciousness, clonic convulsions, and loss of bladder or bowel contents. Postictal confusion can last minutes to hours. The patient will frequently sleep for several hours after the event and complain of headache and possibly injury to the tongue afterward.

   b. Myoclonic seizures are characterized by sudden brief jerking-type movements of one or both sides of the body. These are usually of short duration without a loss of consciousness.

   c. Tonic seizures are accompanied by a brief increase in body tone and may be associated with a change in level of consciousness. Atonic seizures or "drop attacks" are characterized by brief (seconds) loss of body tone and variable changes in the level of consciousness and are frequently associated with falls.

   d. Generalized nonconvulsive seizures (absence seizures) are brief lapses in awareness or consciousness usually lasting around 10 seconds without changes in body tone. These may be characterized as "staring spells" without any symptoms before or after the seizure. There may be associated minor motor activity, such as blinking, eye movements, or facial twitching.

   e. Differential diagnosis for generalized seizures includes syncope, cardiac dysrhythmias, brainstem ischemia, and psychogenic nonepileptic seizure (formerly called *pseudoseizure*).

2. Focal (partial) seizures

   a. Focal seizures with awareness are not accompanied by change in the level of consciousness. They may begin with an aura or warning that is actually part of the seizure. The type of aura depends the area of the brain experiencing the focal seizure. These can be visual changes such as flashing lights (occipital lobe), olfactory symptoms such as an unpleasant smell (mesial temporal lobe), emotional symptoms like fear or déjà vu (limbic area), and sensory or motor abnormalities (Rolandic cortex). The focus of abnormal electrical activity in the brain can spread and produce worsening symptoms. For example, a patient may have isolated hand clonic activity that may spread to include the entire arm and then the entire side of the body, also known as "Jacksonian march."

   b. Focal seizures without awareness (formerly complex partial seizures) may also be characterized by an aura (transient abnormalities in sensation, perception, emotion, or memory), followed by impaired consciousness lasting seconds to minutes. Nausea or vomiting, focal sensory perceptions, and focal tonic or clonic activity may accompany a complex seizure.

   c. Todd's paralysis is a postictal weakness or deficit in a body area affected by a focal seizure or focal to generalized seizure. For example, a patient with a focal seizure causing right arm clonic activity may have postictal weakness in that extremity lasting hours to days. This may be easy to confuse with a TIA or stroke.

   d. Differential diagnosis includes psychogenic nonepileptic seizure, paroxysmal movement disorder, TIA, migraine with aura, and panic attack.

Seizure activity that fails to cease or recurs frequently denotes status epilepticus; initial treatment includes bolus of dextrose, dose of thiamine, and treatment with a benzodiazepine followed by phenytoin.

Focal seizures begin unilaterally and may or may not include altered consciousness.

Electroencepha-lography (EEG), although often normal between seizures, is the best diagnostic tool to confirm abnormal electric activity in the brain.

C. Diagnostic studies

1. In generalized nonconvulsive seizures (absence), EEG typically shows generalized bilaterally synchronous and symmetric 3-Hz spike-and-wave activity.

2. Interictal EEG and imaging studies in generalized convulsive seizures disorders are often normal. Sleep deprivation and other maneuvers may increase the yield of abnormal findings on EEG.

3. In focal seizures with awareness, EEG may show a focal rhythmic discharge at the onset of the seizure, but, occasionally, no ictal activity will be seen.

4. EEG in focal seizures without awareness often reveals interictal spikes or spikes associated with slow waves in the temporal or frontotemporal areas.

5. Laboratory studies, such as CBC, blood glucose, electrolytes, calcium, magnesium, liver and renal functions, and toxicology screen are indicated to evaluate for potential metabolic or toxic causes. Prolactin level and creatine phosphokinase may be elevated after a generalized tonic–clonic seizure.

6. Brain MRI should be completed to rule out a structural abnormality in the patient presenting with the first seizure.

7. LP may be warranted (if infection is suspected) after neuroimaging excludes a tumor or other space-occupying lesion.

D. Treatment

1. Correction of hyponatremia, hypoglycemia, or drug intoxication may be all that is necessary to control seizures.

2. Anticonvulsant therapy is generally not indicated in the setting of a single unprovoked seizure in a patient with a normal neurologic examination, normal brain imaging, and normal EEG. The risk of seizure recurrence is <50% in 2 years even if no treatment is initiated in this setting.

Antiseizure medication is warranted after identification and correction of any underlying cause and the risk of seizure recurrence remains above average.

3. The goal of medical therapy is to prevent seizures by using a single agent, if possible, in progressive doses until seizures are controlled or toxicity occurs. If the medication is unsuccessful owing to persistent seizures or side effects, the initial medication should be stopped and another anticonvulsant tried.

   a. Generalized motor onset and focal seizures are typically treated with lamotrigine, carbamazepine, phenytoin, valproic acid, phenobarbital, or topiramate.

   b. Ethosuximide is frequently used for generalized nonconvulsive (absence) seizures.

   c. Women of childbearing age who need an anticonvulsant medication should be informed about the possible teratogenic potential of medications and advised to take supplemental folic acid. Valproate should be avoided owing to associated fetal risk of malformations.

   d. After 2 years without seizure activity, a plan to discontinue medication with close monitoring over several weeks to months may be considered.

4. Status epilepticus is a medical emergency; it can result in permanent brain damage secondary to hyperthermia, circulatory collapse, or excitotoxic neuronal damage.

   a. Immediate management must ensure a patent airway, including positioning the patient to prevent aspiration of stomach contents.

   b. Management of hyperthermia, related to increased motor activity and high levels of circulating catecholamines, may include a cooling blanket or induction of motor paralysis with a neuromuscular blocking agent.

If seizure activity continues despite full medical treatment, sedation and intubation may be warranted.

   c. First-line therapy for status epilepticus is lorazepam or diazepam administered IV; the second-line IV therapy is phenytoin, fosphenytoin, or valproic acid. If initial IV access is not available, midazolam intramuscular (IM) can be given initially.

   d. If status persists, continuous IV therapy with midazolam or propofol is added.

   e. Metabolic derangements should be corrected, and the patient should have continuous EEG monitoring.

Multiple Sclerosis

A. General characteristics

1. MS onset is usually early in adult life. Symptoms and signs manifest in late teenage years to the mid-forties with some exceptions of earlier and later onset; women are affected about twice as often as men.

2. MS is considered to be an immunologic disorder associated with CNS immunoglobulin production and alteration of T lymphocytes.

3. MS is characterized by inflammation associated with multiple foci of demyelination in the brain and spinal cord with axonal damage. These areas show up on MRI as hyperintense T2 lesions in the characteristic areas affected by MS: periventricular, infratentorial, cortical/juxtacortical, and spinal cord.

4. Most patients (about 85%) are diagnosed with relapsing remitting pattern of disease at onset. Nearly half of these patients will proceed to a diagnosis of secondary progressive MS within 10 years. Primary progressive course is diagnosed in 10% to 15% of patients at disease onset.

5. Based on numerous studies of twins, familial cases, and the association with specific human leukocyte antigen (HLA), specifically HLA-DR2 and HLA-DRB1, a genetic relationship is considered to be likely.

B. Clinical features

1. Most patients present with weakness or sensory complaints in the limbs and/or vision loss.

2. Presenting signs and symptoms can include focal weakness, numbness or tingling, optic neuritis, blindness, blurry vision, diplopia, focal neuralgias, balance problems, fatigue, Lhermitte's sign (feeling of shock that runs down the spine and into the extremities with neck flexion), or urinary symptoms.

3. Bowel and bladder problems become more prominent as the disease progresses. Urinary urgency, hesitancy, and incontinence can occur. Bowel symptoms include constipation and incontinence.

4. Symptoms (or attacks) last days to weeks and affect different areas over different episodes or exacerbations. The symptoms then resolve or remit—hence the name relapsing–remitting pattern.

5. Patients often develop cognitive and psychological deficits.

6. The diagnosis must be questioned if signs and symptoms are not related to multiple areas of the CNS over time.

C. Diagnostic studies

1. The McDonald radiographic criteria are used to diagnose MS. The criteria require at least two lesions consistent with MS (dissemination in time; i.e., simultaneous symptomatic and asymptomatic lesions OR new lesion on follow-up) and clinical objective evidence of at least two lesions (dissemination in space; i.e., periventricular, juxtacortical, infratentorial/brain stem/cerebellum, and/or spinal cord) to confirm the diagnosis. The McDonald criteria also allow for findings on the neurologic examination to count for objective clinical evidence of an MS lesion, even without an MRI. For example, if a patient has optic neuritis in the left eye, and they have new onset of diminished visual acuity in that eye with a corresponding afferent pupillary defect, that is sufficient objective clinical evidence of the lesion to count in the McDonald criteria.

2. MRI of the brain with and without contrast is the preferred initial imaging study to visualize lesions in the CNS in the evaluation of patients with suspected MS.

3. Spinal MRI can also be evaluated if more information is needed to make the diagnosis of MS.

4. CSF can reveal a sterile inflammation with a mild lymphocytosis or slight protein elevation, elevated immunoglobulin G index, oligoclonal bands, and increased myelin

> MS is characterized by demyelination affecting multiple areas of the brain over time; an alternating pattern of relapse and remittance is most common.

> MRI without contrast is best to visualize lesions in MS.

basic protein. Positive oligoclonal bands in the CSF can count in the McDonald criteria to help make the diagnosis.

5. Visual, auditory, and somatosensory-evoked potentials are helpful for assessing nerve transmission. These evoked potentials can be used to support the diagnosis of MS.

D. Treatment

> 💡 High-dose corticosteroids are used for acute MS exacerbations; long-term treatment is with disease-modifying agents and symptom management.

1. Corticosteroids may hasten recovery from acute exacerbations. High-dose IV corticosteroid (methylprednisolone 1 g IV daily for 3 to 5 days) is often used in the setting of significant exacerbations.

2. Disease-modifying agents can decrease the number of relapses and decrease brain lesion buildup and, therefore, are important for long-term therapy.

   a. Interferon-β decreases the frequency of relapses by about one-third. These medications are given subcutaneously or IM.

   b. Glatiramer acetate given with daily subcutaneous injections also decreases the frequency of relapses by about one-third. Interferon-β and Glatiramer are considered tier 1 disease-modifying agents.

   c. Other disease-modifying agents are available and should be considered based on the severity of disease and medication risks. These medications reduce the frequency of relapses more significantly than Interferon-β or Glatiramer, but they are also associated with potentially more serious side effects. These include natalizumab, which has a risk of progressive multifocal leukoencephalopathy (PML) associated with JC virus, fingolimod, mitoxantrone, dimethyl fumarate, and teriflunomide.

   d. Ocrelizumab is the only disease-modifying agent approved for primary progressive MS.

3. Additional symptomatic therapies for MS include the following:

   a. Baclofen or tizanidine help reduce spasticity.

   b. Several agents may relieve urologic dysfunction. Anticholinergics (e.g., oxybutynin) may be effective to relieve bladder urgency. Urinary retention may require straight catheterization.

Dementia

A. General characteristics

1. The fifth edition of the *Diagnostic and Statistical Manual of Mental Disorders* identifies neurocognitive disorders as the umbrella that contains dementia and other cognitive disorders. Neurocognitive disorders can be either major or mild depending on severity. For example, the categorization of Alzheimer's Disease (AD) can be major neurocognitive disorder caused by AD or mild neurocognitive disorder caused by AD.

> 💡 Delirium is sudden and reversible; dementia is more likely progressive and is not reversible.

2. Delirium can frequently be confused with dementia. Delirium is a condition with relatively sudden onset (hours to days) of reduced attention and awareness accompanied by a deficit in memory, language, perception, or other cognitive impairment. This condition is frequently owing to a medical condition (e.g., urinary tract infection [UTI]), substance-related disorder, or metabolic disorder. Delirium differs from dementia in its rapid onset and fluctuating course throughout the day as well as potential for cure.

3. Dementia is characterized by a progressive impairment of intellectual functioning, with compromise in at least one of the following spheres of mental activity: language, learning and memory, complex attention, executive function, social cognition, and perceptual-motor function.

4. AD is the most common form of dementia; other forms include vascular dementia, Lewy body dementia, dementia caused by other degenerative disorders (Parkinson's, Huntington's, etc.), frontotemporal dementia, and dementia caused by infection (HIV, Creutzfeldt–Jakob).

B. AD—may be categorized as mild or major neurocognitive disorder

   1. General characteristics

   a. AD has a characteristic pathology consisting of intracellular neurofibrillary tangles and extracellular neuritic plaques.

   b. AD is the most common cause of chronic dementia, constituting about three-fourths of patients with dementia.

   c. The most significant risk factor for AD is older age; other risk factors include family history and genetics. Apolipoprotein E ε4 allele is a risk factor for AD.

   d. The disease is characterized by steadily progressive memory loss and other cognitive deficits, which typically begin during the seventh or eighth decade of life.

   2. Clinical features

   a. The diagnosis of major neurocognitive disorder owing to AD can be established when an otherwise alert patient exhibits slowly progressive memory and learning loss and at least one other cognitive domain deficit, such as language difficulties, inability to perform complex motor activities (perceptive-motor domain), inattention—especially in environments with multiple stimuli (complex attention domain), poor problem-solving abilities (executive function domain), or inappropriate social behavior (social cognition domain). These domains can be evaluated with history supplemented with tools such as the Mini-Mental Status Examination, Montreal Cognitive Assessment, or with formal neuropsychological testing. The symptoms have to be of a significant severity to interfere with patient's ability to do independent activities and must not be owing to a medical condition such as depression.

   > Alzheimer's is a clinical diagnosis; definitive diagnosis requires brain tissue and is only done postmortem.

   b. The diagnosis of mild neurocognitive disorder caused by AD can be established with slowly progressive decline in one domain—memory and learning. The symptoms must not be owing to another condition such as depression, vascular dementia, or toxic encephalopathy; they must also not be severe enough to interfere with the patient's performance of independent activities.

   c. Formal neuropsychological testing can help to confirm the suspected diagnosis and document the progression of disease.

   3. Diagnostic studies

   a. Initial laboratory tests should include CBC, thyroid-stimulating hormone (TSH), and vitamin B_{12}; additional labs may be indicated in certain patients, such as serum electrolytes, calcium, glucose, renal, and liver function tests. These labs are completed to rule out treatable causes as well as to establish a baseline.

   b. MRI or CT of the head is helpful and indicated to rule out other treatable causes of dementia.

   4. Treatment

   a. Standard medical therapy, initially in low doses, is useful in treating insomnia, agitation, and depression.

   b. Acetylcholinesterase inhibitors, such as donepezil, galantamine, or rivastigmine, may improve symptoms in patients with AD. They do not appear to affect disease progression.

   > AD treatment must start low and go slow; patient supervision is required.

   c. Memantine is an *N*-methyl-D-aspartic acid receptor antagonist that is thought to regulate glutamate and has been approved for use in moderate-to-severe AD. Memantine can be added to an acetylcholinesterase inhibitor (preferred), or it can be used alone in moderate-to-severe Alzheimer's dementia.

   d. Vigilant family supervision is required. Day care centers and respite care are adjuncts to family supervision.

C. Vascular dementia

   1. General characteristics

a. Can be a mild or major neurocognitive disorder. Mild neurocognitive disorder does not limit or affect patient's ability to perform independent activities.

b. Twenty-five percent or more of patients with a chronic dementia have cerebrovascular disease, but only about 10% of dementia patients have purely vascular dementia.

c. Vascular dementia is common. It is the second most common type of dementia.

d. Risk factors for vascular dementia are the same as for stroke: increasing age, physical inactivity, cigarette smokers, hypertension, hyperlipidemia, diabetes mellitus, carotid artery disease (with symptoms), coronary atherosclerotic disease, and the presence of atrial fibrillation.

e. Vascular dementia is frequently associated with history of TIA or stroke followed by dementia symptoms; however, some patients will have MRI evidence of previous silent strokes during imaging workup for dementia. This can be an indication that the patient has vascular dementia or mixed AD and vascular dementia.

> Vascular dementia is differentiated from other causes by its stepwise manner of decline with periods of stability in between.

2. Clinical features

a. Vascular dementia symptoms typically occur in a stepwise manner after strokes and are related to the affected area of the CNS. Two distinct syndromes have been described: cortical and subcortical.

(1) Cortical symptoms include speech difficulty, trouble performing routine tasks, sensory interpretation difficulty, confusion, amnesia, and executive dysfunction.

(2) Subcortical symptoms include gait problems, urinary difficulties, motor deficits, and personality changes.

b. Dementia may be accompanied by focal neurologic findings on physical examination, such as unilateral weakness, Babinski's sign, or unilateral hyperreflexia.

c. Social behaviors may be well maintained, so mental status testing is important to establish the diagnosis.

d. Progression of the disease leads to loss of computational ability, problems with word finding and concentration, difficulty with routine daily activities, and, ultimately, complete disorientation and social withdrawal.

3. Diagnostic studies: CBC, TSH, B_{12}, liver enzymes, electrolytes, BUN, and creatinine. MRI of the brain is preferred to CT to evaluate for evidence of previous strokes.

4. Treatment

a. Control of hypertension, hyperlipidemia, and other metabolic disorders may help prevent new strokes and, therefore, progression of symptoms.

b. Patients may need antiplatelet therapy if indicated by vascular conditions.

c. A trial of anticholinesterase medication is reasonable if the patient might have concomitant AD, but this is not beneficial in patients with strictly vascular dementia.

d. As in AD, standard medical regimens can be used to treat insomnia, agitation, or depression.

e. Caregivers should identify and reduce home hazards and arrange, as necessary, community services or preparation of an advance directive.

D. Frontotemporal dementia

1. General characteristics

a. This clinical syndrome is secondary to degeneration of the frontal lobes of the brain and may include the temporal lobes.

b. Symptoms typically begin at an early age, between 40 and 60 years.

c. Progression of symptoms is more rapid with frontotemporal dementia than with other types of dementia with typical survival after diagnosis of only about 4 years.

> Frontotemporal dementia is distinguished by the prominence of behavioral and personality changes.

2. Clinical features

a. Frontal lobe symptoms include behavioral symptoms (euphoria, apathy, and disinhibition) and compulsive disorders.

b. Other varieties of frontotemporal dementia cause significant speech impairment.

c. Several primitive reflexes (frontal release signs) are often elicited, including the palmomental, palmar grasp, and rooting reflexes.

d. Memory impairment may be spared in contrast to AD.

3. Diagnostic studies

a. MRI often reveals frontal lobe and/or anterior temporal lobe atrophy but, in early cases, may appear normal.

b. Positron emission tomography scans classically show frontal and/or anterior temporal hypometabolism, which helps to differentiate from Alzheimer's associated with biparietal hypometabolism.

4. **Treatment**

a. Cholinesterase inhibitors are not effective in frontotemporal dementia.

b. Supportive care is essential as there is no curative treatment.

c. Behavioral symptoms may require treatment, such as selective serotonin reuptake inhibitors (SSRIs), for depression.

E. **Pseudodementia**

1. General characteristics

a. *Pseudodementia* is a term that describes patients with psychiatric illness who appear to be demented.

b. It is often seen as part of a major depressive episode.

2. **Clinical characteristics**

a. Patients typically complain of memory problems, but, with thorough testing, memory, language, attention span, and concentration appear intact.

b. In true dementia, the patient will often give wrong answers, have poor attention and concentration, and appear indifferent or unconcerned.

3. **Treatment**

a. Antidepressant therapy with an SSRI is the first line of therapy.

b. Acetylcholinesterase inhibitors are not indicated for pseudodementia.

Headache

A. **Tension headache**

1. General characteristics

a. Tension headache is the most common type of headache, but most patients do not seek medical care for these mild-to-moderate headaches.

b. Tension headaches were once thought to be secondary to muscle contraction. Current theory relates tension headaches to abnormal, increased neuronal sensitivity (Table 11-5).

2. **Clinical features**

a. Tension headaches are typified by a bandlike mild-to-moderate pain around the head or generalized head pain. Discomfort is usually reported as steady or aching (nonpulsatile) and is not associated with focal neurologic symptoms. It is typically bilateral and without the symptoms frequently associated with migraine, such as photophobia, phonophobia, nausea, or vomiting.

b. Pain may be episodic or chronic.

c. Insomnia, stress, and anxiety are typical precipitants.

d. There may be tenderness of the temporalis, masseter, posterior cervical, trapezius, sternocleidomastoid, and occipital muscles, but the physical examination generally is normal.

> MRI and PET scan are indicated in the workup for frontotemporal dementia.

> Tension headaches are typically bilateral, nonpulsatile, and without systemic symptoms.

Table 11-5 | Headaches

Type	Place	Quality	Aura	Photophobia/Phonophobia	Other
Migraine	Unilateral	Pulsatile	Migraine with aura Migraine without aura	Typical Prefer to lie still in dark, quiet room	Nausea, vomiting Common triggers
Tension	Bandlike Generalized	Nonpulsatile Tight	±	Not usual	Precipitated by stress, anxiety, insomnia
Cluster	Unilateral Periorbital	Episodic, clusters	None	Autonomic symptoms Unable to stay still	Oxygen for acute treatment

3. Diagnostic studies

a. Routine laboratory tests are helpful only in ruling out concurrent illness or an underlying rheumatologic condition. For example, ESR and/or C-reactive protein may indicate temporal arteritis in the appropriate patient.

b. Imaging studies like brain MRI or CT are usually not indicated and only done if there is an atypical presentation with a high index of suspicion for a structural lesion.

4. Treatment

a. Initial medical treatment is with analgesics, such as aspirin, acetaminophen, or nonsteroidal anti-inflammatory drugs (NSAIDs). If not effective, a trial of antimigraine agents may be employed. These may help if the patient also has migraine headache disorder.

b. Ketorolac IM can be used in the outpatient or hospital setting for more severe tension-type headaches.

c. When appropriate, local heat and muscle relaxants may be employed for muscle-tension discomfort. Physical therapy and stress reduction techniques are also helpful.

d. In the setting of depression or significant stress or chronic recalcitrant tension headaches, antidepressants and/or psychotherapy may be indicated.

e. If headaches are chronic or frequent, prophylaxis with amitriptyline or nortriptyline may be prescribed in an attempt to prevent the headaches.

B. Migraine headache

1. General characteristics

a. Migraine pathophysiology is thought to relate to dysfunction of the trigeminovascular system. Stimulation of this sensitized system results in the perivascular release of substance P and calcitonin gene–related peptide and subsequent neurogenic inflammation with intensified pain.

b. Migraine headaches are typically moderate or severe in intensity, worsen with activity, present unilaterally, and may have throbbing or pulsating discomfort. Patients can often identify migraine triggers, such as red wine, aspartame, hormonal changes, weather changes, changes in sleep pattern, and stress.

c. Patients often relate a family history of migraine disease. Women are affected more commonly than men; migraines often follow the menstrual cycle pattern.

2. Clinical features

a. Migraine with an aura is present in about a quarter of migraine sufferers. The aura commonly involves visual changes, field cuts, or flashing lights. The aura usually lasts several minutes but <1 hour.

(1) The throbbing head pain often occurs during or after the aura.

(2) Migraine with aura can also be associated with transient neurologic deficits and hemisensory loss. It may be mistake for a TIA.

Migraine headache is typically unilateral, pulsatile, and associated with nausea, vomiting, and sensitivity to light and sound.

(3) Less frequently, patients may have an aura of speech abnormalities.

(4) During or after the aura, typical associated migraine symptoms of photophobia, phonophobia, nausea, and vomiting occur.

b. Migraine without aura is a more common presentation of migraine and is frequently accompanied by the same associated symptoms of nausea, vomiting, photophobia, and phonophobia.

c. Headaches typically last 4 to 72 hours.

d. Patients also exhibit irritability and fatigue.

e. Migraine patients often retreat to quiet, dark rooms and prefer to lie quietly. This is in contrast to patients with cluster headaches who tend to move around incessantly.

3. Diagnostic studies

> Headache workup: Labs and brain imaging are performed as indicated by the clinical picture; not routinely required.

a. Routine laboratory tests are done only to help rule out other concurrent disorders such as infection, stroke, seizure, or toxins, if indicated by clinical presentation. Sedimentation rate can be ordered if there is suspicion of temporal arteritis.

b. Imaging studies (i.e., brain MRI) are done only in select clinical settings and then only to rule out causes of secondary headache. Examples of possible indications to image the brain are headache onset after age 50, focal neurologic deficit on examination that does not resolve when the headache resolves, refractory to treatment headaches, headaches increasing in severity and frequency, thunderclap headache, and new headaches in a patient with malignancy or immunodeficiency virus.

4. Treatment

a. Mild-to-moderate migraine headache

(1) Abortive therapy is recommended with acetaminophen or NSAIDs.

(2) Consider a triptan if simple analgesics are not effective.

b. Moderate-to-severe migraine headache

(1) Triptans are the first option (e.g., sumatriptan, zolmitriptan, rizatriptan, naratriptan, almotriptan, frovatriptan, eletriptan).

(2) Triptan plus NSAID is also effective and reduces the need for additional dosages.

(3) For more severe headaches with associated nausea, one option is subcutaneous sumatriptan plus antiemetic (i.e., prochlorperazine or metoclopramide).

(4) Alternative treatment for severe headaches with nausea is IV dihydroergotamine (DHE) 1 mg subcutaneously. Give promethazine 25 mg IV before DHE.

> *Chronic migraine* is defined as pain for 15 days or more per month; chemoprophylactic therapy is warranted.

(5) Another option for severe migraine with nausea is ketorolac 30 to 60 mg IM plus metoclopramide 10 mg IV.

(6) IV diphenhydramine (12.5 to 25 mg) should be given to patients who are treated with antiemetics to prevent extrapyramidal symptoms.

c. In the setting of frequent migraine headache, prophylactic measures may be employed.

(1) Pharmacologic prophylaxis for migraine might include β-blockers, tricyclic antidepressants, calcium channel blockers, NSAIDs (for menstrual-related migraine), valproic acid, or topiramate.

(2) The newest additions to migraine prophylaxis options are the anti–calcitonin gene–related peptide monoclonal antibody medicines: erenumab, fremanezumab, and galcanezumab. These medications are given by subcutaneous injection once a month. Patients typically fail migraine prophylaxis with two or three of the following different categories of medications before trying an anti–calcitonin gene–related peptide medication: an antihypertensive, an anticonvulsant, and/or an antidepressant.

(3) Biofeedback therapy is often employed in migraine patients in the hope of reducing the number of headaches by helping patients deal more effectively with stress.

d. Patients with known migraine triggers should avoid exposure to the trigger.

e. Psychotherapy and stress reduction may be helpful.

C. **Cluster headache**

> Cluster headaches are typically unilateral and dramatic with tearing, sweating, conjunctival hyperemia, nasal congestion, and meiosis.

1. General characteristics

   a. Cluster headache pathophysiology is thought to be secondary to activation of the hypothalamic system, trigeminovascular system, and the autonomic intracranial system.

   b. Cluster headaches are extremely severe, unilateral, periorbital headaches that are short in duration (15 to 180 minutes) and may occur several times a day over a period of weeks to months.

   c. The typical patient with cluster headaches is a middle-aged male. Cluster headaches are three to seven times more common in men.

   d. Onset of headache is usually in the third decade of life.

2. **Clinical features**

   a. The unilateral pain of cluster headache is often accompanied by autonomic symptoms on the same side as the pain: lacrimation, conjunctival injection, nasal congestion, forehead sweating, miosis, and ptosis.

   b. Patients with cluster headache often pace incessantly around the room because the pain is severe and not relieved by rest. This is in contrast to the migraineur who seeks rest in a dark and quiet area.

3. Diagnostic studies

   a. As in other headache syndromes, laboratory studies only help to identify other concurrent conditions and to rule out other causes of acute head and facial pain.

   b. Brain MRI with and without contrast is indicated for the initial diagnosis to rule out other causes of acute cephalgia.

4. **Treatment**

> 100% oxygen is the first-line treatment of a cluster headache.

   a. Abortive and symptomatic therapy of choice for cluster headaches is administration of 100% oxygen at 12 L per minute with a non-rebreathing mask for 15 minutes. The second option is injection of subcutaneous sumatriptan.

   b. Prophylactic therapy of choice for cluster headaches is verapamil. Preventive therapy with a short course of oral corticosteroids may be given for cluster headache periods that are less than a few months.

Movement Disorders

A. **Essential tremor (familial tremor)**

1. General characteristics

   a. The cause of essential tremor is unknown. It is often inherited in an autosomal dominant manner and may thus be called *familial tremor*.

   b. Tremor may begin at any age, but the prevalence is higher with increased age.

   c. It is enhanced by emotional stress; small quantities of alcohol commonly provide dramatic, temporary relief from the tremor.

   d. Although the tremor may interfere with manual skills, it causes only minimal disability initially.

   e. Essential tremor can be easily confused with enhanced physiologic tremor. An enhanced physiologic tremor may not be visible most of the time. It worsens with stress, caffeine, and stimulant medications and may be temporarily relieved with a small amount of alcohol. It does not typically cause disability.

2. **Clinical features**

   a. Patients with essential tremor display a rhythmic to-and-fro movement, usually of the upper extremities. The tremor is an action tremor and can be elicited by having the patient hold out their arms. Sometimes, the head and the voice are involved. The tremor may initially be in only one extremity. The lower extremities are not usually involved.

   b. Speech may also be affected if the laryngeal muscles are involved.

3. **Laboratory studies:** No laboratory testing is needed or warranted.

4. **Treatment**

   a. Low doses of a β-blocker, usually propranolol, may be useful in controlling tremor. This medication should be used with caution in asthmatics and those with bradycardia.

   b. Primidone may be useful in controlling tremor if propranolol fails.

   c. The combination of primidone and propranolol is effective in some patients who are refractory to treatment with one agent.

   d. Patients who progress with persistent disabling upper extremity action tremor and are refractory to treatment can benefit from deep brain stimulation.

B. **Parkinson's disease**

   1. General characteristics

      a. Parkinson's disease is characterized by degeneration of neurons in the substantia nigra, causing a deficiency of the neurotransmitter dopamine and an imbalance of dopamine and acetylcholine. The dopamine deficiency occurs in the basal ganglia. Lewy body deposition in the brain is also associated with Parkinson's disease, but Lewy bodies can also be seen in other neurodegenerative disorders.

      b. Parkinson's disease is a common neurodegenerative disease; only Alzheimer's dementia is a more common neurodegenerative disorder.

      c. The disease occurs in all ethnic groups, with an approximately equal sex distribution, and most often begins between the ages of 45 and 65 years.

      d. Patients generally complain of problems related to their slowed movements, difficulty arising from a seated position, difficulty ascending and descending stairs, trouble with getting dressed, and difficulty with handwriting (micrographia).

   2. **Clinical features**

      a. Early clinical nonmotor symptoms associated with development of Parkinson's disease include anosmia, depression, constipation, and rapid eye movement (REM) sleep behavior disorder.

      b. The essential features that establish a diagnosis of Parkinson's disease are resting tremor, bradykinesia, rigidity, and unstable posture.

      c. The usual presenting complaint is tremor (about two-thirds of patients). The tremor is most noticeable at rest, at 4 to 6 cycles per second, and may be only very slight with voluntary effort. It is characterized as a "pill-rolling" tremor.

      d. Initially, the tremor is confined to one limb or the limbs on one side, but eventually, it may be present in all the limbs and the lips and mouth; it usually does not affect the head.

      e. Bradykinesia, or a generalized slowness of voluntary movements, is evident in the slow, shuffling gait. Other findings are reduced arm swing, slowed rapid alternating movements, infrequent blinking, micrographia, and masklike facies.

      f. Rigidity is found on passive range of motion testing; cogwheel rigidity may be noted.

The tremor of essential tremor is an action tremor, not seen at rest.

The tremor of Parkinson's disease is a resting tremor described as "pill-rolling" and progresses to include all extremities as well as the lips and mouth.

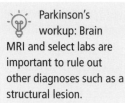
Parkinson's workup: Brain MRI and select labs are important to rule out other diagnoses such as a structural lesion.

g. Postural instability is seen, including difficulty in standing from a seated position, unsteadiness on turning, difficulty in stopping, and a tendency to fall.

h. Depression and dementia develop in >50% of patients over time.

3. Diagnostic studies

a. Generally, no laboratory testing is needed or warranted.

b. Blood tests and imaging studies can be done to rule out other causes of parkinsonism.

c. Brain imaging with MRI is beneficial to identify structural lesions or hydrocephalus.

4. **Treatment**

a. Treatment focuses on symptom management. There is no cure, and the disease is progressive.

b. Therapy should usually be initiated with a monoamine oxidase inhibitor, dopamine agonist, or with levodopa.

c. Selegiline and rasagiline are monoamine oxidase B inhibitors; they inhibit breakdown of dopamine, and some studies indicate that they may alter progression of the disease. These medications are usually used for mild symptoms.

d. Dopamine agonists, such as first-generation bromocriptine or second-generation pramipexole or ropinirole, act directly on dopamine receptors. They have a longer duration of action than levodopa. Currently, dopamine agonists are frequently used in younger patients with Parkinson's disease before levodopa. The benefits of dopamine agonists are not as great as levodopa, but the side effects are less severe. Caution should be used when prescribing this category of medication because of the potential side effect of impulse control disorders. Patients should be screened before prescribing this category medication and asked at office visits about impulsive behavior. If impulsive behavior occurs, the medication should be discontinued.

e. Levodopa is converted to dopamine in the body and initially improves all symptoms of Parkinson's disease. Carbidopa, when added to levodopa in various combinations, allows lower doses of levodopa and reduces the side effect of nausea. With prolonged use of levodopa, motor side effects of dyskinesias (inability to perform difficult voluntary movements) occur. The lowest effective dose should be used to limit side effects.

f. Failure of a patient to initially respond favorably to levodopa should cause question of the diagnosis of Parkinson's disease.

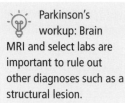
Response to dopamine therapy confirms the diagnosis of parkinsonism; levodopa has the best penetration with fewest side effects.

g. Amantadine, a mild anticholinergic, is often helpful for young patients with tremor, but no disability. Later in the disease progression, amantadine is used to treat dyskinesias.

h. Catecholamine-*O*-methyltransferase (COMT) inhibitors reduce the metabolism of levodopa to 3-*O*-methyldopa and result in more stable plasma levels and more constant dopaminergic stimulation of the brain. Two COMT agents, tolcapone and entacapone, are available as adjuncts to levodopa/carbidopa therapy; these medications may permit a lowering of the total levodopa/carbidopa dose.

i. Physical therapy may help some patients, and quality of life may be improved with household modifications or the availability of special utensils.

j. Psychological support for both the patient and the family is helpful (Table 11-6).

C. **Huntington's disease**

1. General characteristics

a. Huntington's disease is a neurodegenerative disease caused by a trinucleotide repeat in the huntingtin gene on the short arm of chromosome 4. The number of repeats determines how early the onset of disease symptoms will occur.

b. Huntington's disease is an inherited, autosomal dominant disorder that occurs throughout the world in all ethnic groups, with a prevalence of 2.7 per 100,000.

Table 11-6 | Anti-Parkinsonian Medications

Type	Examples	Notes
Monoamine oxidase inhibitors (MAOIs)	Selegiline Rasagiline	For patients with mild symptoms
Dopamine agonists	Bromocriptine Pramipexole Ropinirole	Act directly on dopamine receptors Longer duration of action than levodopa Used in younger patients before levodopa Side effects less severe Warning: impulse control disorders
Levodopa	Levodopa/carbidopa	Carbidopa reduces nausea Dyskinesias with prolonged use
Adjunctive therapies	Amantadine	Used in patients with tremor but no disability Treat dyskinesias
	Catecholamine-*O*-methyltransferase (COMT) inhibitors (tolcapone, entacapone)	Stabilize dopamine levels Adjunct to levodopa/carbidopa
	Physical therapy	
	Psychological support	Patient and family

The prevalence is variable in different populations: In people of European descent, the rate is 5.7 per 100,000.

   c. Symptoms of the disease usually do not develop until after 30 years of age. Often by this time, those who are affected have already had children who may eventually be similarly affected.

2. Clinical features

   a. The disease is characterized by progressive chorea and dementia; it is usually fatal within 15 to 20 years.

   b. The earliest mental changes are often behavioral, with irritability, moodiness, and antisocial behavior that generally progress to an obvious dementia.

   c. The earliest physical signs may be a mere restlessness or fidgetiness, but, eventually, severe choreiform movements and dystonic posturing occur.

3. Diagnostic studies

   a. Genetic testing confirms the diagnosis.

   b. Brain MRI demonstrates cerebral atrophy as well as atrophy of the caudate nucleus.

4. Treatment

   a. Currently, there are no disease-modifying drugs for Huntington's disease. It has no cure, and progression of the disease cannot be halted.

   b. Symptomatic treatment for the disease may include phenothiazines to control dyskinesia and haloperidol or clozapine to control any behavioral disturbances.

   c. Children of Huntington's patients should receive genetic counseling. Genetic testing is very sensitive and specific and can make a definitive diagnosis even in the presymptomatic state.

D. Tourette's syndrome

   1. General characteristics

     a. Tics are the characteristic feature of Tourette's syndrome. Tics can be motor or vocal. Involuntary motor activities like blinking, jerking, or grimacing are common. Vocal tics are involuntary, and they can manifest as grunting, repeating words, or blurting out obscene words (coprolalia).

> Huntington's is autosomal dominant and often manifests with subtle behavioral changes before motor signs are apparent.

b. The onset of symptoms occurs in childhood between the ages of 2 and 10 years; rarely, tics have an onset up to age 21 years.

c. The prevalence of Tourette's syndrome is higher in boys than in girls.

d. Tics resolve or improve in about one-half of the patients by age 18 years.

e. Comorbidities include attention-deficit hyperactivity disorder, obsessive–compulsive disorder, learning problems, and behavior disorders.

> Diagnosis of Tourette's requires the presence of both motor and phonic tics several times per day, nearly every day, for 1 year.

2. **Clinical features**

a. For a diagnosis of Tourette's syndrome, the tics must occur several times per day nearly every day for at least 1 year and vary in number, frequency, and nature.

b. Motor and phonic tics must be present to make the diagnosis. These do not have to be present at the same time. Motor tics that involve the face, head, and shoulders (e.g., sniffing, blinking, frowning, shoulder shrugging, head thrusting) occur initially in most patients.

c. Phonic tics like grunts, barks, hisses, coughing, or verbal utterances are the most common initial manifestation. The percentage of patients with Tourette's syndrome who have coprolalia (involuntary obscene word tic) has been reported as <10% to 40%.

d. Some tics are self-mutilating, such as nail biting, hair pulling, and biting of the lips or tongue.

3. Diagnostic studies

a. Diagnostic evaluation with head CT or MRI is normal.

b. Volumetric MRI may show volume loss in the caudate nucleus.

4. **Treatment**

a. Some patients with mild symptoms may be treated with behavioral therapy, counseling, and education only. Treatment with medication is indicated if symptoms adversely affect relationships, school activities, or work performance.

b. The first-line agents for tics in children are the α-agonists clonidine or guanfacine.

c. The α-agonists clonidine and guanfacine are also good options for those with Tourette's syndrome and concomitant attention-deficit hyperactivity disorder.

d. Patients with Tourette's syndrome and obsessive–compulsive disorder can be treated with cognitive-behavioral therapy. If symptoms persist, an SSRI, such as fluoxetine, can be added to the cognitive-behavioral therapy.

e. Behavior therapy is likely to be beneficial in patients with Tourette's syndrome, especially in those unable to tolerate medications or in those patients who want to avoid medications.

> Cerebral palsy is related to early cerebral injury; presentation and treatment goals vary widely.

E. **Cerebral palsy**

1. Cerebral palsy is often associated with prematurity and/or low birth weight. It is a chronic nonprogressive impairment of muscle tone, strength, coordination, or movements. It is believed to result from cerebral injury before birth, during delivery, or in the perinatal period.

2. Clinical features are widely varied and include spasticity (75% of patients), lack of coordination, fine motor difficulties, ataxia, lethargy, hypotonia, or dystonia. Seizure disorders, cognitive impairment, and disorders of speech, hearing, vision, and sensory perception often accompany cerebral palsy.

3. Physical examination may reveal hyperreflexia, abnormal tone, microcephaly, limb length discrepancies, cataracts, retinopathy, and congenital heart defects.

4. MRI of the brain is indicated to identify the etiology of the injury. This is abnormal in up to 90% of patients with cerebral palsy. Additional diagnostic testing is done to rule out other neurologic disorders, if the MRI findings are atypical, or if the history and physical examination are not consistent with cerebral palsy. Testing for metabolic

disorders includes blood gases, creatine kinase, urine organic acid analysis, blood amino acids, glucose, lactate, pyruvate, and ammonia concentrations.

5. Referral to a geneticist for genetic testing may be indicated if an etiology for the cerebral palsy is not evident, or if indicated by family history.

6. Treatment is supportive, with the goal of attaining maximum function and potential in physical, occupational, and speech ability. Pharmacologic treatment of spasticity and seizures is often required.

F. Restless leg syndrome (RLS)

1. Patients feel a subjective need or urge to move the legs and possibly the arms. Abnormal sensations including tingling, itching, heaviness, burning, coldness, or tension may accompany the urge to move the limbs. Symptoms occur most commonly during periods of prolonged inactivity or rest. Activity or movement relieves the urge to move, but symptoms return upon rest of the limbs.

2. RLS occurs in ~10% of adults.

3. Most cases are primary, although RLS may occur secondary to peripheral neuropathy, uremia, pregnancy, or iron deficiency.

4. The majority of patients also demonstrate frequent involuntary movements during sleep or at rest. Sleep disturbance is common.

5. **Treatment**

   a. In patients with reduced ferritin levels, replacement of iron will help.

   b. Dopamine agonists (e.g., pramipexole and ropinirole) are the drugs of choice. These drugs can cause or worsen impulse control disorder, so caution should be used when prescribing these medications and patients should be informed of this potential side effect.

   c. α-2-δ Calcium channel ligands gabapentin or pregabalin are also effective options.

   d. Benzodiazepines (e.g., clonazepam) may also be effective either alone or in combination with other treatments.

   e. Daily exertional activities such as exercise, warm baths, and leg messages may provide some improvement in symptoms.

> Restless leg syndrome is defined as an abnormal *urge* to move the legs, not any myoclonic activity.

Diseases of Peripheral Nerves

A. Bell's palsy

1. General considerations

   a. The prevalence of Bell's palsy is highest in those between the ages 15 to 45 years, but occurs in all ages.

   b. Bell's palsy is most commonly caused by herpes simplex virus (HSV) activation. Other viruses (e.g., herpes zoster), trauma, neoplasia, or toxins can also be causative. The end result is damage to the myelin layer of the facial nerve.

   c. Unilateral facial muscle weakness and drooping are the primary complaint, with onset occurring over hours and without apparent cause.

   d. There can be a paralysis of all muscles supplied by CN VII (complete palsy) or variable weakness in different muscles (incomplete palsy).

2. **Clinical features**

   a. Facial muscle weakness typically begins abruptly but may progress over a matter of hours to 3 days. Paralysis involves the forehead and lower face; patients cannot close the eye, raise the brow, or smile on the affected side.

   b. Pain about the ipsilateral ear often precedes the facial weakness or is noted concurrently with the weakness.

> In diagnosing Bell's palsy, no abnormality beyond motor function of CN VII is found in this unilateral facial paralysis; no abnormalities in ear or CNS.

> Bell's palsy is a clinical diagnosis; imaging and labs are only indicated if necessary to rule out severe conditions.

    c. Depending on the site of the nerve lesion, patients may demonstrate impairment of taste, lacrimation, or hyperacusis.

    d. Clinical evaluation reveals no abnormality beyond the motor function of CN VII.

    e. The weakness peaks in about 21 days or less, and recovery (partial or complete) occurs within 6 months.

    f. More than 70% of patients fully recover, but some patients have chronic disfigurement or pain.

3. Diagnostic studies

    a. Bell's palsy is a clinical diagnosis. Specific diagnostic confirmation with nerve conduction studies or EMG is only done in patients with atypical or prolonged Bell's palsy.

    b. Appropriate diagnostic procedures, such as brain MRI, may be done to identify other conditions that may produce facial palsy, including stroke, tumors, Lyme disease, AIDS, and sarcoidosis.

4. Treatment

    a. Supportive care such as lubricating eye drops to prevent corneal drying and patching the affected eye at night is recommended.

    b. A course of oral prednisone, if begun soon after the onset of symptoms, has been shown to increase the percentage of patients who completely recover. The dose of prednisone is 60 mg a day for 5 days followed by a 5-day taper.

    c. Antivirals such as acyclovir or valacyclovir can be added to prednisone to improve long-term outcome. Antivirals alone (without corticosteroids) should not be used.

    d. Possible incomplete recovery is associated with patients presenting with severe pain, complete palsy, hyperacusis, or advanced age.

B.   Diabetic peripheral neuropathy

1. General considerations

    a. Peripheral neuropathies become more common with increased age; nearly one-third of the population over age 80 is affected by some type of peripheral neuropathy. Diabetic polyneuropathy causes about one-half of the peripheral neuropathy cases.

    b. Diabetic peripheral neuropathy can cause sensory, motor, or autonomic symptoms. A common presentation is bilateral lower extremity sensory loss, numbness, or pain that progresses proximally over time.

    c. Less commonly, patients may develop mononeuropathies involving specific peripheral nerve or CN.

    d. Neuropathy is generally related to the duration and severity of hyperglycemia, but it may be the presenting symptom in occult diabetes.

2. Clinical features

> The most common form of diabetic neuropathy develops in a "stocking-and-glove" pattern, with symptoms occurring more common in the lower extremity than in the upper extremity.

    a. Symptoms are more common in the lower extremities than in the upper extremities and consist of pain, dysesthesias (burning), paresthesias, numbness, weakness, or anesthesia.

    b. A distal symmetric polyneuropathy can also be diagnosed before the development of any symptoms in the form of reduced deep tendon reflexes (e.g., ankle jerk) or impaired vibratory sensation.

    c. Autonomic complications related to diabetic neuropathy include constipation, gastroparesis, postural hypotension, cardiac arrhythmias, impaired thermoregulatory sweating, and erectile dysfunction. Neuropathy to the level of the calf is correlated with high risk of autonomic neuropathy.

    d. Patients with diabetic neuropathy are at risk for chronic wounds and amputation, especially in those who also smoke cigarettes.

3. Diagnostic studies

   a. Screening for distal symmetric polyneuropathy in diabetics should be accomplished at diagnosis for patients with type 2 diabetes and 5 years after diagnosis for patients with type 1 diabetes. All patients should subsequently undergo annual screening.

   b. Screening in diabetics for distal symmetrical polyneuropathy should consist of asking about symptoms, checking pinprick sensation in the feet, performing proprioception, vibration, and 10-g monofilament testing. Serial nerve conduction studies can be completed to document the presence, severity, and course of the neuropathy, but are generally not needed.

   c. Additional diagnostic workup may be appropriate to rule out other causes of polyneuropathy, including uremia, alcohol abuse, nutritional deficiencies, connective tissue disease, vasculitis, vitamin B_{12} deficiency, hypothyroidism, or amyloidosis.

4. Treatment

   a. Control of hyperglycemia is vital to prevent or slow progression of the disease. Regular inspection of feet, proper food hygiene, and prompt follow-up of any skin changes or pressure are essential.

   b. Duloxetine, gabapentin, pregabalin, or amitriptyline may be useful in controlling deep, constant, aching pain.

   c. Postural hypotension may respond to salt supplementation, lower extremity pressure stockings, or medications, such as fludrocortisone or midodrine.

   d. There are no specific treatments for diabetic peripheral nerve complications, with the exception of an entrapment neuropathy that may respond to a decompression procedure.

> Control of diabetes and frequent monitoring significantly reduce the risk of the development and progression of neuropathy.

C. Guillain–Barré syndrome (GBS)

1. General considerations

   a. GBS is an acute immune-mediated polyneuropathy often following respiratory or gastrointestinal (GI) infections. Other triggers such as immunizations or surgical procedures are much less common, and in many cases, no cause is identified.

   b. GBS is described as progressive ascending flaccid paralysis. There are many varieties of GBS, but the most common in the United States (over 90% of cases) is acute inflammatory demyelinating polyradiculopathy.

   c. Infection with *Campylobacter jejuni* is the most common precipitant. Other viral precipitants are Epstein–Barr virus, cytomegalovirus, and HIV.

2. Clinical features

   a. Symmetrical weakness that begins in the lower extremities and ascends to the upper extremities is typical. Deep tendon reflexes are decreased or absent. Symmetric facial weakness occurs in more than half of the patients.

   b. Symptoms typically worsen over the first few weeks, then level off for several weeks before improvement in symptoms and function.

   c. Sensory abnormalities are common but generally less marked than the motor symptoms. Paresthesias in the distal extremities are common.

   d. Pain is present in most cases and can be severe in a subset of patients.

   e. Significant autonomic dysfunction may be noted, including tachycardia, cardiac irregularities, labile BP, disturbed sweating, impaired pulmonary function, sphincter disturbances, or paralytic ileus.

   f. GBS can be life-threatening if the muscles of respiration or swallowing are involved; nearly one-third of patients may require ventilatory assistance.

> Ascending paralysis is GBS until proven otherwise; it is an acute and life-threatening once the respiratory muscles become involved; one-third of patients require intubation.

3. Diagnostic studies

   a. Patients who have clinical signs and symptoms consistent with GBS should have a diagnostic workup. This should include an LP and nerve conduction studies with EMG.

> 💡 GBS requires hospitalization to maintain adequate respiration.

b. LP with CSF evaluation typically yields an elevated protein with cell counts that are normal.

c. Electrophysiologic studies may reveal marked slowing of nerve conduction velocities, both motor and sensory. These studies may also document denervation or axonal loss.

4. Treatment

a. Patients should be hospitalized with close monitoring of respiratory status with vital capacity. Neuromuscular and autonomic involvement may rapidly result in complications and death from respiratory failure or arrhythmias.

b. Plasmapheresis, instituted as early as possible, is very effective in reducing the time required for recovery and may reduce the likelihood of residual neurologic deficits. In patients who are severely affected, plasmapheresis may also shorten the time on a respirator as well as the length of time it may take to resume walking independently.

c. IV immunoglobulin (IVIG) is also very effective and used in preference to plasmapheresis in adults with cardiovascular instability and in children.

d. Patients benefit from physical, occupational, and speech therapy during rehabilitation.

e. More than half of the patients make a full recovery within 1 year, but some patients have persistent motor abnormalities and disability. The mortality rate in 1 year is ~5%.

D. Myasthenia gravis

1. General characteristics

a. Myasthenia gravis is a disorder of antibodies directed against the acetylcholine receptor on the muscle surface. These antibodies cause an increased rate of receptor destruction, leading to weakness.

b. Myasthenia gravis involves muscle weakness and fatigability, which improve with rest.

c. The onset of myasthenia gravis is usually insidious, but the disorder is sometimes made evident by a coincidental infection that exacerbates the symptoms.

d. The disorder may occur at any age but is more commonly diagnosed in young women and older men.

2. Clinical features

> 💡 Significant improvement after administering edrophonium confirms the diagnosis of myasthenia gravis.

a. Fluctuating weakness is common with myasthenia gravis. There is a tendency to have long-term spontaneous relapses and remissions that may last for weeks.

b. Typical presenting problems include ptosis, diplopia, difficulty in chewing or swallowing, respiratory difficulties, limb weakness, or a combination of any of these; over half of the patients present with ptosis and/or diplopia.

c. Clinical examination confirms the weakness and fatigability of affected muscles, which improves after a short rest.

d. Sensation is normal, and there are usually no reflex changes.

e. Thymus abnormalities are very common in patients with myasthenia gravis. Approximately 10% to 15% of patients with myasthenia gravis will have a thymoma.

3. Diagnostic studies

a. Chest CT or MRI should be obtained to rule out a coexisting thymoma.

b. Electrophysiologic studies may show a decrementing muscle response; these studies are helpful in making the diagnosis of myasthenia gravis. Repetitive nerve stimulation and single-fiber EMG are the two studies frequently used.

c. Serum assay for elevated levels of circulating acetylcholine receptor antibodies is another way of establishing the diagnosis; this assay is positive in 80% to 90% of patients. If negative, antibodies to muscle-specific tyrosine kinase (MuSK) should be checked. MuSK antibodies are positive in nearly half of those with myasthenia gravis and negative acetylcholine receptor antibodies.

d. The diagnosis may be confirmed if marked clinical improvement is achieved by administering a short-acting anticholinesterase (edrophonium).

4. Treatment

a. The mainstay of therapy is administration of the cholinesterase inhibitor pyridostigmine, which produces a transient improvement in strength. This has varying levels of success.

b. Corticosteroids and other immunosuppressive agents are chronic therapies that may be added to pyridostigmine if needed.

c. Acute exacerbations of symptoms can be caused by certain medications, infections, surgeries, or for unknown reasons. Patients with exacerbations can be treated with IVIG or plasmapheresis.

d. Thymectomy often leads to improvement of symptoms and may lead to remission of symptoms.

E. Complex regional pain syndrome (CRPS)

1. General characteristics

a. CRPS usually begins about a month after a fracture, sprain, crush injury, or an operation.

b. The disorder is characterized by regional pain in the affected limb that is greater than expected, restricted mobility, edema, color changes of the skin, and spotty bone thinning.

c. Most patients do not have an identifiable neurologic lesion responsible for the pain.

d. The cause of CRPS is not well understood, but it is thought to be partially secondary to abnormal sensitivity to inflammatory mediators of pain.

2. Clinical features

a. Most cases of CRPS occur following a soft-tissue injury; however, no inciting event is identified in about 10% of cases.

b. The hallmark feature of CRPS is severe burning or throbbing pain with associated allodynia in the affected region/extremity. Cyanosis, abnormal sensitivity to cold and warm exposure, abnormal skin temperature, and atrophy may also be present.

c. Other causes of these symptoms, depending on the presentation, include vasculitis, claudication, nerve root impingement, atrophy from disuse, and progressive systemic sclerosis.

3. Diagnostic studies

a. Bone scintigraphy and plain x-rays can support a diagnosis of CRPS, although the diagnosis is primarily clinical.

b. MRI, although not useful to diagnose CRPS, may be helpful to evaluate for other potential diagnoses.

4. Treatment

a. Early mobilization following an injury may be beneficial in CRPS. Referral to occupational therapy and physical therapy is recommended.

b. Pregabalin, gabapentin, amitriptyline, and nortriptyline are choices for pain relief.

c. NSAIDs may be beneficial in select patients.

d. Bisphosphonates, regional nerve blocks, or dorsal column stimulation may be effective if other treatments fail.

Clinical improvement after administering edrophonium makes the diagnosis of myasthenia gravis.

Most CRPS occurs after an acute injury; early mobilization after trauma can help with prevention.

Allodynia is an extreme sensitivity to touch. It is a hallmark of CRPS.

Central Nervous System Infection

A. Cerebrospinal fluid (CSF)

1. LP with examination of CSF is essential when cerebral infection is considered.

2. CSF findings will aid in securing a diagnosis, identify the etiology of infection, and guide treatment with culture and sensitivities of pathogens (Table 11-7).

3. LP is contraindicated if a mass lesion is suspected.

4. CT scan is indicated before LP in patients who are immunocompromised, have a history of CNS disease (mass lesion, stroke, focal infection), experience new-onset seizure (within 1 week), exhibit papilledema, or have an abnormal level of consciousness or a focal neurologic deficit.

B. Bacterial meningitis

1. General characteristics

a. Patients will frequently have upper respiratory infection (URI), pneumonia, sinus, or ear infection, just before or along with the onset of meningitis symptoms.

b. Meningitis symptoms are based on three processes: inflammation, increased intracranial pressure, and/or tissue necrosis.

c. Bacterial meningitis etiology is different based on the age of the patient. The etiologies are listed below from most common to least.

(1) Patients over age 50: The primary causes are *Neisseria meningitides* (about half of the cases), *Streptococcus pneumoniae* (about 40%), and *Listeria monocytogenes* (around 5%).

(2) Patients from 1 month to 50 years of age: *S. pneumoniae*, *N. meningitides*, and *Haemophilus influenzae*. Meningitis caused by *Haemophilus* has dramatically decreased since the widespread use of the Hib vaccine. Group B *Streptococcus* and *E. coli* occur in the 1- to 23-month-old population.

(3) Patients under 1 month of age: group B *Streptococcus* (*Streptococcus agalactiae*), *E. coli*, other Gram-negative organisms, *S. pneumoniae*, *Enterococcus* species, and *Listeria* species.

2. Clinical features

a. Altered mental status, fever, headache, and a stiff neck are the typical symptoms of meningitis, although all may not be present. A petechial or ecchymotic rash is characteristic of *Neisseria meningitidis*. Patients are often nauseous and may vomit.

b. Symptoms typically are acute, with patients presenting within hours or 1 to 2 days of infection.

c. Careful initial examination may reveal evidence of soft-tissue abscess, otitis, or other parameningeal infection.

> Meningitis in a neonate (<1 month old) is most likely caused by group B *Streptococcus* (earliest weeks, from the birth canal) or *Escherichia coli* (later weeks, from caregiver).

Table 11-7 | CSF Comparisons

CSF	Bacterial Meningitis	Viral (Aseptic) Meningitis	Granulomatous Meningitis
Color	Turbid to grossly purulent	Clear	Variable
Pressure	Elevated	Normal	Generally normal
WBC count	Elevated, increased neutrophils (pleocytosis)	Normal to mildly elevated, lymphocytes or monocytes predominate	Generally mildly elevated, lymphocytes (can be neutrophils)
Protein concentration	Elevated, 100–500 mg/dL	Normal or mildly elevated (<150 mg/dL)	Elevated
Glucose level	Decreased, <40 mg/dL	Normal	Decreased

CSF, cerebrospinal fluid; WBC, white blood cell.

d. Meningeal signs (stiff neck, Kernig and Brudzinski's signs) may be absent or very subtle at the age extremes or be difficult to assess with impaired consciousness.

3. Diagnostic studies

a. Blood cultures should be obtained.

b. Prompt LP and CSF analysis is essential (see Table 11-7).

c. Gram stain and culture of the CSF is diagnostic in >80% of cases.

d. Latex agglutination tests and polymerase chain reaction (PCR) may be the options if a specific rapid diagnosis is needed or if antibiotics are given before blood cultures.

4. Treatment

a. Antibiotic treatment is begun immediately if the CSF is not clear and colorless. Antibiotics should not be delayed if the LP cannot be accomplished or if imaging is necessary. The initial choice of antibiotic is based empirically on the patient's age and the most likely pathogen.

> Empiric treatment of bacterial meningitis over the age of 1 month should include vancomycin plus a cephalosporin and/or ampicillin.

(1) Neonates up to 1 month receive ampicillin plus cefotaxime OR ampicillin plus gentamicin.

(2) Immunocompetent children and adults aged 1 month to 50 years receive cefotaxime or ceftriaxone plus vancomycin.

(3) Adults older than 50 years and those of any age with alcoholism or debilitating illness receive ampicillin plus cefotaxime or ceftriaxone plus vancomycin.

(4) Addition of dexamethasone before or with antibiotics is beneficial, especially for cases caused by *S. pneumoniae* in adults (Gram-positive cocci on Gram stain) and *H. influenzae* type B in children. If given promptly, it will reduce morbidity and mortality.

(5) Supportive care includes fluid management and metabolic/nutritional support.

b. Repeat LP and CSF analysis are crucial to assess response to treatment.

(1) The CSF should be sterile after 24 hours.

(2) A decrease in pleocytosis and the proportion of neutrophils should be seen within 3 days.

C. Viral (aseptic) meningitis and encephalitis

1. General considerations

a. Viral or aseptic meningitis means inflammation of the meninges to include the CSF, arachnoid, and pia mater without a bacterial cause. Encephalitis indicates brain parenchyma is inflamed. The clinical difference between viral meningitis and viral encephalitis is sometimes difficult to distinguish, but patients with viral encephalitis will have abnormal brain function. Patients can have evidence of both these conditions, and the term is called *meningoencephalitis*.

b. Viral meningitis is most frequently (85%) associated with enteroviruses (e.g., coxsackievirus and echoviruses), HSV type 2, and arthropod-borne viruses.

c. Viral encephalitis is most commonly caused by arboviruses, including West Nile virus, equine viruses, and others. Sporadic outbreak of viral encephalitis is most commonly caused by HSV type 1.

d. Aseptic meningitis may also reflect an inflammatory process secondary to systemic diseases, neoplasms, spirochetes, medication hypersensitivity, or fungi.

2. Clinical features

a. Symptoms may include headache, fever, neck stiffness, fatigue, rash, and vomiting. The symptoms are generally not as acute as in bacterial meningitis and may have persisted for several days.

b. Viral encephalitis may present as an acute confused state, especially in children and young adults.

> Fever, stiff neck, and headache indicate meningitis; abnormalities of brain function (confusion, seizures, focal signs) indicate encephalitis.

    c. Examination may reveal a number of systemic manifestations, suggesting a particular causal agent (e.g., rash, pharyngitis, adenopathy, pleuritic pain, jaundice, organomegaly, diarrhea).

    d. Encephalitis involves the brain directly, so there may be markedly altered consciousness, seizures, personality changes, or other focal neurologic signs.

3. Diagnostic studies

    a. Blood cultures should be obtained.

    b. As with bacterial meningitis, prompt LP and CSF analysis are crucial after assessing for evidence of increased intracranial pressure (see Table 11-7).

    c. PCR is faster and more sensitive than viral culture for enteroviruses and HSV. PCR is also the test of choice for most viruses causing meningitis and encephalitis.

    d. Serology is the best test for diagnosis of West Nile virus.

    e. MRI of the brain is likely to show abnormalities in patients with viral encephalitis, but may be normal.

4. Treatment

    a. Suspected herpes virus infection is treated with IV acyclovir. With the exception of infection with HSV, the course of aseptic meningitis is generally benign and self-limited, and no specific therapy is required. Fluids and supportive care may be sufficient.

    b. Mild headaches can be treated with acetaminophen.

    c. Seizures can be suppressed with anticonvulsants.

    d. Breathing should be supported, if necessary.

> 💡 Meningitis caused by herpes virus is typically more dramatic with seizures, altered mental status, and neurologic deficits as well as higher protein and cell counts in CSF compared to other viral causes. This is the only viral meningitis treated with antivirals because of its malignant course.

D. Granulomatous meningitis

1. General characteristics

    a. Pathogens include *Mycobacterium tuberculosis*, fungi (*Cryptococcus, Coccidioides* sp., *Histoplasma*), and spirochetes (*Treponema pallidum, Borrelia burgdorferi*).

    b. Incidence is highest in immunocompromised individuals.

    c. Noninfectious causes include sarcoidosis and other granulomatous conditions.

2. Clinical features

    a. Presentation is less acute than other causes of meningitis; patients typically have symptoms for weeks to months.

    b. Subtle mental status changes are common.

3. Diagnostic studies (Table 11-7)

    a. CSF analysis and culture is key, but results may take weeks depending on etiology.

    b. CT or MRI will show marked enhancement of the meninges and, occasionally, hydrocephalus.

    c. Serologic studies may help confirm suspected etiologies.

4. Treatment depends on cause.

E. Brain abscess

1. General characteristics

    a. Most brain abscesses (90%) occur secondary to another focus of infection in the body. Brain abscess can result from direct spread of infection from sinusitis, mastoiditis, or dental infection when there is a single abscess.

    b. Hematogenous spread to the brain can occur from pneumonia, endocarditis, or pyelonephritis, and this is typically characterized by multiple brain abscesses.

    c. Abscesses may be localized to the extradural (epidural) space, subdural spaces, or the brain parenchyma.

2. Clinical features

   a. Symptoms of a brain abscess may include fever, headache, altered consciousness, hemiparesis, nausea/vomiting, or seizures.

   b. Brain abscess is a space-occupying lesion; focal neurologic signs are possible and vary depending on the location of the abscess. For example, a patient with a cerebellar abscess might present with limb ataxia on the ipsilateral side and gait ataxia.

3. Diagnostic studies

   a. CT or MRI is helpful in identifying brain abscesses, especially if performed using a contrast medium.

   b. LP is contraindicated in patients with focal neurologic symptoms or focal neurologic signs; brainstem herniation may be precipitated by LP in this setting. If meningitis is suspected, empiric treatment can be initiated and imaging accomplished. If negative for a space-occupying lesion, LP can be performed.

   c. The bacteriology of brain abscess is usually polymicrobial and may include both Gram-positive and Gram-negative organisms.

4. Treatment

   a. Brain abscesses are treated with appropriate antibiotics that penetrate brain tissues well: IV penicillin G or ceftriaxone or cefepime plus metronidazole. Vancomycin is added if *Staphylococcus aureus* infection is suspected.

   b. Acute treatment may involve respiratory and circulatory support, airway management, and monitoring of other vital functions.

   c. Surgical excision or decompression may be required in cases of very large lesions or a delayed response to therapy.

> Brain abscess will cause focal signs; the specific manifestation often indicates the location of the lesion.

Central Nervous System Trauma

A. Brain injury

   1. General characteristics

      a. Traumatic brain injury is a phrase frequently used interchangeably with concussion, but a concussion is a type of traumatic brain injury that results in temporary abnormal neurologic function, but without structural changes; so brain imaging is normal in concussion.

      b. Traumatic brain injury is common with about 1.4 to 2.5 million people affected per year; ~52,000 to 56,000 patients die a year owing to traumatic brain injury.

      c. Brain and head injury is frequently associated with spinal injury, so care should be taken to stabilize the spine.

      d. The most common causes of traumatic brain injuries are falls, motor vehicle accidents, and assaults (including intentional self-harm); most traumatic brain injuries in the elderly are secondary to falls.

      e. About half of the brain trauma–related deaths in young people are a result of motor vehicle accidents.

      f. Prognosis is directly related to the site and severity of brain damage. Initial neurologic examination after the injury is the best prognostic indicator. For severe injury, the initial Glasgow Coma Scale score is the best indicator of potential for future recovery.

      g. Traumatic brain injury can be mild, moderate, or severe; a Glasgow Coma Scale score of 13 to 15 correlates with mild injury, 9 to 12 moderate injury, and 8 or less correlates with severe traumatic brain injury.

      h. Contusion of the brain is a focal injury that will be accompanied by abnormal brain imaging.

> The most common traumas in brain injury include falls, MVA, and assaults; prognosis is related to severity and site of trauma.

2. **Clinical features**

   a. Signs and symptoms of mild traumatic brain injury (concussion) may include a brief loss of consciousness or a diminished level of consciousness (dazed feeling), retrograde and/or anterograde amnesia, headache, confusion, vomiting, and somnolence. Patients with more severe injury may experience a longer loss of consciousness, seizures, limb weakness, focal neurologic deficits, pupillary defects, or coma.

   b. The Glasgow Coma Scale assesses initial and ongoing consciousness by objectively scoring eye movement, verbal response, and motor response (Table 11-8).

   c. Physical examination may reveal deficits in the level of consciousness, memory, pupillary defects, CNs (especially III to VII), balance, gait, and extremity strength. Also, signs of basilar skull fracture may be present with traumatic brain injury such as hemotympanum, bruising in the mastoid area (Battle's sign), bruising in the periorbital area (raccoon eyes), and CSF rhinorrhea.

   d. Bleeds owing to traumatic brain injury are most commonly subdural-type bleeds. Contusion or intracerebral hemorrhage may occur on the side of the injury (coup injury) or the contralateral side (contrecoup injury).

   e. Most patients with a concussion recover completely within 1 month. Some patients may have prolonged symptoms after a concussion. Postconcussion syndrome is characterized by persistence of three or more of the following symptoms: headache, amnesia, fatigue, dizziness, phonophobia, irritability, or mood changes. These symptoms follow a head trauma that resulted in concussion with loss of consciousness.

   f. Patients with repeated concussions may develop permanent neurologic damage called *chronic traumatic encephalopathy*. This condition is characterized by changes in behavior, mood, and cognition.

3. Diagnostic studies

   a. Noncontrast head CT is the study of choice to uncover intracranial hemorrhage, show evidence of cerebral edema, and identify displacement of midline structures. Crescent-shaped hemorrhage indicates subdural bleed; biconcave indicates epidural.

> 💡 Traumatic brain injury is more likely to affect CN III (oculomotor), CN IV (trochlear), CN V (trigeminal), CN VI (abducens), and CN VII (facial).

> 💡 The best imaging for trauma to the brain is a CT without contrast.

Table 11-8 | Glasgow Coma Scale

Eye opening	Spontaneous eye opening	4 points
	Eyes open to verbal command	3 points
	Eyes open to pain	2 points
	No eye opening	1 point
Verbal response	Alert and oriented	5 points
	Confused, yet coherent speech	4 points
	Inappropriate words and jumbled phrases	3 points
	Incomprehensible sounds	2 points
	No sounds	1 point
Motor response	Obeys commands	6 points
	Localizes to a noxious stimulus	5 points
	Withdraws from a noxious stimulus	4 points
	Abnormal flexion (decorticate posturing)	3 points
	Abnormal extensor response (decerebrate posturing)	2 points
	No response	1 point

Lowest possible score = 3 points; highest possible score = 15 points.

Minor brain injury: >13 points; moderate brain injury: 9–12 points; severe brain injury: <9 points (coma).

b. CT may detect skull fractures; further studies of the cervical spine should be done to look for related injuries.

c. CTA is done in patients with abnormal brain CT to identify the source and location of the bleed.

4. Treatment

a. For mild concussion, the patient should have a period of 24 to 48 hours of physical and cognitive rest and observation. Athletes who sustained concussion during a sporting activity may then begin a return to play protocol, if asymptomatic, and cleared by a licensed health care provider.

b. For patients with severe brain injury, surgical evacuation may be necessary after acute epidural, acute subdural, and cerebral hemorrhage.

c. Increased intracranial pressure may be relieved by ventricular drainage, elevation of the head of the bed, induced hyperventilation, IV mannitol infusion, and sedation.

d. One week of anticonvulsant therapy is recommended for severe brain injury to prevent seizures.

> Return to play after concussion is a six-step process (limited activity, light aerobic, sport-specific exercise, noncontact training, full-contact practice, return to play) with a minimum of 24 hours between steps.

B. Spinal cord injury

1. General characteristics

a. Severe injury of the spinal cord typically relates to fracture or dislocation causing compression or angular deformity of the cord.

b. Sites of injury may extend from the cervical to the upper lumbar region.

c. Extreme hypotension after acute injury may result in cord infarction.

2. Clinical features

a. Total cord transection

(1) Total cord transection results in immediate, flaccid paralysis and loss of sensation below the level of the trauma.

(2) Reflex activity is lost for a variable time, and there is urinary and fecal retention.

(3) With the slow return of reflex function, spastic paraplegia or quadriplegia develops, with hyperreflexia and extensor plantar responses.

b. Partial cord injury

(1) Patients may be left with mild limb weakness or distal sensory disturbance.

(2) Sphincter function impairment may lead to urinary urgency and incontinence.

c. A unilateral cord lesion produces an ipsilateral motor weakness and impairment of proprioception; the lesion also produces a contralateral loss of pain and temperature sensation below the lesion (Brown–Séquard syndrome).

d. A central cord syndrome can occur with hyperextension of the cervical spine (especially in elderly patients with cervical spondylosis). It is characterized by upper extremity motor impairment greater than lower extremities motor impairment, bladder dysfunction, and sensory abnormalities in the extremities. Younger patients may have this injury owing to trauma and elderly patients owing to falls.

e. A radicular deficit may occur at the level of the injury; if the cauda equina is involved, there may be dysfunction in several lumbosacral roots.

3. Diagnostic studies

a. No laboratory testing is specifically warranted.

b. Imaging studies (plain-film radiography, CT, MRI) are indicated based on signs and symptoms.

4. Treatment

a. Treatment of spinal cord injury involves immobilization as well as decompressive laminectomy and fusion if there is cord compression.

   b. Anatomic realignment of the spinal cord by traction and other orthopedic procedures is important.

   c. Subsequent care of residual neurologic deficit requires therapy for spasticity and care of the skin, bowel, and bladder.

Primary Central Nervous System Neoplasms

A. General characteristics

> *The majority of CNS neoplasms are of glial cell origin (astrocytoma, ependymoma, oligodendroglioma) or meningiomas.*

   1. Approximately one-third of all primary intracranial neoplasms are glial cell origin, and one-third are meningiomas; some other types of primary tumors are vestibular schwannomas, pituitary adenomas, neurofibromas, and CNS lymphomas.

   2. Most glial cell tumors are malignant, and they can be divided into one of several types: astrocytoma, ependymoma, and oligodendroglioma.

   3. Astrocytoma comes in different grades with worsening prognosis. Glioblastoma is grade 4; unfortunately, glioblastoma is the most common primary malignant brain tumor and has a poor prognosis. The mean survival with treatment is 10 to 18 months.

   4. Ependymoma is a primary glial cell tumor that occurs in the ependymal cells that line the ventricles and spinal canal.

   5. Medulloblastoma is the most common primary malignant brain tumor in children. These tumors are located in the cerebellum. The long-term survival with treatment is about 75%.

   6. Certain tumors, especially neurofibromas, hemangioblastomas, and retinoblastomas, may have a familial basis.

   7. The most common sources of intracranial metastasis are carcinoma of the lung, breast, skin (melanoma), kidney, and GI tract. These metastatic brain tumors are more common than primary intracranial tumors in adults.

B. Clinical features

> *Headaches that occur at night awaken patients from sleep or worsen with activity, indicating a need for imaging to identify a tumor.*

   1. Brain tumors may cause headaches that are nocturnal, awaken the patient, or worsen with activities that increase intracranial pressure (i.e., coughing, sneezing, or supine position). The headache is typically located on the same side as the tumor.

   2. Intracranial tumors may produce a generalized disturbance of cerebral function and lead to evidence of increased intracranial pressure (i.e., personality changes, intellectual decline, emotional lability, seizures, headaches, nausea, vomiting, and malaise).

   3. Intracranial tumors may also produce focal deficits depending on their location.

   a. Frontal lobe lesions often produce progressive intellectual decline, slowing of mental activity, personality changes, contralateral grasp reflexes, and, possibly, expressive aphasia.

   b. Temporal lobe lesions may lead to seizures, olfactory or gustatory hallucinations, licking or smacking of the lips, depersonalization, emotional and behavioral changes, visual field defects, and auditory illusions.

   c. Parietal lobe lesions typically cause contralateral disturbances of sensation and may cause sensory seizures, a cortical sensory loss (impaired stereognosis) or inattention, or some combination of these.

   d. Occipital lobe lesions characteristically produce contralateral homonymous hemianopia or a partial field defect, visual agnosia for objects and colors, or unformed visual hallucinations.

   e. Brainstem and cerebellar lesions produce CN palsies, ataxia, incoordination, nystagmus, and pyramidal and sensory deficits in the limbs on one or both sides.

   4. Symptoms of spinal tumors usually develop insidiously, with pain characteristically aggravated by coughing or straining and either localized to the back or felt diffusely in an extremity as motor defects, paresthesias, or numbness, especially in the legs.

5. Physical examination of patients with spinal tumors may reveal localized spinal tenderness.

C. Diagnostic studies

1. MRI of the brain with contrast medium may detect the lesion, define its location and size, evaluate the extent to which the normal anatomy is distorted, and the degree of any associated cerebral edema or mass effect. Head CT with contrast may be performed if MRI is contraindicated.

2. EEG may demonstrate a focal disturbance resulting from the neoplasm or a more diffuse change reflecting altered mental status.

3. CT myelography or MRI of the spine may be needed to identify and localize the site of spinal cord compression.

D. Treatment

1. Complete surgical removal of the tumor may be possible if it is extra-axial or not in a critical or inaccessible region of the brain.

2. Surgical shunting of an obstructive hydrocephalus may dramatically reduce clinical deficits.

3. Radiation or chemotherapy or both increase median survival rates in malignant neoplasms, regardless of any preceding surgery.

4. Anticonvulsants are commonly administered in standard doses.

5. Intramedullary cord lesions are treated by decompression and surgical excision and irradiation.

6. Treatment of epidural spinal metastases consists of irradiation, irrespective of cell type.

> Signs and symptoms for most brain tumors are insidious; any atypical headache pattern or recurring focal symptom should prompt further investigation; MRI is the preferred imaging.

Sleep Disorders

A. General characteristics

1. Sleep consists of two distinct states: REM and non-REM.

    a. REM sleep is predominant when dreaming takes place. During REM sleep, patients are typically paralyzed.

    b. Non-REM sleep is divided into stages 1, 2, and 3.

2. Insomnia complaints include difficulty falling asleep or staying asleep, intermittent wakefulness during the night, early morning awakenings, or some combination of all these. Psychiatric disorders, including depression and manic disorders, are often associated with persistent insomnia. Medications and drugs can also cause insomnia.

    a. Depression is associated with fragmented sleep, decreased total sleep time, quicker onset of REM sleep, and a shift of REM to earlier in the night.

    b. In manic disorders, total sleep time is decreased with shortened REM latency and increased REM activity.

3. Hypersomnia (excessive daytime sleepiness) can be caused by inadequate nighttime sleep, medications, psychiatric illness, sleep apnea, narcolepsy, restless leg disorder, or chronic medical conditions like hypothyroidism or renal failure.

4. Narcolepsy is characterized by excessive daytime sleepiness, sudden brief sleep attacks, cataplexy, sleep paralysis, and hypnagogic hallucinations, which may precede sleep. Type 1 narcolepsy is associated with a low hypocretin (orexin) level in the CSF.

5. Obstructive sleep apnea (OSA) is more common in males and in obese patients. This condition is characterized by daytime sleepiness and excessive snoring. Patients have periods of apnea during sleep that end with a loud snorting or gasping noise; the apneic episodes are a result of obstruction in the upper airway—nasopharyngeal area.

> OSA is more often seen in obese males, with daytime sleepiness and nighttime snoring; management involves weight loss and CPAP during sleep.

6. Parasomnias (abnormal behaviors during sleep) are characterized by sleep terrors, nightmares, sleepwalking, and enuresis.

   a. Sleep terrors and sleepwalking are associated with stage 3 non-REM sleep in the first third of the night.

   b. Childhood enuresis typically takes place within 3 to 4 hours of bedtime but is not limited to a particular stage of sleep. This is a common condition that affects about 15% of 5-year-olds. It may be associated with obstructive sleep apnea in some children.

B. Clinical features

1. Taking a careful history of those with insomnia may reveal depression, abuse of alcohol, heavy smoking (>1 pack/day), inappropriate use of sedatives or stimulants, or a medical history of uremia, asthma, or hypothyroidism.

2. Sleep apnea is often seen in obese, middle-aged, and older men with hypertension and associated congestive heart failure.

C. Diagnostic studies

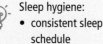 Polysomnography differentiates OSA from other disorders such as periodic limb movement, narcolepsy, chronic insomnia, and REM sleep behavior disorders.

1. Polysomnography (sleep studies) assesses EEG activity, heart rate, respiratory movement, and oxygen saturation. This test is helpful in the diagnosis of obstructive sleep apnea, narcolepsy, sleep movement disorders, and other sleep disorders.

2. Multiple sleep latency test is helpful to determine how long it takes to go to sleep during naps. This test is usually accomplished the day after the polysomnogram in patients with suspected narcolepsy. Patients with narcolepsy typically enter REM sleep rapidly. This test demonstrates the level of daytime sleepiness.

3. Thyroid studies may be helpful if thyroid disease is suggested.

D. Treatment

1. Insomnia

   a. In transient insomnia, de-emphasis and reassurance along with sleep hygiene education are sufficient treatment.

   b. Cognitive-behavioral therapy is helpful for those with chronic insomnia. Part of cognitive-behavioral therapy for insomnia includes educating the patient on a variety of sleep hygiene methods discussed to remove numerous barriers to effective sleep: avoidance of alcohol, caffeine, nicotine, or exercise before bedtime; establishment of regular sleep hours; limiting time in bed; relaxation techniques; and avoidance of prolonged daytime naps. This will increase the sleep needs at night.

Sleep hygiene:
- consistent sleep schedule
- relaxing bedtime routine
- turn off all electronic devices
- cool, dark, quiet place
- go to bed when tired
- limit the bed to sleep and sex
- limit napping
- exercise regularly
- limit caffeine intake
- manage stress

   c. Medications for insomnia should be avoided if possible, but are useful in some patients. Hypnotics like benzodiazepines (e.g., temazepam) and nonbenzodiazepine hypnotics (e.g., zolpidem) may be used for short periods, if necessary. Melatonin agonists (e.g., ramelteon) may also be used for short periods. Other medications may be appropriate in the right patient. For example, a patient with depression and insomnia may benefit from trazodone.

2. Treatment of sleep apnea includes weight reduction (if appropriate) and administration of air under continuous pressure through the nasopharynx during sleep (continuous positive airway pressure).

3. Narcolepsy is managed by administration of modafinil or stimulants, such as methylphenidate.

Practice Questions

Directions: *Each of the numbered items or incomplete statements in this section is followed by a list of answers or completions of the statement. Select the ONE lettered answer or completion that is BEST in each case.*

1. A 24-year-old female presents to neurology clinic for management of new-onset epilepsy. Her seizures are described as beginning with a "funny taste" in her mouth, involving smacking her lips and repeating words, and losing consciousness, but not falling. Overall, each seizure lasts ~2 minutes. She does not become incontinent, and she is otherwise healthy. What is the best choice to classify this type of seizure disorder?
   A. Absence
   B. Focal seizure with loss of consciousness
   C. Myoclonic seizure
   D. Tonic–clonic
   E. Pseudoseizure

2. An EEG of a pediatric patient in epilepsy clinic shows bilateral symmetric and synchronous spike-and-wave activity. What type of seizure is correlated with this pattern?
   A. Tonic–clonic
   B. Atonic
   C. Pseudoseizure
   D. Focal seizure without impairment of consciousness
   E. Absence

3. A 30-year-old female is complaining of fatigue, numbness and tingling in her limbs, feeling unsteady, and intermittent blurry vision for 1 month. She has a mild lymphocytosis, but lab work is otherwise unremarkable. What study should be ordered next to confirm the most likely diagnosis?
   A. CT scan of brain
   B. MRI of the brain
   C. LP
   D. Vitamin D levels
   E. EEG

4. A 76-year-old female with no significant past medical history presents with her son. The son reports that the patient has been increasingly forgetful for the past 6 months, has stopped balancing her checkbook, and recently got lost coming home from her regular supermarket. She is well appearing and neatly dressed. Her physical examination is unremarkable, except for a score of 20/30 on the mental status examination. Which class of medication is the best choice for initial treatment of the suspected diagnosis?
   A. Vitamin E
   B. NSAIDs
   C. Dopamine agonist
   D. Calcium channel blocker
   E. Acetylcholinesterase inhibitors

5. A 45-year-old male presents with unilateral headache rated 9/10 that has occurred for the second time today. He also complains of a "red eye" and tearing on the same side as the headache. On physical examination, he is pacing the room in discomfort, has mildly elevated BP, and a normal neuro examination. What is the initial treatment of choice for the suspected diagnosis?
   A. NSAIDs and IM antiemetic
   B. Trial of oral opioids

   C. Oxygen via nasal cannula and IM triptan
   D. Oral calcium channel blocker
   E. Triptan via nasal inhalation

6. A patient presents for ongoing management of his recently diagnosed migraine headaches, which present with a preceding aura, nausea and vomiting, and photophobia and phonophobia along with unilateral throbbing head pain. Treatment with over-the-counter analgesics has not been effective in reducing the severity and frequency of the migraines. What is the best choice for an abortive treatment option at this stage?
   A. Prescription NSAID
   B. Triptan plus antiemetic
   C. Tricyclic antidepressant
   D. β-Blocker
   E. Topiramate

7. A 20-year-old college student presents with 2 days of worsening fever, stiff neck, and vomiting. Her roommate states she had a "bad earache" earlier this week. She is unable to answer questions and found to have a positive Brudzinski's sign, evidence of possible left-side mastoiditis, and no rash on physical examination. Which choice best represents the likely makeup of her CSF analysis?
   A. Opening pressure: normal; WBC count: mildly elevated with lymphocytes; protein concentration: normal
   B. Opening pressure: normal; WBC count: mildly elevated with lymphocytes; protein concentration: elevated
   C. Opening pressure: elevated; WBC count: normal; protein concentration: normal
   D. Opening pressure: elevated; WBC count: elevated with neutrophils; protein concentration: elevated

8. A 68-year-old patient who has not been seen by a health care provider in many years has experienced cognitive decline. His daughter describes an initial mild decline in his ability to function 6 months ago followed by a period of stability. This pattern has repeated itself twice more. At this time, he continues to live alone, but the daughter is concerned about loss of memory and increasing difficulty completing his usual tasks. During the interview, he is cooperative but displays confusion and some difficulty with memory tasks. Which of the following is most likely present on physical examination?
   A. Elevated BP
   B. Cogwheeling of joints
   C. Resting tremor
   D. Papilledema
   E. Hemiweakness

9. A 66-year-old male woke this morning with left hemiparesis and aphasia. CT scan is negative for bleed. Which of the following is most likely present in his history?
   A. Atrial fibrillation
   B. Cigarette smoking
   C. Family history of hyperlipidemia
   D. Hypertension
   E. Thrombocytosis

10. A 71-year-old overweight female with a history of hypertension and diabetes is brought to the emergency department by her daughter who states her mother was unable to walk without listing to one side and holding onto the wall. The daughter asked her mother what was wrong, but her mother could not articulate. She vomited on the way to the emergency department. What is the most likely diagnosis?
    A. Anterior cerebral artery stroke
    B. Middle cerebral artery stroke
    C. Ruptured berry aneurysm
    D. Subarachnoid hematoma
    E. Vertebrobasilar artery stroke

11. A 36-year-old female has completed a 90-day rehabilitation program for alcohol abuse. She has a fine rhythmic tremor affecting her upper extremities and head. She states her mother had the same tremor. What is the recommended treatment?
    A. Amitriptyline

B. Primidone
C. Propranolol
D. Small amount of alcohol
E. Verapamil

12. A 40-year-old schoolteacher complains of pain and weakness in his legs. He states it began 2 days ago and has progressed to include his pelvis, making it difficult to rise from a chair. This morning his arms feel weak as well. Electrophysiologic studies show marked slowing of nerve conduction velocities. What is the recommended treatment?
    A. Edrophonium
    B. Dopamine agonist
    C. IVIG
    D. Plasmapheresis
    E. Prednisone

Practice Answers

1. **B.** *Neurology; Diagnosis; Seizure Disorders*

   Focal seizure with loss of consciousness is the best classification. She has a characteristic aura with subsequent impaired consciousness and focal seizure activity. This seizure type can also evolve into generalized tonic–clonic. Absence, myoclonic, and tonic–clonic are all types of generalized seizures. Absence is often brief and hard to notice initially. Myoclonic involves brief or repetitive jerking motions, and generalized tonic–clonic involves larger muscle groups of the body demonstrating rigidity and jerking.

2. **E.** *Neurology; Diagnosis; Seizure Disorders*

   Absence seizure is characterized by 3-Hz spike-and-wave activity. Other generalized (tonic–clonic or atonic) seizure EEG activity is characterized by generalized discharges with spike-and-slow wave, or polyspike, activity. A pseudoseizure would not show significant changes on EEG. Focal seizure activity on EEG may show a focal rhythmic discharge at the onset of the seizure, and sometimes no ictal activity will be seen.

3. **B.** *Neurology; Diagnostic Studies; Multiple Sclerosis*

   This patient is presenting with signs and symptoms of MS. MRI is the best study to help conclusively diagnose MS; T1 hypointense areas of axonal damage are diagnostic. CT is not helpful. LP and CSF analysis, as well as vitamin D measurement, may show positive findings but will not be specific for the diagnosis of MS. EEG is not indicated in this patient.

4. **E.** *Neurology; Pharmacology; Alzheimer's Disease*

   An acetylcholinesterase inhibitor is the suggested treatment to slow progression of AD. Vitamin E studies are not yet conclusive in treating or preventing AD. NSAIDs may increase risk of bleeding or MI. A dopamine agonist may be indicated if this patient had concomitant depression. A calcium channel blocker might be indicated in vascular dementia.

5. **C.** *Neurology; Clinical Intervention; Cluster Headache*

   This patient has cluster headache and abortive, immediate treatment includes oxygen and IM triptan. NSAIDs and

opioids are not effective. A calcium channel blocker, such as verapamil, could be beneficial as prophylactic therapy. Triptan via nasal route is abortive therapy for migraine.

6. **B.** *Neurology; Pharmacology; Migraine Headache*

   Triptan plus antiemetic is the best choice for moderate-to-severe migraine abortive therapy. A prescription NSAID could be effective if combined with a triptan, but alone may cause GI upset and not abort the migraine. Tricyclics, β-blockers, and topiramate are all options for prophylactic therapy.

7. **D.** *Neurology; Diagnostic Studies; Meningitis*

   Elevated opening pressure, an elevated WBC count, and elevated protein concentration indicate bacterial meningitis. Option A (normal protein, mildly elevated lymphocytes, and normal opening pressure) describes findings for viral (aseptic) meningitis. Option B (elevated protein, mildly elevated lymphocytes, elevated opening pressure) describes granulomatous meningitis.

8. **A.** *Neurology; History and Physical Examination; Vascular Dementia*

   This patient is presenting a picture of stepwise decline in cognitive function, which is most characteristic of vascular dementia caused by chronic hypertension. This is the second most common cause of dementia. Patients with vascular dementia typically do not exhibit unilateral motor symptoms. Resting tremor and cogwheeling are characteristic of Parkinson's; the cognitive decline typically after motor symptoms. Papilledema is a sign of increased intracranial pressure, which may be present in hypertensive emergencies.

9. **D.** *Neurology; Health Maintenance; Stroke*

   Hypertension is by far the leading risk factor for cerebrovascular accident (stroke). Atrial fibrillation is a very common cause of embolic stroke. Cigarette smoking, hyperlipidemia, and thrombocytosis are risk factors, but with less weight compared to hypertension.

10. E. *Neurology; Diagnosis; Stroke*

Vertebrobasilar artery strokes are more likely to cause nausea and vomiting, vertigo, balance problems, and some motor and sensory deficits. Anterior cerebral artery strokes affect mainly the temporal lobe, causing personality changes as well as lower extremity weakness. The middle cerebral artery is the largest vessel and is most often involved in strokes. Motor deficits are more pronounced, especially in the face, throat, hand, and arm; if the stroke occurs in the dominant hemisphere, speech is also affected. A ruptured berry aneurysm is the most common cause of nontraumatic SAH; patients typically have a severe headache, nausea and/or vomiting, seizure activity, and loss of consciousness.

11. C. *Neurology; Pharmacology; Essential Tremor*

This patient most likely has benign essential tremor, an autosomal dominant disorder. Although small amounts of alcohol will commonly diminish symptoms, because she has a history of alcohol abuse, this is not wise. Primidone may be tried if the patient does not respond to propranolol. Verapamil is a preventive medicine in patients with cluster headache. Amitriptyline is a tricyclic antidepressant that may cause dryness and agitation.

12. D. *Neurology; Pharmacology; Guillain-Barré Syndrome*

This patient is exhibiting signs and symptoms of GBS, a progressive polyneuropathy that may occur after an infection, immunization, or surgical procedure, although most cases are idiopathic. Patients should be hospitalized and monitored closely for involvement of respiratory muscles. Plasmapheresis is the treatment of choice in adults. IVIG is preferred in children or in adults with cardiovascular disease. Edrophonium, an acetylcholinesterase inhibitor, is used to diagnose myasthenia gravis; it prevents the breakdown of acetylcholine and competitively inhibits acetylcholinesterase.

12 | Psychiatry

Nkechi E. Mbadugha and Matthew Wright

Diagnosis of Psychiatric Disorders

> The *DSM* serves to guide all psychiatric diagnosing in the United States.

A. Background

1. Psychiatric diagnoses conform to the *Diagnostic and Statistical Manual of Mental Disorders* (*DSM*) published and periodically updated by the American Psychiatric Association. The *DSM* is widely accepted because professionals from a number of specialties within psychiatry were involved in its conception and development.

2. The *DSM-5*, released in May 2013, set forth a major change in organization from a multiaxial system to a lifelong developmental approach. The multiaxial system for reporting diagnoses used in the *DSM-IV* was removed from the *DSM-5*.

3. The *International Statistical Classification of Diseases and Related Health Problems* (*ICD*) published by the World Health Organization is the official coding system used in the United States. The *DSM-5* is compatible with the *ICD* and contains the code numbers needed for billing and health monitoring purposes.

B. The *DSM* endorses a criteria-based diagnostic approach that requires the following three conditions to be met:

1. The condition is not caused by the direct effects of any drug or external exposure.

2. The psychiatric disorder is not caused by the effects of a medical condition.

3. There is significant impairment of social functioning, occupational functioning, or both.

C. If a patient's signs and symptoms result from a medical condition or substance abuse, the diagnosis should reflect this situation; in this case, the psychiatric symptoms take a secondary role. This relationship holds regardless of the behavior manifested by the patient.

D. In *DSM-5*, the "not otherwise specified" designation is either removed entirely or replaced with "not elsewhere classified (NEC)." NEC categories include a set of specifics that convey additional clinical information.

Schizophrenia and Other Psychotic Disorders

> Psychosis is defined as having symptoms that indicate impaired contact with reality.

A. Definition

1. Brief psychotic disorder, schizophreniform disorder, and schizophrenia present with common symptoms, which are differentiated by severity and duration.

2. Brief psychotic disorder

a. Patients exhibit disordered thought content and thought processes as well as perceptual disturbances, such as illusions or hallucinations, delusions, and impaired reality orientation.

b. Patients' social and occupational functions are disrupted by problems with affect, motivation, perception, and communication or disorganized speech; memory and consciousness are not impaired.

    c. Symptoms are categorized as positive (characterized by an attribute present that should be absent) or negative (characterized by the absence of an attribute that should be present) (Table 12-1).

    d. In brief, psychotic disorder symptoms last >1 day but <1 month and the person gradually returns to premorbid functioning. This disorder often occurs after a traumatic event.

  3. Schizophreniform disorder presents with the same symptoms as seen in schizophrenia, but symptoms last between 1 and 6 months.

  4. In schizophrenia, symptoms last >6 months.

B. Clinical features

  1. Schizophrenia usually runs a chronic and debilitating course. Patients generally lack insight and may not believe they are ill or have abnormal behavior. Prognosis is more favorable with good premorbid functioning, later age at onset, acute (vs. insidious) onset, obvious precipitating factor, and the presence of positive symptoms.

    a. An estimated 0.5% to 1% of the worldwide population is affected; it most commonly manifests in early adulthood. Onset before age 15 years or after age 50 years is rare.

    b. The prodromal phase, which precedes the first psychotic break by months or years, is manifested by subtle behavioral changes, functional decline, social withdrawal, and irritability. Onset of disease tends to be earlier for men (ages 18 to 25 years) than for women (ages 25 to 35 years).

    c. The psychotic phase consists of delusions; hallucinations; disorganized speech; and bizarre behavior, thought process, and content.

    d. The residual phase generally occurs between psychotic episodes. It is characterized by blunted affect, odd thinking or behavior, and other negative symptoms.

  2. At least two of the following five symptoms must be present during a 1-month period, and continuous signs of the disorder must persist for at least 6 months. The presence of hallucinations or delusions is not specifically necessary for a diagnosis.

    a. Delusions: erroneous beliefs based on a misinterpretation of reality, such as paranoia, ideas of reference, thought broadcasting, delusions of grandeur, or guilt. The delusions may be bizarre and have no basis in reality.

    b. Hallucinations: false perceptions in any of the sensory modalities, such as auditory (most common), tactile, olfactory, and visual. To qualify for the diagnosis, the hallucination must not occur as an isolated experience, in a clouded sensorium, or as part of a religious or cultural experience.

> Diagnosis of schizophrenia requires five symptoms to be present for at least 1 month each and overall impairment for at least 6 months.

Table 12-1 | Symptoms of Psychosis and Schizophrenia

Positive symptoms (exaggeration of a normal process)	Hallucinations: auditory visual somatic olfactory gustatory	Delusions: referral grandiose paranoid nihilistic erotomanic	Disorganization: tangential speech circumstantial speech derailment neologism word salad racing thoughts	Movement: agitated body movement catatonia
Negative symptoms (diminution of a normal process)	Avolition/apathy: lack of emotion asociality anhedonia lack of energy difficulty beginning or sustaining activities		Diminished expression: flat affect, alogia	
Cognitive symptoms	Poor executive functions; trouble focusing or paying attention; problems with working memory			

   c. Disorganized speech: used as a marker for disorganized thought processes. The patient is unable to stay on topic (loose associations), unable to provide an answer related to questions (tangential response), or both.

   d. Grossly disorganized behavior: may be exhibited as unpredictable agitation, inappropriate sexual behavior, childlike silliness, catatonic motor behavior, or a reduced level of self-care and hygiene.

   e. Negative symptoms: manifested as blunted affect, poor posture, or lack of goal-directed activities/initiative.

3. The symptoms need to be severe enough to impair an individual's social and/or occupational functioning and ability to communicate effectively.

   a. This impairment may be manifested as an inability to hold a job for an extended period, inability to maintain relationships, or withdrawal from established friends and social relationships.

   b. The patient's educational progress may be disrupted or not completed.

C. The cause of schizophrenia is believed to be an interplay between genetic and prenatal susceptibility and environmental insults.

D. Treatment

1. Hospitalization is recommended for patients who exhibit suicidal ideation or an inability to care for themselves or who pose a threat to self or others.

2. Pharmacotherapy

   a. No therapeutic intervention is totally effective in ameliorating all symptoms, and patients may react differently to the various neuroleptics available. Combined use of antipsychotic drugs and psychosocial treatment is better than either treatment alone.

   b. Neuroleptic and antipsychotic medications

   (1) The serotonin and dopamine antagonists (SDAs), otherwise known as atypical or second-generation antipsychotics, are the drugs of first choice to treat schizophrenia.

   (2) However, clozapine is an atypical antipsychotic that is not considered first line because of the propensity to cause agranulocytosis. Typical antipsychotics (i.e., haloperidol) are an alternative second line.

3. Typical neuroleptic and antipsychotic medications with dopamine antagonist activity (haloperidol, chlorpromazine, thioridazine, loxapine, fluphenazine) are best for decreasing positive symptoms (i.e., delusions).

   a. Side effects such as extrapyramidal symptoms, parkinsonian-like symptoms, neuroleptic malignant syndrome, and tardive dyskinesia are more likely to be encountered with the typical neuroleptics.

   b. If tardive dyskinesia occurs with a typical antipsychotic, stop the offending drug and switch to an atypical neuroleptic.

   c. A 4- to 6-week medication trial is optimal before concluding nonresponse.

4. Second-generation antipsychotics or atypical neuroleptics with SDA activity (risperidone, paliperidone, asenapine, olanzapine, aripiprazole, ziprasidone, quetiapine) generally are preferred for the management of negative symptoms (i.e., withdrawal) and have fewer side effects.

   a. The SDAs are associated with adverse effects such as weight gain, glucose intolerance, and increased lipids.

5. Resistant cases may be treated with an antipsychotic medication combined with another drug such as carbamazepine, valproate, lithium, or benzodiazepines.

Choice of medication in schizophrenia is individual, based on symptoms and patient response.

Tardive dyskinesia typically manifests as involuntary movements, most commonly of the head, tongue, and lips. It is associated with dopamine receptor blocking drugs, most especially haloperidol.

6. Long-active injection (depot) formulations may be helpful in noncompliant patients or those lacking insight.

7. Behavior-oriented therapy targeted toward social skills training (as an adjunct to group and/or family therapy) and illness education may be helpful.

E. Other forms of psychoses

1. **Schizoaffective disorder**

   a. This disorder is defined by major mood symptoms superimposed onto a chronic psychotic disorder. Patients meet the criteria for major depressive episode, manic episode, or mixed episode, during which criteria for schizophrenia also are met, so there is a mixture of psychotic and mood symptoms.

   b. Delusions or hallucinations lasting for at least 2 weeks without mood disorder symptoms help to differentiate schizoaffective disorder from mood disorder with psychotic features.

   c. It carries a better prognosis than schizophrenia but worse prognosis than a mood disorder.

   d. Treatment should target both psychotic and mood symptoms. The second-generation/atypical antipsychotics (i.e., paliperidone) are first line; a mood stabilizer (i.e., lithium or valproate) or an antidepressant can be added. As with schizophrenia, psychosocial support is needed.

2. **Delusional disorder**

   a. This disorder is characterized by the presence of delusions (false beliefs) for at least 1 month. The content of delusions may be bizarre. There are no hallucinations, negative symptoms, or disorganized speech or behavior.

   b. Unlike the other psychotic disorders, the behavior is not obviously odd, and functioning is not significantly impaired.

   c. Types of delusions are delineated in Table 12-2.

   d. The mainstay of treatment is antipsychotics, although systemic study of their effectiveness is lacking. Selective serotonin reuptake inhibitors (SSRIs) can decrease delusional beliefs in some.

> The most frequently encountered hallucinations are auditory.

3. **Substance-induced psychosis** and psychosis owing to another medical condition

   a. Psychotic disorders may be induced by alcohol, illicit drug use, or medications (anticholinergics, antidepressants, hallucinogens, psychostimulants).

   b. Psychotic disorders can be caused by general medical conditions (central nervous system [CNS] disease, endocrinopathies, vitamin deficiency states, HIV/AIDS, systemic lupus erythematosus).

   c. Management of drug- or illness-induced psychosis should target the underlying cause. Antipsychotics may be used to treat acute psychotic symptoms.

Table 12-2 | Types of Delusions

Erotomanic type	Belief that another person, typically a famous or powerful person, is in love with the patient
Somatic type	Belief that the patient has a physical defect or medical condition
Jealous type	Belief that the patient's partner is having an affair
Persecutory type	Belief that the patient or another person is being mistreated or persecuted
Grandiose type	Inflated self-worth, power, knowledge, identity; belief that the patient is a famous person
Mixed type	Characteristics of more than one type of delusion
Unspecified type	A delusion that cannot be clearly determined or characterized

Somatic Symptom Disorders

A. Somatic symptom disorder

    1. General characteristics

        a. Patients present with many vague physical complaints for 6 months or more involving many organ systems that cannot be explained by a general medical condition or substance use. Somatic symptoms are distressing or significantly disrupt the patient's daily life. Visits to health care providers are numerous as are diagnostic tests and procedures, although no medical disorder is found.

        b. Patients commonly complain of symptoms related to the gastrointestinal (GI) tract or to the reproductive or neurologic systems; they may also complain of pain. Periods of increased stress are associated with worsening of the somatic symptoms.

        c. This disorder occurs in females more often than in males and more often in low socioeconomic groups. Onset is most commonly during early adulthood, and 50% of patients have a comorbid mental disorder. The course of illness is often chronic and debilitating. The goal is to improve function not to remove symptoms or reinforce false beliefs.

    2. Treatment

        a. Treatment is regularly (i.e., monthly) scheduled visits with a health care provider.

        b. Patients believe symptoms are caused by a medical illness and are therefore often resistant to seeing a mental health care provider. Group and individual psychotherapy are beneficial to develop coping strategies.

        c. Secondary gain should be minimized and medications avoided.

> Treatment of somatic disorders is difficult; a trusting relationship is paramount to reducing requests for further medical workup.

B. Illness anxiety disorder (formerly hypochondriasis)

    1. General characteristics

        a. This disorder is a preoccupation with the belief of having or the fear of contracting a serious illness. This belief is not of delusional intensity; normal bodily sensations are misinterpreted as manifestations of the disease. Symptoms last 6 months or more and impair functioning. Onset is typically in early-middle adulthood.

        b. Patients exaggerate the significance of every ache or bowel change and monitor their bodies for evidence of disease.

        c. This condition commonly is coexistent with symptoms of anxiety and depression.

        d. The patient's fear persists even though medical investigation reveals no cause.

        e. The course, although generally chronic, is episodic and may be exacerbated after a major stressor.

    2. Treatment

        a. Group and insight-oriented psychotherapy can be helpful, but patients are usually resistant to psychiatric care. Discussing mechanisms for coping with stress without reinforcing their perceived illness behavior is important.

        b. Regularly scheduled appointments with a practitioner are recommended to provide reassurance.

        c. SSRIs can be used if the patient has coexistent anxiety or depression.

> Support and development of coping mechanisms to allay anxiety is first line to reduce illness anxiety disorder.

C. Conversion disorder (Functional neurologic symptom disorder)

    1. General characteristics

        a. This disorder is characterized by one or more neurologic complaints that cannot be explained clinically.

        b. Symptoms are not intentionally produced and may be motor (involuntary movements, tics, blepharospasm, weakness), sensory (paresthesia and/or anesthesia, tunnel vision, deafness), pseudoseizures, or mixed (psychogenic vomiting, syncope, globus hystericus). The most common symptoms are shifting paralysis, blindness, and mutism. Symptoms are inconsistent with known medical or neurologic conditions.

    c. Patients may display an unexpected lack of concern and indifference to their symptoms (*la belle indifference*).

    d. Symptoms tend to be episodic, lasting days to a month, and may remit for a period of time, only to recur during times of stress.

    e. It is most commonly diagnosed during adolescence and young adulthood and is more common in females than in males. A catastrophic event typically occurs before onset of the disorder or will worsen it. With men, there often is an associated occupational or military accident.

  2. Treatment

    a. Psychotherapy, such as insight-oriented or behavioral therapy, is considered first-line treatment. The goal of treatment is to improve function. The spontaneous remission rate is high, so even without intervention most patients will improve.

    b. In general, medication should be avoided. Hypnosis, short-term anxiolytics (i.e., lorazepam), and relaxation therapy may help.

    c. Some patients have responded to amobarbital interviews to uncover underlying psychological factors.

> 💡 Medication should be avoided in conversion disorder; psychotherapy may be helpful.

D. **Factitious disorder**

  1. General characteristics

    a. Patients with this disorder intentionally fake signs and symptoms of medical or psychiatric symptoms. There is no obvious external incentive (e.g., money); the primary motivation is to assume the sick role.

    b. Characterized as factitious disorder imposed on self or factitious disorder imposed on another (formerly factitious disorder by proxy or Munchausen syndrome by proxy). The latter is a form of abuse.

    c. It usually begins in early adulthood and carries a poor prognosis.

    d. Often, patients will seek hospital admission under different names and by feigning different illnesses. When (or if) confronted with their ruse, they usually become angry and abruptly sign out.

    e. Obtaining a reliable past medical history is unlikely. Patients usually are familiar with the disease process that they are feigning; however, true disease processes must be ruled out.

  2. Treatment

    a. Early recognition is paramount in the management of this disorder to avoid unnecessary and/or potentially dangerous procedures.

    b. Once the diagnosis is confirmed, the patient should be confronted in a nonthreatening manner. No specific psychiatric intervention has been notably effective, but psychotherapy (individual, family) is suggested.

    c. SSRIs may be useful to reduce impulsive tendencies seen in acting-out factitious behavior.

E. **Malingering**

> 💡 Malingering, unlike factitious disorders, is motivated by external gain such as attention, money, or interpersonal relationship.

  1. Malingering involves the deliberate production of physical or psychological symptoms, motivated by external gain. Some of these obvious, definable goals are avoiding responsibility, police or legal action, punishment, or dangerous or difficult situations; receiving monetary compensation (e.g., in a lawsuit) or free hospital room and board; and obtaining drugs.

2. Patients tend to express vague, poorly defined complaints and claim that these symptoms cause great distress and impaired functioning. Injuries often are found to be self-inflicted, and history reveals multiple, undiagnosed illnesses or previous injuries and even tampering with laboratory results.

   a. Patients are uncooperative and refuse to accept a clean bill of health.

   b. Their symptoms typically improve when the objective has been met or the ruse has been exposed.

Mood Disorders

A. Definition

1. Mood disorders are a group of clinically distinct entities identified by patterns of mood episodes, which are periods of time (weeks to months) in which some mood impairment is present. The defining feature is a change in mood from a premorbid state. Normally, people feel more or less in control of their moods; however, this sense of control is lost in mood disorders, resulting in a feeling of great turmoil.

2. Mood episodes include major depressive episodes, manic episodes, hypomanic episodes, and mixed episodes.

3. Mood disorders include major depressive disorder (MDD), bipolar (types I and II), dysthymia/persistent depressive and cyclothymic disorder.

4. The cause is largely unknown; however, neurochemical (serotonin, norepinephrine, dopamine, growth hormone, cortisol), genetic, and psychosocial factors (life events) have been implicated.

B. Mood episodes

1. Major depressive episode

   a. Five or more depressive signs and symptoms must be present during the same 2-week period (Table 12-3). This must represent a change from previous functioning and cause significant impairment in functioning.

> A diagnosis of a mood disorder must include a change from previous functional level.

Table 12-3 | Symptoms of a Mood Episode

Depression
Depressed mood (either reported by the patient or observed by others)
Anhedonia
Excessive feelings of guilt
Indecisiveness
Lack of self-worth
Sleep problems such as insomnia or hypersomnia
Cognitive problems (difficulty with memory and concentration)
Psychomotor retardation or agitation
Either decreased or increased appetite or a 5% or greater unintentional change in body weight over a 1-month period
Decreased interest in sex
Either suicidal ideation or thoughts of death without suicidal ideation
Chronic fatigue or decreased energy

Mania
Inflated self-esteem or grandiosity
Irritability
Decreased need for sleep
Pressured speech
Flight of ideas
Distractibility
Impaired judgment, resulting in pursuit of pleasurable activities with a high probability of adverse outcomes
Psychomotor agitation

b. At least one of the symptoms must include depressed mood or anhedonia (loss of interest or pleasure in all activities).

c. Patients should not exhibit manic signs or symptoms (see Table 12-1).

2. The mood episode is not the result of bereavement.

3. Manic episode

    a. Manic episode is characterized by an abnormally and persistently elevated, expansive, or irritable mood that lasts for at least 1 week (or any duration if hospitalization is necessary).

    b. At least three manic symptoms (four if mood is irritable) out of seven are present (see Table 12-3).

    c. Patients may exhibit psychotic features or require hospitalization to prevent harm to self or others.

    d. Mania results in severe social and/or occupational dysfunction.

4. Hypomanic episode

    a. Similar to mania, hypomania is milder and a shorter duration episode characterized by an abnormally and persistently elevated, expansive, or irritable mood. Patients may display unrealistic optimism, poor judgment, pressured speech, increased creativity, and a reduced need for sleep.

    b. At least three manic symptoms (four if the mood is irritable) must be present.

    c. Although the patient's mood and functioning are changed from premorbid functioning, social and occupational functioning is not significantly affected, and there are no psychotic features.

    d. Hypomanic episode does not require hospitalization.

5. Mixed episode

    a. Mixed episode is characterized by rapidly alternating moods, with symptoms of both a manic episode and a depressive episode, which lasts for at least 1 week.

    b. Symptoms typically are severe enough that there is marked impairment in occupational or social functioning.

C. Mood disorders

  1. Major depressive disorder

    a. General characteristics

      (1) MDD has a chronic course with relapses. A simple way to remember symptoms is SIG-E-CAPS: **S**leep (either insomnia or hypersomnia), **I**nterest (depressed mood, anhedonia), **G**uilt (feelings of worthlessness or guilt), **E**nergy (decreased), **C**oncentration (decreased ability to think or make decisions), **A**ppetite (weight changes), **P**sychomotor (retardation or agitation), **S**uicide (or recurrent thoughts of death).

        (a) Premorbid functioning may return between episodes.

        (b) Between 5% and 10% of patients subsequently develop a manic episode.

        (c) MDD is two to three times more common in females than in males. The lifetime prevalence of depressive syndromes is 13% to 20%.

      (2) The suicide rate is estimated at 15%.

        (a) Patients may be at highest risk of suicide after initiating treatment; therapy may bring out the energy that the patient previously lacked to undertake a suicide attempt.

        (b) Higher suicide rates are associated with a previous attempt, white males older than 45 years, a detailed plan, a self-destructive pattern, a recent

> Hypomania is differentiated from mania by the severity of interruption in daily functions.

> In MDD, 5% to 10% of patients develop a manic episode.

severe loss, poor support system, poor health, concurrent substance abuse, psychotic symptoms, access to firearms, and an inability to accept help.

b. Subtypes

(1) Seasonal affective disorder

(a) Seasonal affective disorder is characterized by the predominance of fall or winter onset and likely is caused by the lessening daylight hours; it typically remits in the spring.

(b) It is more common in colder climates and in females; the age range at presentation is 20 to 40 years. Light therapy, SSRIs, and bupropion are effective treatment options.

(2) Atypical depression

(a) Atypical depression is characterized by overeating and weight gain, oversleeping, reactive mood, leaden paralysis (feeling like the arms and legs weigh them down making activities difficult), and oversensitivity to interpersonal rejection.

(b) Monoamine oxidase inhibitors (MAOIs) are useful in this group. SSRIs and atypical neuroleptics may also be effective treatment options.

(3) Catatonic depression

(a) Catatonic depression is characterized by motor immobility or stupor, blurred affect, purposeless motor activity, extreme withdrawal, negativism (i.e., may refuse to cooperate with simple requests for no obvious reason), bizarre mannerisms or posturing, echolalia, echopraxia, or "waxy flexibility" where a patient may assume strange or uncomfortable position and maintain this posture for an extended time.

(b) It often is treated with antidepressants and antipsychotics simultaneously. Adjuncts such as valproic acid, lithium, and risperidone may be beneficial. Electroconvulsive therapy (ECT) and benzodiazepines are also effective treatment options.

(4) Disruptive mood dysregulation disorder

(a) A mood disorder in children that is inconsistent with developmental level and characterized by chronic, severe irritability manifested by verbal and/or physically aggressive outbursts. These tantrums occur at least three times per week for a year or more and in at least two settings.

(b) Between episodes, children display a persistently angry mood nearly every day.

(c) Symptoms need to begin before age 10, and the diagnosis is not made before age 6 or after age 18.

(d) Treatment is individual/family/school therapy; SSRIs or stimulants may be helpful as might an antipsychotic such as risperidone for chronic, severe temper outbursts.

(5) Postpartum depression is characterized by the onset of symptoms within 4 weeks of delivery. SSRIs are the safest treatment. Hormone therapy may be of benefit as well.

(6) Premenstrual dysphoric disorder (PMDD)

(a) A severe form of premenstrual syndrome, PMDD symptoms start in the late luteal phase and dissipate once menses begins. Emotional and mood symptoms predominate lasting about 6 days and interfering with daily function.

(b) SSRIs are first-line treatment (fluoxetine, sertraline, paroxetine, escitalopram) and can be used continuously or instituted the week prior to menses. Birth control, low-dose estrogen, and diuretics may also be beneficial.

Atypical depression is less likely to improve with SSRI treatment.

Chronic, nonspecific irritability and outbursts of behavior are characteristic of DMDD.

c. Pharmacotherapy for mood disorders, in general

(1) If well tolerated, antidepressants should be continued for a minimum of 4 to 6 weeks to determine efficacy. If no response after 4 weeks, increase the dose or switch to a different drug class. Augmentation with another drug may be useful if only partial response to monotherapy. Maintenance treatment should be continued long term (>6 months) both because of the high relapse rate and because future episodes may be more severe.

(2) SSRIs are considered to be first-line therapy as they have minimal adverse effects and are safer than other antidepressant classes.

(a) Selection of a particular SSRI should be based on side-effect profiles and the presenting problems.

(b) Side effects include GI upset, headache, and sexual dysfunction.

(3) Serotonin-norepinephrine reuptake inhibitors (SNRIs) such as venlafaxine or duloxetine, and atypical antidepressants such as bupropion or mirtazapine, are also effective. SNRIs and atypicals have a lower incidence of decreased libido, erectile dysfunction, or anorgasmia, and have a safer side-effect profile than tricyclic antidepressants (TCAs) or MAOIs.

(4) TCAs and tetracyclics cause side effects such as weight gain, orthostatic hypotension, anticholinergic effects, and somnolence. Overdosage with these agents is more lethal than with other antidepressants.

(5) MAOIs require a tyramine-free diet (no wine, beer, nearly all cheeses, aged foods, smoked meats) to avoid serious side effects such as hypertensive crisis.

(6) Precautions

(a) Use of MAOIs with SSRIs, or any combination of drugs that increase serotonin levels, can result in serotonin syndrome, which can cause rapid onset of acute mental status changes, restlessness, nausea/vomiting, diarrhea, diaphoresis, tremor, hyperthermia, blood pressure fluctuations, seizures, muscle rigidity/hyperkinesia, clonus, and, occasionally, coma and death. Serotonin syndrome is managed by stopping the offending agents, IV hydration, aggressive cooling, and benzodiazepines. Cyproheptadine, an antihistamine that blocks serotonin production, can be used in severe cases.

(b) TCAs and MAOIs used concurrently can cause delirium and hypertension.

(c) The serious risks associated with MAOIs make this class of drugs the least likely to be used.

d. ECT

(1) ECT is effective in all types of MDD. Usually, however, it is reserved for severely depressed patients or patients who are unresponsive or intolerant of psychiatric medications or when the clinical picture is so debilitating that rapid improvement is warranted.

(2) ECT can safely be used in pregnant and elderly patients, produces a rapid response, and has very few relative contraindications. Maintenance antidepressant therapy is indicated after ECT is completed.

(3) Common adverse effects include postictal confusion and somatic complaints, such as headache, nausea, and muscle soreness.

(4) The greatest concern is memory loss, which often returns to baseline by 6 months after treatment.

> A safe treatment of acute mood disorders in pregnancy is ECT; it is safe and effective for the mother and does not harm the fetus.

e. Psychotherapy treatment for mood disorders: Most studies indicate that cognitive, interpersonal, and behavioral therapy is effective, especially in combination with pharmacotherapy.

2. Bipolar I disorder

a. General characteristics

A single full manic episode makes the diagnosis of bipolar I disorder, regardless of history of depressive symptoms.

(1) Bipolar I disorder is characterized by the occurrence of one or more manic or mixed episodes, which often cycle with depressive episodes, but the latter is not required for diagnosis. It is commonly known as manic depression.

(2) Manic episodes

  (a) Episodes are characterized by a sudden escalation of mood, which is abnormally and persistently euphoric, expansive, or irritable.

  (b) Patients may go for days without sleep; become excessively talkative or loud, socially outgoing, overly self-confident, hypersexual, or disinhibited; and display a flamboyant clothing style.

(3) Thought processes are difficult to follow because of racing thoughts, flights of ideas, and easy distraction. Judgment is impaired, resulting in spending sprees, promiscuity, or foolish business investments.

(4) Psychotic symptoms (e.g., hallucinations, paranoia, delusions) may be present.

(5) The course usually is chronic with relapses. In general, it carries a worse prognosis and a higher suicide rate than MDD.

(6) Epidemiology

  (a) The lifetime prevalence is about 1%.

  (b) The average age of diagnosis is 30 years, and early onset is correlated with a higher incidence of psychotic symptoms and a poorer prognosis.

  (c) Diagnosis is often delayed because misdiagnosis is very common; the most common misdiagnoses are MDD and anxiety.

  (d) First-degree relatives have an increased incidence of developing the disorder. Monozygotic twin concordance rates are about 75%.

Patients are misdiagnosed an average of 3.5 times before receiving a diagnosis of bipolar disorder.

b. Treatment

(1) Mood stabilizers such as lithium, valproic acid, olanzapine, or carbamazepine are effective. Gabapentin, topiramate, and lamotrigine also show beneficial effects. Second-generation antipsychotics such as risperidone, aripiprazole, quetiapine, and ziprasidone or benzodiazepines are a good choice to treat acute mania.

  (a) Lithium has a narrow therapeutic window, and plasma levels need to be monitored every 4 to 8 weeks.

  (b) Although usually well tolerated, lithium has side effects, including weight gain, tremor, nausea, increased thirst and urination and risk of renal insufficiency, drowsiness, hypothyroidism, arrhythmias, and seizures.

(2) Haloperidol or benzodiazepines (i.e., lorazepam or clonazepam) may be added if agitation or psychotic symptoms are present, especially at the initiation of treatment when acute manic episodes are likely.

(3) Acute depressive episodes can be treated with SSRIs or quetiapine. Olanzapine concurrently with fluoxetine has also been shown to be helpful.

(4) *Caution*: Antidepressant medication may precipitate mania.

(5) Secondary treatment measures include ECT, MAOIs, and TCAs (these two drug classes are least likely used; caution must be exercised because these medications can result in rapid cycling between mood states).

(6) Family, group, supportive, interpersonal, and/or cognitive therapy is essential.

3. Bipolar II disorder

  a. General characteristics

  (1) Bipolar II disorder is characterized by at least one or more major depressive episodes and at least one hypomanic episode. The patient has never experienced a manic episode or a mixed episode. Bipolar II is regarded as a milder form of bipolar I.

(2) Hypomanic symptoms are similar to manic symptoms but are less severe and cause less social impairment. Hypomania usually does not present with psychotic symptoms, racing thoughts, or excess psychomotor agitation.

(3) Prevalence is estimated at 0.5%; it appears to be slightly more common in females than in males.

b. Treatment is the same as for bipolar I disorder.

4. **Persistent depressive disorder (dysthymia)**

   a. General characteristics

   (1) This is a chronic, persistent mild depression that is manifested by pessimism, brooding, generalized loss of interest, decreased productivity, feelings of inadequacy, and social withdrawal.

   (2) There are no psychotic or manic/hypomanic features.

   (3) MDD eventually will develop in 10% to 20% of patients. Bipolar disorder may develop in others, and 25% of patients will have lifelong dysthymic symptoms.

   (4) It is two to three times more common in women than in men; onset is during young adulthood.

   b. Diagnosis

   (1) Patient is in depressed mood for most of the day, for more days than not, for at least 2 years (at least 1 year in children and adolescents).

   (2) During the 2-year period, the person has not been without the symptoms for more than 2 months at a time, and no major depressive episode occurred during the first 2 years of symptoms.

   (3) At least two of the following conditions are noted: poor concentration or indecisiveness, hopelessness, poor appetite or overeating, insomnia or hypersomnia, low energy or fatigue, and lack of self-esteem.

   c. Treatment

   (1) Antidepressants in combination with psychotherapy are most effective.

   (2) SSRIs are the first choice, followed by SNRIs, bupropion, TCAs, or, occasionally, MAOIs.

5. **Cyclothymic disorder**

   a. General characteristics

   (1) Patients are described as moody, erratic, impulsive, and somewhat volatile.

   (2) This disorder (similar to bipolar but less severe) is characterized by recurring periods of relatively less severe depressive episodes and hypomania over a 2-year period, with symptom-free periods lasting for no more than 2 months at any one time. The depressive episodes are not severe enough to be classified as a major depressive episode, and manic or mixed episodes have not occurred.

   (3) It has a chronic course, and there is a 15% to 20% risk of bipolar disorder.

   b. Treatment is similar to bipolar I disorder, with mood stabilizers and antimanic drugs as first-line therapies.

> Dysthymia and cyclothymia shows symptoms but do not meet the criteria for a major mood disorder; over time, many patients will progress either MDD or bipolar disorder, respectively.

Personality Disorders

A. Definition

1. Personality disorders are deeply ingrained, inflexible patterns of relating to others that are maladaptive and cause significant impairment in social or occupational functions.

2. In general, patients lack insight regarding their problems and are not distressed about their maladaptive behavior, so tend to not seek help. These disorders have an impact on two or more of the following categories: affect (how appropriate their emotional

response is in a given situation), impulse control, interpersonal relations, and cognition (how they interpret their environment). Personality disorders are divided into three clusters (Table 12-4).

> 💡 Psychotherapy is the fundamental treatment for all personality disorders.

B. Cluster A personality disorders

1. **Paranoid personality disorder**

   a. General characteristics

      (1) This disorder is characterized by a pervasive distrust and suspicion of others beginning in early adulthood. Patients blame their own problems on others and seem hostile and angry.

      (2) Males are more commonly affected than females.

   b. **Clinical features**

      (1) Suspicion (without evidence) that others are exploiting or deceiving him or her

      (2) Preoccupation with doubts regarding the loyalty or trustworthiness of acquaintances; doubts regarding fidelity causing turmoil in relationships

      (3) Reluctance to confide in others

      (4) Interpretation of benign remarks as threatening or demeaning

      (5) Persistently bears grudges; quick to counterattack

      (6) Emotionally cold with a blunted affect

   c. **Treatment**

      (1) Individual psychotherapy is the key.

      (2) Antianxiety medications or a short course of antipsychotics to decrease paranoia or for transient psychosis may be needed.

2. **Schizoid personality disorder**

   a. General characteristics

      (1) This disorder is characterized by a lifelong pattern of voluntary social withdrawal, often perceived as eccentric and reclusive. Reality testing, however, is intact.

      (2) Patients are quiet and unsociable and have constricted affect. They have no desire for close relationships and prefer to be alone.

      (3) Males are affected twice as often as females.

   b. **Clinical features**

      (1) Patients neither enjoy nor desire close relationships (including family).

      (2) They generally choose solitary activities.

      (3) They show little (if any) interest in sexual activity with another person.

      (4) They are indifferent to praise or criticism.

      (5) An emotional coldness, detachment, or flattened affect is seen.

Table 12-4 | Personality Disorders

Cluster	Description	Types
Cluster A (mad)	Patients are viewed as weird or peculiar; associated with psychotic disorders	Schizoid Schizotypal Paranoid
Cluster B (bad)	Patients are viewed as emotional or inconsistent; associated with mood disorders	Antisocial Borderline Histrionic Narcissistic
Cluster C (sad)	Patients are viewed as fearful or anxious; associated with anxiety disorders	Avoidant Dependent Obsessive–compulsive

c. Treatment

(1) Group therapy and psychotherapy are recommended.

(2) Low-dose, short-term antipsychotics or antidepressants can be given if indicated for comorbidity. Risperidone or olanzapine can help with flattened emotions, and SSRIs or bupropion can alleviate the psychological inability to experience pleasure.

3. Schizotypal personality disorder

a. General characteristics

(1) This disorder is characterized by a pervasive pattern of eccentric behavior and peculiar thought patterns beginning in early adulthood. Of all the personality disorders, schizotypal is most likely to progress to schizophrenia.

(2) The patient often is perceived as strange and eccentric. Their odd behavior and social deficits cause them to have few, if any, friends.

(3) This disorder may become apparent as early as childhood or adolescence.

b. Clinical features

(1) Patients have ideas of reference, which are beliefs or perceptions that irrelevant, unrelated, or innocuous things in the world are referring to them directly or have special personal significance. Ideas of reference are less firmly held or more disorganized beliefs than delusions of reference.

(2) Patients display odd thoughts, speech, beliefs, or "magical thinking" inconsistent with cultural norms; these may include belief in clairvoyance or telepathy, bizarre fantasies or preoccupations, and belief in superstitions or the occult.

(3) Unusual perceptual experiences (e.g., bodily illusions) may be noted.

(4) Patients show suspiciousness, paranoia, and excessive social anxiety.

(5) Inappropriate or restricted affect is seen.

c. Treatment

(1) Psychotherapy with social skills training is the treatment of choice.

(2) A trial of low-dose second-generation antipsychotics (such as risperidone or olanzapine) can help manage symptoms. Antidepressants or benzodiazepines to decrease anxiety can be used if necessary.

C. Cluster B personality disorders

1. Antisocial personality disorder

a. General characteristics

(1) This disorder is characterized by an inability to conform to social norms and a strong tendency to commit unlawful acts. The *DSM* stipulates that the patient must be at least 18 years old for this diagnosis.

(2) A pervasive pattern of disregard for and violation of the rights and feelings of others is characteristic. This disorder is strongly associated with violations of the law.

(3) Patients are described as extremely manipulative, deceitful, impulsive, and totally lacking empathy or remorse. On interview, however, they can act exceedingly charming and seem normal.

(4) It is strongly correlated with childhood conduct disorder.

(a) These children may have a history of physical and/or sexual abuse, starting fires, or harming animals.

(b) Symptoms may decrease with age.

(5) An abnormal electroencephalogram (EEG) may be seen.

(6) Males are affected three times more often than females. There is a familial pattern, and it is common among the homeless and prison populations.

> Schizotypal is differentiated from schizoid by the presence of magical thinking.

> Patients with antisocial personality disorder have no remorse for their behavior.

b. Clinical features

(1) Patients show deceitfulness, lying, and conning others for personal gain.

(2) Irritability and aggressiveness, manifested by repeated physical assaults, are noted, and patients have a reckless disregard for the safety of self or others.

(3) Patients are irresponsible and unable to sustain work.

c. Treatment

(1) Treatment is psychotherapy with socially based intervention.

(2) Pharmacotherapy options include SSRIs, lithium, valproate, second-generation antipsychotics, carbamazepine; propranolol may help to reduce anxiety, impulsivity, and aggression.

2. Borderline personality disorder

a. General characteristics

(1) This disorder is characterized by an unstable and unpredictable mood, affect, and behavior as well as a poorly established self-image. Mood swings and impulsivity are common, and the patient always appears to be in a "state of crisis."

(2) Short and transient psychotic episodes, paranoid ideation, or dissociative symptoms may occur, especially during times of increased stress.

(3) Self-harm and manipulative suicide attempts are very common.

(4) They may be impulsive in terms of spending or sexual behavior.

(5) The patient desperately attempts to avoid abandonment.

(6) Patients cannot tolerate being alone, yet can exhibit intense anger toward their friends.

(a) Splitting (i.e., seeing people as either all good or all bad) is a common defense mechanism.

(b) Patients have volatile and intense relationships.

(c) Inappropriate anger or difficulty controlling anger is seen.

(7) There is a high incidence of MDD with borderline personality disorder; suicide rates peak during early adulthood.

(8) Females are affected twice as often as males. Like antisocial personality disorder, these patients may have an abnormal EEG.

b. Treatment

(1) Treatment includes dialectical behavior therapy. It involves both individual and group therapy encouraging change-oriented strategies and synthesis.

(2) Pharmacotherapy is likely more useful in borderline disorder than any of the other personality disorders. Medication in addition to psychotherapy yields better results.

(a) Low-dose antipsychotics are used to control hostility and brief psychotic episodes.

(b) Antidepressants/SSRIs such as fluoxetine are used to improve mood.

(c) Benzodiazepines can help decrease anxiety but should only be used short term (days to weeks).

(d) Lithium or valproate can be used as a mood stabilizer.

3. Histrionic personality disorder

a. General characteristics

(1) Individuals with this disorder are overly emotional, dramatic, and seductive; they are excitable, with a high degree of attention-seeking behavior and a tendency to exaggerate their thoughts and feelings.

Dialectical behavior therapy, combining both individual and group therapy, was developed specifically for borderline personality disorder.

Histrionic and narcissistic personality disorders are characterized by overdramatic responses to any challenge.

(a) Patients are flamboyant and extroverted, but their rapidly shifting emotions and superficiality render them unable to maintain a deep, long-lasting relationship.

(b) They are easily influenced by others.

(c) They need to be the center of attention and may throw a temper tantrum if the attention shifts. They have a pattern of excessive emotionality and attention-seeking behavior and often are inappropriately seductive or provocative, with exaggerated expression and emotion.

(2) Somatization and substance use disorders are common.

(3) Speech can be excessively impressionistic and lacking in detail.

(4) Histrionic patients may employ the defense mechanism of regression in which they revert to acting like a child.

b. Treatment

(1) Treatment includes psychotherapy, either group or individual.

(2) Antidepressants and/or anxiolytics may be useful but only if specific symptoms warrant their use. Histrionic patients function fairly well in general, so medications do not play much of a role in this disorder.

> Psychotherapy is the mainstay of treatment for histrionic and narcissistic personality disorders.

4. Narcissistic personality disorder

a. General characteristics

(1) Patients have an inflated self-image, pattern of grandiosity, need for admiration, and lack of empathy. They consider themselves to be special and expect to be treated as such, and they may have an arrogant, haughty attitude.

(2) Although they have a sense of entitlement and grandiosity, their self-esteem is quite fragile. They have a need for excessive admiration, and they are prone to depression if criticized.

(3) They have a preoccupation with fantasies of unlimited success, beauty, brilliance, and so forth. Aging is difficult and makes them prone to midlife crisis.

(4) They may be exploitative and take advantage of others to meet their own needs.

b. Treatment

(1) This disorder is difficult to treat. Psychotherapy is key.

(2) Medications are rarely indicated, although lithium can be used if mood swings are prominent. Antidepressants (especially SSRIs) can be a useful adjunct if a concurrent mood disorder is present.

D. Cluster C personality disorders

1. Avoidant personality disorder

a. General characteristics

(1) These individuals have an extreme sensitivity to rejection (inferiority complex).

(2) Patients see themselves as unappealing.

(3) They have intense social anxiety and feelings of inadequacy, which may lead to interpersonal withdrawal and total avoidance of any situation in which they may be criticized.

(4) Although shy, they display a great desire for companionship but with strong guarantees of unconditional acceptance. They may avoid occupational activities that involve interpersonal contact because of fear of rejection.

(5) They show great restraint with intimate relationships because of fear of rejection.

(6) Social phobia (fear of embarrassment or rejection in a particular setting) is common in this group.

b. **Treatment**

   (1) First-line treatment is psychotherapy. Social skills training, group therapy, and assertiveness training may be beneficial.

   (2) β-Blockers and SSRIs (especially paroxetine, sertraline, or escitalopram) are useful for managing anxiety and depression and may help to reduce the patient's sensitivity to rejection. Benzodiazepines can be used short term to decrease anxiety.

2. **Dependent personality disorder**

   a. General characteristics

   (1) These individuals have an enduring pattern of dependent, clinging, and submissive behavior; they cannot make their own decisions without help from others.

   (2) Patients have difficulty disagreeing with others for fear of loss of support or approval.

   (3) They lack self-confidence, avoid positions of responsibility, and have a dislike of being alone. They are passive, self-doubtful, and reliant on others to take care of them.

   (4) Depression may ensue, especially if they experience loss of the person on whom they depend.

   (5) They go to extreme lengths to seek another relationship.

   (6) Social and occupational functioning is impaired; risk for depression is high. Some suffer physical or mental abuse because they fail to assert themselves.

   (7) They feel uncomfortable when alone for fear of being unable to care for self.

   b. **Treatment**

   (1) Psychotherapy, especially insight-oriented, behavioral, group, and family therapy, and assertiveness training may help.

   (2) Anxiolytics and antidepressants may be useful to target symptoms; benzodiazepines and SSRIs are used.

3. **Obsessive–compulsive personality disorder**

   a. General characteristics

   (1) Obsessive–compulsive personality disorder is characterized by a pervasive pattern of orderliness (rules, lists, details), perfectionism, and inflexibility.

   (2) Patients tend to be rigid, stubborn, and emotionally constricted, and they insist that others submit to their ways, causing difficulty with interpersonal and occupational relationships.

   (3) Perfectionism interferes with the ability to complete tasks or form relationships.

   (4) A change in routine threatens to upset their perceived stability and can lead to extreme anxiety.

   (5) The course of this disorder is variable. The disorder may remit, or obsessions and compulsions may develop. Schizophrenia and MDD may develop.

   (6) Obsessive–compulsive personality disorder is egosyntonic (not distressing to the patient), whereas obsessive–compulsive disorder (OCD) is egodystonic (distressing to the patient). There are no recurrent obsessions/compulsions in this personality disorder.

   (7) Patients display excessive devotion to work and productivity to the exclusion of leisure activities; they have a reluctance to delegate tasks unless those tasks are done the way they want.

   (8) Miserly spending or hoarding may be seen.

> Obsessive–compulsive disorder is very distressing to the patient; obsessive–compulsive *personality* disorder is not.

b. Treatment

(1) Psychotherapy and group or behavioral therapy is recommended.

(2) SSRIs can help manage anxiety/depression. Clomipramine is effective as a second-line medication.

E. Personality disorder NEC: This category includes patients who do not meet the full criteria for a specific disorder but who have traits from many different ones.

Anxiety Disorders

A. Definition

1. Anxiety disorders are characterized by excessive amounts of anxiety and heightened arousal that impede daily function and interpersonal relationships.

2. Anxious disorders can result in physical symptoms, such as dizziness, palpitations, perspiration, loss of appetite, nausea, trembling, and other symptoms that cause the patient distress.

B. Generalized anxiety disorder (GAD)

1. General characteristics

a. GAD is characterized by persistent and excessive anxiety regarding general life events. It is not situational (as in phobias) or episodic (like panic disorder).

b. The patient has difficulty coping with the anxiety, which usually is expressed as worry or apprehension, and experiences symptoms more days than not over a period of at least 6 months. However, patients often present to medical providers with somatic complaints, such as racing heartbeat, nausea, epigastric abdominal pain, headaches, fatigue, and muscle tension.

c. GAD is frequently associated with other comorbid psychiatric disorders such as MDD, specific and social phobias, substance abuse, and panic disorder.

d. Diagnostic criteria include at least three of the following: restlessness or hypervigilance, easy fatigability, irritability, sleep disturbance, muscle tension, and difficulty concentrating. Medical and substance abuse disorders, such as thyroid dysfunction, cardiac arrhythmias, stimulant abuse, alcohol withdrawal, and caffeine intoxication, must be ruled out.

e. GAD is common, with the lifetime prevalence estimated around 7% for women and 4% for men. Age of onset is generally in the early 20s, although the diagnosis may develop at any age.

2. Treatment

a. Initial management should include pharmacologic and psychologic therapies.

b. SSRIs, SNRIs, and buspirone are effective; low-dose TCAs also may help but are utilized less frequently secondary to their side-effect profile.

c. Benzodiazepines can be used as an adjunct for short-term management of severe symptoms but are not recommended for monotherapy because of the risk of dependence or abuse.

d. Behavioral therapy and CBT also should be initiated.

> Treatment of anxiety should include cognitive behavioral therapy (CBT) focused on coping mechanisms.

C. Panic attacks and panic disorder

1. Panic attacks

a. Panic attack is defined as a rapid onset of extreme anxiety that peaks within 10 minutes, typically declines within 30 minutes, and rarely lasts for longer than 1 hour.

b. Panic attacks may have a definable trigger or be totally unexpected.

c. Patients may experience palpitations or tachycardia, sweating, trembling, dyspnea/hyperventilation, sensation of choking, chest discomfort, nausea, depersonalization (feel estranged from self and/or the external world), derealization (people, events, and surroundings appear to be changed or unreal), fear of losing control, fear of dying, light-headedness, numbness or tingling, chills, or hot flashes. Four or more of the previous symptoms must be present.

2. **Panic disorder**

   a. Panic disorder is characterized by recurrent panic attacks, and accompanying fears of additional attacks, concern regarding consequences of attacks, or behavioral changes related to attacks.

   b. Panic disorder occurs in 1% to 3% of the population. It is twice as common in females.

   c. Average age at onset is the mid-20s, but panic disorder can occur at any age, including childhood.

3. Diagnosis should specify panic disorder with or without agoraphobia (fear of inability to escape from settings in which attacks may occur).

4. **Treatment**

   a. Ideally, treatment should combine medication and therapy. The most effective psychotherapy for panic disorder is CBT.

   b. Mild cases may be managed with psychotherapy alone.

   c. For acute management of panic attacks, low-dose high-potency benzodiazepines (alprazolam or clonazepam) are acceptable.

   d. For maintenance, SSRIs should be instituted as benzodiazepines are tapered. Paroxetine, fluoxetine, and sertraline are all Food and Drug Administration (FDA) approved for panic disorder. The SNRI venlafaxine is also approved.

D. **Phobias (specific and social)**

   1. General characteristics

      a. Phobic disorders affect up to 8% to 10% of the general population. Phobias generally begin in childhood or early adult life, and become chronic and are not explained by another medical or psychiatric illness.

      b. They are characterized by an irrational and disproportionate excessive fear when presented with an object or a situational event.

      c. Exposure results in an immediate increase in anxiety and can precipitate a panic attack.

      d. Because of the discomfort caused by the increased anxiety, the panic attack, or both, the feared situation or object is avoided.

      e. Except for children, patients with this disorder know that their fear is excessive and unreasonable.

      f. Diagnosis of a phobia is made if the response to phobic stimuli interferes with the patient's daily routine, social functioning, or occupational functioning.

      g. Common comorbidities include MDD, substance abuse, other anxiety disorders, and personality disorders.

   2. Specific phobia

      a. Specific phobias are more common than social phobias. The duration lasts 6 months or more.

      b. Specific phobia and agoraphobia are more common in women than in men; social phobia generally affects men and women equally. Specific phobia typically begins in childhood before age 12, unlike other anxiety disorders and phobias.

      c. Specific phobia refers to the fear of a specific object or situation. There are five types (Table 12-5).

      d. Diagnosis is made if, for a period of 6 months, a patient has marked fear or anxiety of a specific object or situation, exposure almost always causes immediate fear/

> Panic attacks are often misinterpreted as major cardiac events; consider this in a differential for either diagnosis.

> Specific phobias may respond to gradual exposure therapy under supervised conditions.

anxiety, the phobia is actively avoided or endured with extreme anxiety, the fear or anxiety is out of proportion to sociocultural context, and there is clinically significant distress to the patient.

3. Social anxiety disorder (social phobia)

   a. Social phobia is the fear of social or performance situations in which embarrassment or humiliation in front of other people may occur. Feared situations result in an extreme anxiety response. The duration of symptoms is 6 months or more, and generally has an onset in adolescence and early adulthood.

   b. Common inciting events are public speaking, using public restrooms, and eating in public.

4. Agoraphobia

   a. Agoraphobia is closely linked with panic disorder and is described as an intense fear of the inability to easily exit a situation or place where an incapacitating event may occur. The patient may subsequently avoid places where escape is viewed by the patient as difficult or humiliating.

   b. Anxiety-producing situations may include riding on a train or bus; being in any crowded area, mall, supermarket, or theater; or just being alone outside the home.

   c. Agoraphobia generally occurs in patients with a history of panic disorder. If the feared incapacitating event is a panic attack, then panic disorder with agoraphobia is diagnosed.

   d. Diagnostic criteria

      (1) Significant fear or anxiety for 6 months or longer about two or more of the specific situations: public transportation, open spaces, enclosed spaces, standing in line or with a crowd or people, or outside of one's home alone. Patients fear or avoid these situations because of a sense of lack of escape Agoraphobic situations provoke fear/anxiety out of proportion to potential dangers, cause significant distress, and are not related to another psychiatric or medical condition.

      (2) In extreme cases, symptoms may render the patient either unwilling or unable to leave home.

   > The basic underlying pathology in agoraphobia is a fear of inability to escape from an uncomfortable situation.

5. **Treatment**

   a. For social phobias and agoraphobia, SSRIs, particularly paroxetine, fluvoxamine, and sertraline, as well as the SNRI venlafaxine, are considered to be first-line therapy.

   b. TCAs are effective for panic symptoms but are considered second line, given their side-effect profile.

   c. β-Blockers, such as propranolol, have been used successfully to reduce autonomic hyperarousal symptoms and tremor associated with performance situations.

   d. Gabapentin, given its antianxiety properties, is a potential alternative pharmacotherapy for social phobia in dosages of 300 to 3,600 mg per day.

   e. CBT is the first line for phobias. Social phobia, agoraphobia, and other specific phobias may utilize behavioral techniques in therapy such as exposure therapy.

Table 12-5 | Specific Phobias

Animal	Fear of specific animals or insects
Natural environment	Fear of natural phenomena, e.g., storms, heights, water, lightening
Blood-injection-injury	Fear of needles or invasive procedures; a phobic trigger may be the possibility of injury, the sight of blood, or fear of contamination by exposure to bodily fluids, dental procedures, or childbirth
Situational	Fear of specific situations, e.g., fear of bridges, tall buildings, flying, driving, or confined spaces such as elevators
Other	Fear of situations that may lead to choking, vomiting, or an illness in children; fear of loud noises or costumed characters such as clowns

E. **Obsessive–compulsive disorder**

   1. General characteristics

      a. Obsessions are undesired persistent and recurrent thoughts, images, or impulses that are intrusive and inappropriate leading to significant distress.

      b. Compulsions are the ritualistic or repetitive behaviors or thoughts that patients feel compelled to engage in to relieve the aversion caused by obsessions. The behaviors, or mental acts, are excessive and have no realistic connection to the events the patient is trying to avoid.

      c. Patients may or may not have insight and realize that their thoughts and behaviors are irrational and causing distress.

      d. This disorder is egodystonic as opposed to obsessive–compulsive personality disorder, which is egosyntonic (not distressing to the patient). OCD patients are more likely to seek treatment than obsessive–compulsive personality disorder patients.

      e. The majority of patients are diagnosed before age 25 years.

      f. The most common types of obsessions are as follows:

        (1) Contamination: Patients wash their hands excessively or compulsively avoid objects presumed to be contaminated.

        (2) Pathologic doubt: Patients worry about such things as forgetting to lock the door or turn off the stove; these doubts result in repetitive checking.

      g. Other obsessions include the following:

        (1) Intrusive thoughts: Patients have obsessive thoughts without a compulsion; these thoughts may be of a sexual or aggressive nature.

        (2) Need for symmetry: Patients must order and arrange objects, leading to extreme precision and slowness.

        (3) Patients may also have religious obsessions, compulsive hoarding, nail-biting, skin picking, and trichotillomania (compulsively pulling out hair).

      h. The most frequent compulsive rituals include checking and decontaminating, counting, symmetry and precision, hoarding, repeating, and needing to ask or confess.

> Obsessive behavior can take many forms; behaviors to avoid contamination are most characteristic.

   2. **Treatment**

      a. SSRIs (sertraline, paroxetine, fluoxetine, fluvoxamine), in doses often higher than normally prescribed, are considered to be first-line therapy; the TCA clomipramine has shown efficacy, but the side effect profile makes it less frequently utilized.

      b. Adjunctive medication such as clomipramine or a high-potency antipsychotic may benefit patients who only show a partial remission of symptoms with SSRI therapy.

      c. Behavioral therapies including exposure and response prevention should be initiated along with medication.

      d. Neurosurgical interventions such as cingulotomy and deep brain stimulators are a last resort.

F. **Body dysmorphic disorder**

   1. General characteristics

      a. This disorder is characterized by a preoccupation with an imagined defect in physical appearance or an exaggerated distortion of a minor flaw. The most common concerns are facial flaws. Preoccupations cause clinically significant distress and impair normal functioning.

      b. Patients feel self-conscious and fear humiliation; they go to great lengths to hide or correct their perceived anomaly. They frequently perform mirror checking and compare themselves to others.

      c. Visits to medical and surgical offices are common, although the patient usually is still not satisfied with his or her appearance.

> Most body dysmorphic symptoms involve a perception of facial imperfections.

    d. Age of onset is 15 to 20 years; females are affected more often than males.

2. Treatment

    a. Serotonin-modulating drugs (fluoxetine, clomipramine) are efficacious in a majority of patients. SSRI treatment may require higher dosages; treatment response may require 10 to 12 weeks of medication.

    b. CBT has been demonstrated to be effective.

    c. Coexistent psychiatric disorders should be treated appropriately. The most common coexisting disorder is a major depressive episode, followed by anxiety disorder.

Trauma- and Stressor-Related Disorders

A. Post-traumatic stress disorder (PTSD)

    1. General characteristics

        a. PTSD results from exposure to or witnessing a physiologically or psychologically traumatic event that is out of the range of normal human experience. Actual/threatened death, serious injury, and sexual violence are common precipitants.

        b. PTSD is manifested by recurrently experiencing the initial precipitating trauma through dreams, intrusive thoughts or flashbacks, avoidance of provoking stimuli, emotional numbing, and hyperarousal potentially manifest as irritability, and insomnia.

        c. Patients may express a sense of repeatedly reliving the event or may be unable to recall an important aspect of the event secondary to avoidance.

        d. Comorbid depression or panic disorder are common, and there are high concurrence rates with substance abuse.

        e. PTSD can occur at any age. In men, it most often results from combat experience; in women, it most often results from assault or rape.

    2. For diagnosis, each of the following major elements must be present for more than 1 month:

> The diagnosis of PTSD is a combination of symptoms and subsequent withdrawal, avoidant, or extremely reactive behavior.

        a. Exposure to actual or threatened death, serious injury, or sexual violence by direct experience or as a witness

        b. Reexperiencing the trauma through disturbing dreams, intrusive memories, or flashbacks; possibly with physiologic reactions

        c. Persistent avoidance or efforts to avoid internal reminders such as memories, thoughts, or reminders of the event or external reminders including people and places. An increased state of arousal characterized by at least two of the following: insomnia, irritability or angry outbursts, poor concentration, reckless or self-destructive behavior, hypervigilance, or exaggerated startle response.

        d. Negative alternations in mood and thoughts evident by two of the following: dissociative amnesia, negative beliefs about self or the world, distorted cognitions about traumatic events leading to self-blame, chronically negative emotional state, diminished interest, detachment from others, inability to experience positive emotions.

    3. Treatment

        a. SSRIs (sertraline, paroxetine) are considered to be first-line treatment. Short-term benzodiazepines can be used to decrease anxiety. Trazodone is effective for treating insomnia; prazosin may also be used to improve sleep and reduce nightmares as well as other hyperarousal symptoms. Impulsivity may be improved with anticonvulsants such as carbamazepine.

        b. CBT, cognitive processing therapy, exposure therapy and eye-movement desensitization, and reprocessing therapy have all been demonstrated to be effective.

B. **Acute stress disorder**

1. General characteristics

   a. This disorder is similar to PTSD but differs in onset and duration. Symptoms of acute stress disorder occur within 1 month of the traumatic event and last from 2 days to 4 weeks, whereas symptoms of PTSD may develop any time after the event and last for more than 1 month. Acute stress disorder is considered a precursor to PTSD.

   b. It is most prevalent in younger ages. Those most likely affected are victims or witnesses of violent crime or combat experience, survivors of natural disasters, and people involved in motor vehicle accidents.

   c. Common comorbidities include depression, anxiety, substance abuse, and cognitive difficulties (e.g., impaired concentration).

2. **Clinical features**

   a. Either during or after the event, the person has nine or more symptoms from five categories (Table 12-6).

   b. The distressing event is reexperienced in at least one of the following ways: recurrent dreams, images, or thoughts; flashbacks; sensation of reliving the event; or exposure to reminders of the trauma, causing distress.

   c. Distress results in marked impairment in important areas of functioning.

3. **Treatment** is similar to PTSD, including therapy and supportive counseling as well as pharmacotherapy.

C. **Adjustment disorder**

1. General characteristics

   a. This stress-response syndrome is characterized by maladaptive behavioral or emotional symptoms that develop within 3 months after an identifiable stressful life event and end within 6 months after the event.

   b. Among adolescents, precipitants may include parental rejection and divorce, loss of a parent or loved one, leaving home, or beginning college.

   c. Among adults, stressors include marital discord, financial difficulties, or loss of a job, marriage, relocation, retirement, or parenthood. Also included are natural disasters and racial/religious persecution.

> Symptoms of acute stress are similar to PTSD but have been present for <1 month.

Table 12-6 | Symptoms of Acute Stress

Category	Specific Symptoms
Intrusion symptoms	Memories Dreams Flashbacks
Negative mood	Inability to experience positive emotions Inability to be happy
Dissociative symptoms	Sense of numbing or detachment Reduced awareness of surroundings Being in a daze Derealization Depersonalization Amnesia
Avoidance symptoms	Avoidance of stimuli reminiscent of the trauma such as activities, places, or people
Arousal symptoms	Insomnia Irritability Poor concentration Hypervigilance Exaggerated startle response

d. The reaction is either out of proportion to the stressor or causes significant impairment in functioning.

e. Symptoms include tearfulness, depressed mood, vandalism, reckless driving, truancy, fighting, and anxiety.

2. Treatment

a. Adjustment disorder is treated with supportive psychotherapy or group therapy.

b. Short-term benzodiazepines, sleep aids, or SSRIs may be used for associated anxiety, insomnia, or depression but is not a first-line treatment.

Eating Disorders

A. Anorexia nervosa

1. General characteristics

a. Patients have a distorted body image and an intense fear of becoming fat, even though they are underweight.

b. This results in a self-imposed starvation despite normal appetite and craving for food. Patients are categorized by severity based on body mass index (BMI). BMI ≥ 17 kg per m^2 is mild, 16 to 16.99 is moderate, 15 to 15.99 is severe, and <15 is extreme. Patients often feel that losing weight is a desired achievement of self-control, whereas gaining weight is thought of as an unacceptable lack of discipline. Unlike bulimia, this disorder is egosyntonic. Patients deny the seriousness of their low body weight.

c. Patients may exercise excessively, and they commonly have food-related obsessions (e.g., hoarding food, collecting recipes).

d. Approximately 90% of patients are female with a mean age of 17. Anorexia nervosa is more common in developed countries and in professions that require thinness (e.g., modeling, ballet, jockeys, athletes).

e. There are two types of anorexia:

(1) Restricting: The patient eats very little and does not regularly engage in binge eating or purging behavior, such as induced vomiting, abusing laxatives or diuretics, or using enemas.

(2) Binge eating and purging: The patient eats in binges followed by purging behavior.

2. Clinical features

a. Patients exhibit emaciation, orthostatic hypotension, bradycardia, hypothermia, dry skin, lanugo, peripheral edema, constipation, and amenorrhea/delayed menarche.

b. Examination may reveal salivary gland hypertrophy, dental erosion/loss of tooth enamel, calluses, or abrasions on the back of the hand from induced vomiting.

c. Workup may show leukopenia, electrolyte abnormalities (hypochloremia, hypokalemia, elevated blood urea nitrogen [BUN], metabolic alkalosis), and arrhythmias.

d. Osteoporosis and increased likelihood of fractures are of concern owing to decreased estrogen, increased cortisol, and inadequate calcium and vitamin D intake.

3. Treatment

a. Patients rarely seek treatment; family members usually are the first to bring this disorder to attention. A multidisciplinary approach to treatment is essential.

b. The first goal of management is to restore the patient's nutritional state. Hospitalization often is indicated, especially if the patient is more than 20% below the expected body weight. There is a high (10%) mortality rate. Fluid and electrolyte abnormalities must be corrected, and gradual weight restoration is crucial.

> Anorexia nervosa is egosyntonic, patients are not distressed about symptoms; bulimia is egodystonic, patients are distressed and often feel guilty regarding their symptoms.

> **Patients with bulimia nervosa are of normal weight or overweight despite purging behavior.**

　　c. CBT and interpersonal psychotherapies may be helpful in maintaining weight gain and should be maintained for 1 year following weight gain.

　　d. No specific psychopharmacologic medication can induce return to normal eating habits. Antidepressants and antipsychotics may be helpful adjuncts for comorbid depressive or psychotic symptoms. Olanzapine may aid in weight gain. Overall, medications do not play a major role in the treatment of this disorder.

B. Bulimia nervosa

　1. General characteristics

　　a. Patients with bulimia engage in binge eating followed by subsequent purging including vomiting, use of laxatives and/or diuretics, excessive exercise, or other measures to avoid gaining weight. These maladaptive behaviors occur at least 1 day per week for 3 months.

　　b. The binge eating causes emotional distress and a feeling of loss of control.

　　c. Unlike patients with anorexia, those with bulimia commonly maintain normal body weight, or they may even be overweight. Rapid fluctuations in weight are very characteristic in patients with bulimia.

　　d. There is a severity scale for bulimia:

　　　(1) Mild: 1 to 3 episodes per week

　　　(2) Moderate: 4 to 7 episodes per week

　　　(3) Severe: 8 to 13 episodes per week

　　　(4) Extreme: ≥14

　　e. Bulimia is significantly more common in females than in males. Onset is most common between ages 15 and 30 years. It is more prevalent than anorexia. However, patients are more likely to seek treatment because this disorder is egodystonic (upsetting to the patient), unlike anorexia.

　　f. Patients with bulimia tend to be high achievers and respond to societal pressure to be thin.

　　g. There is an increased rate of anxiety and mood disorders, bipolar I disorder, impulse control disorders, and history of sexual abuse.

　2. Physical findings and diagnostic studies include dental erosion, esophagitis, callused or abraded knuckles, salivary gland hypertrophy, gastric distention, and cardiac arrhythmias, hypochloremia, hypokalemia, metabolic alkalosis, hypomagnesemia, hypocalcemia, elevated amylase, and gastric distention.

> **The egodystonia present in bulimia nervosa prompts patients to seek treatment.**

　3. Treatment

　　a. The prognosis for patients with bulimia is better than that for patients with anorexia because they are more likely to seek treatment both because their uncontrolled eating is egodystonic and because there is less denial.

　　b. Restoring the patient's nutritional state is the first treatment. Antidepressants, such as SSRIs (fluoxetine), are useful. Other classes of antidepressants have also been found to be effective, although fluoxetine is the only medication with FDA approval. Bupropion can lower the seizure threshold, so should be avoided in these patients owing to possible coexistent electrolyte abnormalities.

　　c. Behavioral psychotherapy including CBT and interpersonal psychotherapy should be used in conjunction with family therapy. Group therapy with others suffering from bulimia has been shown to be effective. A holistic approach is best.

　　d. Hospitalization usually is not necessary; exceptions are the presence of suicidal ideation or significant metabolic or electrolyte disturbances caused by severe purging.

C. Binge eating disorder (BED)

　1. General characteristics

　　a. Obesity is defined as 20% or more over ideal body weight or a BMI of >30 kg per m^2.

b. Obese patients often suffer emotional distress over their eating binges but do not purge or restrict eating in an attempt to control their weight. They admit to a loss of control over their eating behavior.

2. Diagnostic criteria

  a. Recurrent episodes of binge eating at least once per week for 3 months, characterized by eating a larger amount of food in a 2-hour period than most average people would consume.

  b. The binge-eating episodes are associated with three or more of the following: eating faster than normal; eating until feeling uncomfortably full; eating to excess, even though not hungry; eating alone out of embarrassment; and feeling disgusted, guilty, or depressed after the episode.

  c. Episodes are not associated with any inappropriate compensatory weight loss behaviors (vomiting, fasting, excess exercise, laxatives), and patients are not fixated on body image.

  d. The same severity scale as bulimia in terms of frequency of episodes applies.

3. Treatment

  a. Behavioral therapy with CBT techniques, and behavioral weight loss therapy combined with medication. Nutritional counseling aids in weight loss efforts.

  b. Pharmacotherapy

    (1) SSRIs and venlafaxine appear to reduce binges. Sympathomimetics reduce appetite, and lisdexamfatemine has been approved for short-term use in BED.

    (2) Topiramate may reduce both bingeing behavior and cause weight loss.

    (3) Orlistat (Xenical), a pancreatic lipase inhibitor that decreases fat absorption from the GI tract, can be used as an add-on. However, the unpleasant side effect of oily stool leakage makes this less likely tolerated by patients.

  c. Bariatric surgery should be considered for those with a BMI >35 and comorbidities, and those with a BMI >40.

> BED is driven by a loss of control over eating habits, leading to overeating and GI distress.

Substance-Related and Addictive Disorders Abuse

A. General characteristics

  1. The most commonly abused substances are alcohol, tobacco, and marijuana.

  2. Other substances of abuse include opiates, stimulants, barbiturates, benzodiazepines, and over-the-counter medications.

B. Substance use disorders

  1. This involves the inappropriate use of a substance. Substance use disorder results in significant impairment, as manifested by two or more of the following 11 maladaptive behaviors within a 12-month period.

  a. Tolerance: There is either a decreased effect over time when the same amount of substance is used or a need for an increased amount of a substance over time to achieve a baseline.

  b. Withdrawal: There is a cluster of symptoms that occurs with an onset closely following cessation of the substance necessitating use of the substance to relieve or avoid physical symptoms associated with deprivation of it.

  c. There is use of increasingly larger amounts of a substance or over a longer period than was intended.

  d. There are unsuccessful efforts to stop or decrease the amount of a substance used.

  e. A significantly portion of time spent attempting to acquire or use the substance or to recover from its effects.

> The key to substance use disorder is a pattern of continued use despite ongoing and progressive negative consequences—physical, mental, occupational, and social.

    f. There is social, occupational, or recreational impairment.

    g. There is continued use of a substance despite the awareness that doing so has adverse consequences.

        (1) Patient fails to meet home, school, or work obligations.

        (2) Patient repeatedly uses the substance in hazardous situations (e.g., driving a car).

        (3) Patient has cravings or a strong desire to use the substance.

        (4) Patient continues to use the substance, even though he or she is experiencing interpersonal or social problems as a result.

  2. Substance intoxication refers to maladaptive behavioral or psychological changes attributed to recent ingestion of a substance. Intoxication is reversible and is not caused by a mental disorder or medical condition.

  3. Severity is specified as mild (2 to 3 symptoms), moderate (4 to 5 symptoms), or severe (6 or more symptoms).

C. Epidemiology

  1. Lifetime prevalence of substance abuse or dependence is about 19.5% per 100 persons aged 18 years and older.

  2. Individuals in the United States with substance abuse disorders have nearly a three times greater risk of a comorbid mental disorder (excluding those who use nicotine and caffeine) compared with nonsubstance abusers.

  3. Screening for alcohol or drug use disorder can be assessed in an office setting through use of the CAGE screening (Table 12-7). There are several validated screening tools for general and specific substance use disorders available through the National Institute on Drug Abuse.

D. **Alcohol use/abuse**

  1. Signs and symptoms

    a. Intoxication is often manifested as slurred speech, ataxia, facial flushing, erratic behavior, loss of inhibition, and euphoria.

    b. Chronic abuse may be characterized by acne rosacea, palmar erythema, hepatomegaly, Dupuytren's contracture, testicular atrophy, and gynecomastia in males. Gamma-glutamyl transpeptidase (GGT) is elevated in about 75% of users and may be considered an early sign of alcohol abuse. Also, increased aspartate aminotransferase (AST), alanine aminotransferase (ALT), lactate dehydrogenase, and mean corpuscular volume may be seen on laboratory work in addition to decreased BUN, low-density lipoprotein, and red blood cell volume.

    c. Withdrawal symptoms may ensue on discontinuation of the substance, especially if the use was prolonged or heavy.

        (1) Withdrawal typically begins with tremulousness/shakes/jitters that start approximately 8 to 18 hours after stopping alcohol and peak approximately 24 to 48 hours after cessation.

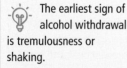 The earliest sign of alcohol withdrawal is tremulousness or shaking.

Table 12-7 | CAGE Screening Test for Alcohol or Drug Abuse

C (cut down)	Have you ever felt you should cut down on your drinking (or drug use)?
A (annoyed)	Have people annoyed you by criticizing your drinking (or drug use)?
G (guilty)	Have you felt bad or guilty about your drinking (or drug use)?
E (eye-opener)	Have you ever had a drink (or used drugs) first thing in the morning to steady your nerves or to get rid of a hangover (eye-opener)?

Reproduced with permission from Ewing JA. Detecting alcoholism: the CAGE questionnaire. *JAMA.* 1984;252(14):1905–1907. Copyright © 1984 American Medical Association. All rights reserved.

(2) Additional manifestations include psychomotor symptoms, abnormal perception, nausea/vomiting (8 to 12 hours after cessation), seizures, hallucinations (within 2 days), and delirium tremens (generally within 2 to 3 days of cessation but can occur a week after cessation).

2. Treatment of alcohol use/abuse

a. Substance dependence is viewed as a chronic relapsing disease by the Substance Abuse and Mental Health Services Administration (SAMHSA). Relapses are not considered to be a failure in the treatment but, rather, a step toward what will, it is hoped, be a complete remission of all symptoms.

b. Nonpharmacologic modalities include education, coping skills, relaxation therapy, family therapy, various kinds of psychotherapy, health and nutritional counseling, lifestyle changes, and aftercare programs. These modalities are indicated for all forms of substance abuse.

c. The 12-step program Alcoholics Anonymous is a popular form of therapy. Family members may benefit from Al-Anon or Al-Ateen.

d. Pharmacologic therapy

(1) Alcohol withdrawal commonly requires the use of benzodiazepines, such as diazepam (Valium) or chlordiazepoxide (Librium), as well as folic acid and multivitamin administration. Thiamine administration is also necessary as it may prevent Wernicke's encephalopathy. An antipsychotic (i.e., haloperidol or risperidone) may be indicated for alcoholic hallucinosis.

(2) Disulfiram (Antabuse) is an alcohol-deterrent medication that causes nausea when alcohol is consumed.

(3) Naltrexone and acamprosate can be used for maintenance therapy as both medications reduce cravings for alcohol.

E. Opioid use/abuse

In 2018, 47,000 people died of opioid overdoses in the United States. Thirty-two percent of these deaths involved prescription opioids according to the Center for Disease Control. Opioids include heroin and many pain control medications such as oxycodone, codeine, fentanyl, and morphine.

1. Signs and symptoms

a. Intoxication manifestations include analgesia, drowsiness, impaired concentration, bradycardia, hypotension, constricted pupils, slurred speech, flushing, respiratory depression, areflexia, and coma.

b. Withdrawal signs/symptoms include lacrimation, piloerection rhinorrhea, sweating, yawning, flushing, anxiety, hypertension, tachycardia, nausea/vomiting, abdominal cramps, and muscle/joint pain.

2. Medication-assisted treatment

a. Naloxone is used to acutely reverse the effects of any opioid. This drug is widely available for acute overdose. Consideration should be given to provide prescriptions for naloxone to those receiving chronic opioid pain management.

b. Opioid abuse and withdrawal also can be managed in several ways, including a slow taper of methadone, buprenorphine, or clonidine along with adjuncts, such as ibuprofen for muscle cramps, loperamide for diarrhea, and promethazine or dicyclomine for GI distress.

c. Ongoing maintenance for dependence often entails methadone maintenance programs. Other medications used are naltrexone, buprenorphine, or a combination of the latter with naloxone.

F. Stimulant use/abuse

1. Stimulants include caffeine, cocaine, amphetamines/methamphetamine, pseudoephedrine, and diet pills.

> Drowsiness, bradycardia, and slurred speech with constricted pupils indicate opioid intoxication; stimulant intoxication presents with tachycardia, euphoria, and dilated pupils.

2. Acute intoxication may be manifested by agitation/aggression, impaired judgment, euphoria, anorexia, elevated blood pressure, chest pain, transient psychosis, tachycardia, dilated pupils, and hallucinations.

3. Some withdrawal signs/symptoms are fatigue, depression, headache, profuse sweating, muscle cramps, and hunger.

4. Treatment with medications for acute withdrawal symptoms is generally not necessary. Benzodiazepines may be utilized to reduce agitation and anxiety. Short-term antipsychotics may be indicated for psychotic symptoms.

G. Nicotine and tobacco cravings can be treated with nicotine transdermal patches, gum, lozenges, or inhaler as well as varenicline and bupropion. Clonidine may also be beneficial.

H. Marijuana, phencyclidine (PCP), and hallucinogen withdrawal usually does not require medication; however, anxiolytics can be used. In the latter two, neuroleptics, such as haloperidol, can be used if acute psychotic symptoms are present.

I. In cases of CNS depressant use or abuse, such as sedatives, benzodiazepines, or hypnotics, treatment is by gradually tapering the medication. Pentobarbital may be used if necessary.

Childhood Disorders

A. **Attention deficit disorder (ADD) or attention deficit hyperactivity disorder (ADHD)**

1. General characteristics

a. ADD and ADHD can manifest as hyperactivity and impulsivity or as inattentiveness. Most children manifest symptoms that result in a diagnosis emphasizing both attention deficits and hyperactivity.

b. Secondary symptoms include emotional immaturity and lability, poor social skills, and, sometimes, motor incoordination. Disruptive behavior may result in peer rejection and deflated self-image. At home, these children often do not comply with parents' requests and can become explosive and irritable.

c. Prevalence of ADHD is between 5% and 8% of school children in the United States, and 2.5% of adults. It is more frequent in boys than in girls and is most common in the firstborn son.

d. A substantial portion of affected children continue to have dysfunctional symptoms into adulthood, most frequently experiencing difficulty with attention.

e. A multifactorial cause is likely, including perinatal complications, genetic and psychosocial factors, and abnormal catecholamine metabolism.

> The diagnosis of ADD/ADHD requires symptoms in at least two different settings such as home and school.

2. Diagnosis

a. The diagnosis is generally established clinically through comprehensive medical, educational, developmental, and psychosocial evaluations.

b. Interviews, observations, and questionnaires with parents and teachers in combination with rating scales, such as the Conners Comprehensive Behavioral Rating Scale and the ADHD Rating Scale IV, are helpful.

c. Diagnostic criteria

(1) Symptoms of hyperactivity, impulsivity, or inattentiveness resulting in impairment must have been present before 12 years of age.

(2) Symptoms must occur in at least two settings (e.g., home, school).

(3) At least six symptoms of inattention, hyperactivity/impulsivity, or both, as listed in Table 12-8, are developmentally inappropriate and present for at least 6 months.

Table 12-8 | Symptoms of Attention Deficit Disorder and Attention Deficit Hyperactivity Disorder Used for Diagnostic Criteria

Inattention Symptoms
Makes careless mistakes and has trouble attending to details
Problems in sustaining attention; does not appear attentive when directly addressed
Does not follow through or complete assigned work
Forgetful
Easily distracted from activities by other things going on at the same time
Loses items critical to accomplishing assigned activities
Avoids activities requiring sustained mental effort
Has difficulty in organizing tasks

Hyperactivity and Impulsivity Symptoms
Fidgets or squirms
Leaves seat often
Restlessness
Difficulty playing quietly
Talking excessively
Blurting out
Difficulty awaiting turn
Interrupts or intrudes on others

3. **Treatment**
   a. Medications are considered a mainstay for ADHD management. Treatment involves CNS stimulants in combination with behavioral therapies, social skills training, and school-based interventions. A multimodal approach is crucial for success.
   b. Pharmacotherapeutic agents, such as methylphenidate, dexmethylphenidate, amphetamine/dextroamphetamine, and lisdexamfetamine have been used successfully and are considered to be first-line treatment. Side effects of stimulants are growth retardation, weight loss, labile mood, tics, and insomnia; patients must be closely monitored. There are long-acting formulations that treat symptoms inside and outside the home.
   c. Atomoxetine is a selective norepinephrine reuptake inhibitor (nonstimulant) approved for the treatment of ADD and ADHD. Efficacy is equal to that of the stimulants, and side effects are similar but less frequent. It is *not* a controlled substance and, therefore, will add convenience to therapy.
   d. Antidepressants, including bupropion, venlafaxine, clonidine, and imipramine, can be used as adjuncts. Guanfacine, a centrally acting antihypertensive, has also been approved for use in ADHD.
   e. Therapy should include behavior modification, educational and classroom management, and family therapy. Group therapy can improve social skills and self-esteem.

> Stimulant pharmacotherapy, with adjunct antidepressant if indicated, plus therapy are the keys to ADHD treatment.

B. Disruptive, impulse control, and conduct disorders
   1. **Conduct disorder**
      a. General characteristics
         (1) This disorder affects boys more often than girls with an estimated ratio of 2:1.
         (2) Conduct disorder is considered a precursor to antisocial personality disorder in adulthood.
         (3) There is high comorbidity with ADD and ADHD, learning disability, mood disorders, and substance abuse disorder.
         (4) Diagnostic criteria: The diagnosis is established on the basis of a pattern of behavior that involves violation of the basic rights of others or of social norms, with at least three acts of the following types: aggression toward people and animals, destruction of property, deceitfulness or theft, and serious violations of rules.

b. Treatment

(1) A multimodal, biopsychosocial approach is used, with the use of pharmacotherapy for specific behaviors.

(2) Stimulants (dextroamphetamine, methylphenidate) have been shown to reduce aggressive/assaultive behaviors. Antipsychotic medications may also aid in the management of aggression.

(3) Guanfacine and clonidine may aid therapy by reducing impulsivity and oppositional symptoms.

2. Oppositional defiant disorder (ODD)

a. General characteristics

(1) This disorder generally begins before age 8 years and has a lifetime prevalence of around 11% for males and 9% for females. ODD may progress to conduct disorder.

(2) There is a high comorbidity with substance abuse disorders, mood disorders, and ADD and ADHD.

(3) Diagnostic criteria: The diagnosis includes at least 6 months of negativistic, hostile, and defiant behavior, including at least four of the following: frequent loss of temper, arguments with adults, defying adults' rules, deliberately annoying others, easily annoyed, anger and resentment, spitefulness, blaming others for mistakes or misbehaviors, and spiteful or vindictive at least twice in the past 6 months.

b. Treatment

(1) Family intervention using training skills in child management for the parents/caregivers is crucial.

(2) Individual psychotherapy, focusing on behavioral modification and problem-solving skills, is recommended. Treat comorbid psychiatric disorders with medications as needed.

> Treatment of ODD must include individual therapy and family intervention to develop skills to manage the child's defiant behavior.

C. Neurodevelopmental (child) disorders

1. Autism spectrum disorder

a. General characteristics

(1) Autism is characterized by impaired social interaction, impaired communication, and repetitive stereotyped patterns of behavior and activities. It is three to five times more common in boys and is generally apparent by age 3 to 6 months. There is a wide spectrum of severity.

(2) Parents are usually the first to note that the child does not respond to cuddling or has not developed a normal pattern of bonding or smiling. These children are often aloof, withdrawn, and lack facial expression.

(3) By age 3, the lack of reciprocal social interaction becomes very apparent including failure to engage in peer relationships. They fail to develop language skills and do not progress through expected developmental milestones.

(4) Absence of spontaneous and varied play activities is prominent. There is usually a restricted repertoire of interests and an intense adherence to specific routines. Autistic children can become very agitated and upset changing focus or activities.

(5) There may be hyper- or hyposensory responses such as seemingly indifferent to painful stimuli or an adverse reaction to sounds or textures. There might be a visual fascination with lights, movement, or parts of toys or objects.

(6) Children with autism may exhibit stereotyped patterns such as repeated motor movements or mannerisms that are not goal directed. Examples are rocking back and forth, hand or finger flapping, or whole body movements.

b. Treatment involves multidisciplinary supportive care.

   (1) Behavioral therapy is most effective. Autism specialists and speech and language pathologists should be consulted. An audiology evaluation and EEG may be indicated as well.

   (2) Pharmacotherapy involving second-generation antipsychotics (e.g., risperidone, aripiprazole), conventional antipsychotics (e.g., haloperidol), or neuroleptics (e.g., carbamazepine) can reduce impulsivity and irritability (such as self-injury and tantrums).

   (3) SSRIs may help improve repetitive behaviors and can be utilized for comorbid anxiety and depression.

2. Tourette's disorder

   a. General characteristics

   (1) Tourette's disorder involves multiple motor and one or more vocal tics several times per day for >1-year duration. Onset is before age 18 years; most are diagnosed between ages 3 and 8 years.

   (2) Tourette is highly familial and comorbid with OCD. Onset of this disorder after a group A streptococcal infection is known as pediatric autoimmune neuropsychiatric disorder associated with streptococcal infections.

   (3) The vocal tics may be socially offensive obscenities or may be grunting or barking noises.

   (4) Motor tics may include tongue protrusion, sniffing, eye blinking, throat clearing, hopping, squatting, or nodding.

   (5) The patient is aware of these tics and is able to exert a mild degree of control over them but ultimately is unable to completely suppress them.

   (6) The tics tend to worsen in times of stress, fatigue, or illness.

   b. Treatment consists of psychological support for the patient and family, as well habit reversal training. Pharmacotherapy may be of benefit and involves first or second-generation antipsychotics (e.g., haloperidol, risperidone, ziprasidone) or low-dose clonidine or guanfacine.

> Presence of vocal tic is required for a diagnosis of Tourette.

Abuse and Neglect

A. Child abuse/maltreatment

1. Considerations

   a. Health care providers are required to alert the appropriate authorities if abuse or neglect of a child is suspected.

   b. When a young patient presents with any condition that appears questionable for physical, emotional, or sexual abuse or neglect, it is best to consult with a mental health professional or family social services.

   c. The child must be protected from further abuse as well as treated for current injuries.

2. Physical signs of abuse

   a. Any injury that cannot be adequately explained or is not consistent with the history given has the potential of being abusive.

   b. Bruises, lacerations, soft-tissue swelling, dislocations, or fractures and spiral fractures are common.

   c. Burns that are doughnut shaped, in a stocking-glove distribution, or symmetrically round (e.g., caused by a lit cigarette) are other signs.

> Injuries, lacerations, or burns that do not align with the given history, or are repetitive, signal an investigation for abuse.

      d. Bruises or injuries that form regular patterns on the face, back, buttocks, or thighs may be the result of abuse.

      e. Retinal hemorrhages or hyphema should alert suspicion of shaken baby syndrome.

      f. Other physical signs are internal hemorrhages, abdominal injuries, bite marks, and injuries that have the shape of the instrument used to make them (e.g., belt, cord, hand).

   3. General characteristics

      a. Psychiatric disturbances resulting from childhood abuse are common and include anxiety, aggressive or violent behavior, PTSD, depression, suicide, substance abuse, poor self-esteem, dissociative disorders, and paranoid ideation.

      b. Abuse or neglect also can be manifested in subtle ways, such as failure to thrive.

      c. Factitious disorder imposed on another

        (1) When involving a child, this is a form of abuse usually perpetrated by the mother. Symptoms are fabricated or clinical signs are induced in a child, resulting in repeated visits to a health care provider for relief.

        (2) The perpetrator induces the various signs and symptoms to receive attention as being either an attentive or a suffering parent.

      d. Neglect can take many forms: inadequate supervision, emotional neglect, nutritional, educational and others potentially leading to child harm.

B. Sexual abuse

   1. General characteristics

      a. Approximately 25% of women and 9% of men report a history of being sexually abused as children.

      b. Factors that may increase risk include poor parent–child relationship, poor parental relationships, lack of a protective caregiver, a nonbiologically related male in the home.

      c. Any of the following should raise the suspicion of sexual abuse in a child:

        (1) Evidence of a sexually transmitted disease

        (2) Bruises, pain, itching, or any trauma of the anal or genital area

        (3) Detailed knowledge about sexual acts that are inappropriate for age

        (4) Child initiates sexual acts with others, especially peers.

        (5) Child exhibits sexual knowledge through play.

C. Intimate partner violence (spousal abuse, domestic abuse)

   1. General information

      a. Intimate partner violence should be suspect when there is an injury and there is also a delay in seeking care from onset of injury, the mechanism of injury does not explain physical findings, overbearing partners, known family history of intimate partner violence, vague and multiple somatic complaints, pregnancy, and substance abuse.

      b. When confronted with a patient who may be a victim of intimate partner violence, the following actions should occur:

        (1) Validation of the abuse—state that violence is unacceptable while avoiding language that blames the victim.

        (2) Determine the patient's current safety—this should include asking if it is safe to go home and if the patient has an emergency escape plan.

        (3) Clearly document the history and physical examination in medical records in case they are necessary for police reports.

        (4) Provide resources and referrals including information about shelters regardless of whether the patient intends to return home as well as information on legal recourse such as restraining orders.

(5) Understand local laws with regard to reporting violence.

   c. Caution is required in dealing with cases of intimate partner abuse.

   d. The patient should be presented with options and allowed to decide which path to take. Do not insist they end the relationship.

   e. The immediate period after leaving an abusive partner is considered high risk for physical violence.

D. Elder abuse

   1. General characteristics

   a. Elder abuse affects 10% of the population older than 65 years of age. Most victims are very old, frail, and vulnerable.

   b. Abuse can be physical, sexual, psychological or emotional, neglect, or financial.

   2. Forms of abuse

   a. Physical or sexual abuse is suspected in the presence of bruises, puncture wounds, fractures, cuts, burns, poor hygiene, soiled clothing, hair loss in clumps, weight loss or poor nutrition, dehydration, lack of eyeglasses or hearing aids, injuries from use of restraints, genital or rectal injuries or bleeding, evidence of excessive drugging, or a lack of or delay in seeking medical attention.

   b. Psychological abuse can be manifested by threats, insults, or verbal abuse or refusal to allow travel, church attendance at social events, or family visits.

   c. Financial abuse may come in the form of misuse of the patient's funds.

   d. Neglect includes the withholding of food, medicine, clothing, routine health care, or other basic necessities.

   e. Violation of basic rights entails the right to open one's own mail or make decisions for oneself.

   3. Clinicians should be aware of the following:

   a. Previous history of abuse by the caregiver

   b. Conflicting accounts of accidents by the caregiver

   c. Unwillingness of a caregiver to agree to implementation of treatment plans

   d. Inappropriate defensiveness by the caregiver

   e. A caregiver who will not allow, or who limits, the patient's responses to questions

   f. Most states have the same reporting requirements for suspected elder abuse as for child abuse.

> Elder abuse can be physical, sexual, psychological or emotional, neglect, or financial. History and physical examination mismatch should triqger an investigation.

Sexual Violence and Rape

A. Definition

   1. Rape is an act of sexual aggression that may be perpetrated on a spouse, a known partner, or a stranger.

   2. Forced participation in any sexual acts can result in psychological sequelae.

   3. A patient who has been raped may experience depression; lack of appetite; sleep disturbances; rage and anger; feelings of worthlessness; enduring patterns of sexual dysfunction; agoraphobia; fear of future violence, death, or contracting a sexually transmitted disease; feelings of being used or dirt. Additionally, PTSD and anxiety disorders are common.

B. Approach to the patient

   1. History and physical examination, including genital and rectal examinations, should be completed as soon after the event as possible.

   a. Rape constitutes both a psychiatric emergency and a legal situation; all procedures should be documented, clothing saved, and samples taken.

b. A rape kit, which has instructions regarding questions to include in the history, how specimen samples are to be collected and under what conditions, and how samples should be handled after collection, is valuable and ensures that the proper evidence is secured.

c. Explain to the patient the purpose of all procedures and inform him or her of what is being done before doing it. This provides the patient with a feeling of some control.

2. Prevention of sexually transmitted diseases and pregnancy: Prophylactic antibiotic therapy, and vaccination against hepatitis B and tetanus if warranted should be initiated. The patient should be given the option of emergency contraception.

3. Counseling: As soon as possible after the event, and preferably before leaving the emergency department (ED), the patient should talk to a mental health professional and follow-up counseling should be scheduled.

Uncomplicated Bereavement

A. Definition

1. Uncomplicated bereavement is defined as a normal response to a major loss. It is usually the clinician's discretion to differentiate a major depressive episode following bereavement from a typical grief reaction.

2. Duration of the reaction depends on the suddenness of the loss, the relationship of the survivor to the deceased, and the age or physical condition of the person who has died.

3. Up to 25% of individuals experiencing uncomplicated bereavement meet the criteria for MDD. Antidepressant treatment is warranted if symptoms are prolonged and/or affect psychosocial functioning.

B. General characteristics

1. The mourner experiences symptoms similar to depression which are considered a normal consequence of loss.

2. Mourners sometimes report illusions, such as briefly seeing or hearing the deceased, or they may deny certain aspects of the death. These are considered to be normal reactions; however, hallucinations that are persistent and/or intrusive, or the belief that the deceased is still alive, are not.

3. Treatment

a. Treatment consists of social contact and reassurance.

b. Patients who meet the criteria for MDD will benefit from antidepressant therapy.

Practice Questions

Directions: *Each of the numbered items or incomplete statements in this section is followed by a list of answers or completions of the statement. Select the ONE lettered answer or completion that is BEST in each case.*

1. A 19-year-old male is accompanied to the office by his mother who is concerned that he has been behaving strangely. The patient dropped out of college and quit his part-time job months ago. She states that he is often silent and stands still staring into space for long periods of time. The patient reveals that he was hearing voices telling him to harm himself for over a month, but they have subsided. During the examination, the patient speaks very little, only giving one-word answers, and his face remains expressionless. What is the preferred treatment for this patient's symptoms?

A. Alprazolam
B. Haloperidol
C. Lithium
D. Risperidone
E. Valproate

2. A 58-year-old male undergoes surgery for a fractured femur after being involved in a motor vehicle accident. On day 2, he becomes irritable, restless. He has a fine tremor of his hands and has experienced episodes of delirium. Which of the following medications should be started for the patient's symptoms?
   A. Chlordiazepoxide
   B. Disulfiram
   C. Fluoxetine
   D. Naltrexone
   E. Acamprosate

3. A 25-year-old female is found lying on the street and incoherent and is subsequently brought to the ED by EMS. On initial assessment, she is arousable but drowsy, her speech is slurred, and her pupils are constricted. Her vitals include a pulse of 51 and blood pressure of 85/60. What is the recommended next step in management?
   A. Atropine
   B. Buprenorphine
   C. Caffeine
   D. Naloxone
   E. Diazepam

4. A 20-year-old female college student just entered senior year. She has a high grade point average (GPA) and takes part in extracurricular activities generally exhibiting high energy and productivity. For the past 2 weeks, however, she reports increased fatigue and lack of interest in studying and participating in her usual activities. She admits to experiencing feeling this way on and off since freshman year. She denies alcohol consumption and use of prescription or recreational drugs. She further denies hallucinations and suicidal ideations. What is the recommended treatment for the most likely diagnosis?
   A. Amitriptyline
   B. Bupropion
   C. Lamotrigine
   D. Paroxetine
   E. Lorazepam

5. A 22-year-old female is taken to the ED after a syncopal episode at her gym. In the ED, physical examination reveals an irregular heartbeat, calluses on the knuckles of the left second to fourth knuckles, bilaterally enlarged salivary glands, and a BMI of 24. What laboratory test is likely to be elevated in this patient?
   A. Amylase
   B. Calcium
   C. Chloride
   D. Magnesium
   E. Potassium

6. A 68-year-old female presents to a new primary care office for an annual wellness examination. She admits it has been several years since any medical examinations. On physical examination, she has a petechial rash, distended veins over the abdomen, hepatomegaly, and palmar erythema. Which of the following laboratory findings is most likely to be found in this patient?
   A. Low ALT
   B. Low ASTC.
   C. Elevated GGT
   D. Elevated BUN
   E. Low MCV

7. A 26-year-old female frequently presents to the office complaining of vague abdominal pain. Her symptoms typically resolve spontaneously during workup without a diagnosis. During her appointments, she is loud and flirts with the provider. She is charming and well-liked by the staff but pouts and whines when she is not the center of attention. What is the recommended treatment for the most likely underlying condition?
   A. Amitriptyline
   B. Cognitive therapy
   C. ECT
   D. Lorazepam
   E. Psychotherapy

8. A 38-year-old male presents to his primary care office complaining of anxiety. He describes five episodes in the past 6 weeks of a feeling of panic occurring with a racing heart, diaphoresis, shaking, and a sensation of choking. His most recent episode was 1 day ago. The episodes start abruptly and peak within a few minutes and then gradually resolve over the next half hour. What is the first step in management?
   A. Prescribe a mood stabilizer
   B. Prescribe an antipsychotic
   C. Prescribe a daily benzodiazepine
   D. Prescribe a short course of benzodiazepine while instituting long-term treatment with an antipsychotic
   E. Prescribe a short course of benzodiazepines while instituting long-term treatment with an SSRI

9. A 25-year-old graduate student's research proposal has been selected for presentation at a prominent, annual biology conference. He was encouraged to submit to the conference by his advisor, and upon hearing he would have to give a presentation he became highly panicked, visibly upset, and refused to speak. What is the most likely diagnosis?
   A. Agoraphobia
   B. Social phobia
   C. Paranoid personality disorder
   D. Pervasive depressive disorder
   E. GAD

10. A 26-year-old complains of insomnia. He states that whenever he tries to go to sleep, he relives his experience in a recent car accident which totaled his car. He is easily startled, he has avoided driving near his accident site, and refuses to discuss it with his family and friends. He reports he has experienced these symptoms for the past 3 weeks. Which of the following is the most likely diagnosis?
    A. PTSD
    B. Acute stress disorder
    C. Agoraphobia
    D. Social phobia
    E. MDD

11. An 18-year-old freshman presents to student health services after being mandated by her university's administration. She was caught vandalizing her dorm's common study room. Upon questioning, she reports she has been skipping classes and has experienced a depressed mood since she arrived on campus. During the interview, she becomes anxious and tearful. What is the most likely diagnosis?
    A. Adjustment disorder
    B. Borderline personality disorder

C. GAD
D. Paranoid personality disorder
E. PTSD

12. A 12-year-old boy has a history of acting physically aggressive toward his teachers and classmates and harming animals. He has run away from home on multiple occasions and was suspended from school for throwing bricks at car windows. This child is at high risk of what personality disorder?

A. Antisocial
B. Avoidant
C. Borderline
D. Narcissistic
E. Obsessive–compulsive

Practice Answers

1. D. *Psychiatry; Pharmacology; Schizophrenia*

Symptoms of schizophrenia typically begin in early adulthood. Bizarre behaviors and hallucinations indicate psychosis. Negative symptoms such as blunted affect, avolition, and alogia are common. Second-generation antipsychotics, for example, and certain atypical neuroleptics such as risperidone, aripiprazole, and quetiapine are preferred for the treatment of negative symptoms. First-generation antipsychotics such as haloperidol are preferred for positive symptoms. For resistant cases, antipsychotics can be combined with other medications such as lithium, valproic acid, or benzodiazepines.

2. A. *Psychiatry; Pharmacology; Alcohol Abuse*

Alcohol withdrawal symptoms appear anywhere from a few hours to a couple of days after cessation of intake. Tremulousness and irritability are the hallmark manifestations that may be followed by hallucinations and psychosis. A long-acting benzodiazepine, such as chlordiazepoxide, is recommended to abate symptoms. Naltrexone is used to reverse the effects of opioid intoxication; it is also used in the maintenance phase of treatment for alcohol or opioid dependence. Disulfiram is an aversion therapy once sobriety has been met. Fluoxetine is an antidepressant, and risperidone is an antipsychotic.

3. D. *Psychiatry; Pharmacology; Opioid Abuse*

Naloxone will acutely reserve the effects of any opioid. The constricted pupils, low blood pressure and pulse, and drowsy state indicate opioid intoxication. Buprenorphine is a partial opioid antagonist used in the treatment of opioid dependence. Atropine stimulates the vagus to increase heart rate, but this would only treat one symptom not the overlying cause. Diazepam (Valium) is used in the treatment of withdrawal symptoms but not during acute intoxication.

4. C. *Psychiatry; Pharmacology; Cyclothymia*

This patient is describing the pattern of mood characteristic of cyclothymia. A subset of patients with cyclothymia will go on to develop a mood disorder, most commonly bipolar II. Cyclothymia is treated in the same way as bipolar disorder: mood stabilizer plus individual and family psychotherapy. Antidepressants, such as fluoxetine and bupropion, may be added if depressive symptoms are severe but should not be used without a mood stabilizer on board; antidepressants, especially when used as monotherapy, may precipitate a mania. TCAs, such as amitriptyline, may cause rapid cycling in a patient with bipolar disorder. Benzodiazepines, such as lorazepam, may be used short term for acute anxiety.

5. A. *Psychiatry; Diagnostic Studies; Bulimia Nervosa*

Patients with bulimia nervosa tend to be of normal weight. The purging behavior leads to calluses on the knuckles (Russell's sign). Amylase is characteristically elevated. Most electrolytes, especially potassium, magnesium, and calcium, tend to be low.

6. C. *Psychiatry; Diagnostic Studies; Alcohol Dependence*

Chronic alcohol abuse leads to liver cirrhosis which is irreversible. Stigmata of liver disease include jaundice, wasting, clubbing, easy bruising, asterixis, and encephalopathy. The high estrogen state that accompanies cirrhosis leads to palmar erythema, spider angioma, gynecomastia, and testicular atrophy. Lab values commonly include elevated ALT, AST, GGT, MCV, and low BUN.

7. E. *Psychiatry; Clinical Intervention; Histrionic Personality Disorder*

Patients with histrionic personality disorder are overly emotional, dramatic, and seductive. They crave attention and often revert to childish behavior if attention is turned away. Somatization is common as it gets them attention from respected members of society. Treatment is a combination of individual and group psychotherapy. Medication is not commonly needed.

8. E. *Psychiatry; Clinical Intervention; Panic Disorder*

Panic disorders start abruptly, last a short time, and gradually subside. Benzodiazepines are helpful during an acute panic attack but should not be used long term. SSRIs, such as fluoxetine or paroxetine, are recommended for long-term treatment. Maintenance therapy should be continued for 8 to 12 months because of the risk of relapse. Counseling should be encouraged.

9. B. *Psychiatry; Diagnosis; Social Phobia*

Social phobia is driven by a fear of embarrassment or humiliation; individuals avoid circumstances where they will be the center of attention. Agoraphobia is the fear of being somewhere without an escape route. Paranoid personality disorder centers on distrust and suspicion of others. GAD is characterized by excessive worry over things that cannot be controlled. Pervasive depressive disorder is milder than MDD but is still characterized by anhedonia.

10. B. *Psychiatry; Diagnosis; Acute Stress Disorder*

Acute stress disorder differs from PTSD in duration and timing of symptoms. With acute stress disorder, symptoms generally begin within 1 month from a traumatic experience and last 2 to 4 weeks in duration. In PTSD, symptoms must be present for >1-month duration, making this the less likely answer for this question.

11. A. *Psychiatry; Diagnosis; Adjustment Disorder*

Leaving home and going to college is a common precipitant of adjustment disorder, characterized by maladaptive behavioral or emotional symptoms. Patients are typically tearful, exhibit a depressed mood, and engage in reckless behavior. Treatment is supportive psychotherapy. GAD is defined as persistent anxiety manifest as excessive worry or apprehension. Paranoid personality disorder is defined as pervasive distrust and suspicion of others. Borderline personality disorder is manifest as an unstable, unpredictable behavior, manipulation, and self-harm, in a desperate attempt to avoid embarrassment. PTSD occurs after a stressful event and is characterized by reliving the event, emotional detachment, and exaggerated startle response.

12. A. *Psychiatry; Health Maintenance; Conduct Disorder*

Conduct disorder is characterized by aggressive behavior without regard for consequences or effect on others. Conduct disorder is considered a precursor to antisocial personality disorder. Comorbid disorders include ADD, mood disorders, and substance abuse. Borderline personality disorder is characterized by unstable and unpredictable movements, impulsivity, self-harm, and manipulative suicide attempts. Avoidant personality disorder is characterized by an extreme sensitivity to rejection and a feeling of inferiority. Narcissistic personality disorder is characterized by an inflated self-image and grandiosity; individuals lack empathy toward others but do not engage in harmful behavior toward others. Obsessive–compulsive personality disorder is characterized by a pervasive pattern of orderliness (rules, lists, details), perfectionism, and inflexibility.

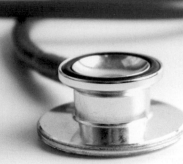

13 | Dermatology

Sheryl L. Geisler

Diagnosis

A. History and physical examination

 1. History

 a. A thorough history is imperative for accurately diagnosing skin diseases. Document the onset, any spread or change in lesions, and associated symptoms such as pruritus, fever, anergy, and so on.

 b. Past medical history, medication history, family history, psychosocial factors, recreational and employment risk, as well as diet and environmental/travel exposures, should be investigated.

 2. Physical examination

 a. A general physical examination, paying particular attention to the skin, hair, nails, and mucocutaneous surfaces, should be carried out under natural or bright light.

 b. A magnifying glass may be useful.

 c. When an abnormality is found, the lesions should be described using the **M-A-D** criteria:

 (1) **M**orphology: lesion type, color, elevation, margination, and other defining characteristics

 (2) **A**rrangement: single, grouped, arciform (arc-shaped), annular (round), serpiginous (wavy or snake-like), or other patterns

 (3) **D**istribution: where on the body (trunk, extremities, etc.); localized versus disseminated, or other patterns

 3. Special signs and tests

 a. Darier's sign: rubbing a lesion causes urticarial flare.

 b. Auspitz sign: pinpoint bleeding when the scale is removed

 c. Nikolsky sign: lateral pressure on a blister causes peripheral extension owing to further separation of the upper skin layers from the underlying dermis.

 d. Photopatch test: documents photoallergy

 e. Patch test: demonstrates hypersensitivity reaction

 f. Koebner phenomenon: minor trauma leads to new lesions at the site of trauma.

 g. Shagreen skin: an oval-shaped nevoid plaque that is skin-colored or pigmented on the trunk or back and is associated with tuberous sclerosis

 4. Diagnostic techniques

 a. Diascopy

 (1) A glass slide or diascope is pressed against the skin.

 (2) Blanching of skin area indicates intact capillaries; extravasated blood (purpura) does not blanch.

> MAD frames the approach to skin disorders: morphology, arrangement, and distribution.

b. Potassium hydroxide preparation (KOH prep)

    (1) Microscopic examination of skin scrapings mounted in KOH, which dissolves keratin and cellular material but does not affect fungi.

    (2) This process will readily identify dermatophyte infections.

c. Scrapings and smears

    (1) Blunt and sharp instruments facilitate specimen collections.

    (2) Various staining techniques and visualization methods (e.g., Tzanck smear, dark-field microscopy) bring out certain characteristics of the lesion or responsible pathogen.

d. Wood's light examination is used to assess changes in pigment or to fluoresce infectious lesions.

e. Acetowhitening (applying acetic acid) is used to facilitate the examination of warts.

f. Biopsy (excisional, incisional, shave, or punch) is indicated if histopathologic confirmation is necessary.

B. Common dermatologic terminology

  1. Common skin lesions are defined in Table 13-1.

  2. The following descriptive terms are also useful:

    a. Telangiectasia: dilated, small, superficial blood vessel; blanches with diascopy

    b. Lichenification: thickened skin with exaggerated skin lines and distinct borders; often a result of excessive scratching or prolonged irritation

    c. Macerated: swollen and softened by an increase in water content; the appearance that skin gets when left in water too long

    d. Verrucous: irregular, rough, and convoluted surfaces, wart-like

Maculopapular and Plaque Disorders

A. Eczematous disorders

  1. The terms *eczema* and *dermatitis* are often used interchangeably. Eczema more commonly denotes endogenous disorders, and dermatitis denotes exogenous disorders.

Table 13-1 | Nomenclature of Common Skin Lesions (Morphology)

Papule	Solid, palpable lesion <5 mm in diameter
Nodule	Solid, palpable lesion >5 mm in diameter
Macule	Flat, circumscribed area of skin color change <10 mm in diameter; nonpalpable
Patch	Macule >10 mm in diameter
Plaque	Plateau-like elevation >10 mm in diameter, may be a group of confluent papules
Vesicle	Circumscribed, elevated lesion containing serous fluid <5 mm in diameter
Bulla	Circumscribed, elevated lesion containing serous fluid >5 mm in diameter
Wheal	Transient, elevated lesion caused by local edema
Petechiae	Minute hemorrhagic spots that cannot be blanched with diascopy
Crust	Hard, rough surface formed by dried sebum, exudate, blood, or necrotic skin
Scale	Flakes of varying size of stratum corneum; may be adherent or loose
Pustule	Vesicle or bulla containing purulent material
Erosion	Defect of the epidermis; heals without a scar
Ulcer	Defect that extends into the dermis or deeper; heals with a scar
Atrophy	Reduction in volume of one or more layers of the skin

2. There are many eczematous disorders, encompassing a wide range of polymorphic inflammatory reaction patterns.

3. **Contact dermatitis: irritant versus allergic**

   a. General characteristics

      (1) Irritant contact dermatitis is commonly caused by chemical irritants, such as cleaners, solvents, and detergents, when in contact with the skin.

         (a) Irritant contact diaper dermatitis, aka diaper rash, is caused by prolonged contact with urine, feces, or harsh detergents from washable diapers.

         (b) Often associated with superimposed *Candida* infection; this fungal infection is characterized by advancing satellite lesions.

      (2) Allergic contact dermatitis denotes an allergic type IV cell-mediated hypersensitivity reaction. Plant exposure (poison ivy, etc.) dust, nickel, and enzymes are common causes of allergic dermatitis. Contact with irritants such as cleaning supplies, solvents, oils, abrasives, oxidizing or reducing agents that the person is sensitive to can be the cause as well.

   b. **Clinical features**

      (1) Patients complain of itching and burning in the affected areas. In diaper rash, the lesions are within the borders of the diaper.

      (2) Acute lesions typically are well-demarcated areas of erythema and, possibly, exudative lesions; vesicles, erosions, and secondary crusts may develop.

      (3) Chronic lesions show plaques and scaling with lichenification. Satellite papules and excoriations (secondary to scratching) are common.

   c. Laboratory studies

      (1) Patch tests resulting in similar reactions support the diagnosis.

      (2) Gram stains or cultures should be done if a secondary infection is suspected.

   d. **Treatment**

      (1) Avoidance or removal of the offending agent is key. If allergic dermatitis owing to poison ivy exposure is suspected, it is critical to wash any item that may have come in contact with the urushiol from the plant leaves, the offending agent, so that additional skin contact with the resin does not occur.

      (2) Topical corticosteroids are sufficient in most cases, and topical calcineurin inhibitors can be used in children. Wet dressings with Burow's solution (aluminum acetate in water) can be used to dry up weeping lesions. For diaper rash, a barrier of petrolatum or zinc oxide is helpful. Keep the area clean and dry with frequent diaper changes and use disposable diapers.

      (3) Severe cases may require systemic steroids.

      (4) Supportive measures include cleaning with mild soaps or oatmeal preparations and antihistamines to help alleviate itching.

4. **Atopic dermatitis**

   a. General characteristics

      (1) This is a chronic relapsing skin disorder that begins in childhood.

      (2) It is a type I immunoglobulin E–mediated hypersensitivity reaction.

      (3) Many patients also have comorbid asthma and/or allergic rhinitis (atopic diathesis).

   b. **Clinical features**

      (1) Papules and plaques, with or without scales, are noted and may be associated with edema, erosion, and crusts.

      (2) Patients complain of pruritus (the "itch that rashes") and dry, scaly skin. Scratching leads to lichenification, fissures, and worsening rash; secondary infections are most commonly caused by *Staphylococcus aureus*.

Satellite lesions indicate *Candida* infection.

The approach to allergic or contact dermatitis include the following:
- avoidance
- topical steroids or calcineurin
- barrier ointment
- antihistamines

(3) The rash is most common on the flexural surfaces, neck, eyelids, forehead, face, wrists, and dorsum of the hands and feet.

c. Laboratory studies: These are not routinely done, although cultures for suspected secondary infection may help to guide treatment.

d. Treatment

(1) Antihistamines help to control pruritus and itching.

(2) Topical corticosteroids are the mainstay of treatment; systemic corticosteroids should be avoided.

(3) Tacrolimus and pimecrolimus are topical calcineurin inhibitors (immunomodulators) approved for moderate to severe atopic dermatitis. There is less skin atrophy with prolonged use when compared with topical corticosteroids.

(4) Hydration and topical emollients are key to management. Soaps, vigorous rubbing, frequent bathing, and irritant clothing such as wool should be avoided as well as low (dry) humidity environments.

(5) Combination of ultraviolet A and ultraviolet B (UVA–UVB) phototherapy is effective.

(6) Rarely, severe systemic cases in otherwise healthy adults may necessitate cyclosporine.

> Lifestyle management in atopy includes avoidance of triggers and irritants along with local emollients and adequate hydration.

5. Nummular dermatitis (discoid eczema)

a. General characteristics

(1) This is a pruritic inflammatory disorder that typically affects young adults and the elderly. It is more common in males than in females.

(2) It occurs more often in winter (low humidity exacerbates); often seen in atopic persons.

b. Clinical features

(1) Small, grouped vesicles coalesce to form coin-shaped plaques with an erythematous base and well-demarcated borders, most commonly on the extremities (Fig. 13-1).

(2) Crusting and excoriations occur.

c. Treatment

(1) This is a chronic disorder that responds to moisturizers and/or topical steroids. Treatment is similar to that of atopic dermatitis.

(2) Psoralen + UVA (PUVA) phototherapy is helpful for refractory cases.

6. Seborrheic dermatitis

> There is a seasonal pattern with seborrheic dermatitis; flare-ups are more common in winter.

a. General characteristics

(1) Seborrheic dermatitis is common during infancy and puberty and in young to middle-aged adults; it may worsen in winter.

(2) It occurs where sebaceous glands are most active (body folds, face, scalp, and genitalia).

b. Clinical features

(1) Scattered yellowish or gray, scaly macules and papules with a greasy appearance, often with background erythema, are noted. Pruritus is variable.

(2) Sticky crusts and fissures are found behind the ears, especially in infants. On the scalp, it manifests as cradle cap in infants and dandruff in adults. Lesions may include the eyelids (blepharitis).

c. Treatment

(1) Cradle cap: Treatment options include ketoconazole shampoo or cream, low-dose topical hydrocortisone, olive oil compresses, and baby shampoo.

(2) Dandruff: Use shampoos containing selenium or zinc and ketoconazole shampoo for acute flare-ups; tar shampoos or topical steroids can be used for severe cases.

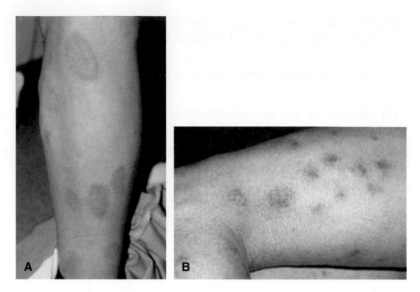

Figure 13-1 ▶ A, B: Coin-shaped lesions of nummular eczema. (**A:** Reprinted with permission from Goodheart HP. *Goodheart's Photoguide of Common Skin Disorders: Diagnosis and Management.* 2nd ed. Lippincott Williams & Wilkins; 2003, Glossary Fig. 28. **B:** Reprinted with permission from Goodheart HP. *Goodheart's Same-Site Differential Diagnosis: A Rapid Method of Diagnosing and Treating Common Skin Disorders.* Lippincott Williams & Wilkins; 2011, Fig. 21-1.)

> 💡 Stasis dermatitis is likely preceded by varicose veins, superficial phlebitis, or venous thrombosis.

(3) Other areas: Use ketoconazole shampoo or topical steroids. Blepharitis is treated with gentle scrubs using baby shampoo.

(4) Maintenance therapy may be necessary with ketoconazole shampoo or cream. Topical pimecrolimus or tacrolimus is also effective.

7. Perioral dermatitis

  a. General characteristics: This disorder typically occurs in young women; often there is a history of prior topical steroid use in the area.

  b. Clinical features: Perioral papulopustules on erythematous bases that may become confluent with plaques and scales (acne-like appearance); vermilion border is spared, and satellite lesions are common.

  c. Laboratory studies: Culture to rule out staphylococcal infection.

  d. Treatment

  (1) Avoid topical steroids because they will aggravate the lesions.

  (2) Use topical metronidazole or erythromycin or oral minocycline, doxycycline, or tetracycline.

  (3) Untreated lesions will fluctuate over time, similar to rosacea.

8. Stasis dermatitis (also see Stasis ulcers, page 424)

  a. General characteristics

  (1) Chronic venous insufficiency owing to valvular incompetency causes serum leakage secondary to venous hypertension. Resulting symptoms include edema, dermatitis, hyperpigmentation, fibrosis, and ulceration.

  (2) Varicose veins, superficial phlebitis, and venous thrombosis commonly develop before skin changes.

  (3) Women are affected three times more often than men. Pregnancy will exacerbate both venous insufficiency and stasis dermatitis.

  b. Clinical features

  (1) Patients complain of leg heaviness or aching, aggravated by standing and relieved with walking.

(2) Dermatitis of the lower legs and feet manifests with inflammatory papules, scales, and crusts. Stippled pigmentation develops, and excoriations are common.

(3) Ulcerations occur in 30% of patients.

c. Laboratory studies

(1) Doppler studies, sonography, or venography will confirm chronic venous insufficiency.

(2) Biopsy of lesions shows dilated vessels, tortuous veins, edema, and fibrin deposition.

d. Treatment

(1) Chronic venous insufficiency is treated with compression stockings.

(2) Sclerosis of varicose veins helps to prevent further dermatitis, but recurrence is common.

(3) Vascular bypass, endothelial thermal ablation, or angioplasty/stenting of obscured veins may benefit severely compromised areas, but results are only fair.

(4) Ulcers require chronic treatment.

B. Lichen simplex chronicus (circumscribed neurodermatitis)

1. General characteristics

a. Lichenification is a long-term manifestation from repetitive scratching and rubbing of a pruritic area. The repeated trauma of the scratching prolongs and worsens the pruritus, setting up an ongoing itch–scratch cycle.

b. It is more common in women than in men.

2. Clinical features

a. Solid, firm, thick plaques with little to no scaling are seen.

b. Light touch precipitates a strong desire to scratch.

c. Lesions can be single or multiple. Common areas include the nuchal area, scalp, ankles, lower legs, upper thighs, exterior forearms, or genital areas.

d. Black skin more typically shows a follicular pattern of smaller papules rather than larger plaques.

3. Laboratory studies

a. A KOH prep is done to rule out fungal infection.

b. Biopsy shows hyperplasia and hyperkeratosis.

4. Treatment

a. Key to management is stopping the itch–scratch cycle.

b. Occlusive dressing with or without low-potency steroids or tar preparations can be used.

c. Antihistamines will reduce itching.

C. Pityriasis rosea

1. General characteristics

a. Pityriasis rosea is characterized by an initial herald patch, an isolated round to oval lesion that precedes a widespread symmetrical papular eruption in most (80%) patients.

b. The cause is unknown but is thought to be viral (possibly human herpesvirus 7).

c. It is most common in teenagers and young adults. Incidence is highest in spring and fall.

2. Clinical features

a. There may be a mild upper respiratory tract infection-like prodrome before the onset of the rash.

> Lichen simplex chronicus is the result of chronic itch-scratch-itch cycle.

> Classic features of pityriasis rosea include a URI prodrome, solitary herald patch, and a broad rash in a Christmas tree-like distribution.

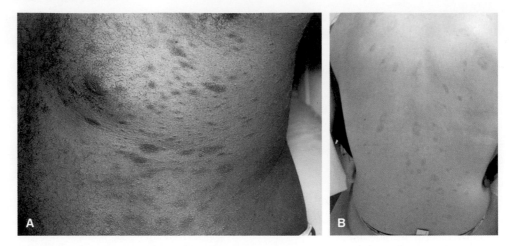

Figure 13-2 ▶ A, B: Pityriasis rosea. (**A:** Reprinted with permission from A from Goodheart HP. *Goodheart's Photoguide of Common Skin Disorders: Diagnosis and Management.* 2nd ed. Lippincott Williams & Wilkins; 2003, Fig. 4-4. **B:** Reprinted with permission from Goodheart HP. *Goodheart's Same-Site Differential Diagnosis: A Rapid Method of Diagnosing and Treating Common Skin Disorders.* Lippincott Williams & Wilkins; 2011, Fig. 15-16.)

    b. The herald patch is a solitary round or oval pink plaque with a raised border, central clearing, and fine adherent scales in the margins (resembles tinea corporis). It usually precedes the rash by a week or so.

    c. The generalized rash begins to appear on the trunk as round or oval, salmon-colored, maculopapular lesions, usually 1 cm in diameter.

    d. The long axis of each lesion typically follows the natural skin folds (cleavage lines or Langer's lines), giving a Christmas tree-like distribution. It is usually confined to the trunk (Fig. 13-2).

    e. Lesions are covered with a fine scale that desquamates, leaving an inverse collarette scale around each lesion.

    f. Pityriasis rosea is self-limited; spontaneous remission occurs in 6 to 12 weeks.

3. Treatment

    a. No treatment is indicated other than symptomatic. Antihistamines may help if itching is bothersome; lotions or emollients will help resolve the scales.

    b. UVB phototherapy may be helpful if started early.

    c. A short course of systemic steroids may be helpful.

D. Molluscum contagiosum

    1. General characteristics

        a. A common viral disease of skin and mucous membranes caused by a DNA poxvirus; more often seen in children but can affect adults. Transmitted by direct contact.

        b. In adults, the lesions are commonly found in the groin areas and on the lower abdomen, often contracted during sexual activity.

        c. In immunocompromised patients (such as HIV), lesions can be larger and more widespread, including predominance on the head and neck.

    2. Clinical features

        a. Manifests as discrete, flesh-colored, waxy, dome-shaped, centrally umbilicated papules over the face, trunk, and extremities.

        b. They range in size from 3 to 6 mm and appear in groups.

        c. A white, curd-like material can be expressed from under the depression of the lesion.

> Molluscum contagiosum is owing to infection with the poxvirus.

3. Laboratory studies: Biopsy may be needed in immunocompromised patients to rule out fungal dissemination.

4. Treatment

    a. Treatment is usually not necessary in healthy individuals because the disease is self-limited and usually resolves within 6 months.

    b. If therapy is indicated, it consists of local destruction of individual lesions by curettage (first-line), cryotherapy, electrodesiccation, or an acid or exfoliative peel (e.g., tretinoin and imiquimod). These treatments can be painful.

E. Lichen planus

    1. General characteristics

        a. This is an acute or chronic inflammatory dermatitis that occurs in adults. Females are more commonly affected than males.

        b. Lichen planus–like eruptions may occur in graft-versus-host disease, malignant lymphoma, and drug reactions.

        c. There is an association with hepatitis C infection in some patients.

    2. Clinical features

        a. Lesions are flat-topped/planar, shiny, violaceous papules with fine white lines on the surface (Wickham striae). Lesions are typically grouped and most commonly occur on the flexor aspect of the wrists, lumbar area, eyelids, shins, and scalp. The Koebner phenomenon is seen.

        b. Mucosal lesions may occur on the vagina, glans, and penis, as well as in the mouth. They are usually very painful and often ulcerate.

        c. Variants include follicular, vesicular, actinic, and ulcerative lesions.

        d. Lesions may affect hair (scarring alopecia) or nails (destruction of nail fold and nail bed with longitudinal splintering).

    3. Laboratory studies

        a. Biopsy and immunofluorescence confirm the diagnosis.

        b. Screening for hepatitis C should be considered. Some studies have found a higher prevalence of anti-hepatitis C virus antibodies in patients with lichen planus.

    4. Treatment

        a. Topical steroids with occlusive dressings for cutaneous lesions.

        b. Intralesional steroids or topical tretinoin is used for severe localized lesions.

        c. Cyclosporine mouthwash is used for oral lesions.

        d. Systemic therapy (cyclosporine, corticosteroids, or retinoids) may be needed in severe, painful cases.

        e. Photosensitizing PUVA therapy is helpful in generalized eruptions.

F. Dyshidrotic eczematous dermatitis (dyshidrosis)

    1. General characteristics

        a. This dermatitis generally develops in people younger than 40 years. Half of the affected have an atopic background.

        b. Eruptions follow stress or occur in hot, humid weather owing to excessive sweating.

    2. Clinical features

        a. Early disease

            (1) Pruritus is common; pain develops if secondarily infected.

            (2) Small, tense vesicles in clusters (tapioca-like appearance) are seen, and occasionally bullae form.

        b. Late disease

            (1) Papules, scaling, lichenification, and erosions from ruptured vesicles are seen.

> 💡 Lichen planus is associated with the 5 Ps: purple, polygonal, planar, pruritic, and papules.

> 💡 When you see clusters of pruritic, small, tense vesicles, think dyshidrosis.

(2) Painful fissures may develop.

c. There is a predilection for the fingers, palms, and soles of the feet.

3. Laboratory studies

    a. Culture can be done if a secondary infection is suspected.

    b. KOH prep will rule out dermatophytosis.

4. Treatment

    a. Topical or intralesional steroids are used for localized lesions and systemic steroids for severe cases.

    b. Apply wet dressings with Burow's solution. Large bullae should be drained but kept intact.

    c. Fissures are treated with topical collodion.

    d. PUVA is recommended in generalized or refractory disease.

    e. Treat secondary infection with systemic antimicrobials.

G. Psoriasis

> Psoriasis is chronic and inflammatory, often found on extensor surfaces, and treatment complexity correlates with severity.

1. General characteristics

    a. Psoriasis affects 2% of the population (3 to 5 million in the United States).

    b. Most patients have localized psoriasis, but more severe forms exist.

    c. A genetic predisposition exists, although only about one-third of the patients have family members with the condition.

    d. Psoriasis is a chronic, inflammatory, scaling condition of the skin that may also involve the mucous membranes. It seems that the earlier the onset of the disease, the more severe it will be. Psoriasis in HIV-positive patients can be very severe and resistant to treatment.

    e. Caused by a greatly accelerated epidermal cell turnover (to a rate 28 times normal), which causes epidermal hyperproliferation.

2. Clinical features

    a. Lesions of psoriasis are usually raised, pink to red papules and plaques with distinct margins and loosely adherent silvery scales (Fig. 13-3). Peeling away the scales produces specks of bleeding from the capillaries (Auspitz sign).

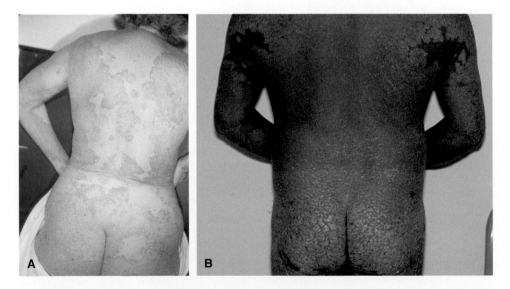

Figure 13-3 ▶ A, B: Psoriasis. (Reprinted with permission from Goodheart HP. *Goodheart's Photoguide of Common Skin Disorders: Diagnosis and Management.* 2nd ed. Lippincott Williams & Wilkins; 2003, Figs. 3-11 and 3-12.)

    b. Patches are most often found on the scalp and the extensor surfaces of the elbows and knees but can be found anywhere on the body.

    c. Pruritus is common. Scratching leads to more lesions (Koebner phenomenon).

    d. Patients with extensive disease also have nail involvement. The nails have tiny pits and ridges, are separated from the nail bed (onycholysis), and have oil staining/spots.

    e. Psoriatic arthritis occurs in 5% to 10% of patients. It involves the distal joints of the hands and feet, typically is asymmetric, and may be present without skin lesions.

    f. Diagnosis is made by history and appearance. The symptoms are usually mild, but the lesions are unsightly and of cosmetic concern.

    g. Variants: Four common variants are described in Table 13-2.

3 **Treatment**

    a. In mild localized cases, treatment consists of topical corticosteroids and topical vitamin D analogs (calcipotriene).

    b. Systemic steroids can be helpful for widespread lesions, but the disease often flares after withdrawal, thereby making it a less desirable treatment option.

    c. Topical coal tar or salicylic acid preparations and occlusive dressings are effective in controlling or removing scales.

    d. Moderate psoriasis may respond to tazarotene gel (topical retinoid).

    e. For more serious widespread involvement, UVB phototherapy, PUVA, and methotrexate have been effective but carry heightened risks for skin cancer, cataracts, and hepatotoxicity. Avoid methotrexate in immunocompromised patients, because it is a potent immunosuppressant.

    f. Pustular psoriasis may respond to acitretin, a synthetic retinoid, used with or without ultraviolet treatment. This is also helpful in erythroderma and psoriatic arthritis but is teratogenic.

    g. Cyclosporine may be effective in severe recalcitrant disease, but recurrence after cessation is common.

> Psoriatic arthritis most commonly affects the distal hands and feet.

Vesiculobullous Disorders

A. Pemphigus vulgaris

    1. General characteristics

        a. This is a serious bullous autoimmune disease; immunoglobulin G antibodies induce acantholysis, resulting in a loss of cell-to-cell adhesion.

        b. The disorder occurs in middle-aged adults. It is more common in people of Jewish or Mediterranean ancestry.

Table 13-2 | Psoriasis Variants

Psoriasis vulgaris	The most common type of psoriasis Involves chronic recurring scaling papules and plaques
Psoriatic erythroderma	Lesions involve the entire skin surface This variant is exfoliative and serious.
Guttate psoriasis	Characterized by acute eruption of teardrop-shaped lesions in a disseminated pattern Spares the palms and soles Often appears after a streptococcal pharyngitis infection
Pustular psoriasis (von Zumbusch syndrome)	Abrupt, life-threatening condition Characterized by widespread pustules that coalesce to form lakes of pus Fever, malaise, and leukocytosis are seen.

2. Clinical features

    a. Lesions usually begin in the oral mucosa; skin lesions occur 6 to 12 months later. There may be pain or burning but not pruritus. Weakness and malaise are common.

    b. Lesions are round vesicles or flaccid bullae that contain clear liquid and easily rupture. There is a positive Nikolsky sign (lateral pressure on the lesions causes the lesion to spread). The lesions are discrete and randomly scattered. Erosions and crusts occur because of the fragility of the blisters.

    c. Secondary infection and fluid and electrolyte imbalance are common causes of morbidity and mortality.

    d. Variants are listed in Table 13-3.

3. Laboratory studies

> Pemphigus vulgaris is Nikolsky-positive.

    a. Immunofluorescence of serum or blister material highlights immunoglobulin G.

    b. Biopsy proves acantholysis.

4. Treatment

    a. Systemic therapy is required. Start with oral prednisone and then add immunosuppressive agents, azathioprine, and/or methotrexate as needed.

    b. Supportive therapies include fluid and electrolyte replacement, cleansing baths, wet dressings, topical steroids, and antibiotics as needed.

B. Bullous pemphigoid

    1. General characteristics

        a. This blistering autoimmune disorder occurs typically in patients in their sixth decade of life or older.

        b. Autoantibodies, complement fixation, neutrophils, and eosinophils cause bullous formation.

    2. Clinical features

        a. There may be a prodrome of urticarial or papular lesions.

        b. Bullae are large, tense, oval, or round and contain serous or hemorrhagic fluid. They rupture less easily than in pemphigus vulgaris (negative Nikolsky sign).

Table 13-3 | Variants of Pemphigus Vulgaris

Pemphigus vegetans	Vegetating plaques composed of excessive granulation tissue and crusting
Pemphigus herpetiformis	Manifests with urticarial plaques and cutaneous vesicles Lesions are arranged in an annular pattern.
Pemphigus foliaceus	Small, scattered superficial blisters Rapidly evolve into scaly, crusted erosions Mucous membranes spared Seborrheic distribution: face, scalp, and trunk
Endemic pemphigus (fogo selvagem)	Clinically similar to idiopathic pemphigus Environmental trigger
Pemphigus erythematosus (Senear–Usher syndrome)	Localized to the malar region of the face
IgA pemphigus	Sudden development of vesicles that evolve into pustules Usually accompanied by erythematous plaques More common on the trunk and proximal extremities
Paraneoplastic pemphigus	Autoimmune multiorgan syndrome associated with neoplastic disease Severe and acute mucosal involvement Extensive, intractable stomatitis Cutaneous blisters, erosions, and lichenoid lesions Life-threatening bronchiolitis obliterans may also develop.
Neonatal pemphigus	Rare, transient condition of a child born to a mother with pemphigus Blisters develop secondary to placental transmission of autoantibodies. Usually resolves with 3 weeks

    c. Typically, bullae collapse and crust; at times, bleeding erosions occur.

    d. Axillae, thighs, groin, and abdomen are commonly affected. Mucous membrane lesions are less severe and less painful than in pemphigus.

3. Laboratory studies: Biopsy and immunofluorescence (+ IgG, C3) will confirm the diagnosis.

4. Treatment

    a. Systemic prednisone may be given at high doses either alone or in combination with azathioprine until remission and then at a lower dose for maintenance.

    b. Rituximab is helpful in some cases.

    c. Mild cases or localized recurrences are treated with topical steroids.

Papulopustular Inflammatory Disorders

A. **Acne vulgaris**

    1. General characteristics

        a. Acne affects all age groups, from neonates to older adults, but is most prevalent in adolescents and more severe in males.

        b. Pathology includes plugged follicles, retained sebum, bacterial overgrowth, and release of fatty acids. Androgens stimulate sebum production.

    2. Clinical features

        a. Acne is an inflammatory follicular, papular, and pustular eruption involving the pilosebaceous apparatus.

        b. The hallmark lesions of acne are comedones, either open or closed, noninflammatory (Fig. 13-4).

            (1) Open comedones are often referred to as "blackheads" because of melanin depositions in a keratin plug.

            (2) Closed comedones, often called "whiteheads," are flesh-colored 1-mm papules.

            (3) Open or closed comedones can become erythematous papules, pustules, nodules, or cysts, ranging in size from 1 to 5 mm.

        c. Sinus tracts occur with nodular acne. Inflammatory lesions can lead to hyperpigmentation and scarring.

    3. Laboratory studies are rarely done. The vast majority of cases do not derive from an endocrine etiology, but if suspected, one would order testosterone, follicle-stimulating hormone, luteinizing hormone, or dehydroepiandrosterone 5 mg levels.

> 💡 Acne is associated with *Propionibacterium acnes* and *Staphylcoccus epidermidis.*

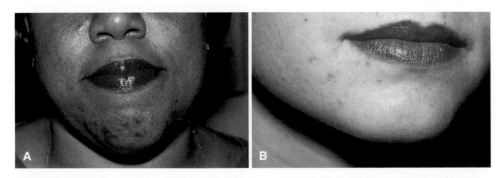

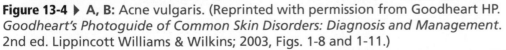

Figure 13-4 ▸ A, B: Acne vulgaris. (Reprinted with permission from Goodheart HP. *Goodheart's Photoguide of Common Skin Disorders: Diagnosis and Management.* 2nd ed. Lippincott Williams & Wilkins; 2003, Figs. 1-8 and 1-11.)

4. Treatment

a. Mild acne can be controlled by keeping the affected areas clean and applying topical preparations such as retinoids, azelaic acid, and salicylic acid.

b. If inflammatory lesions are present, topical benzoyl peroxide, tretinoin, erythromycin, clindamycin, or sodium sulfacetamide is indicated.

c. In more serious or cystic acne, oral antibiotics should be used in conjunction with the topical preparations.

  (1) Tetracyclines were the drug of choice early on and are still effective. Erythromycin, doxycycline, minocycline, trimethoprim-sulfamethoxazole, and clindamycin are also frequently used.

  (2) The bacterium that is involved in acne is becoming resistant to some medications. It is best to treat as conservatively as possible and only for as long as necessary.

  (3) Recurrence after cessation of treatment is common.

d. Oral isotretinoin

  (1) This medication can only be prescribed by a registered dermatologic provider in the iPLEDGE program.

  (2) Isotretinoin is highly teratogenic. Female users of childbearing age must have a negative pregnancy test before starting, use multiple forms of birth control when taking this medication, and have monthly pregnancy tests before receiving a medication refill.

  (3) Side effects can be very serious, ranging from dry eyes, nose, and lips to epistaxis, joint pains, mood swings, and suicidal thoughts.

  (4) Premature closure of the long bones, visual changes, hepatic enzyme elevation, leukopenia, and triglyceridemia also occur.

> Severe acne can be treated with isotretinoin, but all patients need side effect monitoring, and females must have reliable birth control.

B. Acne rosacea

1. General characteristics

a. Acne rosacea is a chronic acneiform disorder mainly affecting females between 30 and 50 years of age.

b. It is a disease of the pilosebaceous units associated with increased activity of capillaries, leading to telangiectasias and flushing secondary to vasodilation.

c. The outbreaks are episodic and typically occur in response to heat, alcohol, sun, or hot, spicy foods. Coffee and tea stimulate outbreaks because of the heat not the caffeine content.

2. Clinical features

a. It is characterized by the insidious onset of scattered, small papulopustules and sometimes nodules; comedones do *not* occur. The face appears red or flushed.

b. There is a symmetric distribution on the face (cheeks, chin, forehead, glabella, and nose). Less often, lesions can appear on the neck, chest, back, or scalp.

c. Later telangiectasia, hyperplasia, and lymphedema develop.

d. Patients often complain of disfiguring appearance.

e. When describing disfiguring effects, the suffix -phyma, meaning "enlarged," is used: rhinophyma (nose), blepharophyma (eyelid), metophyma (forehead), otophyma (ear), or gnathophyma (chin).

> Acne rosacea precipitants include hot beverages or food, hot weather or the sun, alcohol intake, or spicy foods.

3. Treatment

a. Reduce triggers such as alcohol or hot beverages.

b. Topical metronidazole (most effective), sodium sulfacetamide, or erythromycin is often sufficient.

    c. If topical treatment fails, systemic antibiotics, such as tetracycline, minocycline, or doxycycline, can be utilized until remission and then continued at lower doses for maintenance.

    d. Very severe cases may require oral isotretinoin under the care of a dermatologic specialist (see acne vulgaris).

C. Folliculitis

  1. General characteristics

    a. Folliculitis is an inflammation of the hair follicles.

    b. It is most commonly caused by *S. aureus* but can be caused by other organisms as well.

    c. Noninfectious folliculitis is common among people working in hot, oily environments, such as engine workers on ships, machinists, or anyone working in a hot, dirty environment.

      (1) Noninfectious folliculitis can be caused by occlusion, perspiration, and skin rubbing against tight clothes.

      (2) Pseudofolliculitis barbae (razor bumps), another form of noninfectious folliculitis, is caused by ingrown hairs in the beard area from shaving in the direction of hair growth.

> Pseudomonal folliculitis is seen in hot tub users.

  2. Clinical features

    a. The lesions are erythematous papules or pustules. They are usually not painful but may burn.

    b. Sycosis is severe, deep-seated, recalcitrant folliculitis with surrounding eczema and crusting.

    c. Abscesses may form at the site of more severe folliculitis.

  3. Treatment

    a. Gentle cleansing with antibacterial soap and mild compresses help. Protection from offending substances and use of drying agents also help.

    b. Topical application of clindamycin or erythromycin works well on mild cases of infectious folliculitis. Mupirocin ointment may also be used. Correction of the underlying cause is critical to resolving noninfectious folliculitis.

    c. In more extensive cases, oral antibiotics may be necessary.

    d. "Hot tub" folliculitis (*Pseudomonas*) usually resolves without treatment; severe or recalcitrant cases may be treated with an oral fluoroquinolone.

D. Erythema multiforme (EM)

  1. General characteristics

    a. EM can be induced by drugs (e.g., sulfonamides, phenytoin, barbiturates, penicillin, and allopurinol) and infections (herpes simplex virus is common, *Mycoplasma* sp.) or be idiopathic.

    b. Half of all cases occur in patients younger than 20 years of age.

    c. Previous history of EM is a strong risk factor for subsequent cases.

> 90% of erythema multiforme minor is related to HSV.

  2. Clinical features

    a. Lesions begin as macules and become papular and then vesicles and bullae form in the center of the papules. Target or iris lesions are characteristic.

    b. Lesions can be localized to the hands and feet or become generalized.

    c. Mucosal lesions can occur, generally oral, which are painful and erode.

    d. Patients complain of fever, weakness, and malaise. Rarely, lungs and eyes may be affected.

  3. Treatment

    a. Avoid precipitating substances, and control herpes outbreaks with acyclovir.

    b. Severely ill patients are treated with systemic steroids.

> TEN is more severe, covering >30% of body surface area with higher fever and more epidermal loss.

E. Stevens–Johnson syndrome (SJS) and toxic epidermal necrolysis (TEN)

1. General characteristics

   a. This is a mucocutaneous blistering disorder, often caused by a drug reaction with other etiologies of infection or idiopathic. Drugs commonly associated with SJS or TEN include sulfonamides, aminopenicillins, quinolones, cephalosporins, tetracyclines, phenobarbital, carbamazepine, phenytoin, valproic acid, oxicam nonsteroidal anti-inflammatory drugs (NSAIDs), and allopurinol.

   b. SJS (generally <10% body surface area) is thought to be a severe variant of EM, and TEN (generally >30% body surface area) is thought to be a severe variant of SJS.

   c. SJS or TEN may occur in patients of any age or gender.

   d. The pathogenesis is unknown, but it is thought to be an immune-mediated response.

   e. The health dangers are secondary infection, fluid loss, and electrolyte imbalances. TEN can be life-threatening.

2. **Clinical features**

   a. Patients present with fever, photophobia, sore throat, mucosal inflammation, and sore mouth. The cutaneous lesions tend to be concentrated more on the trunk initially. The lesions may be painful or may sting.

   b. Progression occurs over 4 days: diffuse erythema; morbilliform lesions; necrotic epidermis; wrinkled surfaces; sheetlike loss of epidermis; and raised, flaccid blisters (positive Nikolsky sign).

   c. TEN exhibits higher fever and more severe epidermal separation and loss compared with SJS.

   d. Regrowth of skin takes 3 weeks; it is delayed in pressure-point areas.

   e. About 90% of patients have mucosal lesions occurring anywhere from the mouth to the anus, which are painful and eroding.

   f. Other complications include acute tubular necrosis, erosion in the lungs and gut, and bronchitis.

3. Laboratory studies

   a. Labs to evaluate for anemia and lymphopenia or leukocytosis; check C-reactive protein and TNF-α.

   b. Monitor electrolytes.

   c. Blood and wound cultures if infection is suspected.

   d. Biopsy is diagnostic.

4. **Treatment**

   a. Prompt withdrawal of the offending or causative agent is critical.

   b. Extensive necrolysis should be treated in a burn unit; any skin lesions warrant treatment as burns.

   c. Treat patients for fluid and electrolyte imbalance and any complications or infections. Consider tetanus prophylaxis.

   d. Treatment debate

      (1) Treatment with corticosteroids is being debated and has not been conclusively researched. Some studies found that high doses early in the disease are effective, whereas others concluded that steroids may exacerbate the disease.

      (2) Intravenous immunoglobulin is commonly used, but data do not show any improvement in mortality.

> Approach the management of TEN as if the patient has suffered severe burns.

F. Hidradenitis suppurativa

1. General characteristics

   a. Hidradenitis suppurativa is a disorder of the apocrine glands (axilla, anogenital, and scalp).

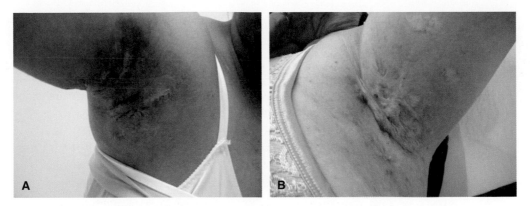

Figure 13-5 ▶ A, B: Hidradenitis suppurativa. (Reprinted with permission from Goodheart HP. *Goodheart's Same-Site Differential Diagnosis: A Rapid Method of Diagnosing and Treating Common Skin Disorders.* Lippincott Williams & Wilkins; 2011, Figs. 11-6 and 11-7.)

    b. It affects females between puberty and menopause (axillary disease) more often than males (anogenital disease).

    c. Predisposing factors include obesity, history of acne, apocrine duct obstruction, and bacterial infection. There appears to be a genetic predisposition.

2. Clinical features

    a. Tender inflammatory nodules or abscess formation is characteristic. Lesions are not related to hair follicles (Fig. 13-5).

    b. Double-ended open comedones and sinus tracts form and may drain purulent material.

    c. Fibrosis, scarring, and contractures may occur. Severity is variable.

3. Laboratory studies include complete blood count, inflammatory markers, and culture for secondary bacterial infection.

4. Treatment

    a. Lifestyle changes include weight loss and reduction of moisture/friction to the area. Smoking cessation if indicated.

    b. Lesions are treated with intralesional triamcinolone, incision and drainage of abscesses, and excision of sinus tracts.

    c. Oral antibiotics are given until lesions resolve; prednisone is added if the lesions are severe and should then be tapered over 2 weeks.

    d. Severe cases, especially in the anogenital area, may benefit from psychological support.

> The key to treating hidradenitis is aggressive local care and reduction in risky behaviors.

Localized Skin Infections

A. **Furuncles and carbuncles**

    1. General characteristics

        a. Furuncles are sometimes referred to as "boils" or "risens." These lesions are deep-seated infections of the hair follicles; *S. aureus* is the most common pathogen.

        b. A furuncle is an infection of a single follicle; a carbuncle includes more than one infected follicle as an interconnected conglomerate mass.

    2. **Clinical features**

        a. Furuncles and carbuncles present as red, hard, tender lesions in the hair-bearing areas of the head, neck, or body. Carbuncles have multiple drainage points.

      b. Lesions progress to become fluctuant and rupture spontaneously, draining pus and necrotic tissue.

   3. Treatment

      a. Treatment should be started with warm, moist compresses.

      b. Topical antibiotic therapy as well as incision and drainage are added as appropriate once the lesion is mature.

      c. Cloths used for warm compresses and/or towels used to clean or dry these lesions should be handled with care to prevent additional infection.

B. Cellulitis

   1. General characteristics

      a. Cellulitis is an acute, spreading inflammation of the dermis and subcutaneous tissue.

      b. Although the causative organism can be identified by culturing any drainage or discharge or by needle aspiration, it is best to begin treatment with antibiotics that will cover *Haemophilus influenzae*, *Streptococcus* sp., and *Staphylococcus* sp.

   2. Clinical features

      a. The area involved is swollen, red, hot, and tender.

      b. The patient may have lymphadenopathy, fever, chills, and malaise.

   3. Treatment

      a. Mild or early infections may be treated with oral penicillinase-resistant penicillin, such as dicloxacillin or a cephalosporin. For patients who are allergic to penicillin, a macrolide or clindamycin is appropriate.

      b. In more severe infections, nafcillin or a third-generation cephalosporin such as ceftriaxone is given intravenously. For penicillin-allergic patients, options are clindamycin or vancomycin. Patients started on parenteral therapy may be switched to oral therapy when the fever, chills, and malaise subside.

      c. It may be appropriate to mark the margins of involvement before treatment to follow the progression or regression of the area.

      d. If there is a poor response to antimicrobial therapy or a necrotizing, soft-tissue infection is suspected, infectious disease consult and surgical intervention are necessary.

C. Abscess

   1. General characteristics

      a. An abscess is a localized infection characterized by a collection of purulent material in a cavity formed by necrosis or disintegration of tissue.

      b. A sterile abscess is one formed without a bacterial pathogen.

   2. Clinical features

      a. Abscess presents as a tender, erythematous, and often fluctuant area, indicating the formation of pus.

      b. The most common locations are axillary and anorectal regions, buttocks, and the head and neck.

      c. Discharge or drainage can be cultured; however, more than one causative organism is the norm.

      d. An abscess may develop at the site of a therapeutic or drug-related injection.

   3. Treatment

      a. Early abscess should be treated with hot soaks for 20 minutes four times daily to bring it to a head. Once the lesion is fluctuant, it can be incised and drained and an iodoform gauze wick can be placed in the wound to facilitate drainage.

Cellulitis is infectious inflammation within the dermis and subcutaneous tissue and may be treated with oral antibiotics against H. influenzae, Streptococcus sp., and Staphylococcus sp.

The most common locations for acute abscess include axilla, anorectal region, buttocks, and the head and neck.

b. Alternatively, hot soaks can be followed by a dressing saturated with a drawing salve.

c. Oral antibiotics, such as dicloxacillin, a cephalosporin, or erythromycin, should be started if the patient has a fever or cellulitis is present surrounding the abscess.

Dermatophytosis

A. General characteristics

    1. Dermatophytosis ("ringworm") is a superficial fungal infection that can affect the hair, nails, and skin.

    2. The three most common dermatophytes affecting humans are *Trichophyton, Microsporum,* and *Epidermophyton* spp.; *Trichophyton rubrum* is the most common dermatophyte in the industrialized world.

    3. When describing the area of infection, the word tinea (meaning "fungal infection") is followed by the affected part of the body (Table 13-4).

B. Clinical features

    1. Generally, dermatophytosis presents as an erythematous, annular patch with distinct borders and a central clearing. A fine scale usually covers the patch.

    2. Symptoms include itching, stinging, and/or burning. Maceration or peeling fissures are common between the digits.

    3. The nails present with a thickening discoloration and onycholysis of the nail bed and nail plate.

    4. In tinea capitis, broken hair shafts are seen as black dots.

    5. A kerion (indurated, boggy, inflammatory plaque studded with pustules) can appear with any of these infections but most commonly is found with tinea capitis. It represents an intense inflammatory reaction to superficial dermatophytes.

C. Laboratory studies: A KOH prep should be done to confirm the presence of fungus.

D. Treatment

    1. There is a wide selection of topical creams, ointments, lotions, powders, and sprays to treat localized dermatophytosis. They should be used twice daily for 4 weeks or more. If vesicles are present, powders help to dry the area and to prevent maceration.

    2. Chronic or resistant infections or nail infections (onychomycosis) may require oral fluconazole, itraconazole, terbinafine, or ketoconazole. Treatment may take 3 months.

    3. Kerions are treated with oral fluconazole or griseofulvin.

    4. Monitoring is very important in treating these infections.

        a. Patients with hepatic disorders should be monitored closely when using oral antifungal medications.

> KOH prep in tinea will show hyphae and arthrospores. In *Candida*, it will show pseudohyphae and budding yeasts.

Table 13-4 | Tinea

Tinea pedis	Foot
Tinea cruris	Groin
Tinea corporis	Trunk, legs, arms, or neck
Tinea barbae	Beard area
Tinea unguium	Nails
Tinea manuum	Hand
Tinea facialis	Face
Tinea capitis	Head

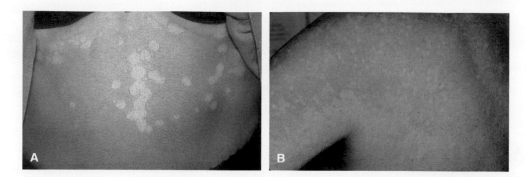

Figure 13-6 ▶ A, B: Tinea versicolor. (Reprinted with permission from Goodheart HP. *Goodheart's Same-Site Differential Diagnosis: A Rapid Method of Diagnosing and Treating Common Skin Disorders.* Lippincott Williams & Wilkins; 2011, Figs. 15-20 and 15-22.)

    b. If the patient will be on these medications for a long period, such as when treating tinea unguium for several months, liver enzymes should be measured at baseline and then monitored periodically.

    c. Patients taking griseofulvin should not use alcohol in any form because it may cause a flushing/headache reaction.

  5. Steroids should be avoided. Long-term use will exacerbate the condition and increase the risk of side effects.

  6. Local measures include keeping the skin clean and dry and wearing cotton socks and loose-fitting underclothes.

E. **Tinea versicolor (pityriasis versicolor)**

  1. Tinea versicolor is caused by *Malassezia furfur*, a normal yeast colonizer of human skin. It is not understood why this yeast manifests in the spore and hyphal form in some patients, causing disease; predisposing factors include warm climates, excessive sweating, and oily skin.

  2. Clinical features

    a. Tinea versicolor consists of hypo- or hyperpigmented macules that do not tan in areas of overgrowth. Most patients are asymptomatic and notice the infection only during the summer when their tan is uneven and spotted owing to localized areas of yeast overgrowth; it is not contagious (Fig. 13-6).

    b. The upper trunk and shoulders are the most common areas involved.

  3. Laboratory studies: KOH prep of scrapings will show hyphae and spores ("spaghetti and meatballs").

  4. Treatment

    a. Treatment consists of daily applications of selenium sulfide shampoo from the neck to the waist; the shampoo is left on for up to 15 minutes for 7 consecutive days. This can be repeated monthly for maintenance therapy as necessary.

    b. Another option is oral treatment with ketoconazole. Patients should not shower for 18 hours after taking oral ketoconazole because it works by being delivered to the skin surface through the patient's sweat.

> 💡 KOH in tinea versicolor will reveal hyphae and yeast cells in a "spaghetti and meatballs" pattern.

Parasitic Infestations

A. **Scabies**

  1. General characteristics

    a. Scabies is infestation with *Sarcoptes scabiei*, an eight-legged mite (Fig. 13-7).

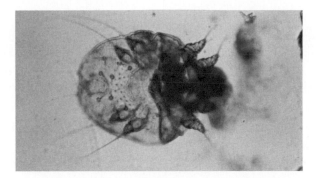

Figure 13-7 ▶ Scabies mite. (Reprinted with permission from Goodheart HP. *Good-heart's Photoguide of Common Skin Disorders: Diagnosis and Management.* 2nd ed. Lippincott Williams & Wilkins; 2003, Fig. 20-12.)

   b. Scabies can be found in patients of any age but rarely in infants younger than 3 months of age.

2. Clinical features

   a. Distribution is most common on the hands, wrists, genitalia, and axillary areas. Lesions are often seen in the web spaces between the fingers and toes, around the belt line, or at the edges of socks.

   b. The lesions are pruritic burrows, vesicles, or nodules with excoriations and crusting.

   c. Secondary infections are typically caused by group A streptococci.

3. Laboratory studies

   a. Look for mites, eggs, or feces in a scraping. A drop of mineral oil before scraping facilitates yield.

   b. Positive microscopy is confirmative but not always successful.

4. Treatment

   a. Topical 5% permethrin (preferred) or 1% lindane lotion or cream is used. It is applied to the skin from the chin to the bottom of the feet and left on overnight (8 hours) and then washed off in the morning. The treatment should be repeated in 7 days.

   b. Antihistamines or topical steroids may help relieve the itching.

   c. Lindane is more toxic and should be avoided in children younger than 2 years of age, people with extensive dermatitis, and those who are pregnant or lactating.

   d. All bedclothes and clothing of infected patients and household contacts should be washed.

   e. All close physical contacts should receive scabicide treatment as well.

B. Spider bites

 1. General characteristics

   a. Although all spiders in the United States are venomous, only a few can puncture the human skin. The most important is the brown recluse (*Loxosceles reclusa*).

   b. Most spider bites occur while the patient is sleeping or dressing in the morning after the spider had crawled into the clothing during the night.

 2. Clinical features

   a. Generally, the patient will begin to feel pain 3 hours after a bite; systemic symptoms begin 4 to 6 hours after the bite.

   b. An acute necrotic injury to the skin lasts 10 to 15 days.

   c. Black widows transmit a neurotoxic venom that can cause neurologic overstimulation (e.g., muscle aches, spasms, and rigidity). These spiders are not prevalent today.

Scabies has a predilection for hands, wrists, genitalia, and axilla.

d. The brown recluse can cause a significant reaction.

    (1) The single bite is accompanied by an infarct of skin caused by rapid blood co-agulation within the vessels that can lead to progressive skin necrosis.

    (2) The lesion is a sinking macule, pale gray in color, slightly eroded in the center, and has a halo of very tender inflammation and hemorrhage.

3. Systemic symptoms such as fever, chills, nausea, and vomiting may be present.

4. The lesion can extend to the muscle and be as large as the palm of the hand.

5. Treatment

    a. Most spider bites can be managed with local care and analgesics.

    b. Neurologic and cardiac manifestations of black widow bites are treated with diazepam and calcium gluconate along with pain management.

    c. Brown recluse bites may be treated locally with wound cleansing and analgesia. Extensive debridement has not proven to be beneficial. Usually, the wound decreases significantly in 5 to 10 days.

    d. Antivenom is rarely indicated and not readily available.

> 💡 Brown recluse spider bites may cause acute cardiac issues; treat with diazepam and calcium gluconate.

C. Pediculosis (Lice)

  1. General characteristics

    a. Lice are 1- to 3-mm flat creatures with three pairs of legs. Females lay 300 nits during a lifetime. Nits are opalescent, found on hair shafts, and hatch in about 1 week.

    b. *Pediculus humanus* var. *capitis* infects the scalp (head lice), and *P. humanus* var. *corporis* infects the body. *Phthirus pubis* infects the pubic area (crabs).

    c. Transmission is from person to person through direct skin contact or sharing of combs, hats, and so on.

  2. Clinical features

    a. Pruritus is variable in severity. Excoriations may become secondarily infected.

    b. Lice are visible but often difficult to find. Nits are more readily seen on the hair shafts.

  3. Laboratory studies: Specimens can be viewed under the microscope to confirm the diagnosis.

  4. Treatment

    a. Prevention is key; avoid sharing contact items such as hats, hairbrushes, and so forth. All contacts should be examined.

    b. Topical insecticides are effective. Permethrin, pyrethrins, and malathion are considered to be first-line treatments; lindane or ivermectin are alternatives.

    c. Special fine-tooth combs help to remove nits; petroleum jelly or other occlusive materials may help to suffocate the lice.

    d. Reapplication in 7 to 10 days is recommended to kill any newly hatched lice.

> 💡 Treatment for lice: topical permethrin and thorough fine-tooth combing.

Warts (Verrucae)

A. General characteristics

  1. Warts are caused by the human papillomavirus (HPV). There are more than 100 known serotypes.

  2. HPV replicates in cutaneous and mucosal epithelium. Growths remain local and regress spontaneously.

  3. Common warts can arise on any skin surface. Genital warts (condylomata) are spread through sexual contact.

B. Clinical features

1. Skin warts can be flat or superficial. Plantar warts are deeper. The surface is rough, resembling tiny heads of cauliflower.

2. Warts of the oral cavity or larynx can be life-threatening if they block the airway.

3. Anogenital warts occur almost exclusively on the squamous epithelial of the external genitalia and perianal area and can be oncogenic depending on the serotype. Men who have sex with men are at increased risk of anal cancer from high-risk serotype infection.

4. Cervical lesions, especially HPV types 6, 11, 16, and 18, are a risk factor for dysplasia, which may progress to cervical or anorectal cancer.

C. Laboratory studies

1. Microscopic study shows characteristic hyperplasia and hyperkeratosis. Koilocytotic squamous cells are present.

2. The presence of HPV is confirmed by immunofluorescence. Molecular probes can detect HPV in cervical tissue.

3. Acetic acid testing enhances abnormal cellular structure for cervical lesion evaluation.

D. Treatment

1. Spontaneous regression is typical over time.

2. Type, location, and age of the patient dictate treatment. The extent of the lesions, the patient's motivation, and the patient's immunologic status also affect treatment choice.

3. Salicylic acid plasters can be effective for common warts. Cryosurgery or electrodesiccation can be effective but risks scarring.

4. Imiquimod is a topical therapy that patients can apply at home, but adherence is a problem.

5. Intralesional interferon may also be effective if other treatments fail.

6. Anogenital warts can be treated with trichloroacetic acid or topical podophyllin, but this may require many applications.

7. Surgical excision is successful, but recurrence is common.

8. Effective vaccines for high-risk HPV types 6, 11, 16, and 18 have been developed and are recommended for preteen girls and boys at 11 to 12 years of age, though vaccination can be given as young as age 9 and up to 26 years of age.

> HPV types 6, 11, 16, and 18 are associated with cervical cancer.

> Type and location of warts, and the age of the patient, dictate treatment options from salicylic plasters (common warts) to topical podophyllin (anogenital warts).

Tumors

A. Benign neoplasm

1. A keratoderma is a generalized thickening of the horny layer of the epidermis.

   a. **Types of keratoderma**

      (1) Punctate keratodermas, found on the palms of the hands and the soles of the feet, and keratodermas, on the digits, are more prevalent in African American patients. The lesions develop central plugs.

      (2) Solar keratosis (actinic keratosis) is a premalignant condition caused by cumulative exposure to the sun and is more prevalent in fair-skinned people. The thickened, rough lesions can progress very slowly to squamous cell carcinomas; therefore, treatment of these lesions is advised if they don't spontaneously regress, and they can also progress to a cutaneous horn.

      (3) Actinic cheilitis is actinic dermatosis of the lip.

      (4) Seborrheic keratosis is a benign plaque, beige to brown or black, with a velvety, warty surface that appears "stuck on." Lesions are more common in older persons.

 b. Treatment

   (1) Liquid nitrogen can be used successfully to treat keratodermas.

   (2) Electrodesiccation and curettage are also effective.

   (3) Mild acid treatments and the application of Monsel's solution (ferric subsulfate solution) have been used.

   (4) 5-Fluorouracil and topical imiquimod are effective, but patients must be warned that the lesions will look worse before they look better.

2. Lipomas (adipose tumors) are benign neoplasms of mature fat cells that pose no harm to the patient. Surgical excision may be appropriate for cosmetic reasons or if the lipoma is located where it is constantly irritated.

3. Pyogenic granulomas (capillary hemangiomas): This term is a misnomer because the lesion does not have an infectious cause.

 a. Clinical features

   (1) These bright red, raspberry-like nodules are usually present on exposed parts of the body, such as the arms, hands, fingers, or legs.

   (2) They often not only appear after an injury or surgery but also can appear spontaneously.

 b. Treatment: Electrodesiccation and curettage or excision is used. Cauterization with silver nitrate and cryosurgery has not proved to be curative.

> Lipomas are fatty tumors between skin and muscle layers, freely movable with finger pressure.

B. Malignant neoplasms: Use the ABCDE method to diagnose and document any suspicious moles (Table 13-5).

1. Melanoma

 a. General characteristics

   (1) Although only about 1% of skin cancers are melanomas, melanoma causes the vast majority of skin cancer deaths.

   (2) The incidence of melanoma continues to rise and is occurring in younger individuals. Since the 1970s, the 5-year survival rate has increased from 25% to 40% to more than 80%.

   (3) Melanomas frequently metastasize widely to regional lymph nodes, skin, liver, lungs, or brain.

 b. Clinical features

   (1) Melanomas are usually a mottled black or dark brown color but can be flesh colored. They sometimes have blue, pink, or red components (Fig. 13-8).

   (2) The lesions have an irregular border, with an outward spreading of pigment. If the lesion changes in size over a relatively short period, malignant degeneration should be considered.

   (3) Although most commonly seen on sun-exposed areas, melanoma can occur anywhere on the body, including the eye; mucous membranes of the genitalia, anus, or oral cavity; subungual areas; and soles of the feet.

   (4) Lesions can be macular to nodular, and four types exist: lentigo maligna melanoma, superficial spreading malignant melanoma (most common), nodular

Table 13-5 | The ABCDEs of Suspicious Moles

Asymmetry	One side of the mole does not mirror the other side
Border	Border or edges of the mole are jagged
Color	Color varies throughout the mole, black or blue
Diameter	Mole diameter is >6 mm
Evolution	Mole appearance changing over time; enlarging

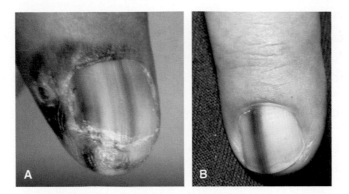

Figure 13-8 ▶ **A, B:** Melanoma. (Reprinted with permission from Goodheart HP. *Goodheart's Photoguide of Common Skin Disorders: Diagnosis and Management.* 2nd ed. Lippincott Williams & Wilkins; 2003, Figs. 22-37 and 22-38.)

malignant melanoma, and acral lentiginous melanomas (palms, soles, and nail beds; more common in darker-skinned persons).

c. Prognosis is strongly related to the depth of the lesion (Breslow depth).

(1) A melanoma entirely within the epidermis carries a very good prognosis.

(2) As the thickness progresses beyond the epidermis, the prognosis diminishes.

(3) The likelihood of survival is further diminished if the melanoma is on the upper back, upper arm, neck, or scalp.

d. Treatment

(1) Early detection is the key to successful treatment and improved outcomes.

(2) Treatment is based on the extent of disease (staging) and metastasis. The mainstay of treatment includes complete, wide excision, regional lynch node dissection, and follow-up with adjuvant therapy as indicated.

2. Squamous cell carcinoma most often arises from a preexisting actinic keratosis. Squamous cell carcinoma in situ is commonly referred to as Bowen's disease.

a. Clinical features

(1) Nonhealing, erosive lesion that is typically slowly evolving and asymptomatic, but may itch or bleed easily.

(2) Lesions most commonly present on sun-exposed areas of the skin (face, head, and neck).

(3) Lesions generally appear as sharply demarcated, scaling, or hyperkeratotic macule, papule, or plaque. Erythema, scaling, erosions, and crusts may occur.

b. Treatment

(1) Complete eradication of the lesion is required. Metastasis to regional lymph nodes does occur in a small percentage of cases.

(2) Treatment is dependent on the location and extent of the lesion. Options include excision with clear margins (preferred), electrodesiccation with curettage, cryosurgery, and radiation therapy.

3. Basal cell carcinoma is the most common cancer in humans.

a. Clinical features

(1) Generally a solitary, slow-growing lesion that can be locally destructive as it spreads to adjacent tissue. Metastasis does not occur.

(2) Found on sun-exposed areas of the skin, the lesion is typically asymptomatic but readily bleeds with minor trauma.

> 💡 Malignant neoplasms are most commonly found on sun-exposed areas, irregular in shape, brown or black, and associated with poor prognosis if thicker than the epidermis.

(3) There are several types of basal cell lesions:

(a) Nodular: translucent or pearly papule or nodule

(b) Ulcerating: ulcer with a rolled border, often covered with a crust

(c) Sclerosing: infiltrating carcinoma; white sclerotic patch with ill-defined borders

(d) Superficial: erythematous, slightly scaly, thin plaques, often with a fine rolled or pearly border

(e) Pigmented: thick, hard area of variegated pigmentation

b. Treatment

(1) Treatment is dependent on the location and extent of the lesion.

(2) Total excision (preferred), electrodesiccation with curettage, cryosurgery, radiation therapy, and laser vaporization. Topical treatment with 5-fluorouracil or imiquimod is also an option.

(3) Table 13-6 compares the features of premalignant and malignant skin tumors.

Ulcers, Burns, and Wounds

A. Ulcers

1. General characteristics

a. Diabetic ulcers, stasis ulcers, and arterial leg ulcers are common in the lower limbs.

b. Decubitus ulcers occur in areas of skin pressure in patients with limited mobility.

2. Clinical features

a. Diabetic ulcers tend to be deep, punched-out lesions over the malleoli, the plantar surfaces of the feet, or the toes. They can be painless in diabetics with associated neuropathies.

b. Stasis ulcers are a result of chronic venous stasis. Stasis dermatitis develops initially followed by ulcers that are wide but shallow develop, with irregular, undulating edges and a clean base. Elevation of the affected limb eases any pain.

c. Arterial ulcers usually do not become as large as venous ulcers and are not preceded by dermatitis. Arterial ulcers are painful, pulses are diminished or absent, and the distal area is cold.

d. Decubitus or pressure ulcers are a result of impaired blood supply caused by localized pressure. The sacrum and hip areas are most commonly affected. Complications include osteomyelitis, bacteremia, and sepsis. There are four stages of pressure ulcers (Fig. 13-9).

Table 13-6 | Comparison of Premalignant and Malignant Skin Lesions

Skin Disorder	Appearance	Location	Treatment
Actinic keratosis (precursor to SCC)	Rough, dry, scale <1 cm; sandpaper feel on palpation	Sun-exposed areas of skin: face, ears, forearms, and scalp in balding males common	Cryosurgery 5-FU Imiquimod
SCC	Variable, eroded papule, or plaque	Sun-exposed areas of skin	Excision
Basal cell carcinoma	Pearly papule w/ erosion, telangiectasias	Head and upper chest	Excision; for superficial: can use 5-FU or imiquimod
Melanoma	Mottled color, size >6.0 mm, irregular border, asymmetry	Anywhere including soles of feet and in the nail bed	Excision

SCC, squamous cell carcinoma; 5-FU, 5-fluorouracil.

3. Treatment

a. All limb ulcers can be difficult to treat.

b. Diabetic and arterial ulcers are treated similarly.

(1) Lifestyle changes include smoking cessation and moderate exercise to enhance blood flow.

(2) Debridement is necessary if the wound is necrotic.

(3) Wet-to-dry dressings or hydrogels are standard treatment because wounds heal better in a moist environment. Hydrocolloids (e.g., DuoDERM) and enzymatic preparations maintain moisture, enhance granulation, promote debridement, and improve rates of epithelialization.

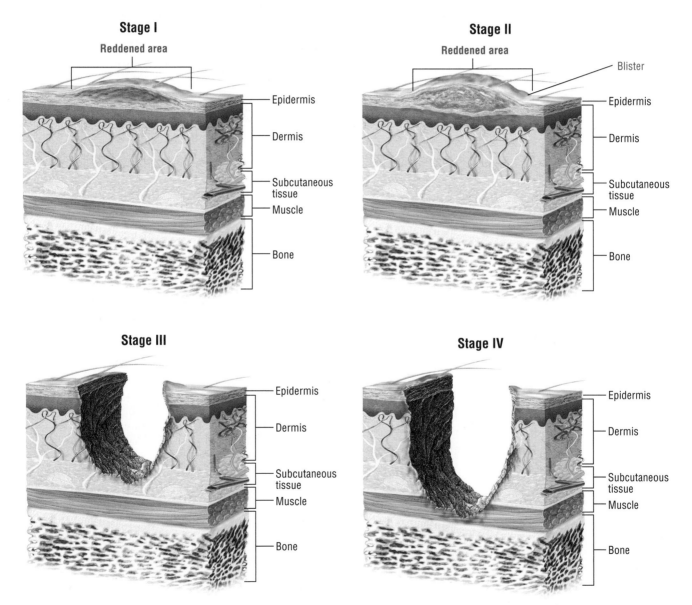

Figure 13-9 ▶ Stages of decubitus ulcer development. **Stage I:** Nonblanching erythema of intact skin. **Stage II:** Necrosis, superficial, or partial thickness involving the epidermis and/or dermis shallow ulcer. **Stage III:** Deep necrosis crater ulcers with full-thickness skin loss damage or necrosis can extend down to, but not through, fascia. **Stage IV:** Full-thickness ulceration extensive damage and necrosis to muscle, bone, or underlying structures. (Reprinted with permission from Werner R. *Massage Therapist's Guide to Pathology*. 6th ed. Wolters Kluwer; 2015, Fig. 2.63.)

    c. Stasis ulcers are treated with elevation and compression to enhance venous return.

      (1) The affected limb should be whirlpooled, the lesion painted with gentian violet, and an Unna boot applied weekly.

      (2) Wraps or support hose may also be used for compression; they should be applied while the leg is elevated and before the veins fill again.

    d. Prevention is the key to managing decubitus ulcers.

      (1) Repositioning, massaging prone areas, and frequent monitoring are essential.

      (2) Efforts to minimize friction, the use of an air mattress to reduce compression, meticulous hygiene, and good nutrition aid in prevention.

      (3) If an ulcer develops, moist sterile gauze (e.g., Gelfoam), hydrocolloid, and/or surgical debridement may be necessary.

    e. Topical and/or systemic antibiotics are indicated for any signs of infections.

B. Open wounds

    1. Tetanus status should be assessed with any open wound.

      a. If the last tetanus booster was more than 10 years ago, an update is needed; if the wound is particularly dirty, a tetanus booster may be given sooner.

      b. If the tetanus status is unknown, the patient should receive tetanus immunoglobulin as well as the vaccine.

    2. Wounds should be cleansed well, irrigated, and closed unless they are more than 8 hours old or signs of infection exist. Dirty wounds may need antibiotic coverage.

C. Burns (see Chapter 15)

> 💡 Tetanus booster is recommended every 10 years, sooner if one sustains a dirty wound.

Hair and Nails

A. Alopecia (loss of hair)

    1. Androgenetic alopecia (male or female pattern baldness)

      a. Male pattern baldness has a genetic component.

      b. Its extent is variable and unpredictable in men; for women, hair loss usually begins at the part line and involves generalized thinning.

      c. Minoxidil solutions are most effective in persons with recent onset and smaller areas of hair loss.

      d. Finasteride may also be effective for men. Side effects include loss of libido and erectile dysfunction.

    2. Alopecia areata is of unknown cause.

      a. It may be seen in thyroiditis, pernicious anemia, systemic lupus erythematosus, or Addison's disease.

      b. Tiny hairs are typically found, which taper near the proximal end (exclamation point hairs). Loss can be patchy, involve only the scalp (alopecia totalis), or include the entire body (alopecia universalis) (Fig. 13-10).

      c. It may respond to systemic steroids, but relapse is common.

    3. Drug-induced alopecia may occur with thallium, vitamin A, retinoids, antimitotic agents, anticoagulants, oral contraceptives, and others.

B. Nails

    1. Onycholysis is the distal separation of the nail plate from the nail bed.

      a. Common causes include excessive exposure to water, soaps, detergents, or alkalis; psoriasis; drugs; or thyroid disease.

      b. Onychomycosis indicates infection with fungi or yeast.

    2. Discolorations and crumbly nails are seen in dermatophytosis and psoriasis.

> 💡 • Alopecia areata: exclamation point hairs
> • Androgenetic alopecia: short, thin, regressing hair
> • Telogen effluvium: short, regrowing normal hairs
> • Trichotillomania: broken hairs of varying lengths

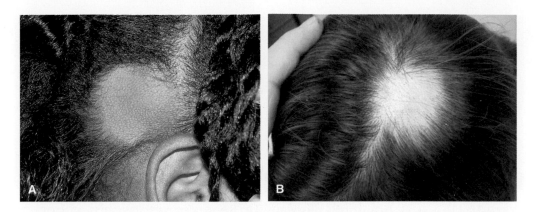

Figure 13-10. ▶ **A, B.** Alopecia areata. (**A:** Reprinted with permission from Goodheart HP. *Goodheart's Photoguide of Common Skin Disorders: Diagnosis and Management.* 2nd ed. Lippincott Williams & Wilkins; 2003, Fig. 10-3. **B:** Reprinted with permission from Goodheart HP. *Goodheart's Same-Site Differential Diagnosis: A Rapid Method of Diagnosing and Treating Common Skin Disorders.* Lippincott Williams & Wilkins; 2011, Fig. 1-4.)

3. Paronychia is an inflammation of the nail fold. Erythema, swelling, and throbbing pain may extend into the proximal nail fold and eponychium.

4. Felon is a subcutaneous infection of the pulp space. This is a closed infection that may rupture or cause osteitis or osteomyelitis; the abscess should be drained.

5. Congenital nail disorders include nail atrophy and clubbed fingers.

6. Systemic disease may cause Beau lines (transverse furrows), atrophy, clubbed fingers, spoon nails, stippling or pitting, and hyperpigmentation.

Pigmentation Disorders

A. **Acanthosis nigricans**

   1. General characteristics

      a. This hyperpigmentation disorder can be hereditary or acquired.

      b. It is commonly associated with obesity, endocrine disorders (most notably insulin resistance), and paraneoplastic syndromes, or it may be drug induced.

   2. **Clinical features**: Acanthosis nigricans develops insidiously. Initially, the skin darkens and appears dirty; later, the skin becomes thickened and velvety, with accentuated skin lines (Fig. 13-11). Commonly affected sites are axillae, groin, and back of the neck.

   3. Laboratory studies: If the disorder is thought to be associated with an underlying pathology, such as diabetes or an internal malignancy, further investigation is needed.

   4. **Treatment**: There is no treatment except that of addressing any underlying predisposing disorder.

> 💡 Acanthosis nigricans is strongly associated with insulin resistance.

B. **Melasma (also known as chloasma)**

   1. Melasma means "a black spot"; it is an acquired hyperpigmentation disorder of sun-exposed areas and is often associated with pregnancy or with oral contraceptives or other medications.

   2. **Clinical features**

      a. Young females are more commonly affected.

      b. Hyperpigmented macular areas evolve rapidly over weeks. The color is usually uniform.

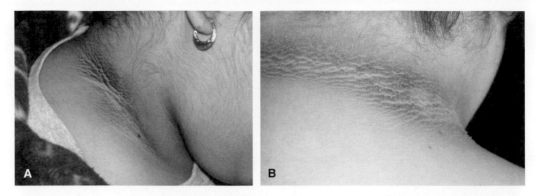

Figure 13-11. ▶ **A, B.** Acanthosis nigricans. (**A**: Reprinted with permission from Goodheart HP. *Goodheart's Photoguide of Common Skin Disorders: Diagnosis and Management.* 2nd ed. Lippincott Williams & Wilkins; 2003, Fig. 14-15. **B**: Reprinted with permission from Baranoski S, Ayello EA. *Wound Care Essentials.* 5th ed. Wolters Kluwer; 2020, Fig. 24-5.)

3. Laboratory studies: Wood's lamp examination accentuates the hyperpigmented macules.

4. **Treatment**
   a. Treatment includes 3% hydroquinone solution in combination with 0.025% tretinoin gel. Alternatively, 4% hydroquinone and glycolic acid in a cream base may be used.
   b. Sunblock is essential in controlling hyperpigmentation.

C. **Vitiligo**
   1. General characteristics
      a. Destruction of melanocytes can be associated with thyroid disease, pernicious anemia, diabetes mellitus, and Addison's disease, or it may be idiopathic.
      b. Vitiligo occurs at any age, in every race, and in males and females equally. About 30% of patients report a family history.
      c. Macules of hypopigmentation may occur focally, segmentally, or in a generalized pattern.
   2. **Treatment**: Sunscreens, cosmetic cover-up products, or repigmentation therapies under the direction of an experienced dermatologist may be used.
   3. Vitiligo can be very psychologically distressing, especially in dark-skinned patients.

Angioedema and Urticaria

A. General characteristics
   1. Urticaria is a group of disorders that can have many causes, most common are food or drug allergies, heat or cold, and stress or infection.
   2. Urticaria affects 15% to 20% of the population.
   3. Hives or wheals are raised red areas on the skin or mucous membranes caused by the release of histamines, bradykinin, kallikrein, and other vasoactive substances from mast cells and basophils in the skin, causing small blood vessels to leak and resulting in intradermal edema.
   4. The wheals may be the size of a pencil eraser or up to the size of a dinner plate, and they may coalesce into even larger areas.
   5. The lesions most commonly are pruritic but may sting or burn.

B. Acute urticaria is often self-limiting, lasting from a few minutes to hours.

    1. Acute urticaria is commonly an allergic reaction to food or drugs. Immunoglobulin E attaches itself to a receptor on the mast cell and causes a chemical release.

    2. Frequent triggers of acute urticaria are things that are ingested: drugs, most notably penicillin or other antibiotics, sulfa drugs, and other medications; shellfish; peanuts; and food preservatives in processed and canned foodstuffs.

    3. Other less common causes include things the skin may contact (e.g., laundry detergents, shampoos, perfumes, and cleaning solvents) or things the patient may inhale (e.g., fabric softeners, perfumes).

C. Chronic urticaria lasts more than 6 weeks. Typically, the lesions wax and wane.

    1. Chronic urticaria is idiopathic; exacerbations can be precipitated by stress.

    2. Females are affected twice as often as males.

D. Physical urticaria can be caused by reaction to heat or cold, water, infection, exercise, or sun exposure. Dermatographism caused by pressure can occur.

E. **Treatment**

    1. Any known triggers should be eliminated, but it is estimated that the cause is not found in up to 80% of cases.

    2. For acute or idiopathic urticaria, an H_1 antihistamine, such as diphenhydramine, hydroxyzine, fexofenadine, or cetirizine, may be used orally.

    3. In chronic urticaria or in acute urticaria which does not initially respond, an H_2 antihistamine, such as famotidine or ranitidine, may be added to the H_1 regimen.

    4. Recurring urticaria or chronic urticaria may require steroids to control.

    5. If there is a concern that urticaria may progress to anaphylaxis, a prescription for an EpiPen should be given to the patient along with education regarding its use.

Practice Questions

Directions: Each of the numbered items or incomplete statements in this section is followed by a list of answers or completions of the statement. Select the ONE lettered answer or completion that is BEST in each case.

1. A 15-year-old male presents complaining of a slowly enlarging lesion on his left thigh. He states that the lesion is slightly pruritic but otherwise nonpainful. He first noticed the lesion about 2 weeks ago and had hoped it would resolve on its own, but instead, it has grown increasingly larger. He denies fever, fatigue, and all other constitutional symptoms. What is the most appropriate treatment?

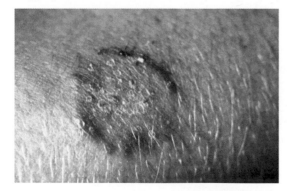

Image courtesy CDC/Dr. Lucille K. Georg. Available at: https://phil.cdc.gov/phil/home.asp. Accessed April 27, 2017.

    A. Oral itraconazole
    B. Oral minocycline
    C. Topical erythromycin
    D. Topical ketoconazole
    E. Topical 5-fluorouracil

2. A 22-year-old college student presents with an acute eruption across his trunk and lower back of salmon pink, teardrop-shaped papules with fine scale on the surface. Scraping of the scale results in pinpoint blood droplets where the scale was removed. A thorough history would likely uncover what recent illness?

    A. Infectious mononucleosis
    B. Lyme disease
    C. Pneumococcal pneumonia
    D. Streptococcal pharyngitis
    E. Syphilis

3. A 32-year-old female complains of pruritic lesions on her lower extremities that have developed over the past several weeks. Examination reveals multiple, sharply defined, violaceous papules of varying size and shape. On close inspection, a fine lacey network of white lines can be seen on the surface of each lesion. What is the most likely diagnosis?

A. Lichen planus
B. Nummular dermatitis
C. Psoriasis
D. Stasis dermatitis
E. Urticaria

4. An 11-year-old female is experiencing a "rash" on her trunk that seems to be slowly spreading. Examination reveals multiple scattered, flesh-colored, shiny dome-shaped papules with central umbilication. What is the likely causative organism?

A. β-Hemolytic streptococcus
B. DNA poxvirus
C. Hepatitis C virus
D. Herpes simplex virus
E. *S. aureus*

5. A 13-year-old male complains of an intensely pruritic eruption in his bilateral antecubital fossae as pictured below. He tells you he has an intermittent history of similar outbreaks, which seem to worsen in winter. On examination, you see areas of dry, scaly skin with some lichenification noted. He is requesting a prescription for a topical steroid because that treatment has helped clear the rash in the past. This patient is at increased risk for having what comorbid disorder in association with this rash?

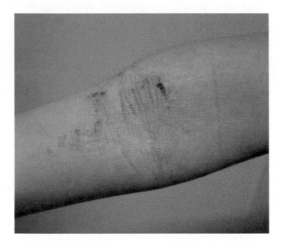

Image courtesy Wikimedia Commons/James Heilman, MD. Available at: https://commons.wikimedia.org/wiki/Category:Atopic_dermatitis#/media/File:Atopy2010.JPG. Accessed April 27, 2017.

A. Acanthosis nigricans
B. Allergic rhinitis
C. Cystic fibrosis
D. Diabetes mellitus
E. Psoriasis

6. A 19-year-old college student is concerned about a rash that has developed on her trunk and seems to be spreading. She states that she first noticed a single, round lesion on her left upper trunk and then about 5 days later a more generalized rash started appearing across her trunk. It is mildly pruritic but otherwise only just a cosmetic concern. On examination, the generalized rash seems to follow the skin lines and consists of multiple salmon-colored, maculopapular lesions. What is the most likely diagnosis?

A. Contact dermatitis
B. Nummular eczema
C. Pityriasis rosea
D. Seborrheic dermatitis
E. Tinea versicolor

7. A 17-year-old male presents with multiple annular, erythematous, iris-shaped papular lesions with central vesicles or bullae on his hands. He reports that the lesions started out as flat, dusky red areas that transitioned over several days to their current state. He also notes several painful erosions in his oral mucosa. What infection would most likely be present in this patient's most recent history?

A. Herpes simplex
B. Influenza
C. *Neisseria gonorrhoeae*
D. Rotavirus
E. Streptococcal pharyngitis

8. A 36-year-old female complains of an intensely itchy rash that started on her wrists and now is spreading to her hands. On examination, there are multiple irregular linear lesions with superimposed excoriations from her scratching. Burrows are present in the interdigital web spaces. What would be the most appropriate treatment for this patient?

A. Oral cephalexin
B. Oral itraconazole
C. Topical ketoconazole
D. Topical metronidazole
E. Topical permethrin

9. A 68-year-old male complains of a "bump" on his face that has been slowly enlarging over the past year and has bled several times without much provocation. On examination, there is a 1 cm nodule with a "pearly" appearance and visible telangiectasias. What is the most likely diagnosis?

A. Basal cell carcinoma
B. Epithelial inclusion cyst
C. Keratoacanthoma
D. Lipoma
E. Melanoma

10. A 20-year-old male complains of a rash that has been present for several months and is becoming more noticeable. There are no associated symptoms reported, but he is embarrassed by the skin's appearance when he is at the beach without a shirt on. His shoulders and upper trunk have numerous hypopigmented macules, some of which have become confluent. Microscopic examination of the macules would likely reveal what finding?

A. Cocci in chains
B. Diplococci
C. Hyphae and budding spores
D. Inclusion bodies
E. Multinucleated giant cells

11. A 42-year-old obese female is concerned about a darkened area of skin in her axillae. She is concerned that it is skin cancer. Examination reveals a dark brown plaque that has a thickened and velvety appearance with exaggerated skin lines. Which of the following laboratory results would most likely be found in this patient?

A. Abnormal liver enzymes
B. Elevated triglycerides
C. Hypokalemia
D. Insulin resistance
E. Normocytic anemia

12. A 74-year-old male has multiple tense pruritic bullae across his abdomen, some of which have ruptured and crusted over. He reports that the lesions started several weeks ago as smaller "bumps" that eventually became fluid-filled. He has no associated constitutional symptoms. On examination, there are multiple bullae that are Nikolsky negative. What is the most likely diagnosis?

A. Bullous pemphigoid
B. Dermatitis herpetiformis
C. Epidermolysis bullosa acquisita
D. SJS
E. Varicella zoster

Practice Answers

1. D. *Dermatology; Pharmacology; Tinea*

The image depicts a classic presentation of tinea corporis with its annular, well-defined, slowly expanding border with central clearing. This is a dermatophyte infection, and KOH microscopic examination of the scales from the border will reveal typical hyphae. Antifungals are the appropriate treatment. Localized infections as seen in this case only require topical treatment. Systemic antifungal treatments such as itraconazole should be reserved for widespread infections or infections involving the nails. Topical erythromycin is an appropriate treatment for mild acne, whereas oral minocycline is useful for treating moderate acne. Topical 5-fluorouracil can be used to treat the premalignant lesions of actinic keratosis and is also approved for the treatment of superficial basal cell carcinoma below the neck and squamous cell carcinoma in situ.

2. D. *Dermatology; Diagnosis; Psoriasis; Guttate*

Guttate psoriasis is characterized by the sudden appearance of teardrop-shaped lesions as described above. There is almost always a history of streptococcal pharyngitis before the skin outbreak. A typical sign seen in various forms of psoriasis is the Auspitz sign: minute bleeding occurring at points of scale removal. A disseminated, benign, and brief rash can appear shortly after initiating treatment for both syphilis and Lyme disease, but the rash would not exhibit the classic teardrop lesions nor the Auspitz sign as seen in guttate psoriasis. That rash is related to the Jarisch–Herxheimer reaction, which is thought to occur as a result of endotoxin-like substances being released from the dying spirochetes. Secondary syphilis is characterized by a diffuse mucocutaneous rash with tender lymph nodes and patchy alopecia.

3. A. *Dermatology; Diagnosis; Lichen planus*

Lichen planus (LP) classically presents as described, with multiple purplish to violaceous, polygonal lesions that are pruritic. The disorder is most commonly idiopathic and can have an acute or insidious onset over several weeks. The lacey, fine white lines of Wickham striae can often be noted on the surface of LP lesions, but would not be seen in any of the other dermatologic disorders listed, nor are the other disorders associated with the 5 Ps as seen in LP: purple, polygonal, planar, pruritic, and papules.

4. B. *Dermatology; Basic Science; Molluscum*

The lesions of molluscum contagiosum are readily identifiable: flesh-colored, dome-like lesions, often with central umbilication which are more commonly seen in children than adults. These benign lesions are caused by a DNA poxvirus.

Autoinoculation can occur. The papules may spontaneously regress over time but can also be treated with cryotherapy or curettage.

5. B. *Dermatology; History; Dermatitis*

The picture and presentation are classic for atopic dermatitis, which has a predilection for involving the flexural folds, although it can also appear on the face, neck, wrists, and dorsum of the hands and feet. Individuals with atopic dermatitis have hyperirritable skin caused by an underlying type I immunoglobulin E–mediated hypersensitivity. Owing to this hypersensitivity, persons with atopic dermatitis are also at increased risk for allergic rhinitis and asthma (atopic diathesis). The other disorders have no relation to atopic dermatitis.

6. C. *Dermatology; Diagnosis; Pityriasis*

The patient is experiencing an outbreak of pityriasis rosea, a benign disorder that occurs most often in teenagers and young adults, more commonly in the spring and fall months. Initially, a solitary "herald patch" occurs that is round with a central clearing and scaly border, which is then followed within about a week by the generalized outbreak. Owing to the pattern following the cleavage lines of the skin, it is often referred to as a "Christmas tree" pattern. The disorder is self-limited, and only supportive treatment (such as antihistamine for pruritus) is indicated. The rash will completely resolve within a few weeks up to a few months.

7. A. *Dermatology; History/PE; EM*

Erythema multiforme (EM) is a self-limited, benign disorder that can be idiopathic or precipitated by drugs or infections. Herpes simplex is the infection most commonly linked to acute eruptions of EM. The hands and feet, including palms and soles, are the most commonly affected body areas. Painful, erosive oral mucosal lesions can occur in conjunction with skin lesions. Owing to the classic appearance of EM, the lesions are often referred to as iris or target-shaped lesions. Unless severely ill, supportive treatment is generally sufficient. The other infections listed are not known to precipitate an EM outbreak although Mycoplasma has been occasionally linked, but not as commonly as herpes simplex. The best prevention of recurrent post–herpes EM outbreaks is prompt treatment of any herpes outbreak with acyclovir or a similar agent.

8. E. *Dermatology; Pharmacology; Scabies*

The patient has contracted a scabies infection, caused by the *S. scabiei* mite. The wrists, hands, genitalia, and axillary areas are most commonly affected. Microscopic examination with mineral oil of scrapings from the end of a burrow will likely reveal mites, eggs, or feces. Scabies is highly contagious, so all bedding, clothing, and so on, need to be washed thoroughly and all close contacts should be treated as well. Topical 5% permethrin cream is highly effective in eradicating scabies. It should be applied to the entire body from the neck down and left on overnight, washed off in the morning, and repeated in 7 days. Antihistamines can alleviate the pruritus.

9. A. *Dermatology; Diagnosis; Basal Cell Carcinoma*

This presentation is classic for a nodular basal cell carcinoma, which is almost exclusively found in the sun-exposed areas of the skin, particularly the head and face. Lesions bleed easily with minor trauma. Basal cell carcinomas do not metastasize but can be locally destructive to the surrounding tissue if left untreated. Treatment varies depending on the location and extent of the lesion as well as patient preference. Melanoma is more often flat, darkly pigmented with mottled coloring and uneven borders but can have an aggressive vertical growth. Lipomas are soft, nontender subcutaneous masses. Keratoacanthoma presents as a rapidly growing firm, rounded, skin-colored papule. An epithelial inclusion cyst is also skin colored, round, and firm.

10. C. *Dermatology; Diagnostic Study*

This patient has tinea versicolor (pityriasis versicolor) which is caused by an overgrowth of *M. furfur*, a lipophilic yeast organism that is a common colonizer of the skin. In favorable conditions, such as oily or sweaty skin, the yeast will overgrow, preventing sun exposure of the affected areas of the skin. In light-skinned individuals, this overgrowth is most noticeable when the surrounding skin becomes tanned and the affected skin areas do not, thereby creating hypopigmented macules. In darker-skinned individuals, the affected areas can appear as hyperpigmented lesions. Scrapings examined microscopically with KOH prep will reveal blunt hyphae and budding spores often referred to as a "spaghetti and meatballs" appearance. Multinucleated giant cells are seen on Tzanck smear of a herpes simplex lesion. Inclusion bodies indicate Chlamydia. Neisseria is characterized by diplococci. Cocci in chains are characteristic of Streptococcal infection.

11. D. *Dermatology; Diagnostic Study; Acanthosis Nigricans*

This is a description of acanthosis nigricans (AN), which most often develops insidiously on the neck, the axillae, or in the groin area. In overweight individuals, AN is often associated with insulin resistance, and patients should be screened for diabetes mellitus. AN at times develops as a cutaneous marker of internal malignancy, most often adenocarcinoma of the gastrointestinal (GI) tract. Correction of the underlying etiology will generally return the skin to a normal appearance.

12. A. *Dermatology; Diagnosis; Bullous Pemphigoid*

Bullous pemphigoid is an autoimmune blistering disorder that almost exclusively develops in elderly patients, with equal occurrence in both males and females. The bullae are Nikolsky negative as opposed to the blisters of pemphigus vulgaris, which are most often Nikolsky positive. Biopsy will confirm the diagnosis. In patients with large areas of involvement, long-term treatment with oral prednisone is required to clear the lesions, initially high dose and then ongoing low-dose treatment to maintain the clearing.

Infectious Disease | 14

Claire Babcock O'Connell

Fever

A. General information

1. The normal range of body temperature is 97°F to 99.5°F (36.0°C to 37.4°C), averaging 98.6°F (36.7°C). There is a normal diurnal variation of 1.25°F to 2.5°F (0.5°C to 1.0°C).

   a. Stimulation of monocyte–macrophage cells elaborates pyrogenic cytokines, which cause an elevation of the set point of the body temperature (i.e., fever). Increased heat production causes shivering; reduction causes peripheral vasoconstriction.

   b. A body temperature of >106.8°F (41.1°C) risks irreversible brain damage.

2. Elevated temperature and the symptoms caused by change in the body temperature are fairly well correlated with illness, particularly infection.

   a. The degree of elevation does not correlate with severity of illness.

   b. Children typically mount high fevers; the elderly and people on chronic medications (e.g., nonsteroidal anti-inflammatory drugs [NSAIDs], steroids) may not mount a fever at all.

B. Fever of unknown origin (FUO) is defined as a temperature of >101.8°F (38.3°C) for 3 weeks with no discernible cause despite at least 1 week of diagnostic workup.

1. The most common causes of FUO are infections, noninfectious inflammatory disorders, and malignancies (Table 14-1).

2. No diagnosis is found in 50% of FUO cases.

C. Diagnostic workup

1. History, physical examination, complete blood count (CBC) with differential, blood cultures, and routine chemistries and urinalysis are routinely completed.

2. Additional laboratory and diagnostic studies should be directed by the suspected differential diagnosis. Avoid ordering a variety of tests without a clear plan.

D. Treatment of fever is mainly for patient comfort. Reduction in temperature is not part of the therapy for the underlying cause.

1. Fevers can be reduced by supportive measures, such as alcohol or cold sponge baths, ice bags, or ice water enemas, or through administration of antipyretics, such as

> ☼ FUO: (1) temp >101.8°F (38.3°C), (2) longer than 3 weeks, and (3) without diagnosis despite workup.

Table 14-1 | Common Causes of Fever of Unknown Origin

Infections	Noninfectious Inflammatory Disorders	Malignancies
Tuberculosis, extrapulmonary	Adult Still's disease	Lymphoma
Abscess	Giant cell arteritis	Leukemia
Osteomyelitis	Polyarteritis nodosa	Renal cell carcinoma
Endocarditis	Takayasu arteritis	Hepatic carcinoma
	Wegener's granulomatosis	

aspirin or acetaminophen. Aspirin products should be avoided in children because of the risk of Reye's syndrome.

2. Empiric broad-spectrum antibiotics are often begun when infection is suspected. Therapeutic trials should be limited to 2 weeks. Overuse or inappropriate use of antibiotics leads to microbial resistance.

3. Therapeutic trials of glucocorticoids should not supplant investigation into specific causes.

Sepsis

A. General characteristics

1. Bacteremia (septicemia) is the multiplication of microbes in the bloodstream. Sepsis is symptomatic bacteremia.

   a. Over 750,000 cases of sepsis occur annually. Incidence has risen because of increased longevity, increased prevalence of immunocompromised, increased microbial resistance, and, most importantly, increase in aggressive interventional procedures.

   b. Mortality is 20% to 50%.

   c. Bacteria are the most common microbe involved, followed by fungi and protozoa.

2. Systemic inflammatory response syndrome (SIRS) is a constellation of signs and symptoms indicating sepsis. The presence of any two of the following defines SIRS: temperature >38.0°C (100.4°F) or <36.0°C (96.8°F); pulse >90 bpm; respirations >20 per minute or $PaCO_2$ <32 mm Hg; white blood cell (WBC) count >12,000 mm³ or <4,000 mm³ (or >10% bands).

3. Severe sepsis is defined as sepsis complicated by organ damage (multiple organ dysfunction syndrome [MODS]).

4. Septic shock is defined as sepsis with circulatory, cellular, and metabolic abnormalities. The hallmark of septic shock is refractory hypotension.

5. The Surviving Sepsis campaign resulted in the development of qSOFA (quick Sequential Organ Failure Assessment) calculation. This bedside prompt uses three criteria (systolic blood pressure [SBP] <100 mm Hg, respiratory rate [RR] > 21/minute, and Glasgow Scale score <15) to identify patients at risk for poor outcome. Score of 2 or more indicates high risk. The use of qSOFA is more accurate in a non–intensive care unit (ICU) setting.

> 💡 Sepsis can be rapidly identified using qSOFA: altered mental status with an abnormal Glasgow Scale score, increased respiratory rate (>22), and low blood pressure (SBP <100).

B. **Clinical manifestations**

1. Most patients will have a fever, although the severity of fever does not correlate with risk or outcome of sepsis.

2. Patients typically exhibit a change in mental status.

3. Specific symptoms may indicate the underlying cause, most commonly infected peripheral or central lines, cardiopulmonary compromise, or gastrointestinal (GI) or genitourinary (GU) infection. Refer to Chapter 3 for cardiogenic shock.

C. Diagnostic considerations

1. CBC, blood cultures, and urinalysis should be done on any patient presenting with suspected sepsis.

2. Imaging studies (chest radiography, abdominal ultrasonography, computed tomography [CT], or magnetic resonance imaging [MRI]) should be chosen based on the possible underlying causes.

3. Low oxygen conditions cause a switch from pyruvate production to lactate production. Lactic acid levels correlate with risk of sepsis. Normal lactic acid is 1 to 2 mmol per L; >2 mmol per L indicates diminished perfusion; >4 mmol per L indicates complete tissue hypoxia.

D. Treatment

1. Airway, breathing, and circulation are of primary concern.
2. Draw labs and maintain cardiopulmonary status with crystalloids and vasopressors. Transfuse whole blood if indicated.
3. Address infection with empiric broad-spectrum antibiotics.
4. Prevent or reverse organ disturbances: oxygen; volume expansion; maintain glucose at 80 to 110 mg per dL; sedate and intubate as needed.
5. Mediate host response and inhibit toxic mediators to reduce mortality and prevent complications.

> Treatment goals include resuscitating from shock, treating underlying infection, and maintaining organ function.

Bacterial Infections

A. Streptococcus spp.

1. General characteristics
   a. Streptococci are a group of Gram-positive, catalase-producing cocci that appear in chains. They can be aerobic, anaerobic, or facultative and are cultured on blood agar media: Incomplete hemolysis is identified as α-hemolytic (*Streptococcus viridans*, *Streptococcus pneumoniae*), complete hemolysis as β-hemolytic (*S. pyogenes*), and no hemolysis as γ-hemolytic streptococci (*Enterococcus*).
   b. The β-hemolytic streptococci are the most common pathogenic type.
      (1) Lancefield classified the β-hemolytic streptococci into groups, labeled A through O.
      (2) The group A β-hemolytic streptococci are the most common of all the pathogenic streptococci.
   c. Humans are the only reservoir of group A β-hemolytic streptococci.
      (1) Asymptomatic carriers are frequent. The highest incidence of infection with group A β-hemolytic streptococci is in patients younger than 10 years.
      (2) Crowded conditions and person-to-person transmission are responsible for its perpetuity.

2. **Clinical manifestations**
   a. Pharyngitis
      (1) An abrupt onset of sore throat and painful swallowing with fever and chills herald an infection.
      (2) There is enlargement of the cervical lymph nodes, edema, hypertrophy of pharyngeal mucosa, and erythema and exudates that may be punctate or confluent.
      (3) The disease is usually self-limited and typically resolves in 3 to 4 days, even without a specific treatment. Untreated infections may lead to nonsuppurative complications.
   b. Scarlet fever is characterized as strep throat with a rash.
      (1) The rash is a diffuse erythema that blanches; superimposed fine red papules may be appreciated only by touch (sandpaper rash). It is described as a sunburn with goosebumps.
      (2) The face is typically flushed, with circumoral pallor and a strawberry tongue.
      (3) The rash fades in 2 to 5 days, with fine desquamation.
   c. Erysipelas is a painful macular rash with well-defined margins; it is characterized by an abrupt onset and rapid progression.
      (1) The rash is typically confined to the face, which becomes fiery red, but it may progress to the extremities. Flaccid bullae may develop.

> Strep infections can manifest in multiple organ systems including oropharynx, skin and soft tissue, and lungs.

(2) The rash desquamates in 5 to 10 days.

(3) Systemic symptoms including fever, chills, severe malaise, and headache may occur.

d. Impetigo (*Streptococcus pyoderma*) is characterized by thick, crusted, golden "honey" yellow lesions.

(1) There is a higher prevalence with poor hygiene and malnutrition.

(2) The bacteria colonize unbroken skin and, with abrasions or bites, inoculate the intradermal space, where lesions develop.

(3) Impetigo can also be caused by staphylococci (bullous impetigo), although it is more likely to present with bullae.

e. Cellulitis manifests with local swelling, erythema, and pain.

(1) The skin is pinkish and indurated.

(2) Group A streptococci are the most common cause of cellulitis in the United States; it is common in patients with lymphedema, chronic stasis, or venous grafts.

(3) Surgical debridement may be necessary if there is poor response to medical treatment.

f. Necrotizing fasciitis (flesh-eating bacteria) is a deep subcutaneous infection that results in destruction of fascia and fat.

(1) Swelling, heat, erythema, and pain spread proximally and distally.

(2) The skin darkens, and blisters and bullae with clear yellow fluid form.

(3) Development of gangrene and necrosis is associated with mental status changes and delirium; mortality is high.

g. Toxic shock syndrome is bacteremia with susceptible strains of toxin-producing streptococci following deep soft-tissue infection. It is also associated with *Staphylococcus aureus* infection.

(1) A viral-like prodrome and a history of minor trauma, surgery, or varicella may be found.

(2) Onset is abrupt with severe pain, typically in an extremity; abdominal infection may mimic peritonitis, pelvic inflammatory disease, myocardial infarction, or pericarditis.

(3) Fever or hypothermia, confusion, combativeness, and coma develop. Patients develop shock and multiorgan failure. A violaceous or blue vesicular or bullous rash is an ominous sign. Mortality is 30% despite treatment.

(4) Complications include endophthalmitis, myositis, peritonitis, septic arthritis, myocarditis, perihepatitis, meningitis, and sepsis.

(5) Common laboratory findings include hemoglobinuria, elevated serum creatinine, low albumin, low calcium, mild leukocytosis and a severe left shift, and low platelet count.

(6) Management includes intravenous (IV) fluids (colloids and crystalloids) and antibiotics as well as vasopressors, mechanical ventilation, and surgical intervention, as needed.

h. Pneumonia (refer to Chapter 2)

i. Nonsuppurative complications of group A β-hemolytic streptococcal infections

(1) Acute glomerulonephritis (see Chapter 6)

(2) Acute rheumatic fever (ARF) is a systemic immune process occurring on an average 15 to 20 days after exposure to streptococcal pharyngitis.

(a) Once rare, it has become more prevalent since the 1980s. The peak age is 5 to 15 years, and the mortality is 1% to 2% despite treatment.

💡 Group A strep is the most common etiology of cellulitis.

💡 Toxic shock syndrome often follows a mild viral syndrome and presents with acute pain, fever, and shock.

Table 14-2 | Jones Criteria for Diagnosis of Acute Rheumatic Fever

Major Criteria	Minor Criteria
Carditis	Fever
Erythema marginatum	Polyarthralgias
Subcutaneous nodules	Reversible prolongation of the PR interval
Sydenham chorea	Rapid erythrocyte sedimentation rate
Arthritis	Elevated C-reactive protein
	History of rheumatic fever

(b) Jones criteria for ARF diagnosis (Table 14-2): The presence of two major criteria or one major and two minor criteria *plus* evidence of recent β-hemolytic streptococci (culture or antistreptolysin O titer) makes the diagnosis.

(c) Complications of ARF

   i. Congestive heart failure, rheumatic pneumonitis, and rheumatic heart disease (RHD) are possible complications. RHD most commonly results in valvular defects, but may also cause arrhythmias, pericarditis, or effusions.

   ii. The 2007 American Heart Association Revised Guidelines no longer recommend prophylactic antibiotics before invasive procedures to prevent endocarditis in patients with a history of RHD.

   iii. Prophylaxis is recommended if a patient has a prosthetic cardiac valve, previous endocarditis, or specific forms of congenital heart disease.

> Since 2007, prophylactic antibiotics are NOT recommended in patients with history of RHD.

(d) Early treatment of streptococcal infection is imperative to reduce the risk of ARF and RHD. Recurrence is common; those at high risk are given prophylactic antibiotics (penicillin, sulfadiazine, or erythromycin) during outbreaks of streptococcal pharyngitis.

(e) Patients with carditis have the poorest prognosis: 30% of patients will die within 10 years, 60% will develop detectable valvular abnormalities, and 10% will have permanent significant heart disease or cardiomyopathy.

3. Diagnostic studies

   a. The diagnosis of streptococcal infection is established by a combination of clinical manifestations, rapid reagent tests, and identification of the bacteria through Gram staining or culture.

   b. The Centor criteria will aid in proper diagnosis of streptococcal pharyngitis.

   (1) There are four possible criteria: tonsillar exudates, the absence of a cough, tender anterior lymphadenopathy, and history of fever. The modified Centor scores add an extra point for the patient younger than 15 years and subtract a point for the patient older than 45 years.

   (2) The presence of three of the four criteria suggests a 40% to 60% chance that the sore throat is caused by group A β-hemolytic *Streptococcus*. Further consideration or testing is warranted in patients with a score <3.

   c. An elevated WBC count, erythrocyte sedimentation rate, and other markers of infection may be found in severe infections or sepsis.

4. Treatment

   a. For the most part, group A β-hemolytic streptococci remain susceptible to penicillins; cephalosporins are also effective.

   b. For patients who are allergic to penicillins, macrolides are recommended.

   c. Supportive care (i.e., fluids, analgesics, antipyretics) should be encouraged as needed.

> First-line medication for streptococcal infections is penicillin.

B. Botulism

1. General characteristics

    a. *Clostridium botulinum*, a strictly anaerobic, spore-forming bacillus found in the soil, may inadvertently be packed in food (home-canned, smoked, or commercial), where toxin is produced and stored until ingested. Botulinum toxin inhibits the release of acetylcholine at the neuromuscular junction.

    b. Infant and wound botulism result from exposure to the bacteria or spores and elaboration of the toxin in vivo. Injection drug users are at an increased risk of wound botulism. Infants should not be fed honey because of the increased risk of botulism.

2. Clinical findings

> Patient with botulism remain awake and aware even as paralysis sets in.

    a. The initial clinical symptom is visual changes, including diplopia and loss of accommodation. Manifestations typically appear 12 to 36 hours after ingestion. Infants display irritability and opisthotonus.

    b. Additional manifestations include ptosis, impaired extraocular muscle movements, and fixed, dilated pupils. Other manifestations include cranial nerve palsies, dysphonia, dry mouth, dysphagia, nausea, and vomiting.

    c. Mental status changes or sensory deficits do not occur.

    d. Respiratory paralysis ensues and, unless mechanical assistance is provided, death results.

3. Diagnostic studies: The toxin can be identified using specific antiserum after mouse inoculation with the patient's serum.

4. Treatment

    a. Botulinum antitoxin is available through the Centers for Disease Control and Prevention (CDC); the CDC will also assist with obtaining assays of serum, stool, or suspect food.

    b. Respiratory failure necessitates intubation and mechanical ventilation. If dysphagia persists, IV nutritional support and hyperalimentation are required.

C. Anthrax

1. General characteristics

    a. *Bacillus anthracis* is a spore-forming, Gram-positive aerobic rod found in sheep, cattle, horses, goats, and swine.

    b. It is transmitted to humans either via inoculation of broken skin or mucous membranes or via inhalation. Farmers, veterinarians, and tannery and wool workers are at high risk.

    c. The organism is a likely candidate for biological warfare.

2. Clinical findings

> The most common form of anthrax is cutaneous; about 5% to 10% will experience hematogenous spread.

    a. Dermatologic (most common form)

        (1) Approximately 2 weeks after exposure to spores, anthrax causes an erythematous papule at the site of inoculation that becomes vesicular with a purple-to-black center, which, in turn, ulcerates, becomes necrotic (eschar), and eventually sloughs. The surrounding skin is edematous and vesicular. The lesion is painless unless secondarily infected with staphylococci or streptococci.

        (2) Regional adenopathy, fever, malaise, headache, and nausea and vomiting may occur. The infection is usually self-limited.

        (3) Hematogenous spread may result in sepsis and hemorrhagic meningitis. This can occur anywhere between 10 days and 6 weeks after exposure.

        (4) Case fatality rate is <1%.

b. Pulmonary

(1) About 1 to 7 days after exposure, a prodrome of fever, malaise, headache, dyspnea, cough, and congestion of the nose, throat, and larynx develops.

(2) Hours to days later, a fulminating hemorrhagic pneumonia or mediastinitis may occur. It is fatal unless antibiotics are begun in the prodromal phase.

c. Gastrointestinal

(1) Ingestion of contaminated meat may lead to fever, diffuse abdominal pain, rebound tenderness, vomiting, and change in bowel habits, which may range from bloody diarrhea to constipation. Ulcerations may lead to hemorrhage, bowel perforation, dysphagia, or obstruction.

(2) Although less common, an overwhelming sepsis may develop, causing delirium, obtundation, meningeal irritation, and hemorrhagic meningitis.

(a) GI anthrax and its complications are very rare in the United States. Case fatality ranges from 4% to 60%.

d. Meningitis may develop after any form of anthrax. Cerebrospinal fluid (CSF) will be grossly bloody with elevated protein and low glucose. Delirium, coma, and death are common. Survival is estimated at 6%.

3. Diagnostic studies

a. Skin lesions yield Gram-positive, encapsulated, box-shaped rods in chains; sputum, blood, CSF, or skin lesion cultures are positive for *B. anthracis*.

b. Chest radiography in cases of inhalation anthrax will classically reveal mediastinal widening secondary to hemorrhagic lymphadenitis. Other manifestations include hilar abnormalities, pulmonary infiltrates or consolidations, and pleural effusions.

c. Any suspected case of anthrax should be reported to the CDC, where immunohistologic testing or polymerase chain reaction (PCR) will be done to confirm.

4. Treatment

a. A combination antibiotic therapy is recommended for inhalation anthrax or disseminated disease or cutaneous infection that involves the head or neck.

b. Ciprofloxacin or another fluoroquinolone is the treatment of choice; meropenem and linezolid are recommended concurrently in severe infection. Antitoxin is also required along with supportive care.

c. An attenuated vaccine is available for persons with a high likelihood of exposure (e.g., laboratory workers, military personnel).

d. Prognosis is excellent in cutaneous anthrax. Prognosis for inhalation or GI anthrax is poor (85% mortality), despite treatment; results are best if treatment is begun early.

D. Cholera

1. General characteristics

a. *Vibrio cholerae* produces a toxin that activates adenylyl cyclase in intestinal epithelial cells of the small intestine. This results in hypersecretion of water and chloride ion and massive diarrhea. Death results from hypovolemia.

b. Epidemics of cholera occur in times of war, overcrowding, natural disasters, and famine, and where sanitation is inadequate. Infection results from ingestion of contaminated food or water.

2. Clinical findings: A sudden onset of severe, frequent, "rice water" diarrhea (gray, turbid, and without odor, blood, or pus); dehydration; hypotension; and electrolyte imbalance develop rapidly.

3. Diagnostic studies: Diagnosis is clinical. Stool cultures will be positive for *V. cholerae*; serum agglutination tests are available.

> Anthrax can infect skin, pulmonary or gastrointestinal systems.

> Ciprofloxacin is treatment of choice against anthrax; antitoxin is also required.

> 💡 The mortality associated with cholera is owing to dehydration, not to the infection.

4. Treatment

a. Replacement of fluids and electrolytes is essential. Oral rehydration with water containing salt and sugar is adequate for mild or moderate cases (1/2 tsp salt, 6 tsp sugar, 1 L water). Oral replacement packets are commercially available to be mixed with clean water. Severe cases require IV hydration.

b. Antibiotics will shorten the duration and reduce the severity of symptoms, but rehydration is vital to survival. Antibiotics should be reserved for the severely ill or those with serious comorbidities.

c. Tetracycline, ampicillin, chloramphenicol, trimethoprim–sulfamethoxazole (TMP-SMX), and fluoroquinolones are effective. Resistance exists, so susceptibility testing is encouraged.

d. The key to prevention is clean water and food sources as well as proper waste disposal. A vaccine is available, but protection is temporary, with boosters needed every 6 months.

E. Tetanus

1. General characteristics

> 💡 Tetanus: tingling, pain, spasticity, hyperreflexia, muscle spasms, seizures, asphyxia.

a. *Clostridium tetani* spores are ubiquitous in soil. The spores germinate in wounds where the bacteria produce a neurotoxin (tetanospasmin), which interferes with neurotransmission at the spinal synapses of inhibitory neurons. The result is uncontrolled spasm and exaggerated reflexes.

b. Puncture wounds are most susceptible. The elderly, migrant workers, newborns, and injection drug users are at a particular risk. The incubation period is from 5 days to 15 weeks.

2. Clinical findings

a. Pain and tingling at the site of inoculation is followed by spasticity of the muscles nearby.

b. Jaw and neck stiffness, dysphagia, and irritability are classic. Hyperreflexia and muscle spasms develop, especially in the jaw (trismus) and face.

c. Painful tonic convulsions, spasm of the glottis and respiratory muscles, and asphyxia develop if the patient is untreated.

d. The patient is typically alert throughout the course.

3. Treatment

a. Tetanus immunoglobulin should be given intramuscularly (IM). A full course of tetanus toxoid should be administered as the patient recovers.

b. Bed rest, sedation, and mechanical ventilation are often necessary to control tetanic spasms.

c. Penicillin is given to all patients to eradicate toxin-producing organisms. The mortality is high.

d. Active immunization is recommended starting in childhood. Three to four initial doses are followed by boosters every 10 years. An additional booster is recommended if a major "dirty" injury occurs and it has been >5 years since the last booster.

e. Passive immunization with tetanus toxoid in addition to vaccine is recommended for patients with major contaminated wounds and uncertain tetanus status.

F. Salmonellosis

1. General characteristics: There are >2,000 serotypes of *Salmonellae*, all of which are members of the species *Salmonella enterica* and are transmitted by ingestion of contaminated food or water.

2. Clinical features: Three patterns are recognized.

a. Enteric fever (typhoid fever)

(1) The incubation period is 5 to 14 days. Organisms enter the mucosal epithelium of the intestines and invade and replicate within macrophages in Peyer's patches, mesenteric lymph nodes, and the spleen; bacteremia accompanies infection.

(2) The onset is insidious, with a prodrome of malaise, headache, cough, and sore throat. Abdominal pain, distention, and constipation and/or diarrhea ("pea-soup") develop as the fever increases. The fever reaches a peak on days 7 to 10; the patient appears toxic and then generally improves over the next 7 to 10 days. Relapses are common (15% of cases). Children often have an abrupt onset.

(3) Physical findings include splenomegaly, abdominal distention and tenderness, and bradycardia. A rash develops during the second week; it appears as pink papules, primarily on the trunk, which fade when pressure is applied.

(4) The organism can be isolated from the blood during the first week of the illness; later, the blood cultures will likely be negative. Stool culture is not reliable.

(5) Complications occur in 30% of the untreated cases. Intestinal hemorrhage can be fatal. Other complications include urinary retention, pneumonia, thrombophlebitis, myocarditis, psychosis, cholecystitis, nephritis, osteomyelitis, and meningitis.

(6) Treatment: Resistance to ampicillin, chloramphenicol, and TMP-SMX is increasing. Resistant strains may be susceptible to ceftriaxone or fluoroquinolones (contraindicated in children and pregnancy). Treatment should be given for 2 weeks.

(7) Prevention: Treatment of carriers is often not effective. Immunization may be provided for household contacts of carriers, travelers to endemic areas, or during epidemics, but it is not very effective. Protection of the food and water supplies as well as proper waste disposal is key to control of the disease.

b. Gastroenteritis

(1) This is the most common form of *Salmonella* infection. The incubation period is 8 to 48 hours after ingestion of contaminated food or drink. Fever, nausea and vomiting, crampy abdominal pain, and bloody diarrhea last for 3 to 5 days. Diagnosis is made through stool culture.

(2) Illness is self-limited, and treatment is symptomatic. Specific treatment with TMP-SMX, ampicillin, or ciprofloxacin is required for severely ill or malnourished patients with sickle cell disease or patients who develop bacteremia.

c. Bacteremia

(1) This is characterized by prolonged or recurrent fevers, with bacteremia and local infection in the bone, joints, pleura, pericardium, lungs, or other sites.

(2) It is most common in immunosuppressed persons.

(3) Blood cultures confirm the diagnosis.

(4) Treatment is fluoroquinolone; carbapenems or azithromycin is used in resistant cases. Abscesses should be drained.

(5) Immunosuppressed patients may benefit from therapy with ciprofloxacin.

G. Shigellosis

1. General characteristics: *Shigella sonnei*, *Shigella flexneri*, and *Shigella dysenteriae* are the most common species that cause dysentery. Transmission is fecal–oral route.

2. Clinical findings

a. Illness starts abruptly with diarrhea, lower abdominal cramps, and tenesmus, accompanied by fever, chills, anorexia, headache, and malaise.

b. Stools are loose and mixed with blood and mucus. Abdomen is tender; dehydration is common.

> Enteric feature is characterized by "pea-soup" diarrhea.

> The incubation period for *Salmonella* gastroenteritis is 8 to 48 hours; manifests with fever, cramping, and bloody diarrhea.

   c. HLA-B27 individuals may mount a reactive arthritis (spondyloarthropathy) because of temporary disaccharidase deficiency.

   3. Diagnostic studies

   a. The stool is positive for leukocytes and red blood cells; a culture yields *Shigella* spp.

   b. Sigmoidoscopy reveals inflamed engorged mucosa, punctate lesions, or ulcers.

   4. Treatment

   a. Replacement of fluid volume is essential.

   b. Antibiotics: Ciprofloxacin is the antibiotic of choice, although another fluoroquinolone may be substituted; amoxicillin is not effective. Susceptibility testing is recommended in light of resistance.

   c. Empiric treatment with a fluoroquinolone is recommended in the severely ill, elderly, malnourished, human immunodeficiency virus (HIV) positive, food handlers, health care workers, and day-care workers.

H. Diphtheria

   1. General characteristics

   a. *Corynebacterium diphtheriae* is transmitted via respiratory secretions. The organism has a propensity for mucous membranes, especially the respiratory tract.

   b. It produces an exotoxin that causes myocarditis and neuropathy.

   2. Clinical findings

   a. Nasal infection produces few symptoms other than nasal discharge.

   b. Laryngeal infection causes upper airway and bronchial obstruction.

   c. Pharyngeal infection is the most common form. A tenacious gray membrane covers the tonsils and pharynx, and patients complain of mild sore throat, fever, and malaise.

   d. Myocarditis and neuropathy involving the cranial nerves may develop; untreated cases exhibit toxemia and prostration.

   3. Diagnosis is clinical; a culture confirms it.

   4. Treatment

   a. A horse serum antitoxin must be administered in all cases of diphtheria. It is obtained from the CDC.

   b. Airway obstruction may necessitate the removal of the membrane via laryngoscopy.

   c. Penicillin or erythromycin is effective. Azithromycin or clarithromycin is an effective alternative.

   d. Patients should be isolated until three negative pharyngeal cultures are documented.

   e. Contacts should be treated with erythromycin to eradicate carrier states.

   5. Diphtheria toxoid is available as a vaccine (diphtheria, tetanus, and acellular pertussis [DTaP]; tetanus and diphtheria toxoid [Td]). Unimmunized persons who are exposed to diphtheria should receive active immunization and antibiotic therapy.

I. Pertussis

   1. General characteristics

   a. *Bordetella pertussis* is a Gram-negative pleomorphic bacillus. Humans are the sole reservoir.

   b. Since the advent of immunization, the United States has seen 99% reduction in cases; however, pertussis remains a disease of importance globally. Vaccination is not lifelong. Sporadic outbreaks in American adults have been reported.

   c. Infection is highest in premature infants and in those with cardiac, pulmonary, or neuromuscular disorders.

   d. Older children and adults tend to have milder disease.

> Characteristic gray pharyngitis with fever and malaise is most common presentation of diphtheria.

2. Clinical findings

   a. Clinical manifestations occur in three stages:

   (1) The catarrhal stage: insidious onset of sneezing, coryza, loss of appetite, and malaise along with a hacking cough most prominent at night. This stage is often misdiagnosed as an upper respiratory viral illness. This is the most infectious stage.

   (2) The paroxysmal stage: spasms of rapid coughing fits followed by deep, high-pitched inspiration (the whoop). Paroxysms may last several minutes. Infants are at risk for apnea.

   (3) The convalescent stage: decrease in frequency and severity of paroxysms; this stage begins usually 4 weeks after the onset of the cough and may last for an additional several weeks.

   b. Adults are often misdiagnosed; any cough persisting for >2 weeks with no other cause should be questioned.

   c. Physical examination is generally unremarkable. Fever is rare.

3. Diagnostic studies

   a. Diagnosis is made by a culture using a special media.

   b. PCR assays may be available through some health departments.

   c. WBC count is usually mildly elevated; a lymphocytosis is characteristic.

4. Treatment

   a. A macrolide (azithromycin, clarithromycin) is the medication of choice. Treatment is aimed at stopping transmission, although it may also aid in reducing the severity of paroxysms. An alternative therapy is TMP-SMX.

   b. A supportive therapy is essential.

   c. Close contacts should also be treated with a macrolide.

5. Prevention

   a. Acellular pertussis vaccine is recommended, beginning in infancy. It is given in combination with diphtheria and tetanus toxoids.

   b. Booster vaccination of adults is now recommended. Tdap (tetanus toxoid, reduced diphtheria toxoid, and acellular pertussis) is the vaccine of choice.

> Pertussis moves through three stages: catarrhal, paroxysmal (whoop), and convalescent.

Viral Infections

A. Epstein–Barr virus (EBV)

1. General characteristics

   a. EBV is a human herpes virus 4, a universal virus transmitted via saliva.

   b. The most characteristic disease is mononucleosis (the "kissing disease"). EBV has also been implicated in Burkitt's lymphoma, nasopharyngeal carcinoma, pediatric leiomyomas, collagen vascular diseases, and other disorders.

2. Clinical findings

   a. After an incubation period of several weeks, patients develop fever and sore throat. Oral lesions include exudative pharyngitis, tonsillitis, gingivitis, and soft palate petechiae. Severe infections also exhibit malaise, anorexia, and myalgias.

   b. Lymph nodes, typically the posterior cervical nodes, are enlarged, discrete, and nonsuppurative, with minimal pain.

   c. Splenomegaly is present in 50% of cases.

   d. A maculopapular and, occasionally, petechial rash develops in 15% of cases; administration of amoxicillin raises the incidence of rash to 90%.

> Sore throat with posterior cervical lymphadenopathy suggests EBV.

    e. Less common manifestations are hepatitis, mononeuropathy, aseptic meningitis, myositis, gallbladder disease, renal failure secondary to interstitial nephritis, and dyspnea and cough ("pseudocroup").

    f. Complications are many; the most common include secondary bacterial pharyngitis (most commonly strep), splenic rupture, pericarditis, myocarditis, aseptic meningitis, transverse myelitis, and encephalitis.

3. Diagnostic studies

    a. An early granulocytopenia is followed by a lymphocytic leukocytosis. Atypical lymphocytes appear as larger cells that stain darker and are frequently vacuolated.

    b. Hemolytic anemia and thrombocytopenia may develop.

    c. Heterophile antibodies and screening mononucleosis tests are usually positive within 4 weeks. A false-positive syphilis test (Venereal Disease Research Laboratory [VDRL] or rapid plasma reagent [RPR]) occurs in 10% of infected patients.

    d. Increased hepatic aminotransferases, increased bilirubin, and decreased cryoglobulins also may be found.

4. Treatment

    a. Treatment is symptomatic, with nonaspirin antipyretics and anti-inflammatories. Antivirals decrease viral shedding, but do not affect the course of the illness.

    b. Patients with splenomegaly should avoid contact sports.

    c. Steroids are indicated for thrombocytopenia, hemolytic anemia, or airway obstruction secondary to enlarged lymph nodes.

    d. Prognosis is good. Although full recovery may take months, 95% recover without specific treatment.

B. Human papillomavirus (HPV)

1. General characteristics

    a. HPV is a group of nonenveloped icosahedral virions. There are 77 known types based on DNA sequence.

    b. HPV invades the cutaneous and mucosal epithelium, proliferates, and causes warts. The local growths commonly regress, but the virus persists, and lesions frequently recur.

    c. Subtypes of HPV are strongly correlated with cancers of the mouth and genitalia.

2. Clinical findings

    a. Common skin warts are ubiquitous and most commonly occur in children and young adults.

        (1) Most are caused by HPV types 1 to 4 and are typically asymptomatic.

        (2) Hands and feet are most commonly affected. Plantar warts may cause pain with pressure.

        (3) Warts vary in size, shape, and appearance; they may be flat and superficial or plantar and deep.

    b. Laryngeal warts are caused by serotype 11.

        (1) They are the most common benign epithelial tumors of the larynx.

        (2) In children, they may be life-threatening if they obstruct the airway and must be removed surgically.

    c. Anogenital warts (condyloma acuminata) occur in the squamous epithelium of the external genitalia and perianal area.

        (1) They are most commonly caused by HPV types 6 and 11 and are sexually transmitted. Condoms reduce the transmission of the virus.

        (2) They rarely turn cancerous, unless the patient is immunosuppressed.

EBV is a common cause of false-positive syphilis testing.

HPV types: 1 to 4, benign warts; 6 and 11, anogenital warts; 16 and 18, cervical neoplasia.

d. Cervical warts are found in 5% of females and may be visible only by colposcopy. (See Chapter 7 for more on cervical dysplasia and screening.)

(1) Between 40% and 70% will regress with time.

(2) HPV types 16, 18, and others have been implicated in intraepithelial cervical dysplasia, neoplasia, and invasive carcinoma.

(3) A vaccine against HPV types 6, 11, 16, and 18 is available. The vaccine is given as a series of three shots. It is recommended for males and females ages 11 to 12 years and approved for ages 9 through 26 years. It is effective against the four most common disease-causing HPV.

> HPV vaccine has reduced cervical cancer by approximately 85%.

3. Diagnostic studies

a. The diagnosis is established by histologic sampling. Hyperplastic prickle cells with excess keratin are found in skin warts. Koilocytotic or vacuolated squamous epithelial cells in clumps on a Pap smear are typical of cervical warts.

b. Molecular probes have been developed to detect HPV DNA in cervical swabs.

4. Treatment

a. Spontaneous remission in months to years is typical of skin warts.

b. The goal of treatment is to reduce the number and frequency of lesions, especially in immunocompromised hosts.

c. Persistent lesions or cosmetically bothersome lesions may be treated medically or surgically.

(1) Medical options include liquid nitrogen, salicylic acid, podophyllum, or topical interferon (imiquimod).

(2) Surgical options include blunt dissection, electrocautery, or carbon dioxide laser.

d. Recurrence is common.

C. Herpes simplex virus (HSV)

1. General characteristics

a. Humans are the only reservoir of HSV. Transmission is either via close contact and inoculation of virus into the mucosal surface or through cracks in the skin. The virus is inactivated at room temperature or by drying.

b. HSV type 1

(1) More than 85% of the US population has evidence of infection with HSV-1. Transmission is via infected saliva.

(2) Primary infection can be asymptomatic or produce severe disease.

(3) Recurrent, self-limited attacks are common.

c. HSV type 2

(1) About 25% of the US population is infected with HSV-2. Transmission is via sexual contact or from the mother's genital tract during delivery.

(2) This virus typically causes genital lesions (vulva, vagina, cervix, glans, prepuce, and penile shaft).

(3) Asymptomatic shedding and painful eruptions can be frequent.

> HSV-1 commonly presents as gingivostomatitis, and HSV-2 predominantly manifests in genital lesions.

d. HSV remains latent within the dorsal root ganglia (HSV-1 has a predilection for the trigeminal nerve and HSV-2 for the sacral root ganglia). Reactivation may be precipitated by fever, stress, menses, trauma, ultraviolet light, weight gain or loss, immunosuppression, or other factors. Reactivation is more frequent and more severe in patients who are immunocompromised.

2. Clinical findings

a. Initial infection has a higher rate of systemic signs, longer duration of herpetic symptoms, and a higher rate of complications.

(1) Acute herpetic gingivostomatitis (HSV-1)

    (a) This typically occurs in individuals from 6 months to 5 years of age.

    (b) The incubation period is 3 to 6 days; acute symptoms last for 5 to 7 days. Lesions heal in about 2 weeks, although shedding may continue.

    (c) Patients present with abrupt onset, fever, anorexia, listlessness, and gingivitis. Mucosa is red, swollen, and friable. Vesicles appear on the oral mucosa, tongue, and lips; these vesicles may rupture and coalesce to form ulcers and plaques. Regional lymphadenopathy is common.

(2) Acute herpetic pharyngotonsillitis

    (a) This is common in adults manifesting initial HSV-1 disease and less common in those manifesting HSV-2 disease.

    (b) Patients present with fever, malaise, headache, and sore throat. Vesicles are formed on the posterior pharynx and tonsils; these vesicles rupture and form shallow ulcers. A grayish exudate may be present over the posterior mucosa.

3. Primary genital herpes (invariably HSV-2)

    a. The initial episode may be asymptomatic or severe, with a prodrome of systemic and local symptoms.

    b. Preexisting antibodies to HSV-1 may have an ameliorating effect on the severity of primary HSV-2 infection.

    c. Fever, headache, malaise, and myalgias are common. Vesicles develop on the external genitalia, labia, vaginal mucosa, glans, penis, prepuce, shaft, or perianal area. Adjoining cutaneous lesions may also occur.

    d. Vesicles rupture and form tender ulcers, which crust over. Mucosa may be red and edematous.

    e. Females tend to have more severe disease and higher rates of complications. The cervix is involved in >70% of female patients, manifesting as ulcerative or necrotic mucosa.

> *Recurrent HSV typically starts with paresthesias before the outbreak.*

4. Recurrence of HSV lesions is heralded by burning or stinging. Neuralgia may also occur, but constitutional symptoms are less likely.

    a. Lesions begin as erythematous papules that rapidly develop into tiny, thin-walled, grouped vesicles, which continue to erupt over 1 to 2 weeks.

    b. Typical locations are the vermillion border (type 1) and the genital area, including the penile shaft, labia, perianal area, and buttocks (type 2).

    c. On an average, HSV-1 infections tend to recur twice per year; maximum shedding is during the first 24 hours of each outbreak. The number of episodes tends to decrease with time.

    d. In 90% of the cases, HSV-2 will reactivate within 12 months. More than 30% of patients have 6 episodes per year, and about 20% have >10 episodes per year. Reactivation can be subclinical; however, viral shedding without visible lesions leads to further transmission of the virus.

5. Complications of HSV infection

    a. Complications include pyoderma, eczema herpeticum, herpetic whitlow (grouped vesicles on the fingers; common in health care workers), herpes gladiatorum (disseminated cutaneous infections; common in wrestlers), esophagitis, keratoconjunctivitis (dendritic corneal ulcers; may cause blindness), and disseminated neonatal infection. Viremia may result in visceral infection with multiple organ involvement, leukopenia, thrombocytopenia, and disseminated intravascular coagulation.

    b. Herpes simplex infection of the central nervous system (CNS) may cause aseptic meningitis, ganglionitis, myelitis, or encephalitis. HSV accounts for 10% to 20% of all encephalitis cases in the United States. Patients develop headache, meningeal irritation, change in mental status, seizures, and focal necrosis syndromes (temporal cortex, limbic system). CSF shows a moderate pleocytosis of mixed cells, mildly elevated protein, and normal glucose. HSV DNA by PCR or MRI confirms an infection. The mortality rate is >70% without treatment; neurologic sequelae are typical even with treatment.

   c. Genital herpes in pregnancy is dangerous to both the mother and the infant. First infection during pregnancy has a high risk of disseminated infection and maternal mortality. Infants exposed to herpes in utero or during delivery have a high rate of visceral and CNS infection. Mortality and sequelae rates are high. Cesarean section is recommended for women with active infection.

6. Diagnostic studies

   a. The diagnosis is usually established clinically, and can be aided by PCR testing of a swab from an ulcer.

   b. Vesicular fluid may be cultured (definitive) or stained (Tzanck smear, immunofluorescence staining), revealing multinucleated giant cells.

   c. Antibodies can be identified in the serum by PCR techniques.

7. Treatment

   a. Local wound care and supportive therapy are recommended.

   b. Treatment is with antivirals (e.g., acyclovir, valacyclovir).

   c. Patients with frequent outbreaks may benefit from suppressive antiviral therapy. Foscarnet is beneficial in immunocompromised patients with resistant infections.

   d. Keratitis is treated with trifluridine.

> Frequent outbreaks of HSV warrant suppressive therapy with acyclovir.

D. Influenza

1. General characteristics

   a. Influenza is caused by an orthomyxovirus. It is readily transmitted through droplet nuclei and occurs in epidemics and pandemics during the fall or winter.

   b. Three strains exist (A, B, and C) and are typed based on the surface antigens hemagglutinin (H) and neuraminidase (N). Influenza A is more pathogenic. Major mutations cause antigenic shifts; minor mutations cause antigenic drifts.

   c. An avian influenza A subtype (H5N1) has caused epidemic infection in birds and has been transmitted from birds to humans. If a mutation occurs to allow human-to-human transmission, this highly virulent and lethal subtype could become responsible for widespread disease.

   d. Public health authorities follow changes in strains to predict new virus and steer vaccine development and monitor outbreaks of influenza and are responsible for alerting the public about emerging influenza strains.

2. Clinical findings

   a. After an incubation period of 18 to 72 hours, patients exhibit an abrupt fever, chills, malaise, muscle aches, substernal chest pain, headache, nasal stuffiness, and, occasionally, nausea. The fever lasts for 1 to 7 days and is accompanied by coryza, nonproductive cough, photophobia, eye pain, sore throat, pharyngeal injection, and flushed faces. Wheezes and rhonchi may be heard, and children often develop diarrhea.

   b. Primary influenza pneumonia may develop in the elderly or those with chronic cardiovascular disease. Patients exhibit progressive cough, dyspnea, and cyanosis.

   c. Complications are especially common in the extremes of age and the chronically ill. Necrosis of respiratory epithelium can result in secondary bacterial infection (*Staphylococcus*, *Streptococcus*, or *Haemophilus* spp.), acute sinusitis, otitis media, and purulent bronchitis.

   d. Reye's syndrome

   (1) Reye's syndrome is defined as a fatty liver with encephalopathy.

> Classic flu symptoms include fever, chills, malaise, aches, cough, and coryza.

(2) It is rapidly progressive, has a 30% fatality rate, and may develop 2 to 3 weeks after the onset of influenza A or varicella infection, especially if aspirin is ingested. The peak age is 5 to 14 years; it rarely occurs in patients older than 18 years.

(3) Clinical manifestations include vomiting, lethargy, jaundice, seizures, hypoglycemia, increased liver enzymes and ammonia levels, prolonged prothrombin time, and changes in mental status.

(4) Treatment is supportive.

3. Diagnostic studies

a. During outbreaks, diagnosis of influenza can be clinical.

b. Leukopenia and proteinuria may be present.

> Rapid molecular assays have high sensitivity and specificity; rapid antigen detection tests have low sensitivity.

c. The virus can be isolated from the throat or nasal mucosa. Viral culture takes 2 to 5 days to return and is not useful for clinical diagnosis. Direct immunofluorescence tests are labor intensive and less sensitive, but recently developed rapid antigen tests are proving to be helpful. Sensitivities range from 50% to 70%; specificities 90% to 95%. Results are most accurate during the first few days of illness.

d. Chest radiography in primary influenza pneumonia typically shows bilateral diffuse infiltrates.

4. Treatment

a. All patients require supportive care with rest, analgesics, and cough suppressants as needed. Isolation will reduce spread.

b. Amantadine and rimantadine are not recommended as single therapy agents because of resistance.

c. Neuraminidase inhibitors (zanamivir inhalation [Relenza] or oral oseltamivir [Tamiflu]) significantly reduce severity if administered within 48 hours of the onset of symptoms. They are effective against both influenza A and influenza B. They are recommended for patients with influenza requiring hospitalization or in patients with high risk of morbidity and mortality.

(1) Patients with uncomplicated disease and at low risk of complications can be treated with oseltamivir, inhaled zanamivir, IV peramivir, or oral baloxavir. Local surveillance monitoring provides a direction for the choice of therapy.

> For influenza management: the annual vaccine is crucial, and for those infected, supportive care is standard with neuraminidase inhibitors as an adjunct early in course of illness.

(2) Neuraminidase inhibitors are contraindicated in patients younger than 12 years. Emergency use with half strength dosing may also be effective in preventing influenza during times of high transmission.

d. Prognosis in uncomplicated cases is very good; patients generally recover in 1 to 7 days. Morbidity and mortality are highest in the very young and the very old. Pneumonia is the cause of most influenza fatalities.

5. Prevention of influenza is through a trivalent influenza virus vaccine.

a. Its configuration is based on the strains isolated during the preceding year. The vaccine should be administered to all the patients yearly in October or November and is especially recommended for all people older than 65 years (some sources suggest all people older than 50 years), children or adolescents on chronic aspirin therapy, nursing home residents, patients with chronic lung or heart disease, and all health care workers.

b. The vaccine is contraindicated in patients with hypersensitivity to eggs or other components of the vaccine, during acute febrile illness, or in cases of thrombocytopenia.

c. Tenderness, redness, and induration at the injection site may occur; myalgias and fever are rare.

d. A nasal spray (FluMist) has been effective in some years. For several years, it was not recommended by the CDC but is now recommended for patients aged 2 to 49 years. It is not recommended in pregnancy or immunocompromised states.

   e. Immunity is set within 2 weeks of the vaccination. Antibodies wane quickly in the elderly and the sick, but the vaccine has been proven to decrease mortality and morbidity from the flu.

   f. Fluzone is a high-dose quadrivalent flu vaccine recommended for patients aged 65 years and older. It has four times the antigen load; it is slightly more effective but with higher frequency of side effects.

E. **Varicella-zoster virus (VZV)**

  1. General characteristics: VZV is a highly contagious member of the herpesvirus family.

   a. Primary infection

    (1) Varicella (or chickenpox) is the primary infection with VZV. Most cases occur in late winter or spring.

    (2) The incubation period is 10 to 20 days; patients are most contagious 1 day before the rash appears. A single attack confers lifelong immunity.

    (3) It is typically a benign illness in childhood, but some cases may be life-threatening, especially in adults or immunocompromised patients.

   b. Reactivation

    (1) Zoster (or shingles) refers to reactivation of varicella virus that has been dormant in ganglionic satellite cells.

    (2) A zoster outbreak may be precipitated by illness, stress, or advancing age.

> Zoster/shingles is commonly precipitated by illness, stress, and advancing age.

  2. **Clinical findings**

   a. Varicella is characterized by a generalized pruritic eruption that follows a centripetal pattern.

    (1) Lesions begin as erythematous macules and papules, form superficial vesicles ("dewdrop on rose petal"), and later crust over.

    (2) Lesions appear in "crops," so at any given time, several morphologies can be identified.

    (3) The mucous membranes may also be involved.

   b. Systemic symptoms are highly variable and include low-grade fever, malaise, myalgias, arthralgias, and headache. Severe, progressive infections manifest with deeper lesions of the lung, liver, pancreas, or brain; the mortality rate approaches 10%.

   c. Complications are varied, including secondary bacterial infection of excoriated lesions, varicella embryopathy, and Reye's syndrome.

   d. Zoster is characterized by a painful eruption, usually following a dermatomal pattern. The thoracic and lumbar areas are the most common sites. Trigeminal eruptions that include the tip of the nose (Hutchinson's sign) risk corneal involvement.

> Zoster outbreaks may cross into adjacent dermatomes but never cross the midline.

  3. Diagnostic studies

   a. The diagnosis is established clinically.

   b. Confirmatory laboratory studies are rarely performed, but, if necessary, serology and fluorescent microscopy confirm the diagnosis.

  4. **Treatment**

   a. Treatment is generally supportive.

   b. Prevention

    (1) Prevention of bacterial superinfection involves good hygiene and trimming of fingernails.

    (2) Immunocompromised patients exposed to varicella should receive acyclovir and varicella-zoster immunoglobulin.

    (3) Prevention of varicella is through a live attenuated vaccine administered at 1 to 2 years of age. Older patients without evidence of immunity should receive two doses, administered 2 months apart. Avoid giving the vaccine during pregnancy.

> Vaccines are available and effective against varicella and varicella-zoster; patients aged 50 years and older should get Shingrix, regardless of history of shingles.

(4) Anecdotal evidence suggests that steroids may prevent postherpetic neuralgia in some patients. Postherpetic neuralgia rates are higher in the elderly and in patients with trigeminal lesions and can be quite debilitating. Treatment is difficult; choices include tricyclic antidepressants, capsaicin cream, narcotic analgesics, or corticosteroids.

(5) Shingrix is a two-dose vaccine indicated in patients aged 50 years or older. It has been shown to be effective in cutting the incidence of shingles and substantially reducing the risk of postherpetic neuralgia. It is contraindicated in patients who are allergic, are immunocompromised, have negative immunity against varicella, or are pregnant.

F. **Rabies (Rhabdoviridae family)**

1. General characteristics

   a. Rhabdovirus is transmitted via infected saliva from an animal bite or an open wound.

   b. Vectors include bats, skunks, foxes, raccoons, and coyotes; rodents and lagomorphs do not transmit rabies. Dogs rarely transmit rabies in the United States but continue to account for a substantial number of cases worldwide.

   c. Incubation period between the bite and the onset of symptoms is from 10 days to years (typically 3 to 7 weeks). A correlation exists between the period of incubation and the distance of the wound from the brain.

2. **Clinical findings**

   a. A history of an animal bite may not be apparent.

   b. Typically, there is pain and paresthesias at the site; the skin is sensitive to changes in temperature and wind.

   c. Patients are restless, with muscle spasms and extreme excitability. They exhibit bizarre behavior, convulsions, and paralysis. Thick, tenacious saliva is produced.

   d. Hydrophobia is defined as painful spasms caused by drinking water.

   e. Less commonly, patients may exhibit an ascending paralysis.

3. Diagnostic studies

   a. Suspected animals should be euthanized so that their brains can be tested for the virus using fluorescent antibody markers.

   b. Domestic animals may be quarantined and observed for bizarre behavior.

   c. PCR tests and genetic probes for use in humans are expensive and often negative early in the disease.

   d. CSF may show rabies reverse transcriptase by PCR. MRI may reveal nonenhancing, ill-defined changes in the brain stem, hypothalamus, or subcortical matter.

4. **Treatment**

> Rabies is universally fatal; prevention is key.

   a. No specific treatment against rabies disease is available. Mechanical ventilation and oxygen therapy should be started. Rabies vaccine immunoglobulin is given along with monoclonal antibodies, ribavirin, interferon-α, and ketamine. It is almost universally fatal within 7 days, most commonly from respiratory failure.

   b. Prevention is the key.

      (1) Control of bat populations is helpful in preventing the spread.

      (2) All household pets should be immunized. Persons who are exposed regularly (veterinarians, park rangers) should also receive active immunization.

   c. After an animal bite, local care with cleansing, debridement, and flushing is recommended. Wounds should not be sutured.

   d. Postexposure immunization includes rabies immunoglobulin (in the wound and IM at a distant site) and human diploid cell vaccine (HDCV). Five injections of 1 mL IM are administered on days 0, 3, 7, 14, and 28. The vaccine may cause pruritus, erythema, and tenderness in 25% of cases, and 20% also develop myalgias, headache, and nausea.

e. If the patient has received active immunization in the past, immunoglobulin is not given; HDCV doses are administered on days 0 and 3 only.

f. Preexposure vaccination of persons at high risk (veterinarians, animal handlers, missionaries to underdeveloped countries, and travelers to endemic areas) is accomplished with IM HDCV doses on days 0, 7, and either 21 or 28. HDCV also can be administered intradermally on days 0, 7, and 28. Rabies antibody titers should be checked every 2 years; boosters are administered to persons who become seronegative.

G. Human immunodeficiency virus (HIV) and acquired immunodeficiency syndrome (AIDS)

   1. General characteristics

   a. HIV was first recognized when a cluster of patients with opportunistic infections was identified in 1981. A human retrovirus that requires reverse transcriptase for replication was later identified as the cause.

   b. Currently, >40 million people worldwide are infected with the virus. The highest prevalence is in Central and East sub-Saharan Africa, where approximately one-third of all adults are infected. An estimated 5 million new cases and 3 million deaths occur per year worldwide.

   c. HIV infects all the cells containing the T4 antigen, primarily the CD4 helper inducer lymphocytes.

   (1) The result is a disordered function of the immune system.

   (2) HIV attaches to the T4 antigen, replicates, and causes cell fusion or cell death.

   (3) Macrophages serve as a reservoir of virus and promote its dissemination to other organs.

   d. HIV is transmitted through bodily fluids. Risk includes sexual contact, parenteral exposure (blood or blood products, including injection drug use and occupational exposure), and perinatal exposure.

   2. Clinical features

   a. The acute HIV syndrome is often not identified. It is a cluster of nonspecific findings similar to EBV infection. Some patients may develop persistent generalized lymphadenopathy without symptomatic HIV disease.

   b. HIV disease is a syndrome of nonspecific and specific diagnoses. It can be progressive and insidious or can be rapidly fatal. The time from infection to symptomatic disease averages 10 years but is quite variable.

   c. Systemic manifestations include fever, night sweats, and weight loss. The wasting syndrome is a result of increased metabolic rate and decreased protein synthesis. There is a disproportionate loss of muscle mass.

   d. Immunodeficiency causes various infections and malignant diseases; common sites include the lungs, upper respiratory system, lymph system, CNS, peripheral nervous system (PNS), mouth, GI tract, eyes, and skin.

   e. AIDS is defined by the CDC as a CD4 count <200 cells per μL or the development of an AIDS indicator disease (Table 14-3). A diagnosis or presumptive diagnosis of AIDS can be made with or without laboratory evidence of HIV infection.

   f. Opportunistic infections and malignancies develop as the CD4 count drops (Table 14-4). Only a few patients in the United States develop opportunistic infections or malignancies because of the success of antiretroviral therapy.

   g. The current World Health Organization (WHO) HIV/AIDS Classification System is based on symptoms: stage I, asymptomatic disease; stage II, minor symptoms; stage III, moderate symptoms; and stage IV, AIDS. In general, as the CD4 count decreases, the viral load increases, and symptoms of infections and malignancies become more frequent and more severe.

> Acute HIV syndrome can present with a nonspecific viral syndrome with nonspecific findings.

> AIDS is defined as a CD4 count less than 200.

Table 14-3 | AIDS Indicator Diseases

I. Definitive AIDS diagnoses (with or without laboratory evidence of HIV infection)

Candidiasis of esophagus, bronchi, trachea, or lungs
Cryptococcosis, extrapulmonary
Kaposi's sarcoma in a patient aged <60 years
Herpes simplex: chronic ulcer(s) (>1 month); bronchitis, pneumonitis, or esophagitis
Cryptosporidiosis, chronic intestinal (>1 month)
Lymphoma of the brain in a patient aged <60 years
CMV disease (other than liver, spleen, or nodes)
Encephalopathy, HIV related
Mycobacterium avium complex or *Mycobacterium kansasii*, disseminated or any site
Pneumocystis jirovecii (nee *carinii*) pneumonia
Progressive multifocal leukoencephalopathy
Toxoplasmosis of brain

II. Definitive AIDS diagnoses (with laboratory evidence of HIV infection)

Coccidioidomycosis, disseminated or extrapulmonary
Histoplasmosis, disseminated or extrapulmonary
Isosporiasis, chronic intestinal (>1 month)
HIV encephalopathy
Kaposi's sarcoma at any age
Lymphoma of the brain at any age
Other non-Hodgkin lymphoma of B cell or unknown immunologic phenotype
Other mycobacterial disease (other than *Mycobacterium tuberculosis*) at a site other than or in addition to the lungs, skin or cervical or hilar lymph nodes
M. tuberculosis, extrapulmonary or pulmonary
Salmonella septicemia, recurrent
HIV wasting syndrome
CD4 count <200 cell/μL *or* a CD4 lymphocyte percentage <14%
Recurrent pneumonia
Invasive cervical cancer

AIDS, acquired immunodeficiency syndrome; CMV, cytomegalovirus; HIV, human immunodeficiency virus.

Table 14-4 | HIV-Related Illnesses by Usual CD4 Count

CD4 Count	Illness
Any time; generally <500	*Salmonella*, recurrent or septicemia *Clostridium difficile* colitis Kaposi's sarcoma *Mycobacterium tuberculosis*, pulmonary, extrapulmonary, or disseminated Herpes simplex; herpes zoster Vaginal candidiasis Hairy leukoplakia
<200	*Candida*, esophagus, bronchi, trachea, lungs HIV encephalopathy; AIDS dementia syndrome *Pneumocystis jirovecii* (nee *carinii*) pneumonia
<100	B-cell lymphoma (non-Hodgkin) Toxoplasmosis *Isospora*; microsporidia Cryptococcosis Coccidioidomycosis Cryptosporidiosis
<50	Histoplasmosis Progressive multifocal leukoencephalopathy *Mycobacterium avium* complex CMV retinitis Lymphoma of the brain

AIDS, acquired immunodeficiency syndrome; CMV, cytomegalovirus; HIV, human immunodeficiency virus.

3. Diagnostic studies

a. Screening for HIV infection detects antibodies; most patients develop antibodies within 6 weeks of exposure. Rapid IIIV antibody tests using either blood or oral fluids are convenient; results are available within 20 minutes. There is also a home kit that provides privacy to the individual. If positive, the rapid test should be followed with an enzyme-linked immunosorbent assay (ELISA) tests followed by a confirmatory Western blot analysis to confirm HIV infection with a sensitivity of >95%.

(1) Persons at high risk for infection, patients in all health care settings, and all pregnant women should be tested for HIV.

(2) Testing is recommended after notifying the patient that it will be done unless the patient opts out.

(a) Written separate consent is no longer recommended by the CDC.

(b) False-positive ELISA may occur after a recent influenza vaccine or in the presence of autoimmune disease.

b. Other laboratory findings may include anemia, leukopenia, thrombocytopenia, polyclonal hypergammaglobulinemia, hypercholesterolemia, and cutaneous anergy.

c. The CD4 count typically decreases as the illness progresses, without treatment. For best accuracy, it should be measured at the same time of day and by the same laboratory. Patients with a CD4 count of >350 cells per μL can have levels measured every 6 months; otherwise, it should be measured every 3 months or with any change in the patient status. Risk of disease progression increases with a CD4 count of <200 cells per μL or CD4 lymphocyte percentage of <20%.

d. The viral load is a measure of actively replicating virus, which correlates with disease progression. Changing viral loads may also support treatment response.

> In HIV management, the CD4 count correlates with immune suppression and related infection risks; testing for viral load correlates with treatment response.

4. Treatment

a. Prevention is essential for the HIV epidemic to end. Primary prevention efforts include safer sex with barrier methods (latex only), harm reduction programs, drug rehabilitation, screening of all blood products, and universal precautions in health care delivery. Development of a vaccine against HIV has been unsuccessful.

b. Secondary prevention efforts include antiretrovirals (Table 14-5) and chemoprophylaxis. Patients should be screened for diseases such as tuberculosis and other infections, and they must be counseled on ways to maintain health and prevent the spread of the virus.

c. Postexposure prophylaxis (PEP) may be offered to individuals with a high probability of exposure, including health care workers who sustain occupational injuries. PEP should be started within 72 hours of exposure.

(1) The chance of contracting HIV from a needlestick injury involving a patient with known HIV disease is 0.3%.

(2) Health care workers who sustain an injury must be counseled. Testing should be done on the health care worker and the patient; retesting is recommended in 6 weeks, 3 months, and 6 months.

(3) Antiretroviral therapy is an option; the decision to begin therapy should be made by the patient. Combination therapy with drugs from different classes should be continued for at least 4 weeks. Full-course PEP reduces the chance of HIV transmission by up to 70%.

d. Preexposure prophylaxis (PrEP) plus counseling is offered to individuals with high risk or with an HIV(+) sexual partner.

e. Pregnant women with HIV disease should be counseled on the risk to the fetus. Antiretroviral therapy to the mother during pregnancy, labor, and delivery and to the newborn reduces the chance of transmission significantly. HIV can also be transmitted through breast milk.

Table 14-5 | Most Common Choices for Prophylaxis of Opportunistic Infections and Malignancies in Patients with HIV Disease

Opportunistic Infection	Drug(s) of Choice, Prophylaxis
Pneumocystis jirovecii pneumonia	Trimethoprim–sulfamethoxazole, pentamidine, atovaquone
Mycobacterium avium complex	Clarithromycin, rifabutin
Toxoplasmosis	Pyrimethamine
Lymphoma	Combination chemotherapy
Cryptococcal meningitis	Amphotericin B, fluconazole
Cytomegalovirus retinitis	Valganciclovir, ganciclovir, foscarnet
Esophageal candidiasis	Fluconazole
Herpes simplex	Acyclovir, famciclovir, valaciclovir, foscarnet
Herpes zoster	Acyclovir, famciclovir, valaciclovir, foscarnet
Kaposi's sarcoma	Combination chemotherapy

    f. Drug treatment of HIV disease includes antiretroviral therapy and treatment of or prophylaxis against opportunistic infections and malignancies (Table 14-6).

        (1) The patient must be counseled to understand the complexity of the treatment. Combination antiretroviral therapy is based on CD4 count, viral load, and overall patient status (nutrition, compliance, access, and acceptance of therapy). Treatment may be aggressive, complex, and toxic.

        (2) Patients should be monitored closely for adherence, effectiveness, adverse effects, and resistance.

        (3) The goal is suppression of the viral load. A rising or persistently high viral load, clinical progression, or continued immunologic deterioration signals treatment failure.

        (4) Prophylaxis against opportunistic infections and malignancies is based on the likelihood of developing disease as judged by the CD4 count and viral load. Discontinuation of prophylaxis after a sustained response to antiretroviral may be considered.

H. **Cytomegalovirus (CMV; human herpesvirus type 5)**

    1. General characteristics

        a. Most infections with CMV are asymptomatic.

        b. Illness occurs in the immunocompromised, especially patients with HIV disease or post-transplant.

    2. **Clinical findings**

        a. Perinatal infection and CMV inclusion disease occur in 10% of babies born to mothers with primary CMV infection during pregnancy.

            (1) The infant may be asymptomatic until later in life.

            (2) Clinical findings include jaundice, hepatosplenomegaly, thrombocytopenia, periventricular CNS calcifications, mental retardation, motor disability, and purpura.

        b. Acute acquired CMV can be transmitted through sexual contact, breast milk, blood transfusion, or respiratory droplets. Patients develop fever, malaise, myalgias, arthralgias, splenomegaly, abnormal liver enzymes, leukopenia, and atypical lymphocytes. It is similar to EBV infection but without pharyngitis, respiratory symptoms, or heterophil antibodies.

        c. Post-transplant patients and those who are otherwise immunocompromised are at risk for myriad clinical manifestations.

CMV can be transmitted via sexual contact, blood, or respiratory droplets, and most cases are asymptomatic.

Table 14-6 | Antiretroviral Medications

Drug Category	Drug	Common Adverse Effects
NRTIs	Zidovudine (AZT; Retrovir)	Anemia, neutropenia, nausea, malaise, headache, insomnia, myopathy
	Didanosine (ddI; Videx)	Pancreatitis, peripheral neuropathy, hepatitis
	Stavudine (d4; Zerit)	Peripheral neuropathy, hepatitis, pancreatitis
	Lamivudine (3TC; Epivir)	Peripheral neuropathy, rash
	Emtricitabine (Emtriva)	Dyspigmentation, especially palms and soles
	Abacavir (Ziagen)	Rash, fever
	Nevirapine (Viramune)	Rash
	Tenofovir (Viread)	Renal insufficiency, hepatitis, GI distress, bone resorption
NNRTIs	Delavirdine (Rescriptor)	Rash
	Efavirenz (Sustiva)	Neurologic manifestations, rash
	Etravirine	Rash, peripheral neuropathy
	Rilpivirine (Edurant)	Mood changes, depression, rash
	Saquinavir (Fortovase, Invirase)	Headache, GI dysfunction
Protease inhibitors	Tipranavir/ritonavir (Aptivus/Norvir)	Hepatitis, rash
	Darunavir/ritonavir (Prezista/Norvir)	Hepatitis, rash
	Ritonavir (Norvir)	Peripheral paresthesias, GI dysfunction
	Indinavir (Crixivan)	Renal calculi
	Nelfinavir (Viracept)	Diarrhea
	Amprenavir (Invirase)	Rash, GI dysfunction
	Lopinavir/ritonavir (Kaletra)	Diarrhea
	Fosamprenavir (Lexiva)	GI symptoms, rash
	Atazanavir (Reyataz)	Hyperbilirubinemia
	Enfuvirtide (Fuzeon)	Injection site pain, allergic reactions
Entry inhibitors	Maraviroc (Selzentry)	Rash, cough, fever
	Enfuvirtide (Fuzeon)	Injection site pain, allergic reaction
Integrase inhibitors	Raltegravir (Isentress)	Diarrhea, headache, nausea
	Dolutegravir (Tivicay)	Rash, hypersensitivities
	Elvitegravir (only in combo)	Elevated creatinine, diarrhea, rash
	Bictegravir (only in combo)	Diarrhea, nausea, headache

AZT, zidovudine, azidothymidine; GI, gastrointestinal; NNRTI, non-nucleoside reverse transcriptase inhibitor; NRTI, nucleoside/nucleotide reverse transcriptase inhibitor.

(1) Retinitis occurs with a CD4 count of <50 cells per μL. Examination reveals neovascularization and proliferative lesions, commonly referred to as "pizza pie." With aggressive treatment of HIV disease, the frequency of retinitis can be reduced.

(2) GI manifestations include esophagitis and odynophagia, small bowel inflammatory ulcers, diarrhea, hematochezia, abdominal pain, weight loss, and cholangiopathy. Diagnosis may require biopsy.

(3) Pulmonary manifestations occur in 15% of bone marrow transplant patients; 80% to 90% of these are fatal.

(4) Neurologic manifestations include polyradiculopathy, transverse myelitis, and encephalitis.

(5) CMV infection is theorized to play a role in the pathogenesis of inflammatory bowel disease, atherosclerosis, and breast cancer.

3. Diagnostic studies

a. Patients may exhibit lymphocytosis or leukopenia.

    b. Culturing is very difficult; antigens can be detected in blood, urine, or CSF via PCR.

    c. Tissue biopsy looks for intracytoplasmic inclusions ("owls' eyes").

4. Treatment

    a. Measures to prevent CMV infection include limiting blood transfusions, filtering to remove leukocytes, and restricting the organ donor pool to seronegative donors. CMV immunoglobulin and IV ganciclovir reduce the risk of pneumonia in bone marrow transplant recipients.

    b. Ganciclovir, valganciclovir, foscarnet, and cidofovir are effective against CMV.

        (1) Initial IV loading therapy is followed by maintenance therapy.

        (2) Sustained-release ganciclovir implants for suppression of retinal infections are effective.

I. Severe acute respiratory syndrome coronavirus 2 (SARS-COV-2, COVID-19)

    1. General characteristics

        a. SARS-COV-2 is a β-coronavirus that gains entry into the cell through angiotensin-converting enzyme 2 (ACE2).

        b. COVID-19 was first identified through a cluster of cases in Wuhan, China, in late 2019 and spread rapidly to pandemic status. As of spring 2021, WHO estimates over 153 million cases and 3.3 million deaths. As of Fall 2021, WHO estimates over 258 million cases and 5.1 million deaths.

    2. Clinical findings

        a. It is estimated that one-third of all infections with SARS-COV-2 are asymptomatic but are believed to be responsible for community transmission. A significant number of asymptomatic cases have evidence of lung abnormalities per CT scan.

        b. The incubation period averages 4 to 5 days but can be up to 14 days. Infected individuals can shed the virus during this time.

        c. The majority of symptomatic infections are mild.

            (1) Initial manifestations include cough, myalgias, and headache. Fever is absent in about 20% early in the illness. The illness progresses characteristically over a few days. Mild cases will last about a week and resolve.

            (2) The course of illness may progress to include fever, sore throat, loss of smell or taste, and GI symptoms, including nausea, vomiting, and diarrhea.

        d. Approximately 15% to 20% of cases are severe.

            (1) The risk of severe disease is increased with age; immunodeficiency including diabetes, obesity, smoking; and underlying cardiac, pulmonary, or renal disease.

            (2) Serious disease is typically heralded by pneumonia, which progresses rapidly to acute respiratory distress syndrome (ARDS). Patients may also exhibit thromboembolic events, acute cardiac or kidney injury, and inflammatory complications (Table 14-7).

        e. Persistent infection manifests with fatigue, dyspnea, chest pain, cough, and cognitive decline. There can be ongoing respiratory impairment and cardiac sequelae.

    3. Diagnostic studies

        a. Lymphopenia is characteristic, and severity is correlated with disease state.

        b. Elevated aminotransferases, lactic dehydrogenase, and inflammatory markers (ferritin, C-reactive protein, erythrocyte sedimentation rate) and abnormalities of coagulation are common.

        c. An elevated procalcitonin and D-dimer are seen in severe cases.

        d. Chest radiography early on is normal. With progressive disease, consolidation and ground-glass opacities are most common. Pathology tends to be bilateral and peripheral. Lung CT is more sensitive.

Initial COVID-19 symptoms can mimic other mild viral illness: cough, myalgias, sore throat, and headache.

Table 14-7 | Common Complications of SARV-COV-2 Infection

Category	Complication
Cardiac	Arrhythmias Myocardial ischemia/infarction Heart failure Cardiogenic shock
Vascular	Venous thromboembolism Deep vein thrombosis Pulmonary embolism Stroke
Neurologic	Encephalopathy Stroke Motor and sensory deficit Ataxia Seizures
Inflammatory	Persistent fever Elevated cytokines Guillain–Barré syndrome Kawasaki-like illness Toxic shock syndrome

4. Management

    a. Risk stratification is imperative, including identification of patients at the highest risk of developing severe disease and allocation of resources.

    b. Most patients can be treated conservatively, as outpatients with careful follow-up. Telehealth capability was instrumental in managing patients during the 2020 pandemic.

    c. Patients should be referred to emergency departments if they exhibit severe dyspnea, oxygen saturation <90%, or altered mental status.

    d. Infection control is paramount in both clinical settings and the community.

    e. Mild-to-moderate cases can be treated with supportive care and consideration of monoclonal antibodies, such as remdesivir. Systemic corticosteroids should not be prescribed to outpatients.

    f. Hospitalized patients are treated more aggressively and may require mechanical ventilation or extracorporeal membrane oxygenation (ECMO). Prone positioning helps improve oxygenation. Patients should receive prophylaxis against venous thrombosis. NSAIDs are recommended for fever. Monoclonal antibodies, high-titer convalescent plasma, and systemic dexamethasone are the most common approach to treatment.

    g. Population testing and public health measures including vaccination are key to control of the pandemic.

Fungal Infections

A. Candidiasis

    1. General characteristics

        a. *Candida albicans* is the most common form of pathogenic *Candida* spp. It is part of the normal flora of human hosts and is an opportunistic pathogen.

        b. Risk factors for disease include neutropenia, recent surgery, chronic illness (especially diabetes mellitus), broad-spectrum antibiotic therapy, IV catheterization (especially total parenteral nutrition), chemotherapy or corticosteroids, injection drug use, and cellular immunodeficiency, as in HIV disease.

> 💡 Candidiasis outside infancy occurs when the immune system is compromised.

2. Clinical findings and treatment

a. Cutaneous disease

(1) Diaper dermatitis commonly is caused by *Candida* spp. and does not indicate immune deficiency in newborns. The diaper area is red, with defined margins. Pustules, vesicles, papules, or scales may be seen, and satellite lesions are characteristic.

(2) Children and adults (particularly adults with diabetes) may develop candidal dermatitis in dark, moist areas, such as axillae or under the breasts or large panniculus, especially if the immune system is stressed. Lesions have distinct borders, and satellite lesions are common.

(3) Treatment is with topical antifungal creams.

b. Mucosal disease of the mouth and esophagus (also see Chapter 5)

(1) Oral mucosal candidiasis (thrush) causes white plaques that can be scraped off, revealing reddened mucosa. In denture wearers, infection may manifest as a painful red palate.

(2) Esophagitis is heralded by odynophagia and dysphagia. Symptoms often resemble gastroesophageal reflux.

(3) Treatment is with oral fluconazole, itraconazole, or amphotericin B if recurrent or recalcitrant.

> Candidal infections manifest in mucosa, skin, genital areas, and endocarditis; more serious fungemia can be fatal.

c. Vulvovaginal disease occurs in 75% of females at least once during their lifetime.

(1) Risk factors include age extremes, pregnancy, uncontrolled diabetes mellitus, antibiotic use, immunosuppression, corticosteroids, and HIV disease.

(2) Symptoms include pruritus, burning, dyspareunia, and a white, cottage cheese or curd-like discharge. Physical examination reveals white plaques on vaginal walls. Association of candidiasis with local contraceptive devices is unclear.

(3) Treatment is with topical azoles or oral fluconazole.

d. Candidal fungemia can be life-threatening.

(1) It occurs in very ill patients with indwelling instrumentation. Any suspect catheters should be removed.

(2) IV amphotericin B is recommended. The mortality rate is >40%.

(3) If disseminated disease develops (positive blood cultures, retinal lesions, or infection of the dermis, brain, meninges, or myocardium), flucytosine should be added; alternatively, fluconazole can be tried.

e. Hepatosplenic candidiasis occurs in patients with very low WBC counts, such as patients with leukemia.

(1) With aggressive chemotherapy, the WBC count begins to rise, and the patient develops fever, right upper quadrant pain and tenderness, and nausea.

(2) An increase in alkaline phosphatase and multiple low-density defects in the liver, spleen, and kidneys develop. The diagnosis is confirmed with biopsy.

(3) Treatment is amphotericin B; once the patient responds, he or she can be switched to fluconazole.

> Candidal endocarditis is often resistant to treatment requiring surgical intervention.

f. Endocarditis occurs through direct inoculation at surgery, in injection drug users, or in late-stage HIV disease.

(1) Approximately 50% of cases involve nonalbicans *Candida* spp. and are resistant to treatment. These organisms cause large vegetations.

(2) Splenomegaly, petechiae, murmur, and large vessel embolization are common.

(3) Treatment is amphotericin B, but infected valves must be surgically replaced. Once the patient has recovered, he or she will typically receive lifelong fluconazole.

B. **Histoplasmosis**

  1. General characteristics

   a. *Histoplasma capsulatum* is a dimorphic fungus found in soil infested with bird or bat droppings.

   b. It is endemic to many areas and is transmitted by inhalation.

  2. **Clinical findings**

   a. Most infections are asymptomatic or mild and unrecognized. Patients with cellular immunodeficiency are at risk for symptomatic infections.

   b. Acute histoplasmosis occurs in epidemics when the soil is disturbed. Patients are prostrate and febrile, with few pulmonary complaints.

   c. Progressive disseminated histoplasmosis may be fatal within 6 weeks. Patients complain of fever, dyspnea, cough, weight loss, and prostration; ulcers may develop in the mouth, pharynx, liver, spleen, adrenals, and elsewhere.

   d. Chronic progressive pulmonary histoplasmosis occurs in older patients, especially those with chronic obstructive pulmonary disease (COPD). It manifests as chronic progressive pulmonary changes with calcified nodes and pericarditis.

   e. Disseminated disease occurs in immunocompromised patients, especially those with late-stage HIV disease. It more likely represents reactivation rather than a new acute infection.

    (1) The highest risk is with a CD4 count of <100 cells per μL. Patients develop fever and multiorgan failure; fulminant disease, septic shock, and death are common.

    (2) Chest radiography shows miliary infiltrates.

  3. Diagnostic studies

   a. Anemia of chronic disease and increased alkaline phosphatase, lactate dehydrogenase (LDH), and ferritin are seen in the severely ill. A pancytopenia may also develop.

   b. A urine antigen assay can confirm the presence of disseminated disease; bronchoalveolar lavage may be helpful in patients with chronic pulmonary disease.

  4. **Treatment**

   a. Itraconazole orally for weeks to months is recommended.

   b. Amphotericin B is recommended for patients who cannot tolerate or fail itraconazole therapy or in patients with meningitis or severe disease.

   c. Lifelong suppressive therapy with itraconazole is recommended for the immunocompromised.

> Histoplasmosis is a fungal infection most concerning in the immunocompromised (HIV, elderly) or those with COPD.

C. *Cryptococcus sp.*

  1. General characteristics

   a. *Cryptococcus neoformans* is an encapsulated, budding yeast found in soil contaminated with dried pigeon dung.

   b. It is transmitted through inhalation and causes illness in patients with cellular immunodeficiency, such as HIV, cancer, or long-term corticosteroid therapy.

  2. **Clinical findings**

   a. Pulmonary disease may develop in patients with COPD, chronic steroid use, or post-transplant. Fever, cough, and dyspnea occur; chest radiography reveals nodules or pneumonitis.

   b. Cryptococcal CNS disease causes headache and meningeal signs. It occurs with a CD4 count of <50 cells per μL. Patients exhibit mental status changes and cranial nerve or visual abnormalities.

> Cryptococcal disease occurs with extremely low CD4 counts, <50.

    c. Cryptococcoma is a rare, intracerebral mass lesion that causes obstructive hydrocephalus.

    d. Disseminated disease, although rare, may affect the skin, prostate, osteoarticular surfaces, eye, lymph tissue, or other sites.

3. Diagnostic studies

    a. CSF shows variable pleocytosis (predominantly lymphocytes), increased opening pressure, increased protein, and decreased glucose.

    b. Budding, encapsulated fungus may be isolated on a culture.

    c. Cryptococcal antigen can be detected in CSF and serum. India ink stain or serology with latex agglutination assay or cryptococcal antigen assay is helpful.

    d. CT or MRI is indicated if cryptococcoma is suspected.

4. **Treatment**

    a. In patients with HIV disease, oral fluconazole is continued for 10 weeks. In severe infections, amphotericin B can be administered for the first 2 weeks, followed by oral fluconazole. Flucytosine may be added in severe disease. Lifelong fluconazole therapy is recommended.

    b. In non-HIV immunocompromised patients, the mortality rate is much higher. Treatment is amphotericin B.

D. ***Pneumocystis jirovecii* pneumonia (PJP; formerly known as *Pneumocystis carinii* pneumonia [PCP])**

1. General characteristics

    a. PJP is caused by a fungus found in the lungs of humans and many animals. Evidence of infection can be found in almost all persons from a young age. It probably is transmitted through the air and lies latent in alveoli.

    b. Premature or debilitated infants in underdeveloped areas are infected during epidemics. Sporadic cases are found in patients with abnormal cellular immunity, which is caused by factors such as cancer, severe malnutrition, immunosuppressive drugs, irradiation, or in those with HIV/AIDS and a CD4 count of <200 cells per µL.

2. **Clinical findings**

    a. Typically, PJP disease presents with fever, shortness of breath, and a nonproductive cough. Physical examination findings are disproportionate to imaging results, which show diffuse interstitial infiltrates that may be heterogeneous, miliary, or patchy. Between 5% and 10% of patients have a normal chest radiograph.

    b. Less commonly, patients may present with spontaneous pneumothorax. Recurrent pneumothorax is often related to previous pentamidine use.

    c. Patients may also develop fatigue, weakness, and weight loss. Infection is likely to recur without treatment of the underlying disease or chemoprophylaxis.

3. Diagnostic studies

    a. Blood gas reveals hypoxia, hypocapnia, and reduced carbon dioxide diffusion. LDH is typically increased, and the WBC count is usually low.

    b. The organism can be demonstrated with specific stains of induced sputum or via bronchoalveolar lavage.

4. **Treatment**

    a. Empiric treatment is recommended for immunocompromised patients presenting with cough or dyspnea. The drug of choice is TMP-SMX.

    (1) Patients often get worse at the start of the treatment. Steroids are added if the partial pressure of oxygen in arterial blood (PaO_2) is <70 mm Hg to prevent deterioration and promote oxygenation.

PJP is the most common opportunistic infection in HIV disease.

TMP-SMX is the drug of choice for both prevention and treatment of PJP.

(2) Hypersensitivity reactions to TMP-SMX (likely because of the sulfa component) manifest with fever, rash, malaise, neutropenia, hepatitis, nephritis, thrombocytopenia, and hyperbilirubinemia. Systematic desensitization is often successful.

b. Dapsone is an alternative treatment and is as effective as TMP-SMX. It is more expensive than TMP-SMX, but it is a good choice for patients who are sensitive to sulfa. Side effects include anemia, rash, and fever. It should not be taken with didanosine.

c. Alternatively, pentamidine can be used either IV or IM. Nebulized pentamidine can be used to prevent PJP. Side effects include rash, neutropenia, abnormal liver function, serum folate deficiency, calcium imbalance, hypoglycemia or hyperglycemia, hyponatremia, and nephrotoxicity. Rarely, fatal pancreatitis occurs.

d. Atovaquone is reserved for patients who cannot tolerate TMP-SMX or pentamidine. It must be taken with a fatty meal and causes mild to minimal side effects.

e. Once a patient is successfully treated for PJP, prophylaxis is continued. All patients with a CD4 count of <200 cells per μL should receive prophylactic treatment. TMP-SMX is the drug of choice.

Parasitic Infections

A. Amebiasis

1. General characteristics

a. Cysts of *Entamoeba histolytica* are viable in the soil and water for weeks to months. Transmission to humans, the only host, occurs through fecal-contaminated food or water, fly droppings, or human-to-human contact.

b. Once ingested, the cysts pass through to the intestines where they hatch. Trophozoites invade the mucosa and induce necrosis. Amebic ulcers are typically flask shaped and occur anywhere in the large bowel or terminal ileum. They are usually limited to the muscularis, but if they penetrate the serosa, they may cause perforation, abscess, or peritonitis.

> Amebiasis is transmitted through fecal-oral route and presents clinically with cramps, fatigue, and colitis.

2. **Clinical findings**

a. Intestinal disease is often asymptomatic.

b. Colitis can be mild to moderate (few semi-formed stools without blood) or severe dysentery (higher number of liquid stools streaked with blood or bits of necrotic tissue).

(1) Patients may have cramps, fatigue, weight loss, and increased flatulence. Cycles of remission and recurrence are typical.

(2) Physical examination may reveal distention, hyperperistalsis, and generalized abdominal tenderness during recurrences.

(3) Patients with severe disease become prostrate and toxic with fever, colic, tenesmus, and vomiting.

(4) Complications include appendicitis, bowel perforation, fulminant colitis, massive mucosal sloughing, and hemorrhage.

(5) Localized ulcerative lesions of the colon and localized granulomatous lesions of the colon (ameboma) result in pain, intestinal obstruction, and hemorrhage.

(6) Amebomas may be single or multiple and must be differentiated from colon cancer, tuberculosis, or lymphogranuloma venereum. Biopsy reveals granulation tissue.

c. Extraintestinal disease

(1) Hepatic amebiasis and amebic liver abscess can be asymptomatic or result in symptoms either suddenly or gradually, over days to months.

(2) Findings include fever, pain, tender hepatomegaly, malaise, prostration, sweating, chills, anorexia, and weight loss.

(3) Pulmonary symptoms (coughing, right lower lung findings) may occur if the abscess is in the superior liver.

(4) Abscesses may rupture and spill into the pleural, peritoneal, or pericardial space; this can be fatal.

(5) Less commonly, amebiasis may metastasize to the lungs, brain, or genitalia.

3. Diagnostic studies

a. Stool specimens reveal cysts or trophozoites. Sigmoidoscopy, colonoscopy, or rectal biopsy shows ulcers; collection of exudates should be examined for trophozoites.

b. Serology can detect antibodies up to 10 years after the infection and, therefore, cannot be used to differentiate the past from the present infection.

c. WBC count is moderately elevated but without eosinophilia. There will be minimal changes, if any, to liver enzymes.

d. Ultrasonography, CT, MRI, or radioisotope scanning reveals the size and location of hepatic abscesses.

4. **Treatment**

a. Asymptomatic infection should be treated with a luminal amebicide (diloxanide furoate, iodoquinol, or paromomycin).

b. Mild-to-moderate infections should be treated with a luminal amebicide plus tinidazole or metronidazole. Alternatives include tetracycline and a luminal amebicide, followed by chloroquine.

c. Severe infection should also be treated with fluids, electrolyte replacement, and opioids to control bowel motility and decrease the risk of toxic megacolon.

d. Hepatic abscess is treated with tinidazole or metronidazole plus a luminal amebicide, followed by chloroquine. If there is no response within 3 days of initial treatment, the abscess should be drained. Complications include bacterial infection, bleeding, and peritoneal spillage.

e. A follow-up with at least three stool examinations at 2- to 3-day intervals starting 2 to 4 weeks after the end of treatment.

(1) Colonoscopy may also be used to confirm treatment success.

(2) Post-dysenteric colitis after severe infection is usually self-limited but may be a trigger for ulcerative colitis.

f. Prognosis with treatment is very good. Without treatment, mortality can be high.

g. Prevention is through adequate control of the food and water supply, proper sanitation, and personal hygiene.

B. **Hookworms**

1. General characteristics

a. Hookworm is endemic to the moist tropics and subtropics.

(1) Sporadic cases occur in the southeastern United States; 25% of the world's population is infected.

(2) Humans are the only host.

b. Eggs are passed in the stool and hatch in moist soil.

(1) The larvae last for hours to weeks. They penetrate the skin and migrate in the bloodstream to the pulmonary capillaries, where they destroy alveoli and are carried by cilia to the mouth. Once swallowed, the larvae attach to the small bowel mucosa and suck blood. Once mature, they release eggs to continue the cycle.

Amebiasis treatment involves intraluminal antibiotics plus systemic treatment as needed, depending on the spread of the organism.

Proper sanitation and protection of the water supply are essential to the control of parasites.

(2) A light infection is defined as 1,000 eggs per g feces and moderate infection as 2,000 to 8,000 eggs per g feces.

2. Clinical findings

a. The site of penetration is pruritic. An erythematous dermatitis with maculopapular or vesicular eruption follows (cutaneous larva migrans); scratching can cause secondary bacterial infections.

b. The pulmonary stage may cause cough, wheeze, blood-tinged sputum, and low-grade fever.

c. With a light infection and adequate iron intake, the patient may remain asymptomatic during the intestinal stage. A heavy infection leads to anorexia, diarrhea, vague pain, and ulcer-like epigastric symptoms. Severe infection causes anemia, protein loss, and malabsorption.

3. Diagnostic studies

a. The eggs can be demonstrated in feces.

b. The stool is positive for occult blood. Hypochromic microcytic anemia and eosinophilia may be found.

4. Treatment

a. Mebendazole (twice/day for 3 days) or either pyrantel or albendazole (once daily for 2 to 3 days) is effective.

b. Pyrantel cannot be used in children younger than 5 years; none of the treatments are recommended in pregnancy.

c. Supportive treatment includes a high-protein diet, vitamins, and ferrous sulfate.

C. Pinworms (enterobiasis)

1. General characteristics

a. Humans are the only host for *Enterobius vermicularis*. There is a worldwide distribution, and children are infected more often than adults.

b. Adult worms are loosely attached to the mucosa, primarily in the cecum. Gravid females pass through the anus to lay eggs on the perianal skin. Each female is capable of producing a large number of eggs. The eggs are viable for 2 to 3 weeks outside the host and are infective within a few hours of ingestion.

c. Infection is easily passed through hands, food, drink, and fomites. The eggs are swallowed and hatch in the duodenum; larvae pass to the cecum and mature in 3 to 4 weeks. The life span is 30 to 45 days.

2. Clinical findings

a. Many patients are asymptomatic.

b. Characteristic symptoms include perianal pruritus (crawling sensation that is worse at night), insomnia, weight loss, enuresis, and irritability. Examination at night may reveal worms in the anus or stool. Scratching causes excoriations and secondary skin infections (i.e., impetigo).

c. Migration can cause vulvovaginitis, diverticulitis, appendicitis, cystitis, and granulomatous reactions.

3. Diagnostic studies: Eggs can be captured on a piece of cellophane tape over the perianal skin; three tries over three consecutive nights yield 90% success rate.

4. Treatment

a. All members of the household should be treated concurrently.

b. Albendazole, mebendazole, or pyrantel is administered in a single dose and then repeated 2 to 4 weeks later.

c. Handwashing after defecation and before meals must be stressed. Bed sheets should be washed thoroughly.

> Mucocutaneous migrans larva is a result of parasitic burrowing under the skin.

> Pinworms are treated with a single dose of medication; repeat in 2 weeks. Practice thorough cleaning to get rid of eggs.

D. Malaria

1. General characteristics

   a. *Plasmodium vivax*, *Plasmodium malariae*, *Plasmodium ovale*, and *Plasmodium falciparum* are endemic to the tropics and subtropics.

   b. There are 300 to 500 million cases per year worldwide, with 1 million deaths. There are 800 cases per year in the United States; almost all are imported.

   c. Transmission is through the bite of the *Anopheles* mosquito.

      (1) The mosquito ingests the parasite, and sporozoites mature and get transferred to humans via saliva. Incubation period ranges between 8 and 60 days.

      (2) The sporozoites invade hepatocytes and mature as tissue schizonts. The schizonts escape the liver and invade red blood cells, where they multiply and cause rupture of the cell within 48 hours.

      (3) The cycle of invasion, multiplication, and red blood cell rupture continues.

2. **Clinical findings**

   a. The typical malarial attack starts with shaking chills (the cold stage), followed by fever (the hot stage), and, finally, diaphoresis (the sweating stage).

      (1) Patients are fatigued between attacks.

      (2) The release of tissue necrosis factors and cytokines contributes to fatigue, headache, dizziness, GI complaints, myalgias, arthralgias, backache, and dry cough.

      (3) There may be liver and spleen enlargement if symptoms continue for >4 days.

   b. Infection with *P. falciparum* can be much more severe and can manifest as cerebral malaria, hyperpyrexia, hemolytic anemia, noncardiogenic pulmonary edema, acute tubular necrosis, adrenal insufficiency, cardiac dysrhythmias, and other complications.

3. Diagnostic studies

   a. Blood films are stained with Giemsa or Wright stain and examined at 8-hour intervals for 3 days during and between attacks. The percentage of infected red blood cells ranges from 5% to 20%.

   b. During attacks, leukocytosis or leukopenia may develop.

   c. Severe infections cause hepatic changes, hemolytic jaundice, thrombocytopenia, marked anemia, and reticulocytosis.

   d. Antibodies appear 8 to 10 days later, which is too late for diagnostic benefit in most cases. Antibodies also persist for 10 years, making the distinction between old and new infection difficult.

4. **Treatment**

   a. Prevention is key to the control of malaria. Evaluation and reduction of risk of exposure and prevention of mosquito bites through proper clothing, mosquito repellant, insect spraying programs, and barriers (mosquito netting and screens) is the first step.

   b. Chemoprophylaxis is recommended for patients traveling to areas of endemicity. Resistance is increasing; travelers should check with the local health authorities. In areas of chloroquine resistance, mefloquine is recommended.

      (1) Chloroquine is the drug of choice for both prophylaxis and treatment. It is generally well tolerated and is safe in pregnancy.

      (2) Transient GI symptoms, headache, pruritus, dizziness, blurred vision, malaise, and urticaria can be reduced if taken with meals or given in divided doses twice per week rather than daily.

   c. Severely ill patients can be treated with parenteral quinine, quinidine, or chloroquine plus either doxycycline, clindamycin, or tetracycline.

> Severe malaria affecting multiple organ systems is invariably due to *P. falciparum*.

d. Alternative drugs include atovaquone and proguanil (Malarone), mefloquine, hydroxychloroquine, atovaquone/doxycycline, or other combinations, especially if resistance to chloroquine is suspected.

e. Prognosis is good if treated, except for cases involving *P. falciparum*, which has a mortality rate of 14% to 17% despite treatment.

Sexually Transmitted Diseases

A. Syphilis

1. General characteristics

a. *Treponema pallidum* is a spirochete that can affect almost any organ or tissue. Transmission occurs most frequently during sexual contact. There has been a rising incidence of the disease in urban areas, particularly among adolescents and young adults as well as injection drug users.

b. Congenital syphilis is transmitted via the placenta from the mother to the fetus and can result in severe birth defects.

2. Clinical findings

a. Early infectious (primary and secondary) and late (tertiary) syphilis are separated by a symptom-free latent phase, during which the infectious stage may recur.

b. Primary syphilis is characterized by chancre, which is a painless ulcer with a clean base and firm, indurated margins. It develops at the site of inoculation, most commonly the genital area. It is associated with regional lymphadenopathy (rubbery, discrete, nontender).

c. Secondary lesions may involve skin, mucous membrane, eye, bone, kidneys, CNS, or liver. There may be relapsing lesions during early latency.

d. Late (tertiary) syphilis includes gummatous lesions involving skin, bones, and viscera; cardiovascular disease; and nervous system and ophthalmic lesions.

(1) Neurosyphilis can result in asymptomatic disease, meningovascular syphilis (chronic meningitis), generalized paresis, or tabes dorsalis (chronic progressive degeneration of parenchyma).

(2) Tabes dorsalis manifests with impaired proprioception, loss of vibratory sense, Argyll Robertson pupil (reacts to light but does not accommodate), or tabes dorsalis crises (severe pain and neurologic decompensation).

e. Congenital syphilis leads to abnormalities in the skin or mucous membranes, nasal discharge (snuffles), hepatosplenomegaly, anemia, and osteochondritis. If infants are not treated, they may develop interstitial keratitis, Hutchinson's teeth (notched, wide-spaced), saddle nose, deafness, and CNS abnormalities.

3. Diagnostic studies

a. *T. pallidum* may be identified using dark-field microscopy, but the technique is difficult. Immunofluorescence staining techniques are somewhat more reliable. The organism cannot be cultured. Serologic testing is the recommended method for diagnosis.

b. Nontreponemal antigen tests detect nonspecific antibodies to lipoidal antigens.

(1) The VDRL and RPR tests become positive 4 to 6 weeks after infection. These tests are positive in 99% of cases during primary and secondary syphilis but may be negative during late forms of syphilis. False-positive results occur, especially in patients with autoimmune disorders.

(2) TRUST (toluidine red unheated serum test) is another nontreponemal test.

(3) The nontreponemal tests measure the amount of antibody present and are used to assess the effectiveness of the treatment.

Syphilitic chancres (ulcers) are painless with a clean base and tidy edges.

    c. Treponemal antibody tests use live or killed *T. pallidum* as an antigen to detect specific antibodies. Once reserved for follow-up after a positive nontreponemal test, treponemal tests are being used frequently for initial testing.

        (1) The fluorescent treponemal antibody absorption test (FTA-ABS) is the most widely used. It is useful in determining whether a positive nontreponemal antigen test is truly positive. Newer, more automated treponemal tests are available, including MHA-TP, TPPA, TP-EIA, and CIA.

        (2) The test is accurate in most patients with primary syphilis and in virtually all patients with secondary syphilis, but it may be falsely positive in patients with Lyme disease, systemic lupus erythematosus, malaria, or leprosy.

    d. Rapid serologic test by fingerstick is available as a Clia-waived office test. The Syphilis Health Check (SHC) is 71% sensitive and 91% specific.

    e. Specific testing for tertiary syphilis includes lumbar puncture, joint fluid analysis, and biopsy as indicated.

4. Treatment

> The first choice medication against syphilis of any stage is penicillin.

    a. Benzathine penicillin G, 2.4 million units IM in a single dose, is the treatment of choice in all stages of syphilis. Late latent and tertiary syphilis require three weekly injections. Patients with penicillin allergy can be treated with tetracycline, ceftriaxone, or azithromycin.

    b. Neurosyphilis is treated with aqueous penicillin every 4 hours for 10 to 14 days. This may be followed with three weekly doses of benzathine penicillin G, as mentioned earlier.

    c. The Jarisch–Herxheimer reaction (fever, toxic state) may occur when there is a sudden massive destruction of spirochetes. To prevent this, antipyretics should be administered during the first 24 hours of treatment.

    d. All cases of syphilis should be reported to the appropriate public health agency for contact tracing. All sexual partners who may have been exposed should be treated.

    e. Careful follow-up, including serologic monitoring, is essential to monitor the effectiveness of treatment and to identify treatment failures. HIV testing and screening as well as treatment of concurrent sexually transmitted diseases should be done.

B. Gonorrhea

    1. General characteristics

        a. *Neisseria gonorrhoeae* is a Gram-negative intracellular diplococcus that is transmitted during sexual activity.

        b. The highest incidence is found in 15- to 29-year-old patients.

    2. Clinical findings

        a. The incubation period is 2 to 8 days after exposure.

        b. Men

> Untreated gonorrhea leads to pelvic inflammatory disease in women, a major cause of infertility.

           (1) Men complain of burning on urination and a serous or milky discharge. Then, 1 to 3 days later, the urethral pain is more pronounced, and the discharge becomes yellow, creamy, profuse, and, occasionally, tinged with blood.

           (2) Without treatment, the infection may regress and become chronic or progress to involve the prostate, epididymis, and periurethral glands with acute, painful inflammation. This may progress to chronic infection, resulting in prostatitis and urethral strictures.

        c. Women

           (1) Women often remain asymptomatic or may develop dysuria, urinary frequency and urgency, and a purulent urethral discharge. Vaginitis, cervicitis, and pelvic pain are common.

           (2) Asymptomatic gonorrhea is a cause of pelvic inflammatory disease and infertility as well as perpetual transmission of the pathogen.

d. Gonococcal bacteremia is associated with peripheral skin lesions or septic arthritis of the knee, ankle, or wrist.

e. Conjunctivitis is caused by direct inoculation. Patients present with copious purulent discharge, which is usually unilateral. Global rupture is a risk if the patient is not treated adequately.

3. Diagnostic studies

a. Gram stain of urethral discharge typically shows Gram-negative intracellular diplococci. Smears are less often positive in women.

b. Nucleic acid amplification testing (NAAT) is the preferred test. This test uses a vaginal swab in females and first-catch urine in males to detect antigen.

c. Cultures are essential in all cases to assess antibiotic susceptibility.

d. Patients should be tested for coinfection with *Chlamydia trachomatis*.

4. Treatment

a. Resistance to penicillin, tetracyclines, and fluoroquinolones is widespread. Currently, the treatment of choice is IM ceftriaxone or oral cefixime. Doxycycline or azithromycin should be administered simultaneously, regardless of coinfection with *Chlamydia*.

b. All sexual partners should be treated.

c. Infection is reportable in most states.

> Neisseria conjunctivitis may cause globe rupture; treat aggressively.

C. **Chlamydia spp.**

1. General characteristics: Chlamydiae are a large group of obligate intracellular parasites, including *Chlamydia psittaci* (psittacosis), *Chlamydia pneumoniae* (respiratory infections), and *C. trachomatis* (trachoma, inclusion conjunctivitis, pneumonia, and genital infections).

2. Clinical findings (GU)

a. Lymphogranuloma venereum starts with a vesicular or ulcerative lesion, which may go unnoticed.

(1) The infection spreads to the lymph nodes, causing inguinal buboes. These may fuse and break down, resulting in multiple draining sinuses and scarring.

(2) Anorectal disease causes tenesmus, discharge, and fistulae.

b. Urethritis and cervicitis

(1) In males, infection with *Chlamydia* spp. is the most common cause of non-gonococcal urethritis. Discharge is less painful than with gonococcal urethritis and is usually watery.

(2) Females are typically asymptomatic or may develop cervicitis, salpingitis, or pelvic inflammatory disease. Infection with *Chlamydia* spp. is a leading cause of infertility.

> Chlamydia in females is often asymptomatic but leads to infertility.

3. Diagnostic studies

a. NAAT is the test of choice using a urine sample or a cervical, vaginal, or anal swab.

b. Gram stain is negative. Complement fixation test or immunofluorescence, ELISA, may help confirm the presence of the disease in certain settings.

c. The diagnosis can be established clinically and treated presumptively. Patients should be tested for coinfection with *N. gonorrhoeae*.

4. Treatment

a. Azithromycin, doxycycline, and erythromycin are effective. Erythromycin is the drug of choice in pregnant women.

b. All partners should be treated.

D. **Trichomonas spp.**

1. General characteristics

a. *Trichomonas* is a flagellated protozoan.

    b. It infects the vagina, Skene's gland, and lower urinary tract of females and the GU tract of males.

  2. Clinical findings

    a. There is pruritus and a malodorous, frothy, yellow-green discharge.

    b. Diffuse vaginal erythema and red macular lesions may be visible on the cervix.

  3. Diagnostic studies

    a. Wet mount reveals motile flagellates.

    b. Other options include NAAT, culture, or rapid antigen testing.

  4. Treatment

    a. Metronidazole in a single 2-g dose; it may need to be repeated if infection does not clear.

    b. All sexual partners should be treated.

Tick-Borne Illnesses

A. Lyme disease

  1. General characteristics

    a. *Borrelia burgdorferi* is transmitted to humans by Ixodides, a small tick that often goes unnoticed. The tick must feed for >24 to 36 hours to transmit the spirochete.

    b. Lyme disease is the most common vector-borne disease in the United States.

    c. Up to 75% do not recall having been bitten by a tick.

  2. Clinical findings

    a. Stage 1: early localized infection (7 to 10 days after bite)

      (1) Erythema migrans, a flat or slightly raised red lesion that expands over several days, typically with central clearing ("bull's eye"; Fig. 14-1). Most common sites are the groin, thigh, or axilla, and it typically resolves in 3 to 4 weeks without treatment.

      (2) About 25% of patients do not either exhibit erythema migrans or recall having a rash. Up to 20% of patients have multiple lesions.

      (3) Flu-like illness occurs in 50% of patients.

> 💡 The most common tick-borne disease is the United States is Lyme; most transmission occurs between May and August.

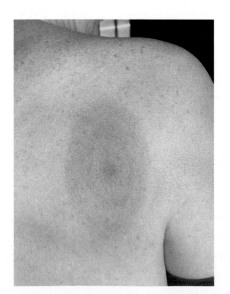

Figure 14-1 ▶ Classic bulls'-eye rash on the upper right back in early Lyme disease.

b. Stage 2: early disseminated infection (days to weeks later)

(1) Manifestations typically involve the skin, CNS (cranial nerve palsies, meningitis, radiculopathies), and musculoskeletal system (arthralgias and arthritis).

(2) Headache, stiff neck, fatigue, malaise, and intermittent musculoskeletal symptoms are common.

(3) Cardiac (pericarditis, arrhythmias, and heart block) or neurologic (aseptic meningitis, Bell's palsy, and encephalitis) manifestations occur in up to 20% of the cases.

c. Stage 3: late persistent infection (months to years later)

(1) Musculoskeletal disease includes joint pain without objective findings, frank arthritis (typically large joints), and chronic synovitis. This most likely is an immunologic rather than an infectious phenomenon.

(2) CNS and PNS manifestations include subacute encephalopathy (memory loss and mood changes), axonal polyneuropathy (paresthesias and encephalopathy), and leukoencephalitis (cognitive change, paraparesis, ataxia, and bladder dysfunction).

(3) Acrodermatitis chronica atrophicans, a bluish red discoloration of distal extremities with atrophy, is seen in Europe, but not in the United States.

3. Diagnostic studies

a. Antibodies can be detected by enzyme immunoassay (EIA) or immunofluorescence assay (IFA). A Western blot assay is used as a follow-up confirmatory test if EIA or IFA is positive. Immunoglobulin M wanes after 6 to 8 weeks; immunoglobulin G may persist indefinitely.

b. Up to 50% of patients with early disease can be antibody negative during the first few weeks. Acute and convalescent titers can be compared for the support of the suspected diagnosis.

c. The test series lacks sensitivity; the probability of a false-positive test may be greater than that of a true-positive test. False-positive tests are common in patients with rheumatoid arthritis, systemic lupus erythematosus, mononucleosis, endocarditis, and other infections. Therefore, diagnosis of early Lyme disease should be based on clinical findings. Late disease is diagnosed by objective evidence of clinical manifestations plus laboratory evidence of disease.

d. Other laboratory tests, such as CSF analysis, synovial fluid analysis, aspirations, or biopsy, may be helpful in patients with discrete manifestations.

4. Treatment

a. Doxycycline is the drug of choice in patients with erythema migrans or a suspicion of Lyme disease based on clinical findings (neurologic, cardiac, and musculoskeletal) and a history of tick bite. Alternatives include amoxicillin, cefuroxime, ceftriaxone, or cefotaxime.

b. Symptomatic treatment with analgesics, such as NSAIDs, may be beneficial in patients with musculoskeletal complaints.

c. Prevention is important. Proper clothing, tick repellent, and a thorough search for ticks after outdoor exposure are essential. Prophylactic therapy (with doxycycline in a single 200 mg oral dose) is indicated if patient meets all CDC criteria: (1) endemic area, (2) tick adhered > 36 hours, (3) therapy begins within 72 hours of tick bite, and (4) no contraindication to doxycycline.

d. The LYMErix vaccine is no longer being manufactured. The vaccine was associated with painful and debilitating side effects in some patients.

B. Rocky Mountain spotted fever

1. General characteristics

a. *Rickettsia rickettsii* is transmitted by the wood tick. The transmission is highest during the late spring and summer.

b. It most commonly occurs in the eastern United States.

> Diagnosis of stage 1 Lyme is clinical; serum studies are unreliable.

> Lyme carditis most commonly manifests as heart block.

> Doxycycline is the drug of choice for Lyme and Rocky Mountain spotted fever (RMSF).

2. **Clinical findings**

   a. Fever, chills, headache, nausea, vomiting, myalgias, restlessness, insomnia, and irritability develop 2 to 14 days after exposure. Less common manifestations include cough, pneumonitis, delirium, seizures, stupor, and coma.

   b. The face is typically flushed and the conjunctiva injected. Faint macules to maculopapules to petechiae develop first on the wrists and ankles and then spread to the extremities and trunk. About 10% of patients do not exhibit a rash.

   c. Less common findings include splenomegaly, hepatomegaly, jaundice, myocarditis, uremia, ARDS, and necrotizing vasculitis.

3. Diagnostic studies

   a. Leukocytosis, thrombocytopenia, hyponatremia, proteinuria, and hematuria are common. A transient rise in aminotransferases or bilirubin is possible.

   b. CSF analysis reveals pleocytosis and hypoglycorrhachia.

   c. A rise in antibody titers appears during the second week of illness.

4. **Treatment**

   a. Mild, untreated cases wane during the second week.

   b. Prompt treatment with doxycycline or chloramphenicol hastens recovery.

   c. Poor outcomes occur in advanced age and in patients with atypical features. Death is caused by pneumonitis or respiratory or cardiac failure.

   d. Sequelae of the disease may include seizures, encephalopathy, peripheral neuropathy, paraparesis, bowel or bladder incontinence, cerebellar dysfunction, vestibular dysfunction, hearing loss, or motor deficits.

   e. Prevention is the key. Protective clothing, tick repellant, and prompt tick removal reduce the incidence of disease.

Practice Questions

Directions: *Each of the numbered items or incomplete statements in this section is followed by a list of answers or completions of the statement. Select the ONE lettered answer or completion that is BEST in each case.*

1. A 21-year-old migrant farmworker presents with a lesion that has not healed. He states it began as what he thought was a bug bite, then became a blister. Now the area is ~2 cm, ulcerative, with black eschar and evidence of necrosis. He denies fever, pain, or discharge. What is the recommended treatment?
   - **A.** Azithromycin
   - **B.** Ciprofloxacin
   - **C.** Clindamycin
   - **D.** Penicillin
   - **E.** Vancomycin

2. Six days after stepping on a nail, a 24-year-old female presents with pain and paresthesias surrounding the wound. She states it feels like the bottom of her foot is tight but it does not look swollen. Without treatment, what symptoms can be expected next?
   - **A.** Delirium and palpitations
   - **B.** Jaw and neck stiffness and dysphagia
   - **C.** Hyporeflexia and loss of muscle tone
   - **D.** Purulent discharge
   - **E.** Severe headache and blurry vision

3. A 33-year-old patient presents for evaluation of abdominal pain, distention, and diarrhea. The diarrhea is thick and has a greenish hue. He describes 3 days of headache and malaise before the development of the pain and diarrhea. Which of the following is most likely to be found on physical examination?
   - **A.** Caput medusa
   - **B.** Nystagmus
   - **C.** Petechiae and purpura
   - **D.** Splenomegaly
   - **E.** Stiff neck

4. A 15-year-old patient presents with a sore throat along with fever and malaise. Examination reveals exudative tonsillitis and soft palate petechiae. Anterior and posterior cervical lymph nodes are enlarged and tender. Presence of which of the following indicates a need for treatment with a corticosteroid?
   - **A.** Allergy to aspirin
   - **B.** Elevated liver enzymes
   - **C.** Splenomegaly
   - **D.** Thrombocytosis
   - **E.** Tonsillar hyperplasia

5. Three patients residing in a local nursing home have been diagnosed with influenza. Which of the following should be recommended to residents as prophylaxis?
   - **A.** Acyclovir

B. Amantadine
C. Oseltamivir
D. Rimantadine
E. Zanamivir

6. A 26-year-old male who is sexually active with men and women presents for evaluation of growths around his buttocks. There are two raised perianal lesions that are hypopigmented with rough surfaces; lesions are nontender. What is the most likely etiology?
   A. CMV
   B. Human herpesvirus 8
   C. HPV 6 or HPV 11
   D. *S. aureus*
   E. *T. pallidum*

7. A 36-year-old patient with a history of asthma since childhood has developed a chronic cough. She states she experienced 3 days of sneezing, coryza, and malaise along with loss of appetite. For the past 3 weeks, she has been experiencing spasms of coughing that lasts several minutes and occurs frequently throughout the day. How should the suspected diagnosis be confirmed?
   A. Bronchial washings
   B. ELISA testing
   C. Sputum Gram stain
   D. Throat culture
   E. WBC count and peripheral smear

8. A 3-year-old girl is brought to the clinic by her mother who states the child woke this morning with a fever. Day care reports several children with fever recently. The child has been lying in bed or on the couch, not wanting to participate in her usual activities or eat any of the foods offered. Examination reveals friable vesicles on the oral mucosa and tongue. Anterior cervical nodes are enlarged and mobile. What is the most likely etiologic agent?
   A. Adenovirus
   B. Coxsackievirus
   C. HSV-1

D. *C. albicans*
E. HPV

9. A 68-year-old female describes local pain and tingling followed by a vesicular eruption. Disease occurring in the distribution of what nerve carries the highest incidence of long-term debility?
   A. Facial
   B. Trigeminal
   C. Thoracic
   D. Lumbar
   E. Sacrococcygeal

10. Several customers who purchased home-canned vegetables at the local farm market have become ill with acute botulism. What was the likely initial manifestation of symptoms?
    A. Diplopia
    B. Impaired extraocular muscles
    C. Dry mouth
    D. Dysphonia
    E. Dyspnea

11. Which of the following patients should not receive the influenza vaccine?
    A. A 9-year-old boy with chronic persistent asthma
    B. An 11-year-old girl with her third upper respiratory infection (URI) of the season
    C. A 16-year-old male with allergy to milk and tree nuts
    D. A 26-year-old female with chronic ulcerative colitis
    E. A 51-year-old male with cirrhosis and thrombocytopenia

12. A mother is concerned about her baby's diaper rash. She has been using zinc oxide cream and keeping the area as clean and dry as possible, but the rash is not improving. Examination reveals beefy red, raised areas as well as a few scattered satellite lesions. What is the most likely cause of the rash?
    A. *Candida* infection
    B. Irritation secondary to urine
    C. Trychophyton
    D. Scabies
    E. Intertrigo

Practice Answers

1. **B.** *Infectious Disease; Pharmacology; Anthrax*

   Cutaneous anthrax is the most common form of the infection. It is a spore-forming bacterium that is transmitted via broken skin. Farmworkers are at increased risk. Fluoroquinolones are the treatment of choice; clindamycin is the second-line treatment.

2. **B.** *Infectious Disease; History and PE; Tetanus*

   Tetanus begins with pain and tingling; jaw stiffness and dysphagia develop next, followed by irritability, hyperreflexia, muscle spasm (especially of jaw and face), painful tonic convulsions, and spasms of glottis and respiratory muscles. The patient remains awake and aware throughout.

3. **D.** *Infectious Disease; History and Physical Examination; Salmonella*

   Enteric fever (typhoid fever) is caused by *Salmonella*-infected contaminated food and water. Fever peaks around days 7 to 10; abdominal distention, "pea-soup" diarrhea, tenderness,

and bradycardia are characteristic. Patients may develop a fine popular rash on the trunk that fades with pressure. Nystagmus indicates a CNS lesion. Stiff neck indicates meningitis. Caput medusa is seen in patients with chronic liver disease or cirrhosis.

4. **E.** *Infectious Disease; Pharmacology; Mononucleosis (EBV)*

   A sore throat with petechiae and enlarged posterior nodes support a diagnosis of mononucleosis. Treatment is supportive; however, corticosteroids are indicated with tonsillar hyperplasia, thrombocytopenia, or hemolytic anemia.

5. **C.** *Infectious Disease; Pharmacology; Influenza*

   The CDC recommends oseltamivir for high-risk persons during influenza outbreaks. Zanamivir may be recommended if prevalence of oseltamivir resistance is a concern. Rimantadine and amantadine are no longer recommended owing to resistance. All residents in long-term care facilities should receive prophylaxis during outbreaks, regardless of immunization status. For the general population, only persons who have not received the annual influenza immunization should be considered for prophylaxis unless the patient has a condition that places him or her at high risk for complications of the flu (i.e., chronic heart or lung disease).

6. C. *Infectious Disease; Scientific Concepts; Anogenital Warts*

Anogenital warts (condyloma acuminata) are caused by HPV, most notably types 6 and 11. Human herpesvirus type 8 is the presumed causative agent in Kaposi's sarcoma. *S. aureus* causes carbuncles and furuncles. *T. pallidum* is the agent of syphilis that presents with a painless ulcer (chancre).

7. D. *Infectious Disease; Diagnostic Studies; Pertussis*

Pertussis (*B. pertussis*) has three phases: the catarrhal stage, the paroxysmal stage, and the convalescent stage. The paroxysmal stage is characterized by spasms of cough, followed by a whoop that may not be heard in adults. Diagnosis is by throat culture; a PCR assay may be available in some areas.

8. C. *Infectious Disease; Scientific Concepts; Herpes Simplex*

Gingivostomatitis is the initial outbreak of oral HSV-1. Lesions are pronounced in the anterior mouth (lips, gums, and buccal mucosa). Herpangina is painful lesion in the posterior mouth, typically due to coxsackievirus. *C. albicans* is the cause of thrush that manifests as white curd-like deposits on the oral mucosa; detachment reveals irritated mucosa underneath. The HPV is responsible for warts and neoplastic disease of the cervix, anal area, external genitalia, and mouth and pharynx.

9. B. *Infectious Disease; Diagnosis; Zoster*

Outbreaks of zoster of the trigeminal nerve carry the highest risk of postherpetic neuralgia. Zoster involving the facial nerve may cause Ramsay Hunt syndrome; pain deep within the ear, facial palsy, and a vesicular rash are characteristic.

10. A. *Infectious Disease; History and Physical Examination; Botulism*

The initial manifestation of botulism is visual changes, typically diplopia and loss of accommodation. Shortly after, patients develop ptosis and impaired extraocular muscles. This is followed by dysphonia, dysphagia, and dry mouth. Respiratory paralysis is the final manifestation, leading to death if not treated with appropriate antitoxin.

11. E. *Infectious Disease; Health Maintenance; Influenza*

The influenza vaccine is contraindicated in patients with allergy to eggs, acute febrile illness, or thrombocytopenia. The vaccine is especially warranted in patients with chronic heart or lung disease, the elderly, residents of institutions, patients on chronic aspirin therapy, and all health care workers.

12. A. *Infectious Disease; Diagnosis; Candida Diaper Rash*

Candida diaper rash is distinguished from irritative contact dermatitis by the presence of satellite lesions. The rash also tends to be more inflamed. Intertrigo is a chronic inflammatory process that commonly also grows *Candida*, but this is found in older patients who tend to be obese and diabetic. Trychophyton is the fungus implicated in tinea. Scabies is more commonly found in the axilla, wrists, finger webbing, waist or belt line, and buttocks; intensive itching and tiny burrows are characteristic.

Surgery | 15

Frank Acevedo

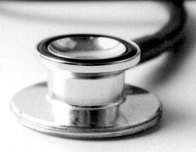

Patient History

A. A comprehensive patient history should be performed when possible. When time and the patient's condition permit, every effort should be made to complete the history. In emergent situations, the mnemonic SAMPLE should be followed:

Symptoms

Allergies

Medications

Past medical history

Last meal

Events preceding the emergency

B. **S**ymptoms need to be thoroughly explored by asking:

  1. Location

  2. Quality of pain

  3. Quantity (how often does it occur)

  4. Timing

  5. Setting (position, relationship to place)

  6. Aggravating/alleviating factors

  7. Associated symptoms

C. **A**llergies inquired about should include not only food and medication reactions but also any history of problems with anesthesia and anesthetic agents. Specific allergies to latex, tape, or surgical appliances should be asked about. Responses may reveal a difficult intubation history, malignant hyperthermia, previous reaction to an anesthetic agent, or other pertinent information.

D. **M**edications should be reviewed for any ingredient that causes increased bleeding tendencies. Drugs such as aspirin, anticoagulants, alcohol, nonsteroidal anti-inflammatory drugs (NSAIDs), chemotherapeutic agents, and antibiotics are the most likely culprits. At particular risk are patients undergoing procedures on the central nervous system (CNS) or in whom spinal anesthesia is being considered. Risk must be reevaluated in the presence of these medications and definitive steps taken to ameliorate it. Herbal medications in particular should be specifically investigated, as many can interfere with normal coagulation and cause an increase in bleeding. These herbal and vitamin supplements include feverfew, garlic, ginger, gingko biloba, ginseng, and vitamin E. The mnemonic DRUGS (**D**ispensed, **R**ecreational, **U**ser, **G**ynecologic, **S**ensitivities) encourages better drug history taking and may help prevent morbidity and mortality associated with medications (Table 15-1).

E. **P**ast medical history that significantly alters surgical risk should be explored. These conditions include significant cardiopulmonary disease (previous myocardial infarction, congestive heart failure, critical aortic stenosis, and chronic obstructive lung disease), endocrine disorders (insulin-dependent diabetes mellitus, thyroid disease, adrenal disease), cirrhosis,

> When language barriers exist, it is essential that the history be obtained by approved translators or translation services.

473

Table 15-1 | Drugs Mnemonic for Taking a Drug History

DRUGS	
D	**Dispensed:** by doctor or other medical or dental provider
R	**Recreational:** alcohol, tobacco, street drugs, anabolic steroids
U	**User:** over-the-counter preparations, herbal supplements
G	**Gynecologic:** birth control preparations, hormone replacement therapy
S	**Sensitivities:** to drugs, food, products, or chemicals

From Hocking G, deMello WF. Taking a DRUGS history. *Anaesthesia.* 1997;52(9):904–905. Adapted by permission of John Wiley & Sons, Inc.

renal disease, immunosuppression, and previous surgical procedures. Assessment of preoperative surgical risk in elective patient populations may require ancillary diagnostic tests such as stress testing, coronary angiography, carotid artery duplex B-mode scanning, and pulmonary function tests (PFTs).

F. **L**ast meal timing and what was ingested should be determined. In emergent procedures, this knowledge allows anesthesia to anticipate the potential for aspiration during induction. In accordance with the American Society of Anesthesiologists (ASA) Practice Guidelines to Reduce the Risk of Pulmonary Aspiration: Application to Healthy Patients Undergoing Elective Procedures (2017), the ingestion of clear liquids is allowed up to 2 hours prior to procedures being performed under general, regional, or procedural sedation and anesthesia. Despite frequently stated concern for gum chewing and sucking of hard candy prior to anesthesia, the literature does not support any specific requirement for the need to avoid these activities. Familiarity with institutional policies is strongly advised.

G. **E**vents leading up to the current presentation should be documented. Determination of the complaint as acute, subacute, or chronic is generally based on the duration of events.

1. Acute is <3 months
2. Subacute is 6 weeks to 3 months
3. Chronic is >3 months

Preoperative Evaluation

A. Routine laboratory assessment

1. No documentation exists linking a reduction in mortality and morbidity to routine laboratory testing in otherwise healthy patients undergoing elective surgical procedures.
2. The routine utilization of preoperative laboratory testing is *not* recommended unless there are clinical indications to do so.
3. Use of laboratory tests performed within a 4-month interval prior to surgery can be relied upon unless there has been a change in clinical status.
4. The history and physical examination are the *most* important preoperative evaluations performed by the surgical team.

B. Selective diagnostic tests

1. The utilization of ancillary tests for further delineation of pre- and perioperative risk should be guided by a thorough history and physical examination tempered by prudent clinical suspicion. About 5% of healthy individuals will have abnormal test results.
2. Complete blood count (CBC): consider performing if the patient has signs and symptoms compatible with anemia, if the loss of blood during the procedure is anticipated to be significant, or if there is a history of hematologic abnormalities.
3. Serum electrolytes
   a. Not indicated for patients without medical problems.

💡 Practitioner guidance should be informed by the Choosing Wisely initiative promulgated by the American Board of Internal Medicine (ABIM) Foundation.

b. Should be considered in patients taking certain medications (e.g., warfarin, digoxin) because of the association with potassium abnormalities and toxicity.

c. More useful as a postoperative laboratory evaluation.

4. Serum creatinine

    a. This is a convenient and inexpensive marker for renal function; creatinine levels decrease with age and decreased muscle mass.

    b. Preoperative creatinine levels should generally be obtained in all patients who are at risk for acute kidney injury (AKI).

    c. Consider following creatinine levels if the patient is going to receive nephrotoxic medications or agents as part of the preoperative workup (i.e., radiologic dyes), if intraoperative hypotension is anticipated, or if cross-clamping of the aorta would be performed.

> In elderly patients, creatinine levels that are in the high normal range may represent significant impairment in renal function requiring adjustment of the dosing of various medications.

5. Blood glucose

    a. Routine testing of serum glucose or HbA1c testing is not required in patients without diabetes. Patient with diabetes undergoing surgery should have a HbA1c if one is not documented within 3 months of surgery.

    b. Patients undergoing vascular and orthopedic procedures, regardless of diabetes history, should undergo HbA1c evaluation because of an increased risk and demonstrated benefit of its use as a screening tool in these patient populations. Additional patients who may benefit from preoperative glucose testing include those undergoing abdominal aortic aneurysm repair or coronary artery bypass.

6. Hepatic enzymes

    a. These are not indicated routinely in healthy patients.

    b. Consider if clinical signs and symptoms indicate hepatic dysfunction or if on any medications that can adversely affect hepatic function.

7. Coagulation studies

    a. The best determinant of bleeding tendencies during surgery is an accurate history detailing coagulation response to minor traumas. Von Willebrand disease is the *most* common genetic bleeding disorder; it will not be picked up with routine coagulation studies.

    b. Coagulation studies do not predict the risk of perioperative bleeding in healthy patients.

    c. Results of coagulation studies should be documented in patients taking anticoagulants or in patients with severe hepatic or biliary dysfunction because coagulation factors may be abnormal.

> Asking patients about duration of bleeding after apparently minor cuts inflicted by accidents or during shaving may help in detecting unrecognized bleeding tendencies.

8. Urinalysis

    a. There is no consensus on the routine use of urinalysis in healthy patients.

    b. The incidence of asymptomatic urinary tract infections (UTIs) is 2% to 7%.

    c. Asymptomatic UTIs are a concern to the surgical team whenever a prosthetic device is to be implanted.

    d. Transient bacteremia during vascular procedures can infect the pseudointimal layer of the graft and may seed to a prosthetic device. The same is true for implanted orthopedic hardware.

9. Electrocardiography (ECG)

    a. An ECG should be obtained in patients undergoing noncardiac surgical procedures if they have a history of cardiovascular disease, arrhythmia, or structural disease of the heart that is considered significant.

    b. Silent myocardial infarctions are more common in elderly patients and in patients with diabetes mellitus.

10. Chest radiography

    a. Little evidence supports or refutes routine chest radiography in patients without significant risk.

    b. Chest radiography may be indicated in patients more than 50 years of age undergoing surgical procedures associated with a high risk, and it should be performed in all patients, regardless of age, who have any history of significant cardiopulmonary disease.

11. Pulmonary function tests

    a. The American College of Physicians (ACP) recommends preoperative PFTs on patients with chronic obstructive pulmonary disease (COPD) or asthma if their baseline status cannot be clinically evaluated. In addition, those patients with dyspnea or diminished exercise tolerance that is not clarified by the clinical evaluation should undergo PFTs for further delineation.

    b. The *most important* determinant of postoperative pulmonary complications is the proximity of the surgical site to the patient's diaphragm.

12. Arterial blood gas (ABG)

    a. ABGs are not routinely indicated for preoperative evaluation. Perform if there is any indication of severe underlying cardiopulmonary disease that is not optimized, or to confirm a suspected acid–base disturbance.

    b. Pulse oximetry should be used before considering an ABG; often, the oxygen saturation information is enough in the preoperative patient.

13. Pregnancy test: the ASA position statement on pregnancy testing is that "testing may be offered to female patients of childbearing age and for whom the result would alter the patient's management." The careful practitioner should inquire about the sex assignment at birth as transgender men may identify as male but still have female reproductive organs and the potential to be pregnant.

C. Risk assessment for postoperative complications: The goal of this crucial assessment is to identify factors that increase morbidity and mortality.

1. General history and physical examination

    a. Determine presence and time frame of previous myocardial infarction, heart failure, chronic pulmonary disease, diabetes mellitus, peripheral vascular disorders, and hepatic or renal impairment.

    b. Evaluate for jugular venous distention, cardiac murmurs, irregular pulses, pulmonary rales, abnormal aortic pulsations, and peripheral edema.

    c. Many rating systems have been developed to stratify patients into risk categories, particularly with regard to cardiac disease. One risk index is Detsky's Modified Cardiac Risk Index (Table 15-2).

2. Pulmonary complications

    a. Pulmonary complications include atelectasis, pneumonia, respiratory failure, hypoxemia, and exacerbation of underlying pulmonary conditions such as COPD and asthma.

    b. Obstructive sleep apnea (OSA) incidence has risen in association with the obesity epidemic in the United States and may be as high as 7% to 10% in the general patient population. Development of desaturation and respiratory failure is higher in this patient population, highlighting the need to screen for OSA by history or via application of a questionnaire. Anesthesia screens patients using the STOP-bang questionnaire (Table 15-3).

3. Cardiac complications

    a. Cardiac complications, particularly perioperative myocardial infarction, occur with an alarming frequency in certain surgical patients. More than 1.5 million patients in the United States suffer some perioperative cardiovascular morbidity. The

The use of pulse oximetry may be inaccurate in patients who are cold, have decreased perfusion, have marked bradycardia or tachycardia, or are wearing fake nails or nail polish. Pulse oximetry does not provide any information on a patient's ventilation status.

A thorough evaluation of pulmonary and cardiac function provides a good assessment of operative and anesthesia risks.

Table 15-2 | Detsky's Modified Cardiac Risk Index

Risk	Points
Age >70 years	5
Myocardial infarction	
Within 6 months	10
After 6 months	5
Canadian Cardiovascular Society Angina Classification[a]	
Class III	10
Class IV	20
Unstable angina within 6 months	10
Alveolar pulmonary edema	
Within 1 week	10
Ever	5
Suspected critical aortic stenosis	20
Arrhythmia	
Rhythm other than sinus or sinus plus atrial premature beats	5
More than five premature ventricular beats	5
Emergency operation	10
Poor general medical status[b]	5

Class	Points	Cardiac Risk
I	0–15	Low
II	20–30	Intermediate
III	31+	High

[a]Canadian Cardiovascular Society Classification of Angina: 0, asymptomatic; I, angina with strenuous exercise; II, angina with moderate exertion; III, angina with walking one- to two-level blocks or climbing one flight of stairs or less at a normal pace; IV, inability to perform any physical activity without the development of angina.

[b]As defined by Goldman risk index.

Data from Goldman L, Caldera DL, Nussbaum SR, et al. Multifactorial index of cardiac risk in noncardiac surgical procedures. *N Engl J Med*. 1977;297(16):845–850; Detsky AS, Abrams HB, McLaughlin JR, et al. Predicting cardiac complications in patients undergoing non-cardiac surgery. *J Gen Intern Med*. 1986;1(4):211–219; Karnath BM. Preoperative cardiac risk assessment. *Am Fam Physician*. 2002;66(10):1889–1896.

incidence of perioperative myocardial infarction, as assessed by Goldman Criteria, is 3.2%, with cardiac death occurring in 1.7% of surgical patients. Postoperative deaths occurring within 30 days of surgery account for 7.7% of all global deaths causing approximately 4.2 million deaths (*Lancet*).

b. The Lee's Revised Cardiac Risk Index (1999) has been thoroughly validated as a way to predict risk in patients who undergo elective noncardiac surgical procedures, although it does not perform well in patients undergoing vascular surgical procedures. This prediction of cardiac risk is based on the presence or absence of six predictors. The greater the number of risk factors, the higher the risk of adverse outcomes (Table 15-4).

c. Further prediction of postoperative risks, including cardiac, can be evaluated utilizing the American College of Surgeons National Surgical Quality Improvement Program (NSQIP). Use of this method is more complicated and is not as thoroughly validated as other tools (https://riskcalculator.facs.org/RiskCalculator/).

4. Anesthesia complications

a. ASA classification (Table 15-5): Although performed by anesthesiologists since 1941, the ASA classification does *not* predict operative risk; instead, it was developed as an aid to assess the physical status of the patient before a surgical procedure and help make the choice of the anesthetic used.

Table 15-3 | STOP-bang Questionnaire

Yes	No	
		Snoring? Do you snore loudly (loud enough to be heard through closed doors or your bed partner elbows you for snoring at night)?
		Tired? Do you often feel tired, fatigued, or sleepy during the daytime (such as falling asleep during driving)?
		Observed? Has anyone observed you stop breathing or choking/gasping during your sleep?
		Pressure? Do you have or are being treated for high blood pressure?
		Body mass index (BMI) more than 35 kg/m²?
		Age older than 50 years?
		Neck size large (measured around Adam's apple)? For male, is your shirt collar 17 inches or larger? For female, is your shirt collar 16 inches or larger?
		Sex = male?

Scoring criteria (for general population): low risk of obstructive sleep apnea (OSA), yes to 0–2 questions; intermediate risk of OSA, yes to 3–4 questions; high risk of OSA: yes to 5–8 questions, yes to 2 of 4 STOP questions + individual's sex is male, yes to 2–4 STOP questions + BMI >35 kg/m², yes to 2 of 4 STOP questions + neck circumference (male) 17 inches/(female) 16 inches.

From Toronto Western Hospital, University Health Network. *STOP-Bang Questionnaire*. http://www.stopbang.ca/osa/screening.php. Copyright © 2012, University Health Network.

Table 15-4 | Lee's Revised Cardiac Risk Index

Criterion	Point Value
High-risk surgery	1
Coronary artery disease	1
Congestive heart failure	1
Cerebrovascular disease	1
Insulin-dependent diabetes mellitus	1
Elevated serum creatinine >2 mg/dL	1
Interpretation: Scoring	
Points = 0: Class I, very low (0.4% complications) Points = 1: Class II, low (0.9% complications) Points = 2: Class III, moderate (6.6% complications) Points = 3: Class IV, high (>11% complications)	

Reprinted with permission from Lee TH, Marcantonio ER, Mangione CM, et al. Derivation and prospective validation of a simple index for prediction of cardiac risk of major noncardiac surgery. *Circulation*. 1999;100(10):1043–1049.

Table 15-5 | Classification by the American Society of Anesthesiologists

Class 1	Healthy patient, no medical problems
Class 2	Mild systemic disease
Class 3	Severe systemic disease but not incapacitating
Class 4	Severe systemic disease that is a constant threat to life
Class 5	Moribund, not expected to live 24 hours regardless of operation

The letter e is sometimes added to the class designation to designate an emergency operation.

b. Difficulty associated with airway intubation as well as some complications associated with liberation from ventilation can be predicted by applying the Mallampati scoring system. This system is applied by having the patient open their mouth and assessing visible pharyngeal structures (Table 15-6).

c. The Cormack–Lehane airway assessment system can also be utilized and is based on an assessment of laryngeal structures visualized during direct laryngoscopy (Fig. 15-1).

D. Deep vein thrombosis (DVT) prophylaxis

  1. General characteristics

    a. Classically, the triad of stasis, intimal damage, and hypercoagulability described by Rudolph Virchow has been used to identify patients at risk.

    b. DVT can commence at the induction of anesthesia at the start of elective surgical cases, so attempts at prophylaxis should be started preoperatively.

    c. Specific surgical populations are at varying risk. The 2016 American College of Chest Physicians (ACCP) recommends that treatment be based on risk assessment and stratification using the Modified Caprini Risk Assessment Model (Table 15-7). Recommendations for treatment are based on the overall risk of DVT faced by each patient population (Tables 15-8 and 15-9).

> 💡 DVT prophylaxis decisions is a balance of patient risk assessment and the type of surgery planned.

    d. Prophylaxis using agents that alter blood coagulability should *not* be considered during the immediate postoperative period for procedures within the CNS.

    e. Some high-risk patient populations (orthopedics, bariatric surgery) may require DVT prophylaxis for up to 30 days after hospital discharge.

  2. Prophylaxis options

    a. Unfractionated heparin, 5,000 units subcutaneously (SQ) every 8 or 12 hours, should be started preoperatively and continued until the patient is fully ambulatory.

      (1) Every-8-hour dosing is associated with a higher incidence of wound complications, such as hematoma formation.

      (2) Heparin therapy is a cost-effective and efficacious method of prophylaxis.

    b. Enoxaparin (a low-molecular-weight heparin), 40 mg SQ daily, should be started 12 hours before or soon after the procedure and continued until the patient is

Table 15-6 | Modified Mallampati Scoring

Class I	Soft palate, uvula, fauces, pillars visible
Class II	Soft palate, uvula, fauces visible
Class III	Soft palate, base of uvula visible
Class IV	Only hard palate visible

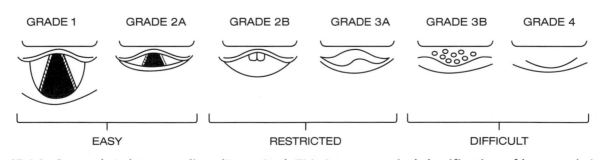

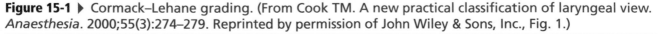

Figure 15-1 ▶ Cormack–Lehane grading. (From Cook TM. A new practical classification of laryngeal view. *Anaesthesia*. 2000;55(3):274–279. Reprinted by permission of John Wiley & Sons, Inc., Fig. 1.)

Table 15-7 | Caprini Score

Score	Risk Factor
1 point each	Age 41–60 years Swollen legs (current) Varicose veins Obesity (BMI >25 kg/m^2) Minor surgery planned Sepsis (<1 month) Serious lung disease including pneumonia (<1 month) Acute myocardial infarction Congestive heart failure (<1 month) Medical patient currently at bed rest History of inflammatory bowel disease History of prior major surgery (<1 month) Abnormal pulmonary function (COPD) Oral contraceptives or hormone replacement therapy Pregnancy or postpartum (<1 month) History of unexplained stillborn infant, recurrent spontaneous abortion (3), premature birth with preeclampsia or growth-restricted infant
2 points each	Age 61–74 years Arthroscopic surgery Malignancy (present or previous) Laparoscopic surgery (>45 minutes) Patient confined to bed (>72 hours) Immobilizing plaster cast (<1 month) Central venous access Major surgery (>45 minutes)
3 points each	Age ≥75 years History of DVT/PE Positive factor V Leiden Elevated serum homocysteine Family history of thrombosis Positive prothrombin 20210A Positive lupus anticoagulant HIT (Do not use heparin or any LMWH) Elevated anticardiolipin antibodies Other congenital or acquired thrombophilia
5 points each	Stroke (<1 month) Multiple trauma (<1 month) Elective major lower extremity arthroplasty Hip, pelvis, or leg fracture (<1 month) Acute spinal cord injury (paralysis) (<1 month)

BMI, body mass index; COPD, chronic obstructive pulmonary disease; DVT, deep vein thrombosis; HIT, heparin-induced thrombo-cytopenia; LMWH, low-molecular-weight heparin; PE, pulmonary embolism.

Table 15-8 | Risk Stratification

Total Risk Factor Score	Risk Level	Incidence of DVT
0–1	Low risk	2%
2	Moderate risk	10%–20%
3–4	Higher risk	20%–40%
5 or more	Highest risk	40%–80% (1%–5% mortality)

DVT, deep vein thrombosis.

Table 15-9 | Summary of Current Deep Vein Thrombosis Recommendations

Type of Surgery	Caprini Score	Prophylaxis
General, abdominal–pelvic	0 Low risk	None
General, abdominal–pelvic	1–2 Low risk	LMWH, LDUH, or MP
General, abdominal–pelvic	3–4 Moderate risk	MP
General, abdominal–pelvic	≥5 High risk (−)	LMWH, LDUH, or MP
Abdominal or pelvic surgery for cancer	≥5 High risk (−)	LMWH 4 weeks
General, abdominal–pelvic	5 High risk (+)	MP
General, abdominal–pelvic	5 High risk (−) LMWH/LDUH contraindicated	Low-dose ASA, fondaparinux, or MP

Key: (−) or (+): low or high risk of bleeding.

ASA, acetylsalicylic acid; LDUH, low-dose unfractionated heparin; LMWH, low-molecular-weight heparin; MP, mechanical prophylaxis.

Data from Kearon C, Akl EA, Ornelas J, et al. Antithrombotic therapy for VTE disease CHEST guideline and expert panel report. *Chest.* 2016;149(2):315–352.

fully ambulatory or up to 14 days following the surgery. Trauma patients without contraindications to anticoagulant use should have enoxaparin administered as a 30 mg dose 2×/day.

(1) Enoxaparin is more expensive per dose than unfractionated heparin, but it may be cost-effective when factoring in other requirements of dosing with unfractionated heparin.

(2) The dosage may need to be adjusted in cases of renal impairment. Adjusting enoxaparin in renal impairment: creatinine clearance (CrCl) >30 mL/min: 30 mg SQ 2×/day or 40 SQ q 1×/day; CrCl <30 mL/min: 30 mg SQ 1×/day.

(3) Enoxaparin is the preferred prophylaxis for high-risk trauma patients or those with abdominal or pelvic cancer.

(4) In high-risk trauma patients, factor Xa levels should be monitored and enoxaparin adjusted accordingly.

c. Warfarin has been used primarily in orthopedic patient populations after the initial use of heparin.

(1) The dosing of warfarin varies from patient to patient; an optimal international normalized ratio (INR) of between 2 and 3 should be the target.

(2) The use of warfarin is associated with a higher incidence of bleeding complications.

d. Fondaparinux is associated with a lower incidence of DVT in hip surgery.

(1) It works by blocking activated factor X. The dose is 2.5 mg SQ daily, starting 6 hours postoperatively.

(2) Adjustment is necessary in patients with renal insufficiency.

e. Nonfitted thromboembolic stockings are not recommended. Only fitted stockings should be used, if at all; their benefit in preventing thromboembolism in surgical patients is questionable.

f. Sequential compression devices are beneficial in all patient populations.

(1) Application is usually to both lower extremities in the operating room, and they are continued until the patient is fully ambulatory. In lieu of bilateral

> Warfarin carries the highest risk of bleeding complications; monitor INR closely.

lower extremity application, they may be used on one lower and one upper extremity. Foot pump pneumatic devices are an option as well when devices cannot be applied to an extremity.

(2) These devices are the prophylactic measure of choice for patients in whom anticoagulation is contraindicated.

g. Greenfield filter insertion (retrievable)

(1) This is an invasive procedure that allows prophylaxis only from clots that form in the lower extremities but does not protect against clots forming in the upper extremities.

(2) A filter is indicated in some patients with a history of DVT: those who have bled while on anticoagulation; those in whom anticoagulation is contraindicated because of procedure or adverse reaction; those in whom a thromboembolic event has developed while on prophylaxis or full anticoagulation; and those undergoing CNS procedures. After Greenfield filter insertion, anticoagulation should be continued if there are no compelling contraindications because of the risk of inferior vena cava (IVC) thrombosis and insertion site thrombosis.

(3) The use of IVC filters has been associated with complications because of device migration, embolization, perforation of the IVC, and filter structural failure such as filter fractures. The 2019 American Society of Hematology guidelines recommended against IVC filters as prophylaxis because of low certainty of evidence of its efficacy.

E. Surgical nutrition

1. General characteristics

a. A malnourished patient is defined as someone who has lost more than 10% of their lean body mass and/or has not had adequate nutritional intake for more than 7 days.

b. Expected risks of malnutrition include greater incidence of infection, immune dysfunction, wound complications, and perioperative morbidity and mortality.

c. Increased nutritional requirements will be present because of the hypermetabolic hypercatabolic response seen in the systemic inflammatory response syndrome (SIRS). Tumor necrosis factor-α (TNF-α) has been shown to enhance muscle catabolism and promote patient cachexia in metabolic stress.

d. Surgical nutrition is particularly important in the critically ill surgical patient admitted to an intensive care unit.

e. Unless contraindications exist, the enteral route is the preferred method of administering nutritional support.

2. Clinical features

a. Weight loss, reduction of subcutaneous fat stores, and wasting may be apparent.

b. Severe malnourishment may be associated with decreased cognitive function.

c. Subtle changes in skin and hair occur, especially when essential fatty acid deficiency syndromes may be present involving α-linolenic (ω-3) or linoleic (ω-6) acids.

d. The American Society of Parenteral and Enteral Nutrition (ASPEN) recommends calculation of the intake Nutritional Risk Screening (NRS) or Modified Nutrition Risk in Critically Ill (mNUTRIC) scores as well as investigation of comorbidities, gastrointestinal (GI) tract function, and aspiration risk.

3. Physiologic impact

a. Cardiovascular system develops decreased myocardial mass, stroke volume, and cardiac output.

b. Respiratory system undergoes catabolism of major muscles of respiration, with decreased vital capacity and difficulty in liberation from ventilation of patients.

c. GI tract develops atrophy of villi, with overgrowth of bacteria. Overgrowth of bacteria plus mucosal dysfunction may result in bacterial translocation and subsequent

Patients at highest risk and those with recurrent lower extremity clots are candidates for filter placement.

Enteral feedings are preferred whenever possible.

multisystem organ dysfunction. Depletion of the amino acid glutamine has been linked with the occurrence of bacterial translocation from the gut.

   d. The immune system develops both impaired cell-mediated and humoral immunity.

   e. Ultimately, poor wound healing develops, with an increased incidence of wound infection, dehiscence, and evisceration.

   f. In severe malnutrition, marasmus or kwashiorkor may develop.

4. Diagnostic studies

   a. Serum creatinine, creatinine height index, total lymphocyte count, albumin, prealbumin, and/or transferrin may be abnormal.

   b. Both the Society of Critical Care Medicine and ASPEN recommend that energy requirements be calculated by using indirect calorimetry (IC).

5. Treatment

   a. Treatment goals are replacement of caloric and nitrogen requirements necessary to maintain nutritional homeostasis or a prevention of catabolism and promotion of anabolism.

   b. Critically ill patients, according to ASPEN, should have energy requirements calculated by IC (preferred if available) or by the use of a formula that provides 25 to 30 kcal/kg/d.

   c. Patients who are elderly; have marasmus, kwashiorkor, anorexia nervosa; or are undergoing chemotherapy are at risk for the development of refeeding syndrome. The refeeding syndrome is associated with abnormal glucose and lipid metabolism, thiamine deficiency, hypophosphatemia, hypomagnesemia, and hypokalemia. In this patient population, limit initial feedings (enteral or parenteral) to no more than 20 kcal/kg during the first week.

   d. Preferred nutritional replacement is always via the enteral route to maintain GI integrity and aid in the prevention of multisystem organ dysfunction. Second-line options include the use of peripheral or central catheters and the infusion of intravenous (IV) hyperalimentation.

6. Complications

   a. Aspiration prevention

   (1) Measurement of residual volumes is not recommended. Positioning of the patient with the head at >30 degrees can assist with the prevention of aspiration.

   (2) Gastrostomy tube feedings have better outcomes than nasoenteric tube feedings but are still associated with aspiration.

   (3) Jejunostomy tube feedings are a preferred enteral alternative to prevent this complication, especially in patients with pancreatitis.

   (4) Use of prokinetic agents such as metoclopramide and erythromycin (oral or IV) may be indicated to help with gastric motility dysfunction. Caution should be utilized as both agents can increase the QTc.

   b. Diarrhea

   (1) Diarrhea caused by osmotic loading is a common complication and can be controlled by limiting the concentration or rate of infusion.

   (2) Never assume that diarrhea is solely from enteral feedings, and always consider *Clostridium difficile* pseudomembranous enterocolitis as a potential etiology.

   (3) The administration of oral contrast for the performance of computerized tomography (CT) may also cause diarrhea.

   c. Hyperalimentation complications can be broken down into those related to catheter insertion and those related to the infusion of the solution

   (1) Catheter-related problems include air embolus, sepsis, pneumothorax, hemothorax, hydrothorax, and cardiac rupture.

Marasmus is owing to severely low caloric intake; weight loss, dehydration, and chronic diarrhea occur. Kwashiorkor is caused by protein deficiency; edema, abdominal bulging, and inability to gain weight result.

The use of erythromycin as a prokinetic agent can result in cardiac toxicity and tachyphylaxis and stimulate bacterial resistance.

(2) Infusion complications include severe hyperglycemia (including nonketotic hyperosmolar coma), hepatic steatosis, electrolyte abnormalities, and trace element and vitamin deficiencies.

(3) Hyperalimentation should be reserved for those situations where there are absolute contraindications for utilizing the GI tract for feeding.

Trauma

A. General characteristics

1. Unintentional and violence-related injuries are the leading cause of death between the ages of 1 and 44 years (Centers for Disease Control and Prevention).

2. Motor vehicle accidents are the leading cause of accidental deaths in the United States. Worldwide, more than 1 million people die from motor vehicle collisions each year. Alcohol is linked to at least half of all the fatal motor vehicle incidents.

3. In children <1 year of age the leading cause of death is suffocation, whereas in children between 1 and 4 years of age the leading cause of death is drowning.

4. In-field emergency medical services, rapid transport to trauma centers, and application of Advanced Trauma Life Support (ATLS) guidelines generate the best results. There is some evidence supporting rapid transport without aggressive field resuscitation as a means to use permissive hypotension. Permissive hypotension prevents the dislodgment of "fresh clot" and further exsanguination.

> Primary survey starts with ABCDE: Airway, Breathing, Circulation, Disability, and Exposure/environmental control.

B. Primary survey: Airway, Breathing, Circulation, Disability, and Exposure/environmental control (ABCDE) are assessed along with initial resuscitation:

1. Assuring a patent and functioning airway is the first priority.

   a. Cervical spine stabilization should be provided by a hard (Philadelphia) collar.

   b. Altered mental status is the most common indication for intubation; evaluate Glasgow Coma Scale (GCS) score and pupillary reaction (Table 15-10).

Table 15-10 | Glasgow Coma Scale

Eye Opening	
4	Spontaneous
3	To voice
2	To pain
1	None
Verbal	
5	Oriented
4	Confused
3	Inappropriate words
2	Incomprehensible words
1	None
Motor	
6	Obeys commands
5	Localizes pain
4	Withdraws
3	Abnormal flexion
2	Abnormal extension
1	None

A score of 15 is normal. A score of 13–15 indicates mild head injury, 9–12 moderate head injury, and <9 severe head injury.

    c. Orotracheal intubation is the preferred modality.

    d. Nasotracheal intubation requires that the patient be awake.

    e. Cricothyroidotomy can be performed in emergent situations but only by experienced operators and not in patients under the age of 12 years because of the risk of developing secondary subglottic stenosis. This contraindication becomes relative when a patient cannot be intubated or ventilated.

2. Breathing is the next priority in the trauma patient evaluation

    a. Evaluate the work of breathing to differentiate an airway issue from a ventilation issue.

    b. Clinicians should look for the presence of tension pneumothorax, open chest wounds, or flail chest.

    c. Tension pneumothorax is associated with hypotension, tracheal deviation away from the side of injury, jugular venous distention, lack of or decreased breath sounds on the affected side, hyperresonance on the affected side, and subcutaneous emphysema. The diagnosis of tension pneumothorax is based on clinical parameters and not on a chest radiograph. When suspected, emergent needle decompression should be undertaken.

    d. Open chest wounds should never be completely occluded with dressings because this may convert the wound into a tension pneumothorax. Flail chest is characterized by paradoxical breathing:

        (1) Segmental rib fractures cause free-floating segments that move opposite to normal respiratory patterns.

        (2) The major problem is not the fractures but, rather, the underlying pulmonary contusion.

3. Circulatory status is assessed once airway and breathing have been secured:

    a. Assess organ perfusion by evaluating patient's level of consciousness, skin color, and temperature (core temperature preferred).

    b. Cardiopulmonary resuscitation may be necessary.

    c. IV access with at least two angiocatheters ($\geq$16 gauge) should be established.

    d. Initial infusion of balanced solutions, such as Ringer's lactate or normal saline, should be started (fluids should be warmed if large quantities are to be infused). After infusion of 1 L of crystalloid, consider an early blood transfusion as the primary method of resuscitation. Resuscitation with Ringer's lactate has in the past been decried because of a belief that the potassium in it would worsen or cause hyperkalemia; however, this concern is unfounded. Infusion of Ringer's lactate will prevent hyperchloremic non-anion gap acidosis.

    e. Persistent hypotension requires the exclusion of tension pneumothorax, myocardial contusion or infarction, or cardiac tamponade. Beck's triad (jugular venous distention, hypotension, and muffled heart sounds) characterizes cardiac tamponade.

4. Disability must be assessed by performing a neurologic evaluation with the GCS (see Table 15-10).

        (1) Exposure/Environmental Control is addressed by removing all clothing so a complete survey can be performed while paying attention to the development and treatment of hypothermia.

C. Secondary survey: After the completion of the primary survey and assurance of ABCDEs, a secondary survey should be performed.

    1. Head to toe evaluation

    2. Complete history and physical examination

    3. Reassess vital signs.

    4. Delay completion of the complete history and physical examination if patient needs to go to operating room emergently but complete it within 24 hours.

5. Primary rationale for secondary survey is to detect occult injuries. Thoracic or abdominal injuries, neurologic deficits, lacerations or hematomas, or musculoskeletal injuries must be identified.

6. Progressive changes or additional clinical manifestations are important indicators of ongoing pathology.

7. Some major injuries may not be apparent at first inspection.

8. Continued monitoring of the trauma patient is essential.

9. The digital rectal examination (DRE) was once a mandatory evaluation in trauma; however, new guidelines no longer consider it a mandatory part of the physical examination. Data show that DRE rarely changes trauma management and is unreliable as a screening tool because of its low sensitivity. The DRE, however, may be helpful in determining and classifying spinal injuries.

10. Caution must be exercised with cerebrospinal fluid rhinorrhea or suspected cribriform plate fractures and the insertion of nasogastric tubes. If a cribriform plate injury is suspected, only an orogastric tube should be used if warranted.

D. Penetrating chest trauma

1. Most cases (95% of penetrating chest trauma) can be managed by tube thoracostomy alone.

2. The remaining cases (5%) must be evaluated regarding clinical indications for operative intervention (Table 15-11).

E. Blunt abdominal trauma

1. The **F**ocused **A**ssessment with **S**onography for **T**rauma (FAST) examination has largely replaced diagnostic peritoneal lavage as the diagnostic test of choice for detecting intra-abdominal injury. Some clinicians also scan the thorax using the lung sliding technique, to look for associated pneumothorax. This is referred to as an extended FAST or eFAST.

   a. FAST examination evaluates the abdominal cavity for air or fluid collection in the perihepatic (right flank), perisplenic (left flank), pericardial, and pelvic (retrovesical) regions.

   b. A specific diagnosis of an injured organ does *not* have to be made.

2. CT may be added as needed to clarify the FAST result:

   a. CT or any other diagnostic study that involves the transport of a trauma patient should only be undertaken in patients who are hemodynamically stable and *must* be performed under constant hemodynamic and clinical monitoring by a provider.

   b. Evaluate renal function prior to the CT scan with contrast. CT scans ordered for the initial evaluation of head trauma do not need to be performed with contrast agents, as blood is self-enhancing.

F. Penetrating abdominal trauma

1. Immediate laparotomy is indicated if a patient exhibits any signs of shock, peritoneal irritation, or evisceration.

> DRE is no longer routine protocol in trauma patient workup. It remains indicated for assessment of possible spinal injuries.

Table 15-11 | **Indications for Thoracostomy in Penetrating Trauma**

Caked hemothorax unable to drain via thoracostomy tube
Evacuation of 1,500 mL of blood in an injury <3 hours old
Evacuation via tube thoracostomy of 200 mL of blood for 3 consecutive hours
Signs of cardiac tamponade
Signs of esophageal perforation
Bowel sounds in the chest, indicating diaphragmatic injury
Persistent leakage of air
Development of a bronchopleural fistula

2. Selective laparotomy can be done in the hemodynamically stable patient without any of the above signs after the performance of a FAST examination. If the FAST examination reveals free intraperitoneal air or fluid, laparotomy is indicated.

G. Penetrating flank trauma

   1. Workup in the stable patient includes CT with oral and IV contrast. Penetrating flank trauma is difficult to assess because many injuries in this region may be retroperitoneal.

   2. Wherever sequential clinical examinations are required, a team approach that uses practitioners who are involved with the initial care of the patient is best. Analgesia, with opioids or NSAIDs and tailored to the diagnosis, should be considered in every patient. Withholding appropriate analgesia for fear of changing the findings during sequential clinical examination is unfounded and can cause severe physiologic and psychological consequences in patients.

> Gunshot wounds are more likely than stab wounds to penetrate the peritoneum and injure internal organs.

H. Vascular trauma

   1. Look for signs of arterial injury, such as a pulsatile mass or hemorrhage, expanding hematoma, significant hemorrhage, presence of a thrill or bruit, or acute ischemia to the involved extremity.

   2. The presence of a pulse distal to the injury does *not* rule out significant vascular injury.

   3. Arteriography and the ankle–brachial index are useful adjunct diagnostic tests for determining arterial injury.

I. Head trauma

   1. GCS (see Table 15-10)

      a. The GCS score should be calculated in all the trauma patients and repeated frequently as part of their neurologic monitoring.

      b. It is useful for triage and prognosis.

      c. The initial GCS correlates to the severity of the brain injury. Patients with a score of 3 or less have an extremely poor prognosis for significant recovery.

      d. The avoidance of secondary insults to the brain as caused by hypotension and hypoxemia is paramount in determining the outcome and reducing the severity of the injury.

      e. According to traumatic brain injury management guidelines, in all patients with head trauma, an abnormal CT scan of the head, and who also have a GCS score of 8 or lower should be managed with intracranial pressure monitoring and intubation to protect their airway.

> Raccoon eyes or Battle sign is indicative of a basilar skull fracture; a CT will confirm. Most patients heal with supportive care only.

   2. Basilar skull fractures

      a. Basilar skull fractures may be associated with rhinorrhea, otorrhea, or ecchymosis of the eyelids (raccoon eyes).

      b. Be vigilant for ecchymosis behind the ear (Battle's sign).

   3. Epidural hematomas (Fig. 15-2)

      a. Epidural hematomas are usually caused by injuries to the middle meningeal artery.

      b. The patient may experience a brief period of loss of consciousness followed by a lucid interval and subsequent obtundation.

      c. Brain herniation may develop and is heralded by a triad of coma, fixed and dilated pupils, and decerebrate (extensor) posturing.

      d. Diagnosis is established by CT and requires emergent craniotomy.

   4. Subdural hematomas (Figs. 15-2 and 15-3)

      a. Subdural hematomas usually result from injuries to bridging veins.

      b. They are associated with severe head injuries and can result in significant axonal injury even after evacuation. Severe shearing of axons is referred to as a diffuse axonal injury (DAI).

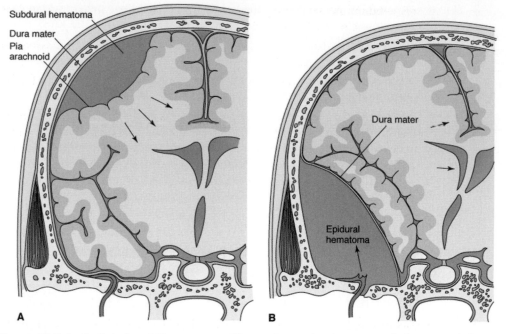

Figure 15-2 ▶ **A:** Subdural hematoma. The red area in the upper left area of the drawing is the hematoma. Note the shift of structures. **B:** Epidural hematoma. The red area in the lower left area of the drawing is the hematoma. Note the broken blood vessel and the shift of midline structures. (Reprinted with permission from Silbert-Flagg J, Pillitteri A. *Maternal & Child Health Nursing: Care of the Childbearing & Childrearing Family*. 8th ed. Wolters Kluwer; 2018, Fig. 52.2.)

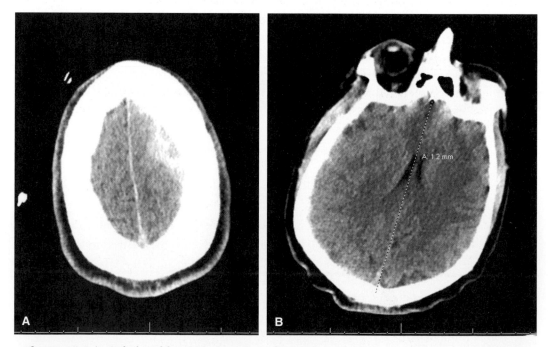

Figure 15-3 ▶ Subdural hematoma. **A:** Left subdural hematoma. **B:** Right subdural hematoma with shift.

c. Chronic subdural hematoma is more common in alcoholics and elderly patients and presents as a hematoma of varied densities.

d. Subdural hematoma can occur after an apparently minor trauma and is associated with mental status changes or focal neurologic deficits.

e. CT is diagnostic; once the diagnosis has been established, burr holes over the hematoma are indicated to evacuate the clot.

f. Patients on anticoagulants and antiplatelets are at an increased risk of intracranial bleeding even with minor head trauma. Evaluation of fall risk should be undertaken and risk versus benefit of continuing anticoagulation determined in each patient. Reversal of anticoagulant effect should be undertaken utilizing the appropriate agent. The use of platelet transfusion in head trauma patients on preinjury antiplatelet therapy is controversial.

g. Indications for surgical intervention include: clot thickness >10 mm, 5 mm or greater midline shift, decrease in GCS by 2 points or greater from baseline, persistent ICP >20 mm Hg despite treatment, and change in pupillary responses.

> 💡 Epidural hematomas are associated with middle meningeal artery. Subdural hematomas are associated with bridging vein injury.

Burns

A. General characteristics: Burns generally are classified as first, second, third, or fourth degree (Fig. 15-4). The classification of burns into a fourth degree is controversial, and many use only a three-tiered classification schema.

1. First-degree burns involve minor damage to the epidermis.

2. Second-degree burns are subdivided into superficial partial-thickness burns that extend to the papillary dermis and deep superficial burns that extend into the reticular dermis.

3. Third-degree, or full-thickness, burns involve and destroy the epidermis and the dermis including the dermal appendages.

4. Fourth-degree burns destroy the skin and subcutaneous tissue, with further involvement of fascia, muscle, bone, or other structures.

B. Incidence

1. More than 486,000 people are treated throughout the United States on an annual basis for burns of all types.

2. Approximately 3,275 deaths/year occur among the approximately 40,000 patients who are hospitalized for burn injuries. Of the 40,000 patients, 30,000 are hospitalized at burn centers.

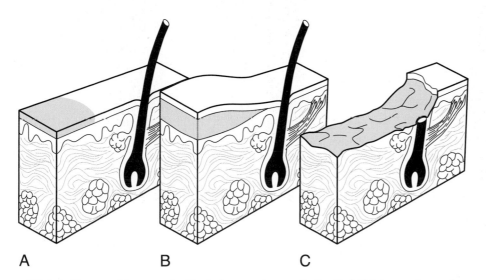

A   B   C

Figure 15-4 ▶ Types of burns. **A:** First-degree burn. **B:** Partial-thickness burn (second degree). **C:** Full-thickness burn (third degree).

> **Assess burn injuries in a child for evidence of child abuse.**

3. Fire or flame burns are the most common types of burns in adults, whereas scald burns are the most common type of burn in children.

4. Always keep in mind that burn patients are trauma patients and they may have associated blunt force injuries secondary to falls while jumping to get to safety, or other penetrating injuries.

C. **Clinical features**

1. First-degree burns are characterized by erythema, tenderness, and the absence of blisters.

2. Second-degree burns (partial-thickness burns)

   a. Superficial second-degree burns have thin-walled, fluid-filled blisters; are moist; blanch with pressure; and are painful.

   b. Deep second-degree burns have thicker-walled blisters (many of which are ruptured), exhibit a mixture of erythema and pallor, and are painful with application of pressure.

3. Third-degree burns (full-thickness)

   a. Third-degree burns give the skin a white, leathery, or charred appearance.

   b. The skin is characteristically dry and without the presence of sensation.

4. Fourth-degree burns

   a. Fourth-degree burns are characterized by significant charring and exposure of muscle, fascia, tendons, and ligaments.

   b. The extensive damage to nerves results in little to no sensation of pain.

5. Fifth-degree burns exist for billing and coding purposes and are those burns that result in amputation or loss of a body part.

6. Any burn that occurs on the face, on the upper torso, or in an unconscious patient should raise the suspicion of associated upper airway involvement.

7. In cases where burns are caused by electrical energy, the findings on the skin do not correlate with the extent of the clinical injury.

8. Children who bite extension cords may suffer delayed rupture of the labial artery.

D. Diagnostic studies

1. In patients with moderate to severe or extensive burns, required laboratory studies include hematocrit, electrolytes, blood urea nitrogen (BUN) and creatinine, urinalysis, and chest radiography.

2. Depending on the extent of the injuries and patient status, also consider obtaining an ABG, ECG, carboxyhemoglobin, and glucose levels contingent on the history obtained.

> **Carboxyhemoglobin levels often underestimate the degree of CO intoxication; interpret in conjunction with other values.**

3. Direct further laboratory and imaging studies once the secondary survey has been performed. Remember that burn patients may have significant associated trauma from falls or blunt injuries.

E. **Treatment**

1. Maintain ABCs (see previous discussion).

2. Estimate the percentage of burn:

   a. Many formulas are available: rule of nines, Lund and Browder, and Berkow. PEARL: The palm of a burn *victim's* hand is roughly equal to the area of a 1% burn.

   b. Rule of nines (Fig. 15-5)

      (1) The major body areas are divided so that each area is a multiple of nine:

         (a) The head represents 9% of the body surface and each arm is 9%.

         (b) The front of each leg (extending to the groin) is 9%, and the back is 9%.

         (c) The front of the torso is 18% and the back of the torso is 18%.

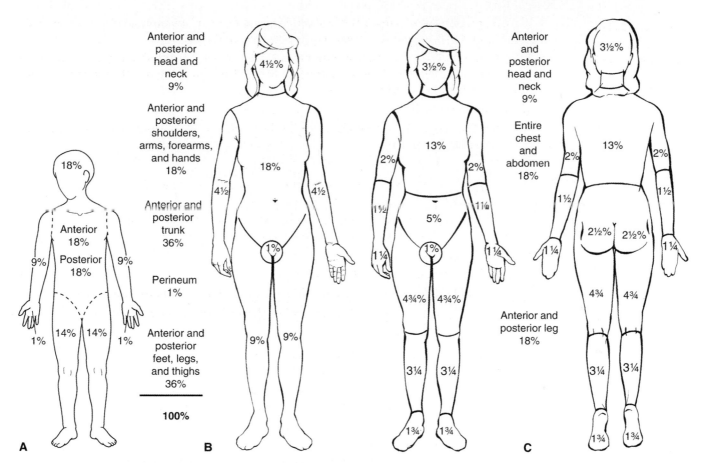

Figure 15-5 ▶ **A:** Rule of nines (child). **B** and **C:** Rule of nines (adult). (**A:** Reprinted with permission from Thorne CH, Gurtner GC, Chung K, et al. *Grabb and Smith's Plastic Surgery*. 7th ed. Wolters Kluwer; 2013. **B** and **C:** Reprinted with permission from Harwood-Nuss AL, Wolfson AB, Linden C, et al. *The Clinical Practice of Emergency Medicine*. 3rd ed. Lippincott Williams & Wilkins; 2001.)

(2) This formula is accurate for adults only; the larger head size and smaller thighs in children make their percentages different.

3. Stop the burning process:

   a. Sterile water is usually sufficient, but first look for powders if dealing with a chemical substance, as pouring water on a chemical may activate it and cause further burn damage. If dealing with a chemical substance, identification of the substance in question is important because specific neutralization measures may be required.

   b. Burns that are caused by white phosphorus may require neutralization with 1% copper sulfate solution and administration of calcium gluconate to address concomitant hypocalcemia.

   c. Hydrofluoric acid burns will require copious lavage for at least 30 minutes, with concomitant application of calcium gluconate gel to the affected area.

4. Manage shock by aggressive fluid resuscitation:

   a. Many formulas exist; choose one and become familiar with it.

   b. Parkland formula: Percentage of burn area × body weight (kg) × 4 mL/hr equals the total amount of fluid needed in the next 24 hours.

   (1) Half the calculated fluid is given during the first 8 hours, with the rest over the remaining 16 hours. Be prepared to adjust fluid resuscitation based on end points such as urine production.

   (2) Ringer's lactate solution is recommended.

> Avoid applying water if a chemical burn is known or suspected.

(3) Colloids can be introduced during the second 24 hours. However, their use remains controversial because thermal injury of capillaries may make them particularly prone to leakage. Administration of colloids to patients with leaky capillaries may cause fluid loss from, rather than retention within, the intravascular space.

(4) Monitor urine output as a measure of adequate circulation and hemodynamic stability. Frequent adjustments to IV fluid rate may be more advantageous than frequent bolus infusions to correct oliguria.

(5) Insert a nasogastric tube because gastric distention can be problematic and, in severe cases, may cause non–fluid-respondent hypotension because of mediastinal shift from an overly distended stomach.

(6) A Foley catheter should be inserted early and used for monitoring urine output.

   (a) Maintain a urine output of at least 0.5 mL/kg/hr in an adult.

   (b) Maintain a urine output of at least 1 mL/kg/hr in a child.

(7) Address the need for escharotomy in circumferential burns of extremities or the anterior trunk, as these burns can cause a compartment syndrome and make ventilation difficult.

(8) Sulfadiazine (Silvadene) is the most commonly used topical burn ointment. Other preparations, such as mafenide, may be used. Care must be taken when using mafenide, because in large amounts, it can block the action of carbonic anhydrase and lead to severe metabolic acidosis.

(9) Deep dermal burns and full-thickness burns typically are excised on or about day 3.

   (a) Coverage is attained by numerous methods. Autograft is the best method, but allograft of skin is acceptable.

   (b) Other alternatives include epidermal cell culture, artificial skin, and porcine xenograft.

   (c) Tissue expanders may also be used to assist with coverage.

(10) Complications

   (a) Common complications of severe burn trauma include inhalation injury, hypovolemic shock, neurogenic shock secondary to pain, renal failure, multiorgan system dysfunction, and gastric or duodenal ulcerations (Curling ulcers).

   (b) The most common complication associated with all burns is infection of the burn wound, which has the potential for hematogenous spread. Infection though is a late complication and antibiotics do not have a role in the initial management of burn patients.

   (c) Pneumonia is a potential complication.

   (d) Chronic healing burn wounds can undergo malignant transformation into a squamous cell carcinoma (Marjolin ulcer).

> Patients with extensive burns who require air transport to a burn center should have nasogastric tubes placed to prevent gastric distention and hypotension caused by an expanding stomach on the mediastinum. Gastric expansion is most commonly seen as a result of decreased cabin pressures and expansion of intraluminal gasses during air transport.

> Silver sulfadiazine is oculotoxic and should not be used near the eye.

Orthopedic Injuries

See Chapter 9.

Postoperative Complications

A. **Postoperative fever**

  1. General characteristics

    a. Most early postoperative fever is caused by cytokines (interleukin [IL]-1, IL-6, TNF-α, and interferon-γ), released as part of the systemic inflammatory response to tissue trauma, and resolves without intervention.

   b. Mnemonic of the five Ws is useful to aid in determining the cause of fever (Table 15-12): **W**ind, **W**ater, **W**ound, **W**alking, and **W**onder drugs/**W**hopper.

2. Clinical features

   a. Wind (atelectasis)

   (1) Wind refers to the probable cause of fever in the first 24 to 48 hours postoperatively.

   (2) Examination may reveal bronchial breathing and, in cases of significant atelectasis, the trachea may be deviated toward the affected side.

   (3) The actual fever is postulated to be primarily caused by cytokine secretion of IL-1 and TNF-α.

   b. Water (UTIs)

   (1) Postoperative UTI most commonly develops 48 to 72 hours after surgery.

   (2) Many cases are caused by indwelling urinary catheters or genitourinary instrumentation.

   (3) Patients may complain of dysuria, frequency, or urgency.

   (4) Foley catheters should be removed as soon as possible.

   c. Wound infections

   (1) Wound infections are the most common cause of postoperative fever after 72 hours.

   (2) *Staphylococcus aureus* is the most common pathogen.

   (3) Mild change in the vital signs is seen early, and pain may or may not be present at the site of infection.

   (4) Superficial infections involve the skin and subcutaneous tissue; deep infections involve areas below the fascia.

   d. Walking (thrombophlebitis)

   (1) Superficial thrombophlebitis is most commonly associated with intravascular catheters. Purulent drainage around an indwelling catheter with induration of the vein may be detected on physical examination.

   (2) Deep thrombophlebitis can be associated with indwelling central lines or DVT.

> Fever in the first 24 hours post-op is most likely respiratory; enhanced breathing should be encouraged to prevent collapse.

Table 15-12 | Mnemonic of the Five Ws

Five Ws	Timing	Notes
Wind (atelectasis)	First 24–48 hours postoperatively	Bronchial breathing Shift of trachea toward affected side
Water (UTI)	48–72 hours postoperatively	Irritative voiding symptoms Cloudy urine Positive urine cultures
Wound (wound infection)	After 72 hours postoperatively	Early postoperatively, mild elevation in vitals is possible Undue pain at wound site with erythema and/or drainage *Staphylococcus aureus* is the most common pathogen
Walking (thrombophlebitis)	After 72 hours postoperatively	Unilateral edema Homans (low specificity) Cellulitic streaking indicates streptococcal infections; local abscess formation indicates staphylococcal infections
Wonder drugs/**W**hopper (drug fever/abscess)	Fever after 1 week is a serious complication unless caused by drug allergies	Persistent fever with negative cultures should raise an index of suspicion for drug fever. Intra-abdominal abscesses may present with blood cultures that are polymicrobial

UTI, urinary tract infection.

(3) Thrombophlebitis of the lower extremity may be associated with Homans' sign; however, this test has a very low specificity. Unilateral edema of an extremity is a more specific indicator of deep vein thrombophlebitis.

e. Wonder drugs

    (1) Wonder drugs (such as anesthetics, sulfa-containing antibiotics, and others) often are implicated in drug fever that develops 1 week postoperatively.

    (2) This is a diagnosis of exclusion and should be considered when faced with a negative sepsis workup in a postoperative patient with fever.

f. Whopper (significant infection)

    (1) Whopper refers to the presence of a postoperative abscess.

    (2) In the case of intra-abdominal fluid collections, an ileus may develop as a sequela of an occult abscess.

    (3) Blood cultures may be polymicrobial, indicating anastomotic leakage in GI surgery.

3. Imaging studies

a. A directed workup may include CBC with differential, wound cultures, sputum cultures, blood cultures, chest radiography, and abdominal CT. Intra-abdominal abscesses, if intraloop (i.e., situated between two loops of the small bowel), can be associated with a 5% to 33% false-positive rate while performing CT evaluation.

b. Chest radiography in patients with atelectasis may reveal shifting of the mediastinum toward the affected side, with evidence of loss of lung volume (raised diaphragm) on the affected side.

c. When deep vein thrombophlebitis is suspected, B-mode real-time ultrasonography can be used to reveal thrombi. Venography, once the gold standard for DVT, is invasive, can lead to DVT formation, and has been largely replaced by spiral CT scanning.

4. Treatment

a. Atelectasis

    (1) Atelectasis is best addressed by prevention:

        (a) Patients should be instructed to stop smoking at least 6 to 8 weeks (ACP recommendation) before any thoracic or abdominal procedure.

        (b) Instruction in using an incentive spirometer should be given and its use encouraged as a preventive measure.

    (2) When atelectasis develops postoperatively, incentive spirometry, mucolytics, expectorants, and inhaled β-agonists are beneficial.

b. UTIs

    (1) UTIs are the most common nosocomially acquired infection.

    (2) UTIs should be treated based on culture and sensitivity reports.

    (3) Antibiotics chosen should be based on urinalysis and Gram stain results. Foley catheter use should be selective, avoided where possible, and removed promptly when feasible.

    (4) Daily use of Foley catheter "bundles" is a protocol designed to increase safety via proper technique; these protocols will assist in determining continued need for bladder catheterization.

    (5) In critically ill patients already on multiple antibiotics, a UTI with *Candida* spp. may be suspected.

c. Superficial thrombophlebitis

    (1) Superficial thrombophlebitis requires termination of the IV line at the site of inflammation and use of warm compresses.

Post-op fever necessitates a prompt and systematic workup to find the cause and direct treatment.

Post-op UTIs are most common in the elderly and in those undergoing surgery of the GU or GI systems.

(2) If systemic signs and symptoms are present or if the patient is immunocompromised or diabetic, antibiotics that cover Gram-positive organisms, both *Staphylococcus* spp. and *Streptococcus* spp., are indicated.

d. Septic thrombophlebitis requires vein stripping of the affected site because it will behave like an abscess and make antibiotic penetration difficult.

e. DVT

(1) DVT should be treated with anticoagulation using either heparin or low-molecular-weight heparin.

(2) For patients in whom anticoagulation is contraindicated, DVT progresses while on anticoagulation, or pulmonary embolism (PE) occurs while on anticoagulation, vena caval interruption with a Greenfield filter should be considered.

f. Intra-abdominal abscesses

(1) Intra-abdominal abscesses require either surgical debridement or percutaneous drainage, both in combination with appropriate antibiotics.

(2) Percutaneous drainage by an interventional radiologist can be performed as either a CT-guided or an ultrasound-guided procedure.

(3) Uniloculated abscesses are amenable to percutaneous drainage.

B. **Keloids and hypertrophic scars**

1. General characteristics

> There are little data to predict the development of keloids; treatment is often unsatisfactory.

a. Both keloids and hypertrophic scars represent abnormal healing and an imbalance between collagen deposition and degradation.

b. Keloids are more common in those with African and Asian heritage.

2. **Clinical features**

a. Keloids tend to extend beyond the original wound or trauma, whereas hypertrophic scars are usually limited to their original boundaries.

b. Hypertrophic tissue usually regresses without intervention, whereas keloid tissue requires intervention.

c. Diagnosis is established based on clinical findings.

3. **Treatment**

a. No single treatment modality has been shown to be effective across the board in all patients.

b. Topical triamcinolone (Kenalog), 40 mg/mL in a dosage of 2 mL every 6 to 8 weeks, has been shown to be effective. In addition, intralesional steroid injections have proven to be effective. However, side effects may include dermal atrophy, telangiectasia, and hypopigmentation.

c. Excisional surgery also can be used but is associated with a very high recurrence rate unless combined with other treatment modalities.

C. **Pressure ulcers**

1. General characteristics (see also Chapters 13 and 16)

> Pressure sores develop owing to immobility, moisture and shearing forces on the skin and underlying structures.

a. Pressure ulcers are linked to pressure and shear forces over bony prominences.

b. Most patients who develop pressure ulcers have an inability to change position and, thus, sustain long periods of uninterrupted pressure, with subsequent tissue ischemia.

c. Risk assessment can be performed by completing the Braden Risk Assessment Scale: sensory perception, moisture, activity, mobility, nutrition, and friction/shear.

d. Risk factors for the development for pressure ulcers include: poor mobility/immobility, poor nutrition, impaired blood flow, neuropathy or impaired sensation, darker skin pigmentation, type of surface the patient lays on, excess sedation or pain medication administration, older age, impaired mental status, urinary or fecal incontinence.

e. Patients with spinal cord injury are at the greatest risk of developing these types of ulcerations.

2. **Clinical characteristics:** Follow the National Pressure Ulcer Advisory Panel (Table 15-13).

3. Diagnostic procedures: Swabbed cultures are not routine as they only reflect surface colonization. Deep-tissue biopsy or deep-tissue cultures are the standard in differentiating between colonization and true infection.

4. **Treatment**

a. The most effective approach to pressure ulcers is prevention by frequent positioning of the patient, consideration of shear and friction when moving the patient, adequate nutrition, and removal of moisture.

b. Risk assessment identifies the most vulnerable patients. Utilization of advanced static mattresses or overlays is helpful.

c. Treatment should encompass a multimodal approach that includes the removal of the pressure source, supplemental nutritional support, and surgical intervention.

d. Reconstructive procedures are performed only after tissue cultures show that there is no evidence of infection.

e. Treatment can include skin grafts or rotational flaps. In some cases, diverting colostomies may be needed in order to heal extensive sacral pressure ulcers though their use is controversial and not universally accepted.

f. Sacral ulcers may be particularly challenging as they require that the surrounding tissue be kept free of urine and feces. Use of Foley catheters should be avoided where possible; Texas condom catheters should be utilized in males, and females can have urine collected by external catheter systems. Incontinence to stool may require use of fecal collection devices if the stool is liquid; in severe cases, patients may require colonic diversion to keep the sacral area free of fecal contamination.

g. Antibiotics should be reserved for patients who manifest clinical signs of septicemia.

> Prevention is best; once pressure ulcers are identified, coordination between wound care, surgery, and nutrition consultations can assist in the appropriate multimodal treatment.

D. **Necrotizing fasciitis**

1. General characteristics

a. Necrotizing fasciitis is a rare postoperative complication; it is more common in patients with diabetes mellitus, alcoholics, and IV drug abusers. The Food and Drug Administration (FDA) has identified the use of sodium-glucose cotransporter-2 (SGLT2) inhibitors as cause of necrotizing fasciitis of the perineum (Fournier's gangrene). Some case series have identified patients with diabetes mellitus as accounting for 20% to 30% of identified cases.

b. It is associated with mortality rates ranging from 25% to 70% in some studies.

c. It can be polymicrobial or caused by group A streptococci or clostridial infections. Saltwater necrotizing fasciitis is typically caused by *Vibrio* spp.

2. **Clinical characteristics:** Patients can present with a multitude of symptoms, including rapidly progressing erythema, tissue crepitus, marked tissue tenderness, high temperatures, tachycardia, hypotension, and an altered mental status.

Table 15-13 | **Classification of Pressure Ulcers**

Stage I	Intact skin with erythema that blanches
Stage II	Partial-thickness skin loss; may present as abrasion, blister, or shallow ulcer crater
Stage III	Full-thickness skin loss extending to the subcutaneous tissue but not beyond the fascia; crater with or without undermining of adjacent tissue
Stage IV	Full-thickness skin and subcutaneous tissue loss with extension into muscle, tendons, bone, or joint capsule

See also Figure 13-9

3. Diagnostic procedures

   a. Look for the triad: elevated white blood count (>14,000 cells/µL), elevated BUN (>15 mg/mL), and hyponatremia (<135 mmol/L). This triad is not found in all patients, but if present should prompt a heightened index of suspicion.

   b. Ultrasonography, CT, and magnetic resonance imaging (MRI) have been used to demarcate the affected regions before surgical intervention.

   c. Plain film radiographs are of use only if gas is present within the affected tissues.

4. **Treatment**

   a. Aggressive surgical debridement is the mainstay of therapy.

   b. Antibiotic therapy should cover all possible pathogens.

      (1) An initial therapeutic choice of a carbapenem of β-lactam/β-lactamase inhibitor along with clindamycin, as well as an agent effective against methicillin-resistant *S. aureus* (MRSA), such as vancomycin, daptomycin, or linezolid, is acceptable.

      (2) Hypersensitivity to antibiotic agents may require substitution with an aminoglycoside or fluoroquinolone, plus metronidazole.

      (3) It is important to monitor renal function and adjust dosages accordingly, because renal impairment is a major hallmark of this disease.

> Necrotizing fasciitis must be treated aggressively with both surgical and medical interventions to reduce mortality.

Laparoscopic and Bariatric Surgery

A. **Laparoscopic surgery**

   1. Currently, there are more than 4.8 million laparoscopic procedures performed annually in the United States.

   2. In many areas of surgery, it has been accepted as the "gold standard" of care without randomized prospective trials evaluating results. The laparoscopic approach is generally believed to reduce length of stay and risk of complications compared with the standard open approach.

   3. Complications of laparoscopic surgery can be broken down into those associated with access, creation of the pneumoperitoneum, and directly related to the proposed operative procedure.

   4. Access complications

      a. Perforation of bowel or vascular structures can occur during the introduction of the trochar. Risk is increased with the use of the closed technique of trochar insertion versus the open technique.

      b. Abdominal wall hematomas may develop.

      c. Complications also include umbilical wound infection or hernia formation.

   5. Pneumoperitoneum complications

      a. Intra-abdominal pressures >15 mm Hg during insufflation of CO_2 can impact on all organs and make ventilation difficult during anesthesia.

      b. CO_2 can be absorbed during the procedure and cause acid–base disturbances.

      c. The establishment of pneumoperitoneum with CO_2 can result in subcutaneous/mediastinal emphysema, pneumothorax, hypoxia, hypotension, CO_2 embolism, cardiovascular failure, and various cardiac arrhythmias of which bradycardia is most common.

   6. Cardiac output can decrease by up to 30% with an increase in systemic vascular resistance; therefore, arterial blood pressure is compensated for and maintained.

   7. Cardiac monitoring in borderline-risk cardiac patients may require preoperative and intraoperative monitoring.

> Suspected air embolism is managed by placing the patient in a Trendelenburg and left lateral decubitus position with 100% oxygen.

💡 Subtle
subcutaneous
emphysema may
only be detectable
during palpation or
auscultation of the
chest while performing
a postoperative physical
examination.

💡 Biliary tract
disease may
affect absorption of the
fat-soluble vitamins A,
D, E, and K, with vitamin
K deficiency causing
bleeding tendencies
requiring pre- or
perioperative vitamin K
administration.

💡 Iatrogenic ureteral
injuries can be
lessened by the use of
ureteral stents placed
preoperatively.

8. DVT can be associated with the establishment of pneumoperitoneum. Calf vein DVT is seen in 40% of the patients, and 15% have been found to have axillary vein DVT on follow-up examinations.

9. Subcutaneous emphysema of the anterior chest wall may be seen postoperatively as a normal variant. If associated with pneumothorax, the patient may show signs of desaturation or respiratory distress.

10. Complications associated with specific operative procedures:

   a. Cholecystectomy

      (1) Biliary injury is the most important complication of laparoscopic cholecystectomy. It is most commonly caused by misidentification of the hepatic ductal system.

      (2) Delayed stricture of the common bile duct because of thermal injury during dissection may occur.

   b. Antireflux surgery

      (1) Perforation of the stomach or esophagus is the most common complication.

      (2) Postoperative dysphagia, paraesophageal hernia, atelectasis, and pneumonia are common complications.

   c. Inguinal hernia surgery

      (1) Transabdominal preperitoneal herniorrhaphy is the most commonly used method of repair.

      (2) During dissection, potential intraoperative complications include injury to the epigastric vessels, bladder perforation, and injury to the spermatic cord.

      (3) Postoperative complications include wound hematoma or seroma, mesh infection, and neuralgia.

      (4) Urinary retention occurs in 3% to 7% of these patients.

      (5) Recurrence of the hernia can occur as a postoperative complication.

   d. Laparoscopic appendectomy: The most common complication in laparoscopic appendectomy is intra-abdominal abscess. For open appendectomy, the most common complication is wound infection.

   e. Laparoscopic colectomy

      (1) Mortality and morbidity are similar to that of open techniques.

      (2) Intraoperative complications include enterotomy, bleeding from the mesentery, and iatrogenic ureteral injuries.

      (3) Anastomotic leak is more common in patients who have had episodes of intraoperative or perioperative hypotension or who have had intraoperative or perioperative pressor utilization.

B. **Bariatric surgery**

   1. There are several types of bariatric surgeries including gastric bypass surgery, laparoscopic adjustable gastric banding (LAP-BAND), gastric sleeve, and biliopancreatic diversion.

   2. Bariatric surgery patients typically have many comorbidities: diabetes mellitus, OSA, hypertension, gastroesophageal reflux disease, and cardiovascular disease. Morbid obesity is in itself a significant risk for pulmonary postoperative complications.

   3. All the patients undergoing bariatric surgery should be closely monitored for at least 24 hours after the procedure. Particular attention should be paid to blood pressure, heart rate, and oxygen saturation.

   4. Short-term complications of bariatric procedures include: pneumonia; desaturation from OSA or hypoventilation syndrome; DVT; and bleeding from the anastomosis leading to unexplained tachycardia, hypotension, and desaturation. The single most important prognosticator for a postoperative bariatric complication is a persistent heart rate that remains >120 bpm for more than 4 hours.

5. Long-term complications of bariatric procedures are numerous:

a. Marginal, anastomotic, and stomal ulcers present as abdominal pain, nausea, and vomiting. Severe presentations include bleeding, obstruction, and perforation. All patients who have had bariatric surgery and present with vague abdominal symptoms should be carefully evaluated for the presence of one of these ulcers.

b. Postoperative ventral hernia is more common in open procedures.

c. Vitamin and mineral deficiencies associated with impaired vitamin B_{12}, calcium, and vitamin D absorption may be observed. Common manifestations include anemia, renal stones, and osteopenia or osteoporosis.

d. Because of the small size of the gastric pouch, patients may become dehydrated because they cannot take in large amounts of water and need to become accustomed to drinking water more frequently.

e. For the first 3 months after the procedure, patients may complain of nonspecific symptoms including body aches, dry skin, and hair loss or thinning.

f. Noninsulinoma pancreatogenous hypoglycemia syndrome may occur in patients as they experience symptoms related to hypoglycemia.

Practice Questions

Directions: Each of the numbered items or incomplete statements in this section is followed by a list of answers or completions of the statement. Select the one lettered answer or completion that is best in each case.

1. A 27-year-old woman with a history of gestational diabetes (2 years ago) and recurrent cholecystitis presents for preoperative clearance prior to a laparoscopic cholecystectomy. Which of the following would *not* be indicated as part of her preoperative lab workup?
A. Complete blood count
B. Serum creatinine
C. Arterial blood gas
D. Hepatic enzymes
E. Glucose

2. A 71-year-old man undergoes left hip repair surgery after a motor vehicle collision. Which of the following is the best choice for DVT prophylaxis in this patient?
A. Enoxaparin
B. Warfarin
C. Thromboembolic stockings
D. IVC filter

3. A 75-year-old woman sustained a mechanical fall from standing and comes to the emergency department for evaluation via ambulance. Her primary survey reveals GCS score of 14 with decreased breath sounds, hyperresonance, and subcutaneous emphysema in the right thorax. What is the next step in immediate management?
A. Arterial blood gas
B. Chest CT
C. Chest MRI
D. Needle decompression
E. Thoracotomy

4. A 31-year-old man comes to the emergency department via ambulance after having fallen from his bicycle. Friends who accompanied him provide information that he was not wearing a helmet. Currently he is muttering about an elephant he saw at the circus; opens his eyes only to sternal rub; and can localize the injury in his right elbow region and his head. What is the GCS rating at this moment?
A. 15
B. 13
C. 10
D. 9

5. A 55-year-old man comes to the emergency department with severe burns. He has varying second- and third-degree burns to the head, both arms, and the entire chest and stomach from a gas grill accident. What is the approximate surface area of his injury?
A. 18%
B. 27%
C. 36%
D. 45%
E. 54%

6. A 58-year-old man develops a fever of 100.9°F, 12 hours after orthopedic shoulder surgery. The patient has been properly dosed with prophylactic anticoagulation and has no leg pain. Physical examination reveals bronchial breath sounds at the left base; the surgical site is appropriately tender but without drainage. What is the best next step in the management and treatment of his fever?
A. Sequential compression devices and early mobilization
B. Abdominal CT and consideration of drain placement
C. Chest x-ray and incentive spirometry
D. Empiric antibiotics to cover nosocomial UTI
E. Empiric antibiotics for *Staphylococcus aureus* wound infection

7. An 82-year-old nursing home patient presents with head trauma after a fall. She has an altered mental status and cranial nerve deficits on examination; cardiovascular and pulmonary examinations are unremarkable. What is the most likely diagnosis?

A. Ischemic stroke
B. Hemorrhagic stroke
C. Basilar skull fracture
D. Epidural hematoma
E. Subdural hematoma

8. A 36-year-old woman is brought to the emergency department via ambulance after being rescued from a house fire. She has 36% of her body surface area covered in second- and third-degree burns. Her arms and legs are characterized by a white leathery appearance and no response to light touch. What is the description of these burns?

A. First-degree burns
B. Superficial second-degree burns
C. Deep second-degree burns
D. Third-degree burns
E. Fourth-degree burns

9. A 40-year-old woman presents for evaluation 1 year after a surgical procedure with complaints of fatigue and occasional nausea. She had often become dehydrated, but this has improved in the last few months. In addition, she states that she has had significant weight loss in the past year. Her recent lab work reveals a macrocytic anemia. What is the most likely type of surgery that she underwent?

A. Bariatric surgery
B. Cholecystectomy
C. Appendectomy
D. Colectomy
E. Inguinal surgery repair

10. According to ASPEN criteria, surgical nutrition goals for an intensive care unit patient are in what range?

A. 10–15 kcal/kg/d
B. 15–20 kcal/kg/d
C. 25–30 kcal/kg/d
D. 30–35 kcal/kg/d

11. A 68-year-old man underwent a left total knee replacement 2 days ago. Today, he has a fever of 101.2°F and increased erythema and tenderness around the surgical site. You suspect a surgical site infection. What pathogen is most likely involved?

A. *Enterobacter* species
B. *Escherichia coli*
C. *Staphylococcus aureus*
D. *Pseudomonas aeruginosa*
E. *Candida albicans*

12. A 74-year-old man has been bedbound for 16 days after surgery for multiple injuries sustained in a motor vehicle collision but is overall stable and improving. Skin examination reveals an area of erythema with an abrasion-like appearance overlying his sacrum. What staging best describes this pressure ulcer?

A. Stage I
B. Stage II
C. Stage III
D. Stage IV

Practice Answers

1. **C.** *Surgery; Diagnostic Studies; Preoperative Clearance*

Complete blood count (C), serum creatinine, and hepatic enzymes are indicated as routine labs for a patient undergoing GI surgery and receiving anesthesia. With a gestational diabetes history, glucose should be checked as well. ABG would only be necessary if the patient had an underlying cardiopulmonary disease.

2. **A.** *Surgery; Health Maintenance; DVT*

Enoxaparin or other low-molecular-weight heparin is the preferred anticoagulation for trauma patients. Warfarin is appropriate in many orthopedic cases, typically nontrauma. Stockings are not sufficient anticoagulation prophylaxis. An IVC filter is indicated in patients with recurrent emboli or a contraindication to anticoagulants.

3. **D.** *Surgery; Clinical Intervention; Pneumothorax*

Needle decompression is indicated. Decreased breath sounds, hyperresonance, and subcutaneous emphysema describe a tension pneumothorax in this trauma patient. Clinical diagnosis is made, and imaging is not the appropriate next step in management because of the time-sensitive nature of the required treatment. ABG is not immediately necessary to diagnose or treat this condition.

4. **C.** *Surgery; History and PE; Head Injury*

This patient's GCS score is 10, indicating a moderate head injury. He opens eyes to pain—score of 2; he is mumbling

inappropriate words—score of 3; and he can localize pain—score of 5.

5. **D.** *Surgery: History and PE; Burns*

Using the rule of nines: the head represents 9%; each arm is 9%; and the front of the torso is 18%. The final calculation is: $9 + (9 \times 2) + 18 = 45\%$.

6. **C.** *Surgery; Diagnostic Studies; URI; Atelectasis*

Atelectasis is the most common cause of low-grade fever in the first 24 hours postoperatively. He should be evaluated with radiography and encouraged to perform incentive spirometry. DVT may cause fever but would likely be associated with leg pain; the use of compression devices and early ambulation help prevent this. Abdominal CT and consideration of a drain placement is appropriate after abdominal surgery if an abscess forms, which could cause a fever. Nosocomial UTI and wound infection with *Staphylococcus aureus* could cause fever but would present with dysuria or pain at the infection site, respectively.

7. **E.** *Surgery; Diagnosis; Subdural Hematoma*

Subdural hematomas are more likely in elderly (and alcoholic) patients, resulting from trauma to bridging veins, often from a fall. Epidural hematoma typically presents with a lucid interval, and often with more significant neurologic findings. Her physical examination findings do not support a diagnosis of stroke (hemiplegia) or a basilar skull fracture (raccoon eyes, lid ecchymosis).

8. D. *Surgery; Diagnosis; Burns*

Third-degree burns are characterized as skin with a dry, white, leathery, or charred appearance, with no sensation. First-degree burns involve erythema, pain, and no blisters. Superficial second-degree burns are moist with thin-walled, fluid-filled blisters that blanch with pressure and are painful. Deep second-degree burns have thicker-walled blisters, exhibit a mixture of erythema and pallor, and are painful. Fourth-degree burns are characterized by significant charring and exposure of underlying structures.

9. A. *Surgery; Clinical Intervention; Bariatric Surgery*

Bariatric surgery often results in B_{12} deficiency and related anemia, typically months to a year after surgery, because of removal or shortening of the ilium where intrinsic factor–cobalamin complex is absorbed. Short-term complications result from the smaller size of the gastric pouch and can include body aches, dry skin, dehydration, and symptoms related to hypoglycemia.

10. C. *Surgery; Health Maintenance; Nutrition*

The goal for caloric intake is 25 to 30 kcal/kg/d. In a patient at risk for developing refeeding syndrome, the goals are closer to 20 kcal/kg/d.

11. C. *Surgery; Basic Science; Wound Infection*

Staphylococcus aureus is the most common pathogen found to infect surgical sites. The other species are causative agents for infection but not as commonly as *S. aureus*. For treatment, antibiotic coverage should include MRSA until wound culture results can guide a narrow spectrum.

12. B. *History and PE; Diagnosis; Pressure Ulcer*

Stage II pressure ulcer represents partial-thickness skin loss, with an appearance similar to an abrasion, or blisters. Stage I is limited to skin with blanching erythema. Stage III is full-thickness skin loss typically with a crater of an ulcer. Stage IV is full-thickness skin loss including subcutaneous tissue resulting in visualization of underlying structures.

16 | Geriatrics
Kathy Kemle

Background

A. The number of years that an individual can expect to live at birth has been increasing in all industrialized and many developing countries. But in the United States in 2017, life expectancy fell for the first time. Overall life expectancy was impacted by a decrease for white males as the statistics did not change for females or nonwhite populations.

B. In general, it is estimated that persons who reach age 65 will have an average life expectancy of an additional 18 to 20 years. The exceptions to this are black males for whom life expectancy is shorter and Hispanic females for whom it is longer.

C. Longer life expectancy coupled with a declining birth rate results in overall aging of the population. The number of persons >65 years of age worldwide is estimated to be 1.6 billion or 17% of the population by the year 2050.

D. This aging phenomenon brings with it a new focus on geriatrics owing to higher burdens of chronic disease and greater use of health care resources. About half of persons 85 and older have difficulty walking or climbing stairs. In 2014, those aged 65 and older comprised 15% of the U.S. population but accounted for 33.6% of total U.S. health care expenditures.

Patient Care

A. **Normal changes of aging**

    1. Individuals and their organ systems age at varying rates, making the elderly the most heterogeneous group in the population.

    2. Clinically significant aging changes by system are listed in Table 16-1.

B. **Comprehensive geriatric assessment**

    1. Comprehensive geriatric assessment has been shown to improve patient placement and functional status, and it provides a baseline for comparison of future status changes. Even with a greater number of diagnoses discovered, fewer medications are used in patients who are followed by a comprehensive geriatric team.

    2. Assessment encompasses cognitive status, physical evaluation, functional status, psychological status, nutritional status, and socioeconomic status. Table 16-2 lists some commonly used assessment instruments.

    3. Functional status includes activities of daily living and instrumental activities of daily living (Table 16-3).

    4. Assessment of driving skills is difficult because of the multidimensional nature of the tasks involved and the lack of easily administered standardized assessment tools. The Clinician's Guide to Assessment and Counseling Older Drivers, developed by the National Highway Transportation Safety Administration and the American Geriatrics Society, focuses on visual acuity, visual fields, testing of muscular strength and range

> Assessment for driving ability is multidimensional: visual acuity, visual fields, muscle strength and range, reflexes, cognitive ability, and maze testing.

Table 16-1 | Common Changes in Aging

Dermatologic	Loss of rete pegs (intermittent regular protrusions of the epidermis layer); thinning skin; loss of subcutaneous fat; fragile skin; decrease in collagen and elastin; increased photoaging
Pulmonary	Decline in forced vital capacity; less effective cough; decline in forced expiratory volume; increased fibrosis; less elastin; decreased chest wall compliance
Immune system	Decline in B- and T-cells function (most changes result from decreased nutrition rather than aging alone)
Cardiovascular	Decline in compliance; increased wall thickness; decreased maximal heart rate; decreased cardiac output; increased systemic vascular resistance; increased reliance on atrial contraction for ventricular filling; baroreceptor dysfunction
Endocrine	Impaired glucose tolerance; decreased testosterone and estrogen
Gastrointestinal	Impaired swallowing; slower transit time; decreased gastric acid; slight gallbladder duct dilation
Genitourinary	Vulvar and vaginal atrophy; prostatic hypertrophy; increased uninhibited bladder spasms; urethral atrophy
Musculoskeletal	Loss of fluid in collagen; decreased elasticity; decrease in myocytes
Neurologic	Slower response times; decline in vibratory and proprioceptive senses; decline in righting reflexes
Vision	Increased lens opacity; decreased peripheral vision; decreased accommodation
Hearing	Loss of cochlear cells; increased and stickier cerumen
Renal	Variable decline with aging

Table 16-2 | Instruments for Geriatric Assessments

Cognition	Mini-Mental Status Examination Clock Drawing Test Yesavage Geriatric Depression Scale Blessed Dementia Scale Categorical Word Fluency Short Portable Mental Status Questionnaire Montreal Cognitive Assessment (MOCA) Scale Saint Louis University Medical Status Exam (SLUMS)
Function	Physical Self-Maintenance Rating Scale Lawton–Brody Function Scales (ADLs, IADLs) Performance of Activities of Daily Living
Nutrition	Mini-Nutritional Assessment Tool and its Short Form; anthropomorphic metrics
Mobility	Tinetti Get-Up-and-Go Test; 4-stage balance test

ADLs, activities of daily living; IADLs, instrumental activities of daily living.

Table 16-3 | Activities of Daily Living and Instrumental Activities of Daily Living

Activities of Daily Living	Instrumental Activities of Daily Living
Bathing	Telephoning; email
Grooming	Meal preparation
Dressing	Shopping
Mobility	Finances
Toileting	Stairs
Eating	Reading
Transferring	Laundry
	Housework
	Transportation
	Medications
	Employment

of motion, and on cognitive assessment tools: the Montreal Cognitive Assessment Test, Trails B, and the maze.

C. Prevention

1. Medicare provides for an Initial Preventive Physical Examination done only once within 12 months of Medicare Part B enrollment. If the provider accepts Medicare assignment, there is no charge for the beneficiary.

2. Medicare provides payment for annual wellness visits for beneficiaries, which are designed to establish a personalized health plan. Under the traditional Medicare plan, there is no cost (no deductible or copay) to the beneficiary for this visit. It is *not* a routine physical exam but is meant to improve individual health by identifying risk factors and assisting the patient to develop their own plan for good health. Physician assistants (PAs) may perform these screenings and counsel patients on their individual preventive needs. See Table 16-4 for required elements of the encounter. Please be aware that these visits do not include routine laboratories, and beneficiaries may be responsible for their own deductibles and copays. Only one visit may be billed per 12 months. See Medicare Learning Network at CMS ICN 905706 August 2018.

3. The efficacy of many preventive services in older adults has not been defined.

4. Table 16-5 lists routine tests recommended for the elderly as well as screening procedures that are generally not appropriate.

   a. The Tdap (tetanus, diphtheria, and pertussis) vaccine (if not previously vaccinated) followed by the tetanus and diphtheria toxoid (Td) booster is recommended every 10 years.

   b. The pneumococcal vaccine (indicated once after age 65 years) and yearly influenza vaccines should be strongly encouraged in the elderly because they are at greater risk for poor outcomes from these diseases.

   c. Currently, the 23-valent (PPSV23) pneumococcal vaccine is recommended to those eligible and vaccine-naive (one dose). In 2016, the 13-valent pneumococcal conjugate vaccine (PREVNAR) was initially recommended. In those with additional underlying conditions and/or who previously received the PREVNAR vaccine, the 23-valent version is then given 12 months later.

   d. The herpes zoster vaccine is indicated once on reaching 50 years, primarily to reduce the incidence of postherpetic neuralgia. Shingrix, in a two-dose series, is recommended as the first line. Zostavax is no longer available in the United States.

   e. The clinician should monitor the Centers for Disease Control and Prevention website or download their app for the latest information as recommendations change frequently.

D. Pharmacology

1. General

   a. The geriatric population is particularly vulnerable to adverse effects of medication; therefore, any new symptom should provoke a careful review of the patient's drug

> 💡 Immunization for geriatric patients: yearly influenza, single-dose pneumococcal, single-dose zoster, and tetanus/diphtheria/pertussis booster.

Table 16-4 | **Medicare Annual Wellness Checklist of Required Services**

Updated medical, family, surgical, and social history
Medication review including over the counter and supplements
Completion of Medicare Preventive Physical Examination form
Functional ability and safety screening
Completion of counseling and referral form (copy to patient)/personalized for individual
Completion of Geriatric Depression Scale (may be done by office staff)
Completion of Mini-Mental Status Examination or other cognitive screening
Advance care planning

Table 16-5 | Recommended Screening Procedures for Older Adults

Height/weight	At least annually
Blood pressure	At least annually
Vision	Annually
Hearing	Annually
Depression	Annually
Alcohol questionnaire	Periodically; base frequency on patient history
Lipids	Every 5 years; more often in CAD, DM, PAD, prior stroke
Bone density	Women: at least once after age 65 years; men: at least once after age 70 years
Glucose (diabetes screening)	Every 3 years in patients with BP >135/80 mm Hg
Mammography	Every 2 years in women age 50–74 years
Pap smear	Every 3 years; may cease if all Pap smears have been normal until age 65 years; if never tested, stop after two negative annual smears. Women without a cervix should not undergo Pap smears.
Stool hemoccult	Annually
Colonoscopy	Every 10 years from age 50 to 75 years
Smoking cessation	Every visit
Dental care	At least annually
Calcium intake	At least annually
Exercise	Each visit
Safety counseling	At least annually
Immunizations	Pneumococcal—23-valent at least once after age 65 years; evaluate for PREVNAR 13; influenza—annually; tetanus, every 10 years; zoster—once at age 50 years or older, with Shingrix
Aspirin	81 mg by mouth daily if history of CAD unless contraindicated
Annual blood chemistry panel	Based on clinical presentation
Annual complete blood count	Based on clinical presentation
Annual electrocardiography	Based on clinical presentation
Annual chest radiography	Based on clinical presentation

[a]Consider chest CT scan for individuals with a smoking history of ≥30 years; covered by Medicare.

BP, blood pressure; CAD, coronary artery disease; DM, diabetes mellitus; PAD, peripheral arterial disease.

Private insurers may have other quality metrics that require more frequent or different screenings. The clinician should use appropriate tests based on the history and expected life expectancy, as well as, most importantly, the patient's wishes.

list, including over-the-counter, herbal, or homeopathic preparations, as well as prescription medications.

b. Adverse drug reactions (ADRs) or events are the most common unintended negative medical events, accounting for up to one-third of hospitalizations in older adults. The most common drugs associated with ADR-related hospital admissions are shown in Table 16-6.

c. All clinicians who care for older adults should be familiar with and refer to the "Potentially Inappropriate Medications for the Elderly According to the Revised Beers Criteria (2019)."

> Up to one-third of hospitalizations in the elderly are caused by adverse drug events; medications with anticholinergic effects are most commonly implicated.

2. Pharmacokinetics (absorption, distribution, metabolism, and excretion) is altered during the aging process, which results in a higher frequency of drug-related adverse events.

a. Altered absorption from the gastrointestinal (GI) tract is not a certainty of aging; however, a decline in gastric acid may affect the absorption of those drugs that require a low pH for full absorption.

b. Interstitial and skin perfusion declines, resulting in slower absorption of topical preparations and subcutaneous or intramuscular injections.

Table 16-6 | Drugs Commonly Implicated in Adverse Drug Events

α-Blockers	Cyproheptadine
α-Agonists	Glyburide
Barbiturates	Megestrol Disopyramide
Reserpine	Cyclobenzaprine (and other relaxants)
Diphenhydramine	Indomethacin (all NSAIDs)
Doxepin	Dicyclomine
Diazepam	Chlorpropamide
Amitriptyline	
Meperidine	Meprobamate
Trazodone	Metoclopramide
Digoxin	Chloral hydrate

NSAIDs, nonsteroidal anti-inflammatory drugs.

Table 16-7 | Medications with Unexpected Anticholinergic Effects

Furosemide (all loop diuretics)	Digitalis
H$_2$-blockers	NSAIDs Cox 1 > Cox 2*
Clonidine	Amantadine
Opioids	Some antiarrhythmics, especially disopyramide
SSRIs	β-Blockers, especially propranolol
Benzodiazepines	Most antipsychotics
Tricyclic antidepressants	Fluoroquinolones
Antituberculin drugs, especially isoniazid and rifampin	Amiodarone
Cox 2 associated with increased CV risk	

CV, cardiovascular; SSRI, selective serotonin reuptake inhibitors; NSAIDs, nonsteroidal anti-inflammatory drugs.

> Regarding altered pharmacokinetics, watch for altered absorption issues and decreased hepatic or renal clearance problems.

c. Metabolism of drugs (biomedical modification and degradation mostly as a result of enzymatic processes) is not changed significantly by aging but may be affected by the disease.

d. Moderate reductions in free water and serum proteins occur with aging, resulting in higher active drug concentrations. Malnutrition adds to the decline in serum proteins, magnifying this effect.

e. Decline in liver mass and hepatic blood flow, as well as declines in renal clearance, affect drug clearance. Dosages of many agents should be reduced. Renal insufficiency may be present even in persons with normal serum creatinine levels, so doses should be based on known or estimated creatinine clearance. Glomerular filtration rate is a more sensitive and accurate indicator of renal function but is less readily available.

3. Pharmacodynamics (the effect of medication on targeted tissue) is difficult to measure in the elderly because of altered pharmacokinetics. The elderly are more sensitive to the effects of some drugs, such as warfarin, and centrally acting drugs, such as benzodiazepines.

a. Certain drugs and drug combinations with high risk of adverse consequences should be used with caution and used rarely in the elderly (Tables 16-6 to 16-8).

b. Any drug with anticholinergic properties is likely to produce confusion in the elderly, and effects of multiple drugs are cumulative. Many commonly prescribed agents have anticholinergic effects (Table 16-8).

c. Side effects and drug interactions may be readily apparent (rash and vomiting) or more subtle (change in personality, somnolence, delirium, and weight loss).

Table 16-8 | Medications Associated with Delirium

Antibacterials	Cardiovascular
Antithrombotics	Corticosteroids
Anticonvulsants	Hypoglycemic
Antineoplastics	Nonsteroidals
Antipsychotics	

4. About 30% (or in some estimates more than 50%) of community elderly use some form of alternative therapy, such as saw palmetto for prostatism, glucosamine, or chondroitin for osteoarthritis, and melatonin for insomnia. Because there may be impurities or drug interactions with prescription pharmaceuticals, clinicians should ask about *all* of these and ideally inspect the bottles brought by the patient.

E. **Assessment and management of the hospitalized older adult**

1. Older age alone is not a contraindication to surgical procedures, but mortality or morbidity rates are higher for those with comorbidities.

2. Iatrogenic problems, especially delirium, are more common in older adults.

   a. Delirium is characterized by alteration of consciousness, waxing and waning of symptoms, psychomotor retardation or agitation, and decreased attention span.

   b. Delirium is a *medical emergency and should be evaluated promptly*. It is associated with poor outcomes. The risk of mortality remains high, with rates ranging from 35% to 40% even at 1-year postdischarge from acute care settings.

   c. Delirium is most common with surgical admissions, especially orthopedic and urologic procedures.

   d. Evaluation and management of delirium includes the following requirements:

      (1) Maintain a high index of suspicion because delirium is underrecognized and undertreated.

      (2) Perform a complete physical examination, including neurologic and rectal examination.

      (3) Identify and treat reversible factors (unnecessary medications, pain, infection, anemia, dehydration, congestive heart failure (CHF), electrolyte imbalance, central nervous system oxygenation, sensory deprivation, fecal impaction, and urinary retention); these are often additive, so all must be considered and addressed.

      (4) Encourage family visitation; remove or avoid restraints when possible; mobilize the patient; assist with feeding; reduce noise; and provide familiar surroundings, including assistive devices such as eyeglasses and hearing aids.

      (5) Recommend lorazepam or preferably haloperidol in small doses if medication is necessary to permit thorough evaluation. Be aware of potentially lethal side effects such as prolonged QT, potentially leading to fatal arrhythmias.

   e. Hospital programs that use volunteers to offer companionship and support for the hospitalized elderly, such as Hospital Elder Life Program (HELP; http://www.hospitalelderlifeprogram.org), have been effective in preventing delirium, reducing its rate from 16% to 9% in one study.

> The key to managing delirium is *prevention*: identification and resolution of any reversible triggers including medications, infection, pain, illness, or sensory deprivation.

F. **Rehabilitation**

1. Sites of care include rehabilitation hospitals, subacute placements in long-term care facilities, outpatient facilities, and home.

2. Premorbid function is the best predictor of outcome after stroke or serious fracture.

3. Mobility aids, such as canes and walkers, as well as functional assistive devices are helpful, especially if used in conjunction with education on their use by a physical or occupational therapist.

G. Palliative care

1. As it becomes clear that a disease process is not amenable to further treatment or cure, the focus needs to shift to more intense concern with symptom amelioration.

2. Older adults and demented persons experience pain just as younger individuals do but may have more difficulty in expressing their sensations or describing them as painful. For example, chest pain owing to myocardial infarction may be felt as tightness or soreness.

   a. Nociceptive pain arises in somatic or visceral tissues and is usually described as aching, stabbing, or intense pressure and pain.

   b. Neuropathic pain originates in disordered central or peripheral nerves and is described as electrical, burning, shooting, or stinging.

   c. Pain management involves pharmacologic and nonpharmacologic modalities.

      (1) Pharmacologic

         (a) Dosing of pain medication should be titrated in the elderly because these patients are often very susceptible to side effects and interactions.

         (b) Pain is best managed by constant dosing of small amounts rather than less-frequent larger doses. This produces better control of discomfort while minimizing side effects. Sustained-release preparations are useful in those with stable pain patterns and should be started after titration of shorter-acting formulations.

         (c) Nociceptive pain

            i. Mild pain should be managed with acetaminophen. In general, unless treating bony metastases, avoid nonsteroidal anti-inflammatory drugs (NSAIDs) because of the risk for GI bleeding and renal toxicity. Topical NSAIDs may be useful for mild arthritic complaints. Avoid acetaminophen doses higher than 3 g per day in robust persons and 2 g per day in the frail.

            ii. Moderate to severe pain should be managed with hydrocodone or acetaminophen, oxycodone, morphine, transdermal fentanyl, or methadone. In general, avoid tramadol as it can cause delirium in older adults and is not very effective.

            iii. Opioid-induced nausea can be minimized by avoiding rapid administration of large doses in those who are opioid-naive. It will predictably be resolved in 48 hours. If antiemetic medication is needed, haloperidol or prochlorperazine is preferable. Haloperidol has fewer extrapyramidal symptoms (EPS) if it is given in IV rather than oral form. They may even be started prophylactically. This type of nausea is mediated in the chemoreceptor trigger zone via dopamine and serotonin systems and does not respond well to antihistamines. Another potential agent is mirtazapine, which is active at multiple receptor sites and is usually well tolerated.

            iv. Sedation occurs with opioid use but fades with time.

            v. Respiratory depression caused by opioid use can be avoided by starting at low doses with slow titration. It does not occur until sedation, loss of reflexes, and lack of pupillary response develop sequentially.

            vi. Unlike the other opioid side effects, constipation will not decrease with time. It must be treated by initiation of stimulant laxatives when the opioid is started. Another option when stimulants fail, μ-opioid receptor antagonists, such as methylnaltrexone bromide (Relistor) and similar agents, are designed to reduce constipation induced by opioids. They have been approved for patients with advanced disease who require continuous opioid treatment to manage pain.

> Pharmacologic pain management in palliative care centers on frequent, small, and low doses.

vii. A rare but frightening side effect of opioids is a fine red pruritic rash, which is caused by histamine release and is often mistaken for allergy. The rash rapidly dissipates without treatment, but pruritus may require antihistamines.

(d) Neuropathic pain

i. Neuropathic pain should be managed with anticonvulsant medication (especially the pentin agents, such as gabapentin, or pregabalin), duloxetine, or lidocaine topical patch. The pentins may be associated with excess sedation and respiratory depression especially if used with opioids. Avoid older anticonvulsants if possible because of sedation and other toxicities. Duloxetine may have unacceptable side effects in the elderly.

ii. Methadone is also highly effective for this type of pain but must be dosed very carefully, as its metabolism is highly variable, and overdose is more likely with this agent. Its use should be limited to those with experience in palliative care.

iii. Avoid tricyclic antidepressants because of their potential for delirium and other anticholinergic effects. Rarely, low doses may be useful for those who do not respond to less toxic agents.

> 💡 Neuropathic pain in the elderly can be managed with anticonvulsants, i.e., gabapentin.

(2) Nonpharmacologic control of pain can be achieved through many means (music, relaxation techniques, aromatherapy, and massage), cold or warm applications, positioning, splinting, electrical stimulation, hypnosis, acupuncture, or biofeedback. For most patients, it should be the first therapy and/or added to opioids or other pharmaceuticals.

3. Nonpain symptoms of chronic disease may be just as distressing as pain symptoms.

a. Nausea, dyspnea, fatigue, and anxiety are common.

b. Treatment of underlying cause and supportive measures are key to management.

c. Dyspnea is the subjective sensation of breathlessness and does not always correlate with pulse oximetry. It responds well to low-dose opioids, a circulating fan, oxygen, and other treatments directed at its cause(s).

d. Fatigue is common in advanced disease and is managed by advising rest and occasionally using steroids and stimulants.

H. Geriatric syndromes

1. Syndromes are multifactorial and require aggressive, multifaceted investigation.

2. Immobility is a great disabler.

a. Encouraging the elderly to be active in even a limited exercise program is imperative. Exercise improves balance, has cognitive and physical benefits, and preserves functional capacity.

b. Table 16-9 lists the most common consequences of immobility.

Table 16-9 | Consequences of Immobility

General deconditioning	Depression
Cardiac deconditioning	Dementia
Renal lithiasis	Delirium
Pressure wounds	Hyperglycemia
Deep venous thrombosis	Worsened chronic disease
Pulmonary embolism	Constipation
Urinary retention, urinary tract infection	Fecal impaction
Atelectasis	Pneumonia
Reflux disease	Osteoporosis

Table 16-10 | Common Drug Classes Frequently Associated with Falls

Anticonvulsants
Antihypertensives (especially central acting)
Benzodiazepines (especially long acting)
Tricyclic and other antidepressants
Hypnotics
Diuretics
Vasodilators
Opioids

3. Accidents are the fifth leading cause of death in the elderly, and two-thirds of these are falls. Community dwellers should be asked yearly about any falls. If a fall is reported, further evaluation should be completed, including physical examination and medication review. A simple method to evaluate for fall risk is to ask the patient to arise from a chair without using their arms. Ability to complete this maneuver indicates adequate proximal muscle strength and balance.

   a. Falls are the result of disordered interaction between the individuals and their environment.

   b. Age-related changes in gait, balance, vision, and hearing as well as disease predispose older adults to falling.

   c. Falls may be a sign of acute illness or delirium, most often urinary tract infection (UTI), exacerbation of CHF, or pneumonia.

   d. Evaluation of a fall should include a full history, physical examination including orthostatic blood pressure measurements, assessment and management of any injuries, and a search for the factors that may have precipitated the fall. Many medications are associated with falls (Table 16-10).

4. Urinary incontinence (see Chapter 6)

   a. Incontinence is *not* a normal part of aging; new onset requires evaluation and may indicate infection.

   b. Falls are often the result of an overactive bladder, which may cause the individual to rush to the bathroom.

   c. Medications used for urge pattern incontinence are anticholinergic and, therefore, of limited use in the elderly population. A new agent, with less anticholinergic potential, mirabegron (a β-adrenergic agonist), is another option. It has not been fully studied in older adults and has been associated with elevated blood pressure and tachycardia; thus, careful monitoring is imperative.

   d. Diuretics and drugs such as caffeine and other xanthine derivatives may exacerbate incontinence.

   e. Behavioral techniques such as frequent or prompted voiding are often useful for urge incontinence. Acupuncture has proven effective for some patients.

5. Cognitive impairment

   a. Impairment of cognition is *not* a normal part of aging.

   b. Mild cognitive impairment

      (1) Mild cognitive impairment is characterized by deficits in cognition, especially memory, without deficiencies in activities of daily living.

      (2) It may progress to dementia in susceptible individuals, especially those with other risk factors such as lower educational level, history of head trauma, sedentary lifestyle, lack of cognitive or social stimulation, or history of diabetes/metabolic syndrome or hypertension.

Fall risk is elevated by changes in gait, balance, vision, hearing, medication use, underlying illness, and psychosocial state.

(3) Treatment with acetylcholinesterase inhibitors has not been shown to retard progression to dementia.

c. Dementia (see Chapter 11)

(1) Dementia is a progressive decline in cognitive function with associated deficits in instrumental and activities of daily living. Unlike delirium, dementia is generally irreversible.

(2) There are many recognized causes of dementia and all result in loss of intellectual capacity, eventually involving all activities of daily living.

(3) Chronic dementia progresses to a terminal phase that is characterized by immobility, eating difficulties, and frequent infections.

d. Behavioral complications of dementia

(1) Troubling behaviors are common in dementia and cause a great burden for caregivers and safety issues for patients.

(2) Medications may modify some target behaviors but not all; medications can be associated with undesirable side effects.

(3) Behaviors are managed best by environmental manipulation.

(4) Antipsychotic medications are *not* approved by the U.S. Food and Drug Administration (FDA) for this purpose and carry a black box warning for increased mortality in these patients.

(5) No drug therapy works well.

(a) Acetylcholinesterase inhibitors and memantine as well as anticonvulsants and β-blockers may be helpful, but studies on efficacy for behavior are conflicting.

(b) Benzodiazepines, especially lorazepam in small doses, are the recommended agents for sedation if drugs must be used.

(6) Table 16-11 describes common behaviors seen in dementia and their management.

> Unlike delirium, dementia is progressive and irreversible; management of patient environment is crucial.

6. Dizziness

a. One of the most common complaints in primary care, dizziness is a sensation of light-headedness, spinning, or impending syncope. It is encountered frequently in older adults because age-related changes in balance predispose them to this disorder. Older adults rely on vision more than younger people and invariably have loss of proprioception and vestibular function.

b. Dizziness is classified as vertigo (the sensation of rotational movement of self or surroundings) or non-vertigo (presyncope, disequilibrium, unsteadiness, floating, or light-headedness).

Table 16-11 | Behaviors Seen in Dementia and Their Management

Behavior	Management Options
Wandering	Provide a safe place to wander Patient identification system (bracelets, MedAlert) Identify and avoid precipitants Sedatives (last resort)
Screaming	Search for cause and remove or ameliorate Distraction; Consider pain and therapeutic trial of an analgesic
Aggression	Identify and avoid precipitants Sedatives
Poor impulse control	Anticonvulsants; mood stabilizers
Restlessness/agitation	Consider depression
Hallucinations	If bothersome, use atypical antipsychotics If Parkinson's or Lewy body disease, use pimavanserin, quetiapine

    c. Historical accuracy is the key to successfully establishing the diagnosis.

    d. Examination should include orthostatics, observation of gait, a check for nystagmus, as well as cardiac and neurologic examinations.

    e. Treatment varies with the cause.

    f. Prognosis for recovery is good in three-fourths of patients.

    g. Non-vertiginous

        (1) Disequilibrium is a sensation of unsteadiness and is caused by vestibulopathies, visual and musculoskeletal disorders, and neuropathies or anxiety or depression disorders. Canes or walkers often are useful.

        (2) Presyncope is the sensation that a faint is imminent and is caused by decreased cerebral perfusion, usually because of orthostatic hypotension or vagally mediated cardiac events. Advise the patient to arise slowly, and correct reversible causes.

        (3) Light-headedness is a vaguer sensation and often is psychiatric in origin. A trial of antidepressants may be warranted.

7. Syncope

    a. Syncope is defined as a sudden, transient loss of consciousness not resulting from trauma. The occurrence of syncope increases with age.

    b. Common causes include arrhythmias, aortic stenosis, carotid sinus hypersensitivity, myocardial infarction, hypoglycemia, orthostatic hypotension, postprandial hypotension, psychogenic disorders, pulmonary embolus, and vagal fainting.

    c. History and physical examination are key to diagnosis.

    d. Diagnostic tests should be chosen based on the history and physical examination.

    e. Tests include electrocardiography, ambulatory monitoring (Holter), echocardiography, tilt-table test, electrophysiologic studies, and possibly computed tomography (CT) or magnetic resonance imaging (MRI) of the brain.

    f. Treatment varies with the cause.

8. Sensory impairment

    a. Vision

        (1) Declines in accommodation and peripheral vision occur with aging.

        (2) Age-related clouding of the lens occurs even without disease.

    b. Hearing

        (1) Cerumen impaction and presbycusis are common causes of hearing loss in the elderly.

9. Malnutrition

    a. Undernutrition is the most common disorder, but overweight and obesity also are problematic.

    b. Undernutrition (macronutrients)

        (1) The cause is most often "pre-mouth" (i.e., problems with the inability to shop for or prepare meals or inadequate assistance with feeding).

        (2) Other causes include mouth disorders such as edentulous state, xerostomia, or oral candidiasis; dysgeusia (abnormal taste); dysphagia; mesenteric ischemia; gastritis; generalized fatigue; endocarditis; malignancy; depression; and pain anywhere in the body.

        (3) Water deficit is common because the elderly lack a thirst response and often are on diuretics, increasing water loss.

        (4) Evaluation should include a complete history and food diary, especially regarding medications, food availability and preferences, and pain referable to the GI tract, as well as a search for other medical causes. Medications are especially common sources but are often overlooked.

> **Common causes of syncope:** cardiac (arrhythmias, other), hypoglycemia, orthostasis, postprandial, psychogenic disorders, emboli, vagal event.

> **Top 10 root causes of weight loss in the elderly:** dementia, depression, disease, dysphagia, dysgeusia, diarrhea, drugs, dentition, dysfunction, and thyroid.

(5) Laboratory studies that may be useful include complete blood count, electrolytes, renal and liver function, thyroid-stimulating hormone, erythrocyte sedimentation rate, C-reactive protein, and urinalysis; chest radiography may be useful as well. Other studies may be needed as suggested by the evaluation.

(6) Treatment is geared toward the cause.

c. Undernutrition (micronutrients)

(1) Vitamins C, D, B_{12}, and the other B vitamins are the most common deficiencies in older adults. Supplementation should be based on levels and adjusted as needed.

(2) Vitamin D deficiency is an underrecognized cause of myalgias, arthralgias, and sarcopenia in older adults. Supplementation has been shown to reduce fall risk in those who are deficient but not in healthy older adults. The American Geriatrics Society consensus statement, released in 2014, recommends that a level of 30 ng per mL or 75 nmol per L is appropriate for older adults to reduce fracture risk. Higher doses are recommended for other forms of vitamin D deficiency, such as osteomalacia and hypoparathyroidism. It is important to recognize that the recommendations are changing rapidly. Readers should consult the most recent guidelines and apply them on an individual basis.

> Undernutrition can be subtle; most common deficiencies are vitamins C, D, and B_{12}.

(3) For most, undernutrition results from reduced intake but declines in gastric acid and intrinsic factor render the elderly especially vulnerable to vitamin B_{12} deficiency. An increasingly used drug, metformin, is associated with B_{12} deficiency as well. It is important to recognize that serum levels are not necessarily coincident with central nervous system levels. Oral replacement with 1,000 mg daily is preferred to parenteral dosing.

10. Pressure wounds (see Chapter 13)

a. Predisposing factors in elderly skin consist of loss of subcutaneous fat, loss of the rete pegs (projections of dermis into the epidermis that help prevent shearing off of the epidermis), and a decline in elasticity.

b. Predisposing factors, in general, include diseases that reduce perfusion or delivery of nutrients to tissue, increased shearing force, moisture (such as fecal or urinary incontinence), dehydration, and immobility.

> Patients with limited mobility or self-care ability should be monitored closely for early signs of pressure on the skin: erythema and warmth.

c. Treatment primarily consists of paying attention to systemic factors, including hydration, nutrition, adequate oxygenation and carrying capacity, frequent repositioning or turning, pressure-relieving devices, optimal management of related diseases, and pain relief.

11. Vertebral compression fractures

a. Associated with osteoporosis, vertebral fractures usually occur in the thoracic or lumbar spine and present as deep pain over the site of the fracture, sometimes radiating in the appropriate nerve root distribution.

b. Trauma may be minimal or absent.

c. Diagnosis is established by radiography. MRI is indicated in cases where neurologic damage is suspected by history and/or physical exam.

d. Treatment is symptomatic with analgesics and vertebroplasty or kyphoplasty.

e. Complications include kyphosis with possible restrictive lung disease as a result, immobility, chronic pain, and even death.

I. **Psychiatric disorders**

1. General characteristics

a. Older adults tend to be self-reliant and satisfied with life.

b. Stoicism and present focus are typical.

c. They often deny mental illness.

2. Common disorders

   a. Depression is characterized by sadness, withdrawal from previously enjoyed activities, and anhedonia, but the elderly concentrate on somatic complaints more than on mood. Typical presentations also include memory impairment, agitation, anxiety, and displaced anger.

      (1) Diagnosis is established by clinical suspicion and completion of a screen, such as the Yesavage Geriatric Depression Scale. One must also rule out depression induced by medical disease, such as indolent cancer, or medication.

      (2) Although effective, older adults may be reluctant to participate in psychotherapy; thus, pharmaceuticals are the usual therapy.

         (a) Fewer side effects make selective serotonin reuptake inhibitors and agents like mirtazapine the drugs of choice.

         (b) Occasionally, stimulants in low doses, such as methylphenidate, are useful for a short time, especially in patients with psychomotor retardation.

         (c) Avoid tricyclic antidepressants because of sedation and anticholinergic effects (blurry vision, constipation, dry mouth, urinary retention).

      (3) Some patients are resistant to medications. Electroconvulsive therapy has been shown to be very effective and safe even in frail elderly patients.

   b. Anxiety

      (1) Avoid benzodiazepines if possible; if they must be used, shorter-acting agents are preferable. Although both long-acting and short-acting agents are associated with increased fall risk, long-acting ones are more often implicated.

      (2) Avoid antihistamines and use buspirone. Consider antidepressants because anxiety is often caused by depression in older adults.

   c. Psychosis

      (1) Senile psychosis is characterized by hallucinations and delusions.

      (2) It is associated with isolation, sensory impairment, and dementia.

      (3) It should not be treated unless it is bothersome to the patient or prohibits the caregivers from providing care.

      (4) Newer antipsychotics in low doses are the agents of choice; however, some dispute their risk–benefit ratio because of higher risk of cardiovascular disease, diabetes, and falls.

   d. Substance abuse

      (1) Tobacco use is common and should be discouraged even in the very aged individual; tobacco cessation may be beneficial even in the extremes of age.

      (2) Ethanol produces intoxication with ingestion of lesser amounts.

         (a) Hidden sources of ethanol may be consumed, such as household cleaners, tonics, and personal hygiene products.

         (b) Withdrawal is more lethal in the elderly.

      (3) Other agents, including prescription drugs, are often misused unintentionally but are rarely directly abused in the elderly population to produce euphoria.

> 💡 Mood disorders are often denied by elderly patients; depression often presents as somatic complaints.

Selected Common Diseases and Disorders with Unique Features in the Elderly

A. **Xerosis**

   1. Xerosis is characterized by dry skin, pruritus, and cracking skin.

   2. Treatment consists of decreasing the frequency of bathing and using tepid or cool water followed by emollients.

B. Oral disorders

1. Oral disorders frequently result in weight loss.

2. Dysgeusia may be related to dental disease or sinusitis, but it is often secondary to drugs. Common drugs that cause taste disturbances include any anticholinergic agent, digitalis, and angiotensin-converting enzyme (ACE) inhibitors.

3. Xerostomia (dry mouth) is common and may result from age-related reduction in saliva production, although medications are more often responsible. It is associated with tooth decay and gingivitis or periodontitis. Avoid anticholinergic drugs and promote oral hygiene. Saliva substitutes may be helpful but are expensive and many patients prefer frequent small sips of water or other beverages.

4. Toothlessness commonly reduces mastication. Dentures may contribute to decreased taste and lead to denture ulcers.

5. Oral candidiasis is common and should be considered in any elderly patient who decreases oral intake, especially if the patient is on steroids or antibiotics, has diabetes or another immunodeficiency disorder, or who is wearing dentures as they may harbor organisms.

   a. White patches are common, but red mucosa or angular cheilitis may be the only sign, especially in patients with dentures.

   b. Treatment is with topical or oral antifungal agents.

> In patients who wear dentures, candidiasis is more likely to appear as red mucosa rather than white patches.

C. Infectious diseases

1. Decline in B- and T-cells immunity related to aging increases vulnerability to infection.

2. Fever typically indicates bacterial infection, but sometimes is the result of malignancy or medication intake. Elderly often do not mount a fever even with serious infections.

3. Pneumonia (refer to Chapter 2)

   a. Predisposing factors include decreased ciliary activity, less effective cough, and decreased vital capacity.

   b. Presentation may be atypical, with less cough, absent fever, and absent or unimpressive leukocytosis. Often, only confusion and tachypnea are seen. Chest x-ray does not always show typical infiltrates, particularly early in the course of illness.

   c. Aspiration pneumonia is more common in the elderly. Although antibiotics are often used, they are not very effective. The risk is not reduced by use of a percutaneous endoscopic gastrostomy tube; in fact, it is increased.

> To reduce the risk of aspiration pneumonia, avoid endoscopic feeding lines.

4. UTI (refer to Chapter 6)

   a. UTI often presents with vague symptoms or confusion.

   b. It is difficult to distinguish from asymptomatic bacteriuria, which is common and should not be treated because inappropriate antibiotic use leads to resistance and exposes patients to unnecessary risk.

   c. Diagnosis of a UTI requires urinalysis and culture and correlation with signs and symptoms.

   d. Treatment consists of appropriate antibiotics, increased fluids, and attention to hygiene.

   e. Although UTI may cause delirium, it should *not* be assumed to be the etiology until other potential causes are ruled out.

D. Respiratory diseases (refer to Chapter 2)

1. Pulmonary fibrosis

   a. There is increased incidence with aging; limited fibrosis is a part of normal aging.

   b. Fibrosis is characterized by shortness of breath and bibasilar rales.

     c. Newer agents such as nintedanib and pirfenidone have slowed progression, but their use in older adults is controversial.

     d. Treatment is largely symptomatic, including supplemental oxygen.

2. Chronic obstructive pulmonary disease (see Chapter 2): Avoid theophylline because of the high risk of side effects and interactions. Be cautious with β-agonists in patients with CHF, as they may exacerbate it.

3. Pulmonary embolus

     a. Presentation often is less specific, with confusion, arrhythmia, or fever.

     b. Diagnosis and treatment are the same as those in younger adults. Spiral CT may not be appropriate, however, because many older persons suffer from chronic renal insufficiency, limiting the use of contrast material. Consider renal protective agents such as acetylcysteine.

E. **Cardiovascular disease (see Chapter 3)**

1. Ischemic heart disease

     a. Ischemic heart disease is common in the elderly but frequently presents atypically, often with shortness of breath or fatigue, weakness, or confusion rather than with chest pain or tightness.

     b. Elderly patients are more likely to have severe or multivessel coronary disease.

     c. Cardiac enzymes may not rise as much or may be difficult to interpret secondary to renal disease.

     d. Elderly patients who present with myocardial infarction are more likely to die compared to younger individuals.

     e. Treatment is the same as in younger adults; be mindful of comorbidities that may affect treatment options.

     f. Age alone is not a contraindication to invasive or surgical therapies.

> 💡 Ischemic heart disease in the elderly can present atypically, often without chest pain but only dyspnea and fatigue.

2. Hypertension

     a. Hypertension is common in older adults.

     b. It should be treated aggressively but cautiously in older adults diagnosed with primary hypertension. Evaluation of side effects (e.g., falls secondary to orthostatic hypotension) may preclude lowering the systolic pressure to recommended levels.

     c. Diagnosis and treatment are the same as in younger individuals.

     d. Renal artery stenosis, contributing to secondary hypertension, is more common in the elderly.

     e. Systolic hypertension should be treated because it is more closely associated with stroke than diastolic hypertension. Thiazide diuretics are the first choice for systolic hypertension but have numerous side effects including dehydration, hyperuricemia, hyponatremia, and hypokalemia. The dose in an older adult should not exceed 25 mg per day of hydrochlorothiazide as more of it only results in side effects not blood pressure control.

     f. Avoid centrally acting agents because of the high risk of sedation, dry mouth, and depression.

3. Valvular disease

     a. Aortic sclerosis

          (1) Aortic sclerosis results from thickening of the aortic leaflets.

          (2) It causes a systolic murmur similar to that of aortic stenosis from which it cannot be distinguished on physical examination alone.

     b. Aortic stenosis

          (1) Elderly patients may not exhibit the classic pulsus parvus et tardus (slow, late pulse) or the typical radiation pattern to the carotids and axillae. Presentation is more likely to be falls with syncope, CHF, or fatigue.

(2) Age alone is not a contraindication to surgical repair, especially with endoscopic techniques that carry acceptable risk even in the very frail. Recent recommendations are predicated on evidence that earlier intervention prevents cardiac decompensation.

c. Mitral regurgitation may cause heart failure or death. Treatment is surgical.

4. CHF

a. Diastolic dysfunction (aka heart failure with preserved ejection fraction [HFpEF]) is more common in the aged than in younger persons and results in poor compliance and poor filling, leading to heart failure.

b. Presentation is often sudden shortness of breath and pulmonary edema.

c. Diagnosis is established clinically and supported with echocardiography. Cardiac catheterization remains the preferred method to evaluate coronary vascularity; however, its usefulness in older adults may be lessened because of potential renal toxicity from the dyes used in the procedure.

d. Treatment is with ACE inhibitors, angiotensin receptor blockers (ARBs), β-blockers, and calcium channel blockers. Diuretics should be used judiciously because of the high probability of renal insufficiency as well as the risk of dehydration and hypotension.

e. Pacemakers have been shown to optimize diastolic function in patients with refractory heart failure by cardiac resynchronization therapy and reducing pacing rates. Automatic implantable cardioverter-defibrillator (AICD) may reduce the rate of sudden cardiac death but at the potential cost of trading a relatively symptomless event for one with burdensome discomfort. Age alone is not a contraindication to either therapy.

f. Systolic heart failure (reduced ejection fraction [HFrEF]) is generally treated as in younger individuals with a few caveats. ARBs are better tolerated in the elderly compared to ACE inhibitors. Aldosterone antagonists are problematic because of the effects of aging on renal function and higher incidence of hyperkalemia. The clinician should closely monitor renal function and electrolytes.

F. **Endocrine disorders (refer to Chapter 10)**

1. Hypothyroidism

a. Hypothyroidism is a very common problem, especially in elderly women, and may present in a typical fashion or quite atypically.

b. Thyroid dysfunction often mimics changes associated with aging itself. These symptoms include a general slowing of mental and physical functions, tendency to low body temperatures and cold intolerance, weight gain, constipation, hardening of the arteries, hearing loss, elevation of serum lipids (cholesterol), elevation of blood pressure, and anemia.

c. Evaluation is via thyroid function testing; thyroid-stimulating hormone typically is elevated.

d. Treatment

(1) Treatment is with levothyroxine, with a goal of restoring the thyroid-stimulating hormone to high normal or just above normal. Be cautious with rapid titration in those with heart disease.

(2) Dosage should be low, 12.5 to 25 mg per day and increased at 4- to 6-week intervals. Because the half-life of levothyroxine in the elderly is variable, assessing levels at less-frequent intervals may lead to overdose.

> Hypothyroid must be ruled out in an elderly patient presenting with signs of depression or cognitive decline.

2. Hyperthyroidism

a. Hyperthyroidism may present as hypothyroidism (apathetic hyperthyroidism), atrial fibrillation with a rapid ventricular response, or dementia.

b. Evaluation is via thyroid function testing.

c. Treatment is the same as in younger patients.

G. **GI disorders (refer to Chapter 5)**

1. Reflux disease is evaluated and treated as in younger adults; however, prokinetic agents, such as metoclopramide, should be avoided, if possible, owing to the risk of centrally acting side effects.

2. Peptic ulcer disease is more likely to present with failure to thrive, nausea, or melena rather than with dyspepsia or pain.

3. Consider H_2 receptor blockers as first-line therapy as proton pump inhibitors (PPIs) have been associated with unacceptable side effects. Choice of agent should be based on the overall clinical picture but avoid cimetidine because of its high anticholinergic effects. Beware of large doses of magnesium-containing antacids in patients with renal dysfunction.

4. Constipation

a. Aged individuals are predisposed to bowel dysfunction owing to changes of aging, immobility, inadequate hydration, and medications.

b. Diagnosis is established by history and physical examination and, occasionally, by abdominal flat plate.

c. Treatment is increasing fluids and activity, improving mastication, increasing dietary fiber, and using stool softeners and laxatives or enemas, if necessary. Avoid anticholinergic drugs as much as possible. Aggressively manage opioid-related constipation with stimulant laxatives or with μ-opioid receptor antagonists such as methylnaltrexone in the terminal patient.

d. If unrelieved, complications may ensue: impaction, stercoral ulcers (ulcerations of the colon because of pressure and irritation from retained feces), obstruction, and death.

> 💡 Manage the risk of constipation with aggressive supportive measures including fluids, fiber, and stool softeners or laxatives; prevention is key to reducing complications.

H. **Neurologic disorders (refer to Chapter 11)**

1. Subdural hematoma

a. Subdural hematomas may be chronic (developing over weeks) or acute (caused by a single, identifiable traumatic event).

b. Chronic subdural hematomas are common and may arise with little or no trauma.

c. Presentation usually is confusion, decreased level of consciousness, and perhaps focal findings but may appear to be dementia.

d. Diagnosis is established via CT.

e. Treatment may be surgical (burr holes) or, if the hematoma is small and not progressing, watchful waiting.

f. Chronic subdural hematomas frequently recur even after surgery.

I. Cerebrovascular disease (see Chapter 11)

Legal, Ethical, and Financial Issues

A. Competence is a legal term and is determined by a judge.

B. Decisional capacity is determined by a physician and may change depending on circumstances and cognitive ability.

C. Elder mistreatment

1. Suspicion of abuse requires a report to legal authorities.

2. Abuse may take many forms including neglect; exploitation; and verbal, psychological, or physical mistreatment.

3. Abuse often is associated with caregiver stress, especially if the caregiver is financially dependent on the elderly person and has psychological or substance abuse problems.

4. Patterns of injury that are not consistent with the history should raise suspicion.

D. Financing and costs

   1. Elderly patients account for about one-third of U.S. health care dollars. Medicare pays for most of these expenditures.

   2. Eligibility for Medicare depends on social security status, which is determined by enrollment in the system, aging and/or disease (end-stage renal disease and amyotrophic lateral sclerosis [ALS] confer automatic status), or disability. Table 16-12 describes Medicare coverage.

   3. Hospice is covered under Medicare Part A and is accessed when the enrollee chooses comfort care and two physicians certify a life expectancy of ≤6 months.

   4. Prescription medications are covered under Part D, but it has many coverage gaps. Beneficiaries can visit the Medicare website and input their prescription drugs to ascertain which plan may be best for them during the annual enrollment period.

   5. Nursing home care for subacute rehabilitation is covered for up to 100 days after a 3-day qualifying hospital stay (20 days fully and 80 days with a copay). Managed Care Plans (Part C) can enroll beneficiaries in long-term care (LTC) rehabilitation without a qualifying hospital stay.

   6. Informal caregivers, usually family members, provide the majority of daily care for those in the community who require assistance.

   7. An increasing number of Medicare recipients are enrolling in Medicare Part C, which is offered by private insurers, often at little or no cost to beneficiaries. It may offer other services such as dental or hearing aids, making it particularly attractive. The Plans must cover everything that is covered by traditional Medicare; however, there is no stipulation that they must cover rehabilitation with little likelihood of success, so an LTC stay may be denied or the patient may be declined by a facility.

   8. Many of the plans recognize the efficacy of using nurse practitioners (NPs) or PAs for preventive services within the home, reducing the need for more expensive emergency centers or hospital visits.

Table 16-12 | Medicare Coverage

Plan	Eligibility	Coverage
Traditional Medicare		
Part A	Age 65 or SS disability; ESRD or ALS	Hospitalization Long-term acute care Subacute nursing home Hospice care Home care Durable medical equipment
Part B	Social security eligible + premium	Physician, PA/NP visits Laboratory tests OT/PT outpatient care Emergency care Ambulance Outpatient mental health Does not cover eyeglasses or hearing aids
Part D	Social security + premium + copay	Prescription drugs Beneficiary chooses plan Formularies vary
Medigap/supplemental	Eligibility + premium	Cover "gaps" such as blood transfusions; deductibles, copays
Nontraditional Medicare		
Part C Medicare Advantage Plans	Same as traditional	Usually 100% coverage but varies; may cover dental, glasses, hearing aids; often also have Part D

ALS, amyotrophic lateral sclerosis; ESRD, end-stage renal disease; OT/PT, occupational therapy/physical therapy; PA/NP, physician assistant/nurse practitioner. SS, social security.

Practice Questions

Directions: *Each of the numbered items or incomplete statements in this section is followed by a list of answers or completions of the statement. Select the ONE lettered answer or completion that is BEST in each case.*

1. A 79-year-old complains of bilateral knee pain that worsens with activity. Examination reveals mild crepitus, reduced range of motion, and no edema or effusion. What is the recommended first-line oral analgesic?
   A. Acetaminophen
   B. Gabapentin
   C. Hydrocodone/acetaminophen
   D. Ibuprofen
   E. Ketorolac

2. An elderly female was started on medication for urinary incontinence. A week later, she is brought to the clinic owing to excessive dry mouth, dysphagia, and blurred vision. What medication was she *most* likely prescribed?
   A. Dicyclomine
   B. Tolterodine
   C. Cimetidine
   D. Pseudoephedrine
   E. Mirabegron

3. An 81-year-old female with a history of Alzheimer's dementia has become more agitated over the past few months. Occasionally, she becomes combative with the staff in her assisted living facility. Staff has tried nonpharmacologic interventions such as distraction without efficacy. Evaluation did not reveal a medical cause except possibly a UTI with 50 to 100,000 gram-negative rods on a clean catch culture specimen. Which of the following medications is considered best to reduce her aggressive behavior?
   A. Haloperidol
   B. Lorazepam
   C. Memantine
   D. Midazolam
   E. Trimethoprim/sulfamethoxazole

4. A 69-year-old female describes myalgias and arthralgias that have interfered with her ability to ambulate. She has fallen twice in the past month but denies any loss of consciousness or injuries. She lives alone and spends most of her day inside. She avoids caffeine but has a shot of whiskey each evening. She is thin and prefers not to eat meat more than once per week. A deficiency of which of the following is most likely present?
   A. Calcium
   B. Parathyroid hormone
   C. Vitamin B_{12}
   D. Vitamin D
   E. Zinc

5. A 78-year-old female presents to the emergency department with acute severe back pain. She states the pain started suddenly when she was shopping. Examination reveals a kyphotic spine with tenderness in the thoracic area. Radiography confirms a fracture of T10. What is the next step in the workup of this patient?
   A. Bone density
   B. Bone scan
   C. Vitamin B_{12} level

D. Adjusted calcium level
E. MRI of spine

6. An 81-year-old male has been increasingly anxious since the death of his wife last year. He denies any thoughts to hurt himself or others. After referral to a psychologist, he returns for follow-up. Although he admits that the counseling is helping, he is still anxious, losing weight, and having trouble sleeping. Which of the following is the recommended treatment?
   A. Buspirone
   B. Chlordiazepoxide
   C. Fluoxetine
   D. Lorazepam
   E. Atenolol

7. A 73-year-old patient with a history of moderate emphysema is brought to the emergency department with fever and obtundation. Examination reveals a thin female with dry mucous membranes, tachypnea, and scattered rhonchi and wheezes. Abdomen is soft, bowel sounds are hyperactive, she winces with deep palpation of the suprapubic area. Remainder of the exam is unremarkable. What is the most likely diagnosis?
   A. Cerebral vascular accident
   B. Encephalitis
   C. Pneumonia
   D. Rupture abdominal viscus
   E. UTI

8. An 82-year-old female with no significant medical history has had blood pressure readings of 162/78, 166/80, 158/72, and 170/82. What is the recommended management?
   A. Clonidine
   B. α-Blocker
   C. Restrict salt intake
   D. Thiazide diuretic
   E. Workup for renal artery stenosis

9. The daughter of a 92-year-old patient is concerned that her previously very active mother has lost interest in all her usual activities. She has been sleeping more and eating less but has not lost weight. Examination reveals a pleasant woman with slow responses. She is wearing multiple layers of clothes although the ambient temperature is mild. She complains of constipation and impaired hearing. She has no significant medical history and is not on any prescription medications. Vitals include T 97.4°F, P 66, R 14, BP 150/88. What is the recommended treatment for the most likely diagnosis?
   A. Buspirone
   B. Dexamphetamine
   C. Diuretic
   D. Iron supplements
   E. Levothyroxine

10. A 90-year-old male has had two presyncope events. Vitals are T 98.2°F, P 90, R 16, and BP 120/100. S1 is soft; S2 is split. There is a III/VI low-pitched systolic murmur that follows a crescendo–decrescendo pattern. It is best heard in the second

intercostal space and radiates to both carotids. What is the most likely diagnosis?
A. Aortic regurgitation
B. Aortic stenosis
C. Mitral regurgitation
D. Mitral stenosis
E. Pulmonary stenosis

11. A 77-year-old female presents for routine care. She had a stroke 4 years ago with mild residual left-sided paresis. She lives with her daughter and is active with the local senior group. She takes a thiazide diuretic for hypertension X12 years. She smoked a half-pack per day for 20 years, quitting before her 40th birthday. Which of the following should be included in preventive care?
A. Colonoscopy
B. Bone scan

C. Lipid panel
D. Mammography
E. Chest CT scan

12. A 90-year-old female presents with stocking-glove distribution pain described as burning and stinging. She cannot identify any precipitating factors, but it is more bothersome at night, preventing her from sleeping. What should be your first choice for medication in this patient?
A. Amitriptyline
B. Gabapentin
C. Oxycodone
D. Acetaminophen
E. CBD oil

Practice Answers

1. A. *Geriatrics; Pharmacology; Osteoarthritis*

When prescribing for elderly patients, one must remain vigilant regarding pharmacokinetics as well as potential impact of side effects. Mild nociceptive pain should be treated with acetaminophen. NSAIDs (ibuprofen and ketorolac) should be avoided owing to the risk of GI bleeding or effects on the kidneys. Ketorolac is a strong NSAID that should be limited to a very short duration of use. Acetaminophen combined with hydrocodone or other narcotic analgesics should be reserved for moderate to severe pain that is not relieved by less-potent means. Gabapentin can be helpful in cases of neuropathic pain but is only approved for postherpetic neuralgia.

2. A. *Geriatrics; Pharmacology; Urinary Incontinence*

Dicyclomine is an anticholinergic medication that relieves urinary frequency, urgency, and nocturnal enuresis; however, the anticholinergic side effects can be dangerous and cause the side effects noted in the question. Tolterodine is also an anticholinergic, but it is selective for bladder over salivary glands and therefore, less risk of side effects. Pseudoephedrine is an α-adrenergic agonist effective in stress incontinence. Cimetidine is an H_2-blocker with prominent anticholinergic side effects.

3. B. *Geriatrics; Pharmacology; Alzheimer Dementia*

The best treatment for a patient who has become combative is to distract them or provide another activity until they calm. The positive urine culture most likely has nothing to do with the aggression because the behavior is intermittent and associated with care provision. If a medication must be used, most recommend a low dose of an intermediate-acting benzodiazepine. Lorazepam has an intermediate onset and a half-life of 10 to 20 hours. Midazolam has a very fast onset, but its half-life is also very short (1 to 3 hours). Oxazepam has a short half-life, but a very slow onset. Memantine may slow the progression of the disease, but its effectiveness in alleviating specific behaviors is mixed. Haloperidol is a typical antipsychotic; it quickly sedates the patient, but it has a very long half-life with anticholinergic and other adverse effects. It also carries a black box warning from the FDA.

4. D. *Geriatrics; GI/Nutrition; Vitamin Deficiency*

Deficiency of vitamin D is common in the elderly, especially those who do not get outside often. It is a common cause of myalgias and arthralgias in the elderly, and adequate supplementation is associated with a significant reduction in fall risk, but only in those proven deficient. Deficiency in calcium and vitamin D causes osteoporosis, which can lead to pathologic fractures. Her lack of meat intake may cause a deficiency of vitamin B_{12}, but that would usually manifest as macrocytic anemia with psychotic features and neuropathy. Lack of parathyroid hormone is usually caused by injury to the glands; effects include muscle cramps. Zinc deficiency causes poor neurologic functioning, weakened immune system, diarrhea, thinning hair, and GI disturbances.

5. A. *Geriatrics; Diagnostic Studies; Osteoporosis*

Pathologic fractures in the elderly are most commonly caused by osteoporosis or malignancy with metastasis. Vitamin B_{12} deficiency severe enough to cause pernicious anemia has been associated with osteoporosis but is not a recommended first test. Calcium deficiency contributes to osteoporosis but does not confirm the diagnosis. A bone density scan (densitometry) will confirm osteoporosis. A bone scan would be appropriate if bony metastasis was likely. An MRI might be warranted if the fracture was not visible on plain radiographs but is not likely to give additional information.

6. A. *Geriatrics; Pharmacology; Anxiety*

Of those listed, buspirone is the best choice for anxiety in the elderly. It has a good track record and few side effects. Benzodiazepines should be avoided in the elderly; if necessary, a short-acting medication is preferred. Antidepressants are recommended because anxiety is often related to depression.

7. C. *Geriatrics; Diagnosis; Pneumonia*

The two most common causes of fever and mental status changes in the elderly are pneumonia and UTI. The history of emphysema and lung sounds supports a diagnosis of pneumonia. Suprapubic tenderness may indicate a UTI or urinary retention, but it is less likely in this patient. A ruptured viscus would cause pain and rigidity of the abdomen. Encephalitis or a stroke would likely cause focal neurologic findings.

8. D. *Geriatrics; Pharmacology; Systolic Hypertension*

A thiazide diuretic is the first choice for the treatment of systolic hypertension. Patients should be cautioned to maintain hydration, and renal function should be monitored. A β-blocker would risk lowering the diastolic pressure which may cause syncope. Clonidine is a centrally acting antihypertensive that may cause sedation, dry mouth, and depression and is almost never used in older adults. Salt restriction is not effective in isolated systolic hypertension. Renal artery stenosis causes elevation of both systolic and diastolic pressures.

9. E. *Geriatrics; Pharmacology; Hypothyroidism*

The elderly are very prone to hypothyroidism. Depressive features and/or a slowing of mental and physical function may be the initial manifestation. Other manifestations include cold intolerance, constipation, dryness of skin and hair, hearing loss, elevated blood pressure, elevated lipids, and anemia, among others. Treatment is with thyroid replacement. Buspirone might be appropriate if this proved to be depression rather than an organic disease. Diuretics would be appropriate to treat hypertension if no other cause of elevated blood pressure is found. Iron deficiency anemia causes fatigue, weakness, and pallor; it is readily apparent through routine labs. Stimulants should be avoided in the elderly owing to dangerous side effects.

10. B. *Geriatrics; Diagnosis; Aortic Stenosis*

Aortic stenosis is common in the elderly. The systolic murmur described is characteristic. Aortic regurgitation would include a diastolic blowing murmur. Mitral stenosis is associated with a loud S1, opening snap, and diastolic rumble. Mitral regurgitation is associated with a high-pitched, blowing murmur heard best at the apex with radiation to the axillae. Pulmonary stenosis is associated with a split 2 and a systolic ejection murmur with or without a click. Aortic sclerosis is possible but not likely, given the presyncope.

11. C. *Geriatrics; Health Maintenance; Screening*

A lipid panel should continue to be screened in the elderly, especially in patients with a history of coronary artery disease, peripheral artery disease, diabetes mellitus, or a previous stroke. A bone density should be done at least once after age 65 years in women or 70 years in men; a bone scan is not considered routine screening. Recommendations for screening colonoscopy, mammography, and Pap smear stop at age 75, unless there are compelling reasons. A chest radiograph is not recommended as screening at any age: A chest CT should be considered in patients with a smoking history of 30 years or more. Additionally, all screening in the elderly should be considered based on life expectancy and functional status and discussed with the patient and/or family (if the patient lacks decision-making capacity).

12. B. *Geriatrics; Treatment; Neuropathic Pain*

Although a recent review indicated that it may not be effective and it is only indicated for postherpetic neuropathic pain, of those listed, gabapentin is the agent of choice for neuropathic pain. As a tricyclic antidepressant, amitriptyline is not recommended because of anticholinergic side effects. Acetaminophen is not likely to be effective, nor is oxycodone. CBD oil has been used but has little evidence of efficacy.

Pediatrics | 17

Claire Babcock O'Connell and Thea Cogan-Drew

Examination of the Newborn

A. Examination at birth

1. Begin with observation, auscultation of the heart and lungs, and inspection for birth trauma or deformities.

2. Apgar score is assessed at 1, 5, and 10 minutes (see Table 8-14). Apgar scoring is completed in the delivery room; low serial scores alert the clinician of the need for resuscitation efforts.

3. The New Ballard Score is a more complex assessment of activity, position, and tone, which is used to evaluate neuromuscular and physical maturity. This rubric estimates the gestational age (Fig. 17-1). Growth charts plot the number of weeks to birth weight to help determine if the newborn is small for its gestational age, large for it, or of normal weight.

   a. An infant born small for its gestational age may be a result of maternal drug use, chromosomal abnormalities, exposure to intrauterine viral infection, multiple gestation, advanced maternal age (>35 years), placental insufficiency, or lack of maternal weight gain.

   b. Most often, the cause of an infant being large for gestational age is maternal diabetes.

A. Nursery examination

1. The complete newborn examination should be completed within 24 hours of birth.

2. Skin: Check for color, temperature, rashes or lesions, edema, and hair distribution.

   a. Erythema toxicum

      (1) Common; first appears 3 to 5 days after birth as small pustules on erythematous bases (halos).

      (2) Normally, the rash spreads centripetally and spontaneously; resolves within 1 to 2 weeks.

   b. Milia

      (1) Very small, white papules concentrated on nose, cheeks, forehead, and chin

      (2) Resolve without intervention in 1 to 2 months

   c. Miliaria

      (1) A flushed macular appearance frequently involving the neck, face, scalp, and diaper area; it is caused by blockage of eccrine sweat glands.

      (2) Light clothing and decreased humidity speed resolution of this "prickly heat" or "heat rash" phenomenon

   d. Mongolian spots

      (1) Common in dark-skinned infants and involve small to large, blue–black macules concentrated on the back and buttocks; these macules are frequently misdiagnosed as bruising.

NEUROMUSCULAR MATURITY

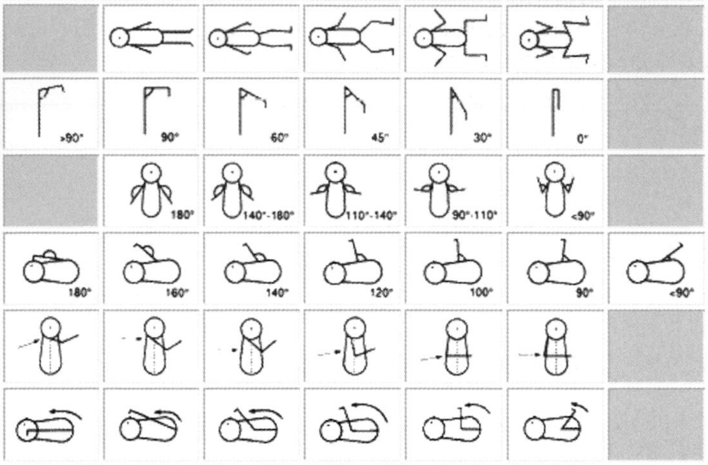

SIGN	SCORE							SIGN SCORE
	-1	0	1	2	3	4	5	
Posture								
Square Window	>90°	90°	60°	45°	30°	0°		
Arm Recoil		180°	140°-180°	110°-140°	90°-110°	<90°		
Popliteal Angle	180°	160°	140°	120°	100°	90°	<90°	
Scarf Sign								
Heel To Ear								
						TOTAL NEUROMUSCULAR SCORE		

MATURITY RATING

TOTAL SCORE	WEEKS
-10	20
-5	22
0	24
5	26
10	28
15	30
20	32
25	34
30	36
35	38
40	40
45	42
50	44

SIGN	SCORE							SIGN SCORE
	-1	0	1	2	3	4	5	
Skin	Sticky, friable, transparent	gelatinous, red, translucent	smooth pink, visible veins	superficial peeling &/or rash, few veins	cracking, pale areas, rare veins	parchment, deep cracking, no vessels	leathery, cracked, wrinkled	
Lanugo	none	sparse	abundant	thinning	bald areas	mostly bald		
Plantar Surface	heel-toe 40–50 mm: -1 <40 mm:-2	>50 mm no crease	faint red marks	anterior transverse crease only	creases ant. 2/3	creases over entire sole		
Breast	imperceptible	barely perceptible	flat areola no bud	stippled areola 1–2 mm bud	raised areola 3–4 mm bud	full areola 5–10 mm bud		
Eye / Ear	lids fused loosely: -1 tightly: -2	lids open pinna flat stays folded	sl. curved pinna; soft; slow recoil	well-curved pinna; soft but ready recoil	formed & firm instant recoil	thick cartilage ear stiff		
Genitals (Male)	scrotum flat, smooth	scrotum empty, faint rugae	testes in upper canal, rare rugae	testes descending, few rugae	testes down, good rugae	testes pendulous, deep rugae		
Genitals (Female)	clitoris prominent & labia flat	prominent clitoris & small labia minora	prominent clitoris & enlarging minora	majora & minora equally prominent	majora large, minora small	majora cover clitoris & minora		
						TOTAL PHYSICAL MATURITY SCORE		

Signature of Examiner

Gestation by Dates

	weeks

Birth date	Hour	
		am pm

APGAR	1 min	5 min

Scoring

Gest. Age by Maturity Rating	_____weeks
Time of Exam	Date_____ am Hour_____ pm
Age at Exam	_____hours

_____

_____   M.D. / R.N.

Figure 17-1 ▶ New Ballard Score.

(2) Most resolve spontaneously within 4 years, although they may persist for life.

e. Nevus simplex (stork bite)

(1) Light red macules frequently found on the eyelids, nape of the neck, and forehead; occur secondary to areas of surface capillary dilation.

(2) These almost always resolve spontaneously by age 2 years, although some may persist into adolescence, at which time they may be treated with laser therapy.

f. Vernix caseosa (greasy covering) and lanugo (fine hairs) are more frequently seen in preterm infants.

g. Dry, cracked, and peeling skin is more likely in post-term infants.

3. Head or face

a. Craniosynostosis

(1) This refers to premature fusion of one or more sutures (sagittal is most common).

(2) Referral to a neurologist is necessary to ensure proper growth and development.

b. Fontanelles

(1) Anterior: 1 to 4 cm in size in either direction; closes around 10 to 26 months of age

(2) Posterior: 1 cm in size on average; closes around 1 to 3 months

(3) A third fontanelle along the sagittal suture may be present and may be associated with trisomy 21.

c. Hematomas and hemorrhages

(1) Caput succedaneum is fluid accumulation under the scalp secondary to birth trauma. Swelling is palpable crossing the midline.

(2) Hematomas frequently appear contained within suture lines (cephalohematoma).

(3) Subgaleal hemorrhages occur beneath the scalp; they are uncommon but may result in enough blood loss to cause hemorrhagic shock.

d. Unusual appearing facies beyond the edema and bruising secondary to delivery may represent an underlying syndrome.

4. Ears

a. Posteriorly rotated or low-set ears should prompt suspicion of other congenital anomalies such as Down or Turner's syndrome.

b. Preauricular pits and tags are common and are usually benign when they appear in isolation. Infants with a family history of preauricular pits associated with deafness should be followed serially for hearing loss. Other auricular malformations may be linked to underlying genitourinary anomalies, and these infants should be screened with renal ultrasonography.

c. Hearing is best assessed during the newborn period by auditory brain stem response (ABR) or evoked otoacoustic emission (OAE) testing. All states in the United States have required universal newborn hearing screening using at least one of these methods. A follow-up test should utilize the method (ABR or OAE) not used for screening. All infants should be screened regularly during development.

5. Eyes

a. Abnormalities or asymmetry of red reflex warrants immediate referral to a pediatric ophthalmologist. Congenital cataracts, glaucoma, or retinoblastomas present as absent red reflex in the infant.

> Signs for possible various syndromes or abnormalities in the newborn examination include unusual facies, posteriorly rotated ears, auricular malformations, cleft soft palate, large tongue, webbed neck, prune belly, or gluteal cleft pits.

   b. Brushfield spots (gray or pale yellow spots at the periphery of the iris) are associated with Down syndrome.

   c. Subconjunctival hemorrhages are common benign findings associated with the trauma of delivery; generally resolves with time.

   d. Strabismus, or crossing of the eyes, almost always is present during the newborn period and does not represent pathology unless it is fixed or persists past 4 months of age.

6. Nose and mouth

   a. Nose

   (1) Nasal patency is best assessed by testing the nares individually. This may be accomplished by placing a cold metal object below the nose to check for fogging or using a cotton wisp to look for air movement.

   (2) Choanal atresia or stenosis presents with unilateral or bilateral obstruction. Symptoms can include the inability to pass a small-caliber catheter may be helpful in establishing the obstruction, which is then confirmed with axial computed tomography (CT) with intranasal contrast. Bilateral obstruction results in respiratory distress because infants are obligate nasal breathers.

   b. Mouth

   (1) Esophageal atresia presents as excessive drooling.

   (2) Epstein pearls appear as small, pearly nodules along the midline of the hard palate and are benign retention cysts.

   (3) Cleft lip or palate deformities are easily identified via inspection. A bifid uvula indicates a submucosal cleft.

   (4) Pierre Robin syndrome may first be recognized by the observation of a small mandible and tongue as well as a clefted soft palate. Prone positioning often controls respiratory difficulties caused by the tongue occluding the airway.

   (5) Infants with trisomy 21 frequently have large tongues that often seem to be larger than the mouth.

   (6) Natal teeth may need to be extracted, if loose, to eliminate the possibility of aspiration.

   (7) Short frenulum may present with difficulty feeding. Lactation consult is the first step in the evaluation of this condition.

7. Neck

   a. Webbed or redundant skin of the neck may suggest Turner's syndrome.

   b. Masses

   (1) Midline: thyroid. Thyromegaly is associated with congenital hypothyroidism and requires immediate attention to prevent growth failure or cretinism.

   (2) Anterior to sternocleidomastoid: brachial cleft (also may see sinus tract remnants)

   (3) Posterior to sternocleidomastoid: cystic hygroma

   (4) Within sternocleidomastoid: torticollis, hematoma

8. Lungs and chest

   a. Fractures resulting from birth trauma may be palpated in the clavicles; examine for tenderness, crepitus, bruising, or decreased range of motion of one arm, usually the right. Treatment may include short-term immobilization but is usually not necessary.

   b. Decreased, asymmetric, or abnormal breath sounds

   (1) Grunting, intercostal retractions, tachypnea (>60 breaths/min), and cyanosis are all signs of respiratory distress. The differential diagnosis for respiratory distress is varied, including respiratory, cardiac, and noncardiopulmonary causes. Urgent evaluation and testing is indicated for an etiology requiring immediate intervention.

(2) Unilaterally decreased breath sounds may indicate pneumothorax or diaphragmatic hernia. A mediastinal shift supports the diagnosis of pneumothorax.

(3) The most common causes of infant respiratory distress are aspiration, congenital pneumonia, and TTN. TTN occurs in the immediate newborn period to term or later births and more frequently to infants born by cesarean delivery. Infants born to diabetic mothers are at a higher risk for TTN. Symptoms of increased work of breathing usually resolve within 72 hours. Infants should be provided supplemental oxygen and, if the condition is severe, tube feedings to decrease the work of breathing.

(4) Breast buds are common in the newborn period and typically resolve by 1 month of age.

9. Heart

   a. Heart rate is rapid (average, 140 beats/minute [bpm]). See Tables 17-1 and 17-2 for age-specific heart and respiratory rates.

   b. Murmurs are common and not always associated with pathology.

   c. Cyanosis, congestive heart failure, and diminished peripheral pulses are the most common serious presentations of heart disease in the infant.

10. Abdomen

    a. Prune belly or absence of abdominal musculature may be associated with renal anomalies.

    b. Severely scaphoid belly plus respiratory distress suggests diaphragmatic hernia.

    c. Prominent kidneys are suggestive of hydronephrosis or cystic kidney disease.

    d. The liver may be palpable up to 1 cm below the right costal margin. If larger, evaluation should be initiated.

> Newborn grunting, intercostal retractions, tachypnea, and cyanosis are all signs of respiratory distress, which is commonly caused by aspiration, pneumonia, or transient tachypnea of the newborn (TTN).

Table 17-1 | Age-Specific Heart Rates

Age	Average Rate (beats/min)	Range (beats/min)
0–30 days	140	90–190
1–6 months	130	80–180
7–12 months	116	75–155
1–2 years	110	70–150
2–6 years	102	68–138
6–10 years	94	65–125
10–14 years	84	55–115

Table 17-2 | Age-Specific Respiratory Rates

Age	Rate (breaths/min)
0–2 months	30–60
2–12 months	40–50
1–8 years	20–40
8–15 years	15–25

11. Genitalia and anus

a. Anus

(1) Inspect the gluteal cleft for pits, birthmarks, or tufts of hair, as these findings may represent an underlying neurotubular defect or spina bifida. Follow up with x-rays and appropriate referral.

(2) Anal patency is easily verified with the use of a lubricated thermometer or direct observation of stooling. Delayed stool (>24 hours after birth) may indicate Hirschsprung's disease.

b. Male genitalia

(1) Hypospadias

(a) Hypospadias refers to an abnormal placement of the urethra where the meatus is proximal and ventral to its normal or anterior location. Epispadias, dorsal displacement, is less common.

(b) Do not circumcise; bilateral renal ultrasonography is warranted to rule out ascending pathology.

(c) Refer to a pediatric urologist.

(2) Empty scrotal sac

(a) Testes usually descend by the third month of life; more than 80% descend by 9 months of age. If not descended by the age of 1 year, refer to a pediatric urologist for surgical intervention.

(b) Testicular cancer and infertility are significant concerns for such children. Bilateral absence of testes should raise suspicion of an infant not fully virilized. A referral to a pediatric endocrinologist is warranted.

(3) Inguinal hernias

(a) Inguinal hernias are more common in premature male infants.

(b) Observe and palpate for an extra full scrotal sac after an episode of crying. Transillumination of scrotal masses is helpful in the differentiation of hernia and hydrocele.

> 💡 Transillumination is helpful in evaluating any scrotal masses in the newborn; and most hydrocele masses resolve without any intervention.

(4) Hydrocele

(a) Observed in about 80% of newborn males, hydrocele refers to a collection of fluid in the scrotum owing to patency of the process vaginalis. Hydroceles transilluminate whereas sold masses (e.g., hernia) do not.

(b) The majority resolve without any intervention within 18 months.

(c) Hydrocele may be associated with hernia.

c. Female genitalia

(1) Vaginal leucorrhea or bloody discharge along with edematous labia is the result of maternal estrogens. These features usually resolve in 7 to 10 days, but they may resolve more slowly in the breastfed infants.

(2) Vaginal adhesions (fused introitus). Application of estrogen or beclomethasone cream for 5 to 10 days or refer to a pediatric urologist.

d. Ambiguous genitalia are most often associated with rare conditions, such as chromosomal anomalies and adrenal hyperplasia, affecting the action of testosterone. Examination findings include microphallus, absence of testes, clitoromegaly, posterior labial fusion, and palpable gonads within the labial folds. These findings require immediate attention. Initially, evaluate for life-threatening congenital adrenal hyperplasia. Families should be counseled by a clinician knowledgeable about ambiguous genitalia (disorders of sexual development) urgently. Sex chromosomal testing is now widely available; thus, atypical genitalia can be appropriately categorized in infancy.

12. Skeletal

a. Developmental dislocation of the hip (DDH)

(1) Occurs as frequently as 1 in 500 infants and at higher rates for female infants delivered from the breech presentation.

(2) Examination techniques

(a) The Barlow maneuver is performed with the infant fully relaxed; it attempts to dislocate the hip via posterior pressure. The examiner adducts the fully flexed hips while pushing the thighs posteriorly. If during this maneuver the femoral head is felt to dislocate or leave the acetabulum, it is considered a positive Barlow maneuver.

(b) The Ortolani maneuver attempts to identify the hip that is dislocated or subluxed. Grasp the medial aspect of the flexed knee with the thumb and fully abduct the hips. As the hips are brought to full abduction, feel for spasm or a clunk (not a click sound) for a positive finding.

(c) Positive Barlow and/or Ortolani maneuvers require bilateral ultrasonography of hips and referral to a pediatric orthopedic surgeon to prevent a lifelong disability.

(d) When DDH is suspected, it should be followed with ultrasonography and plain films of the hips at 6 months of age. Continued monitoring is recommended until the child is successfully ambulating.

> DDH can be identified using the Barlow or Ortolani maneuvers and requires pediatric orthopedic intervention.

b. Extremities

(1) Inspect for skin tags at the lateral borders of hands and feet, which represent rudimentary digits (polydactyly). Consider other malformations when these are present.

(2) Clubfoot, or talipes equinovarus, is a fixed, severe eversion of the plantar surface and warrants immediate orthopedic referral.

c. Spinal deformities, such as tufts of hair or hemangiomas that cross the midline as well as deep sinus tracts in the gluteal cleft, may represent spina bifida occulta or a tethered spinal cord.

13. Neurologic (reflexes)

a. Sucking and rooting

(1) These two are the earliest reflexes.

(2) Stroking the face elicits turning of the head toward the stimulus; when offered a nipple or the examiner's finger, the infant instinctively suckles.

b. Moro or startle reflex

(1) Allow the infant's head to suddenly drop 1 to 2 cm and observe for abduction at the shoulders and elbows along with spreading and extending of the fingers, followed by adduction and flexion of the same.

(2) This reflex disappears by 3 to 4 months of age.

c. Palmar and plantar grasp: Placement of the examiner's finger in the infant's palm or sole should elicit the grasping reflex, which disappears by 4 months of age.

d. Traction response: Pull the infant by the arms to the sitting position, and observe the head lag initially, finally coming briefly to midline before falling forward.

e. Placing reflex

(1) This reflex is noted when the infant is dangled above the bed, allowing the toe to have minimal contact with the surface.

(2) The extremity responds with flexion or a stepping response.

> A positive Babinski (upgoing plantar) reflex is a normal finding present in the newborn.

f. Deep tendon reflexes are brisk; clonus may be noted.

g. A Babinski (upgoing plantar) is normal and may be noted as late as 2 years of age.

Problems Common to the Term Newborn

A. Hypoglycemia

1. General characteristics
   a. Healthy term infants born after an uncomplicated pregnancy and delivery should *not* be routinely screened for hypoglycemia.
   b. Infants at risk for hypoglycemia (preterm, diabetic mother, small for its gestational age, perinatal distress, symptomatic) should be fed within the first hour of life and then have their blood glucose measured. Monitoring of blood glucose should take place every 3 to 6 hours over a 24- to 48-hour period and should be timed before the next feeding.
2. Physical examination
   a. Infant may be asymptomatic or present with poor feeding, lethargy, jitteriness, tremulousness, irritability, apnea, or seizures.
   b. In cases associated with hyperinsulinemia, cardiac failure may develop.
3. Laboratory testing
   a. Heel blood and bedside glucometer readings are adequate for screening.
   b. Abnormal results should be confirmed with whole-blood testing.
   c. Normal glucose level should be maintained at >50 mg per dL for <48 hours of age and at >60 mg per dL for >48 hours of age. These goals are only for infants with identified risk factors or symptoms of hypoglycemia.
4. **Treatment**
   a. Hypoglycemia is treated with a bolus of dextrose and water ($D_{10}W$) and intravenous (IV) glucose as needed. Infant feeding is an option as well.
   b. Continue to monitor; resolution usually occurs by the fifth day of life.
   c. Failure to resolve should prompt investigation for underlying likely causes.

B. Neonatal jaundice

1. General considerations (Table 17-3)

Table 17-3 | Characteristics and Management of Neonatal Jaundice

Type	Onset	Laboratory Tests	Treatment
ABO incompatibility	First 24 hours after birth	Coombs' (+)	Transfusion
		Reticulocytes ↑	Phototherapy
		Hct/Hgb ↓	
Rh isoimmunization	First 24 hours after birth	Coombs' (+)	Transfusion
		Reticulocytes	Phototherapy
		Hct/Hgb ↓	
Hereditary spherocytosis	First 24 hours after birth	Coombs' (−)	Transfusion if severe
		Reticulocytes ↑	Phototherapy
		Spherocytes on peripheral smear	
G6PD deficiency	First 24 hours after birth	Coombs' (−) Specific test for G6PD	Phototherapy
Physiologic jaundice	Appears after 24 hours	Bilirubin increases by <5 mg/dL/day, peaks at 3–5 days	Phototherapy when bilirubin is >15 mg/dL or not descending
Breastfeeding jaundice	Second to third day of life	Bilirubin ↑ and may persist for 6–8 weeks	Supplement breast milk with formula; feed or pump breast milk every 2 hours until an adequate supply is established. Phototherapy when bilirubin is >15 mg/dL

Hct/Hgb, hematocrit/hemoglobin; G6PD, glucose-6-phosphate dehydrogenase.

a. More than 65% of infants experience a bilirubin level of >5 mg per dL in the first week of life. Literature supports transcutaneous bilirubin screening in all infants before 24 hours of age to determine the need for further testing.

b. Most common causes of unconjugated hyperbilirubinemia are physiologic jaundice, prematurity, and breastfeeding jaundice.

c. Common etiologies are divided into two categories: overproduction of bilirubin and decreased rate of conjugation.

> In neonatal jaundice, etiologies with excess production are correlated with elevated reticulocyte counts; and etiologies with decreased conjugation present with a normal reticulocyte.

(1) Excess production of bilirubin may result from hemolysis secondary to blood group sensitizations (Coombs' test–positive incompatibilities such as Rh and ABO) or hereditary spherocytosis or glucose-6-phosphate dehydrogenase (G6PD) deficiency (Coombs' test negative). Sepsis and nonhemolytic anemia (extravascular hemorrhage) are other possible causes. Reticulocyte counts are elevated.

(2) Decreased rate of conjugation with normal reticulocyte counts commonly results from physiologic jaundice and uncommonly from Gilbert or Crigler–Najjar syndrome. Reticulocyte counts remain normal.

d. Kernicterus results from toxic bilirubin levels of higher than 20 to 25 mg per dL and is associated with encephalopathy.

e. Hyperbilirubinemia in the first 24 hours of life should be evaluated immediately.

2. Physical examination

a. Jaundice begins at the head and extends to the chest and extremities as bilirubin levels rise.

b. Scleral icterus and jaundiced oral mucosa help distinguish this in a darkly pigmented infant.

c. Splenomegaly may be present in hereditary spherocytosis.

3. Laboratory tests

a. Laboratory tests should include prenatal maternal blood type, Rh, and antibody testing. Baby's blood type should be performed if the mother is type O or Rh-negative with direct antibody testing.

b. Direct and indirect bilirubin levels should be obtained. Complete blood count (CBC), reticulocyte count, and blood smear should also be considered.

c. Conjugated hyperbilirubinemia (direct bilirubin >2 mg/dL and >10% of the total) may be caused by biliary obstruction or atresia, choledochal cyst, hyperalimentation, α_1-antitrypsin deficiency, hepatitis, sepsis, infections (especially urinary tract infections), hypothyroidism, inborn errors of metabolism (IEMs), cystic fibrosis, and red blood cell abnormalities.

d. Monitor hematocrit and hemoglobin in cases of hemolysis or hemorrhage.

(1) Initiate sepsis workup as indicated.

4. **Management and treatment**

a. Transfusion is necessary if the cause is ABO incompatibility, Rh isoimmunization, or nonimmune hemolysis (Coombs' test negative).

b. Phototherapy benefits all types of jaundice.

(1) Phototherapy may be started as early as 12 hours of age. In term babies, bilirubin levels fall up to 2 to 3 mg per dL in 4 to 6 hours and should be monitored regularly using total serum bilirubin levels. Generally, you can expect a 6% to 20% drop in the total bilirubin in an 18- to 24-hour period with phototherapy.

(2) Decision to begin phototherapy depends on the baby's weight, age, risk factors, and the level of bilirubin (Table 17-4).

(3) Phototherapy reduces the risk that total bilirubin concentration will reach a level at which exchange transfusion is recommended. There are several Food and Drug Administration (FDA)-approved phototherapy devices available that use narrow-band LEDs (blue or blue–green) as the light source. Correct

Table 17-4 | Guidelines for Phototherapy in Neonatal Jaundice

Weight (g)	Bilirubin Level (mg/dL)
500–1,000	12–15
1,000–1,500	15–18
1,500–2,500	18–20
>2,500	>20

selection of the light source protects the infant from ultraviolet (UV) radiation exposure. Protect the eyes.

   c. Sunlight exposure is not recommended for severe hyperbilirubinemia as it can be dangerous to infants. Infants can easily sunburn and overheat in direct sunlight. If sunlight is to be used in mild jaundice, it should be filtered through a tinted window and the infant should be placed well away from direct sunlight.

C. **Respiratory distress in the newborn**

   1. General considerations: Respiratory distress may be owing to pulmonary, cardiovascular, or other causes (Table 17-5).

   2. Physical examination

      a. The infant typically appears cyanotic in room air.

      b. Respiratory rate is higher than 60 bpm.

      c. Grunting as well as intercostal and sternal retractions is common.

      d. Cyanosis resolving with supplemental oxygen supports either a pulmonary or a noncardiovascular cause. This is known as the hyperoxia challenge test.

Table 17-5 | Common Causes of Respiratory Distress Syndrome

Pulmonary causes	Unilateral or bilateral choanal atresia Transient tachypnea of the newborn (resolves in 24 hours) Fluid aspiration (blood or meconium) Hyaline membrane disease (especially in premature infants) Congenital pneumonia (rectal flora pathogens)
Cardiovascular causes	
1. Cyanotic lesions	Valvular pulmonary stenosis (only when severe) Pulmonary atresia with ventricular septal defect (the most extreme form of tetralogy of Fallot) Tricuspid atresia Transposition of the great arteries Total anomalous pulmonary venous return Truncus arteriosus (<1% of cases)
2. Mild cyanosis resulting from left-sided outflow tract obstruction	Hypoplastic left heart syndrome (usually involving atresia of mitral valve, aortic valve, or both) Aortic stenosis Coarctation of the aorta
Other causes	Hyperthermia or hypothermia (hypothermia is especially troublesome for a preterm infant) Intrauterine exposure to cocaine Metabolic acidosis Hemorrhage or asphyxia resulting in damage to the CNS (can occur as a result of traumatic delivery)

CNS, central nervous system.

3. Laboratory and imaging studies

    a. Chest radiography, pulse oximetry, and arterial blood gases provide the basic information.

    b. CBC and blood cultures should be monitored if appropriate.

    c. A complete metabolic profile typically is performed on all cyanotic infants.

    d. Echocardiography or CT of the head and chest may be warranted by the suspected cause.

4. Management

    a. Provide immediate supplemental oxygen with close monitoring.

    b. Begin IV fluids (glucose or saline, as the situation warrants).

    c. Provide intubation if true respiratory failure is present.

    d. Determine the underlying cause and manage appropriately.

> The hyperoxia challenge test in newborn respiratory distress: Cyanosis that resolves when supplemental oxygen is applied supports either a pulmonary or a noncardiac cause.

Developmental Milestones and Disorders

A. Developmental milestones

    1. General considerations

        a. Typically, developmental surveys are carried out at each well-child examination; these examinations usually correspond to the typical vaccination schedule.

        b. Developmental screenings are done frequently between birth and 3 years of age and then each year thereafter.

        c. Parents and caregivers are important sources of information regarding the child's abilities.

        d. It is important to distinguish between a child whose pattern of development has slowed or regressed and a child who has always been developmentally slow because the causes generally are quite different.

    2. From birth to 5 years of age, the areas that are typically surveyed are gross and fine motor skills, personal and social behaviors, and language; assessment of older children shifts to higher cognitive functions and sexual maturation.

        a. Table 17-6 highlights the milestones for children from birth to 5 years of age.

        b. Table 17-7 highlights milestones for children from 6 to 10 years of age.

        c. Between 10 and 19 years of age, the focus shifts from developmental milestones to physical maturation and psychological development. The classical and most efficient way to gauge sexual maturation in males and females is by using Tanner stages (Table 17-8).

B. Developmental disorders

    1. General considerations

        a. Disorders of development are often first noted by parents or caregivers when a child fails to meet one or more milestones in development. Areas of concern include motor, visual–spatial, verbal, attention, behavioral, and social abilities.

        b. The most common neurodevelopmental disorder is attention-deficit hyperactivity disorder (ADHD); the most severe (in terms of affecting all areas of development) is intellectual disability.

    2. Evaluation of developmental disorders

        a. A comprehensive history should include a detailed prenatal history, labor and delivery, complications during pregnancy as well as the immediate postnatal period, major illness or hospitalizations, history of metabolic disease, and family history.

Table 17-6 | Typical Developmental Milestones: Birth to 5 Years of Age

Age/Skill	Gross Motor	Fine Motor	Personal/Social	Language
0–2 months	Turns head side to side	Clenched fist Eye contact	Recognizes human face	Cries Startles at loud noise
2–3 months	Lifts head	Tracks object past midline Hands open	Smiles responsively	Vocalizes in play
4–5 months	Head steady in supported position	Hands together	Shows displeasure through vocalization	Looks for source of sound
6–8 months	Rolls over Sits leaning forward on arms	Reaches for objects Raking grasp	Responds to own name Holds own bottle	Imitates speech sounds Vocal imitation
9–11 months	Stands while holding on	Passes object from hand to hand	Feeds self Imitates waving	Understands *no* May say *mama*
12–14 months	Stands alone for 2 seconds	Bangs two objects together Places pellet in bottle	Hugs dolls or stuffed animals Routinely gestures to meet needs	Uses one or two words with meaning
15–17 months	Stoops and recovers Walks well	Builds tower of two or three cubes	Attempts use of spoon	Waves bye-bye Uses four or five words
18–21 months	Runs well Kicks a large ball Walks backward	Scribbles Turns pages of book	Drinks well from a cup Feeds self Uses a spoon well	Follows simple commands (e.g., *give me*) 20–50 words
24 months	Throws ball overhead Jumps	Turns doorknobs Builds towers of six to seven blocks	Washes and dries hands Little spilling during self-feeding	Two or three words combined Points to body parts
36 months	Stands on one foot for at least 2 seconds	Copies circle	Takes turns Toilet trained	Uses pronouns (*I, me, you*) Gives name
48 months	Hops on one foot	Wiggles thumb Copies cross	Dresses self	Knows colors Asks questions
5 years	Skips using alternate feet	Holds a pencil correctly	Brushes teeth without help	Easily carries on a conversation May count or recite part of the alphabet

Table 17-7 | Typical Developmental Milestones: 6 to 10 Years of Age

Skill/Age	6 Years (Grade 1)	7 Years (Grade 2)	8 Years (Grade 3)	9 Years (Grade 4)	10 Years (Grade 5)
Language	Speaks using correct sentence structure	Defines words Compares and contrasts Speech reaches adult proficiency	Defines more words Recites days of the week	Comprehends absurdities in sentences	Understands abstract words
Hand–eye coordination	Draws more precisely	Legible printing Ties own shoelaces	Begins to learn cursive writing	Draws people, with detail	Draws people, with greater detail
Calculation and reading	Reads one-syllable words Counts to 20 Later reads simple sentences, adds and subtracts primary numbers	Reads two-syllable words Counts to 100 Adds and subtracts two-digit numbers	Reads many more two-syllable words Performs simple multiplication	Reads three- and four-syllable words Alphabetizes Does simple division Comprehends fractions	Able to read more complex words Easily uses addition, subtraction, fractions, division, multiplication, and estimation

Table 17-8 | Typical Tanner Stages for Males and Females from 11 to 17 Years of Age

Tanner Stage	2	3	4	5
	Ages 11–12	**Ages 13**	**Ages 14–15**	**Ages 16–17**
Males	Straight hair at base of penis	Coarse, dark, and curly pubic hair	Hair is almost completely full	Pubic hair achieves adult appearance
	Age 11	**Age 12**	**Age 13**	**Ages 14–15**
Females	Minimal, straight pubic hair	Increased pubic hair that is dark and coarse	Hair approaches normal adult appearance	Pubic hair reaches adult appearance and forms inverted triangle

b. A complete physical examination is essential, especially the neurologic examination and careful inspection for dysmorphic features.

c. Referral to appropriate specialists, including speech and occupational therapists, psychologists, and educational specialists, should be made as dictated by the child's needs.

3. Speech and/or language delay

a. Causes are many, with the most common being conductive hearing loss secondary to chronic middle ear effusion. Other causes include prematurity, neglect, autism, and congenital syndromes.

b. Language delay may be characterized by omitted sounds, difficulty pronouncing certain letters, dysfluency, or failure to have appropriate language skills by 2 or 3 years of age. Language should be assessed as expressive language and receptive language.

c. Hearing should be carefully assessed, especially when speech delay appears to be the only impairment.

d. Management includes referral to speech and language specialists for specific diagnosis, development of a treatment plan, and monitoring during development.

> Hearing should be thoroughly assessed in any speech or language delay.

4. ADHD (see Chapter 12)

5. Pervasive developmental disorders, including autism (see Chapter 12)

6. Intellectual disability

a. Intellectual disability is defined as an IQ of <70, with disturbances in adaptive behavior.

b. Physical examination

(1) Abnormal muscle tone is seen at 6 months.

(2) Motor delay is apparent by 1 year.

(3) All spheres of development are affected to some degree by 2 years.

c. Laboratory testing is carried out to uncover possible causes and contributing factors and includes CBC to rule out anemia; lead screen; chromosomal studies, especially if the child is dysmorphic; metabolic testing; thyroid studies; electroencephalography; and magnetic resonance imaging as appropriate.

d. Treatment includes referral to special programs for social, occupational, and cognitive support.

7. Spina bifida (myelomeningocele)

a. Two forms exist.

(1) Aperta is when the neural tube defect involves the overlying skin.

(2) Occulta appears as hairy tufts, dimples, or dermal sinus noted in the lumbosacral region.

b. Risk factors include insufficient intake of folic acid during pregnancy and maternal use of valproate.

c. Characteristic findings

(1) Neurological: hypotonia, sensory deficits, paralysis, hydrocephalus, or macrocephaly

(2) Extremities: contractures, tethered cord (which may cause back pain), clubfeet, scoliosis, or hip dislocations

(3) Urinary: frequent urosepsis, incontinence

> Adequate intake of folic acid during pregnancy reduces the risk of spina bifida significantly.

d. Treatment includes prompt intervention for hydrocephalus through shunting and referral for supportive services.

8. Cerebral palsy (see Chapter 11)

Inborn Errors of Metabolism, Chromosomal Abnormalities, and Common Dysmorphic Syndromes

A. Inborn Errors of Metabolism (IEMs)

1. General considerations

    a. All states screen infants for phenylketonuria (PKU), congenital adrenal hyperplasia, galactosemia, and hypothyroidism. These disorders are treatable, and testing generally is inexpensive.

    b. In general, more expansive and/or selective screening should be considered under the following conditions:

    (1) Acutely ill infant or neonate

    (2) Developmental delay (index of suspicion is higher with regression of development)

    (3) Failure to thrive

    (4) Intellectual disability

    (5) Organomegaly

2. **Management and treatment**

    a. Better outcomes are associated with early identification and when families both understand and can adhere to treatment regimens.

    b. Table 17-9 describes the specific characteristics, special tests, and management principles for PKU, congenital adrenal hyperplasia, galactosemia, and hypothyroidism.

B. Chromosomal abnormalities

1. General considerations

    a. Chromosomal abnormalities are found in 1 in 200 live births and approximately 7% of spontaneously aborted conceptuses.

    b. Occurrence of one or more of the following should prompt further evaluation: certain dysmorphology, metabolic disorder, degenerative disorders, ambiguous genitalia, multiple congenital anomalies, retinoblastoma, Wilms' tumor, developmental delay, abnormal stature, and primary amenorrhea.

> In recognizing an IEM, a delay or regression of a developmental milestone should trigger evaluation.

Table 17-9 | Common Inborn Errors of Metabolism: Epidemiology, Signs, Symptoms, Testing, and Management

Condition	Signs and Symptoms	Specific Evaluations	Treatments
Hypothyroidism (1:4,500 live births)	Lethargy, intellectual disability, eczema, failure to thrive; rarely goiter, thick tongue; up to 75% of newborns are asymptomatic during the first 2 months of life	Serial TSH, free T_4	Replacement therapy with L-thyroxine
Congenital adrenal hyperplasia (1:5,000 live births)	Virilized female; males may have ambiguous genitalia; infants may present early in life with salt-wasting, adrenal crisis	17-Hydroxyprogesterone	Corticosteroid replacement
Phenylketonuria (1:12,000 live births)	Moderate to severe intellectual disability, hyperactivity, seizures, autism, and hypopigmentation	Test after 24 hours of protein intake and then quantitative serum phenylalanine determination	Lifetime of low-protein diet; avoid products with phenylalanine
Galactosemia (1:60,000 live births)	Neonatal nausea and vomiting, jaundice, hepatic dysfunction and liver enlargement, intellectual disability, cataracts, and death	Galactose-1-phosphate uridyltransferase electrophoresis after galactose intake	Lactose- and galactose-free diet

TSH, thyroid-stimulating hormone; T_4, thyroxine.

c. Types of chromosomal anomalies

(1) Structural: deletions, duplications, translocations, inversions

(2) Numerical: triploidy and tetraploidy (both lethal), trisomy, monosomy, aneuploidy of sex chromosomes, and mosaicism

d. Initial evaluation when chromosomal abnormalities are suspected should include karyotype and fluorescent in situ hybridization. Evaluation is based on clinical suspicion, DNA analysis, and bacterial artificial chromosome–comparative genomic hybridization arrays.

e. Management is specific to the disorder and may include supportive care, environmental and educational programs, physical therapy, and other modalities.

2. Selected chromosomal abnormalities

a. Trisomy 21 (Down syndrome)

(1) Incidence is 1 in 700 live births.

(2) It is frequently associated with advanced maternal age.

(3) Common characteristics:

(a) Diagnosis is made if any six of the following characteristics are seen: hypotonia, poor Moro reflex, hypermobility of joints, flattened facies and occiput, excess skin on the posterior neck, anomalous auricles, upward-slanting palpebral fissures, pelvic dysplasia, dysplasia of the middle phalanx of the fifth finger, and a single transverse palmar crease (simian crease).

(b) Other features may include macrosomia, intellectual disability, hearing loss, Brushfield spots in the eyes, thyroid disease, gastrointestinal (GI) atresia, and atlantoaxial instability.

(c) Congenital heart disease is present in up to 40% of cases; atrioventricular septal defects are most common.

b. Klinefelter syndrome (XXY)

(1) Incidence is 1 in 600 live male births.

(2) Common characteristics

(a) Initially tall, thin, and long limbed; become obese in the adult years. Scoliosis is frequent.

(b) Ataxia, expressive language disorders, learning disabilities, and usually mild developmental delay are characteristic.

(c) Males exhibit small penis, hypogonadism, oligospermia or azoospermia, scant pubic and facial hair, and gynecomastia.

(d) Behavior concerns are frequent including poor self-esteem and substance abuse.

c. Turner's syndrome (monosomy X)

(1) Incidence is 1 in 2,000 female live births.

(2) Common characteristics

(a) Features include short stature, webbed neck, prominent ears and low posterior hairline, broad chest with widely spaced nipples, increased carrying angle, and congenital lymphedema.

(b) Other characteristics may include hearing impairment, visual and spatial perceptive disabilities, primary amenorrhea, ovarian dysgenesis, absence of secondary sex characteristics, coarctation of the aorta, horseshoe kidney, and aortic stenosis.

d. Fragile X syndrome

(1) Incidence is 1 in 7,000 male live births and 1 in 11,000 live female births.

> Turner's syndrome presents in females, with short stature, wide neck, and congenital lymphedema; Klinefelter syndrome presents in tall males, thin boys with hypogonadism, and often language disorders and developmental delays.

(2) Common characteristics: The range of clinical manifestations is very wide. All males will have some degree of manifestations, with 80% exhibiting cognitive and intellectual disability. Female carriers can be free of symptoms, although up to 50% may have some mild cognitive impairment.

  (a) Pale blue irises, long narrowed facies, large protruding ears, large protruding jaw, flat feet, and hyperextensible fingers

  (b) Prepubertal large gonads

  (c) Autism with disorganized speech patterns

  (d) Mitral valve prolapse

e. Beckwith–Wiedemann syndrome (chromosome 11p15)

  (1) Incidence is 1 in 15,000 live births.

  (2) Common characteristics

    (a) Large-for-gestational-age infants, hypoglycemia during infancy, creases and pits in earlobes, asymmetric limbs, organomegaly, and large tongue

    (b) At risk for Wilms' tumor and hepatoblastoma

f. Prader–Willi syndrome (chromosome 15q11)

  (1) Incidence is 1 in 25,000 live births.

  (2) Common characteristics

    (a) Infants are often small for gestational age and exhibit hypogonadism, small hands and feet, almond-shaped eyes, and hypotonia.

    (b) Intellectual disability, short stature, polyphagia, and eventually obesity are characteristic.

    (c) Diabetes and obesity hypoventilation syndrome (Pickwickian syndrome) are common complications.

g. Angelman syndrome (chromosome 15)

  (1) Incidence is unknown but estimated at between 1 in 15,000 and 1 in 30,000 live births.

  (2) Common characteristics

    (a) Severe intellectual disability, marked developmental delay, poor language skills, paroxysmal laughter, and tongue thrusting

    (b) Prognathism, seizures, and abnormal gait and posturing

C. Common dysmorphic syndromes

  1. General considerations

    a. Dysmorphic syndromes may result from a chromosomal anomaly or single-gene defects. Some are multifactorial; others may result from a combination of genetics and environment.

    b. Characteristics of these chromosomal or genetic anomalies include the following:

      (1) Multiple anomalies are common.

      (2) Abnormal growth patterns, both pre- and postnatally, are seen.

      (3) A child typically exhibits characteristics not seen in parents or siblings.

      (4) An infant may present with intellectual disability, abnormal muscle tone, seizures, sensory deficits, and motor and speech delay.

    c. Testing is specific for the syndrome under consideration.

    d. Treatment involves detailed genetic counseling and, in some cases, surgical intervention.

> Two common autosomal dominant dysmorphic syndromes are Ehlers–Danlos (affecting collagen and connective tissue) and Marfan syndrome (connective tissue defect with cardiac complications).

  2. Common dysmorphic syndromes

    a. Ehlers–Danlos syndrome is primarily an autosomal dominant condition (10 clinical types or disorders are known).

(1) The primary defect involves collagen and connective tissue, resulting in joint laxity, hyperelastic skin, pectus deformity, and excessive bruising.

(2) Death often results from a ruptured aneurysm.

b. Marfan syndrome is an autosomal dominant mutation.

(1) The primary defect involves a connective tissue protein, resulting in tall, lanky stature; joint laxity; high arched palate; long digits; and myopia.

(2) Complications result from mitral valve prolapse, aortic root dilation, aortic insufficiency, aneurysms, and spontaneous pneumothorax.

c. Fetal alcohol syndrome is related to maternal alcohol use.

(1) These children are born small and may remain small. Characteristics involving the head and facies include microcephaly, long and smooth philtrum, thin upper lip, small palpebral fissures, and small distal phalanges.

(2) This syndrome is complicated by developmental delay, hyperactivity, moderate intellectual disability, and involvement of internal organs (congenital heart disease, cleft lip or palate, and renal anomalies).

d. Neural tube defects

(1) Causes may include genetics and environment.

(2) Defects may be as severe as anencephaly or as mild as a small spina bifida.

(3) Folic acid supplementation before and throughout pregnancy may be protective.

e. Cleft lip and palate

(1) Typically, the cause is multifactorial, but cleft lip and palate may result from autosomal dominant, autosomal recessive, or X-linked disorders.

(2) Various degrees of severity are seen, involving specific deformities of the lip, hard palate, and soft palate.

(3) Look for other malformations because, in many cases, this will not be an isolated defect.

(4) Many cases are amenable to surgery.

f. Osteogenesis imperfect (*COL1A1* or *COL1A2* mutations)

(1) This autosomal dominant defect involves type 1 collagen, resulting in bone fragility and pathologic fractures.

(2) Some cases result in blue-tinted sclera and varying degrees of deafness.

(3) In its severest form, fetal demise may occur.

Failure to Thrive, Growth Delay, and Selected Nutritional Disorders of Childhood

A. **Failure to thrive**

1. General characteristics

a. Failure to thrive is defined as a child aged 2 years or younger with weight plotting below the fifth percentile for age on more than one occasion or whose weight crosses two major percentiles downward on a standardized growth grid.

b. Exceptions to this definition are genetic short stature, small-for-gestational-age infants, preterm infants, and overweight infants with a decreased rate of weight gain and increased rate of height gain.

c. Failure-to-thrive presentation affects approximately 10% of infants and children. It is most commonly associated with environmental and/or behavioral factors. Some specific factors to consider are prematurity, congenital anomalies, intrauterine exposure to toxins, developmental delay, anemia, lead poisoning, gastric reflux, renal tubular acidosis, and acute or chronic infections.

> Failure to thrive has numerous etiologies including ingestion problems, social or psychological barriers to food access, malabsorption causes, metabolic problems, or infection. Workup should be guided by history with these causes in mind.

2. Specific causes to be considered include
   a. Lack of appetite (caused by anemia, psychosocial problems, central nervous system [CNS] pathology, chronic infection, or GI disorder)
   b. Difficulty with ingestion (caused by psychosocial problems, feeding difficulty, cerebral palsy or other CNS disorders, dyspnea, craniofacial abnormalities, myopathies, or congenital syndromes)
   c. Lack of or low availability of food (consider inappropriate feeding techniques, inadequate access to or volume of food, inappropriate food for age, abuse, or neglect)
   d. Vomiting (caused by reflux, obstruction of the intestinal tract, or increased intracranial pressure)
   e. Malabsorption (cystic fibrosis, biliary disease, disorders of metabolism, immune deficiency, inflammatory bowel disease, or celiac disease)
   f. Diarrhea (caused by bacterial gastroenteritis, parasitic infection, or starvation)
   g. Inadequate absorption of calories (caused by hepatitis or Hirschsprung's disease)
   h. Increased metabolism or increased use of calories (chronic or recurrent infection [most common is urinary tract infection], chronic pulmonary insufficiency, congenital or acquired heart disease, neoplasm, lead poisoning, chronic anemia, or endocrinopathies)
   i. Defective use of calories (IEMs, renal tubular acidosis [uncommon], cyanotic heart disease)

3. Laboratory tests
   a. Investigation centers on uncovering the cause.
   b. Observation by a team or in a hospital setting is desired if a behavioral or psychosocial cause is suspected.
   c. Specific laboratory testing is needed as per history and physical examination. Initial laboratory should include:
      (1) CBC with differential and erythrocyte sedimentation rate (ESR)
      (2) Urinalysis with culture and sensitivity
      (3) Serum electrolytes, blood urea nitrogen (BUN), and creatinine
      (4) Thyroid-stimulating hormone (TSH) with thyroxine (T_4)
      (5) Tuberculin skin test
      (6) Radiography of wrists for bone age

4. **Treatment**
   a. Identify and treat the underlying cause.
   b. Remove the child from the home if indicated and necessary.
   c. Increase feedings for infants from 100 kcal to 150 kcal per kg per day.

B. Selected causes of growth delay
   1. **Familial short stature**
      a. General characteristics
         (1) Familial short stature is apparent before the second year of life that manifests as a deceleration in height.
         (2) Height is hereditary and closely matches the parental height.
      b. Physical examination: The child has normal development without other signs or symptoms of disease.
      c. Special testing: It is rare that additional workup is necessary.
         (1) Further testing to rule out other causes may include CBC; ESR; urinalysis; BUN and creatinine; serum electrolytes, including calcium and phosphorus; examination of stool for fat content; karyotype; and intrinsic growth factor (IGF)-1 and IGF-binding protein 3.

(2) Radiography of the distal radius reveals bone age equal to chronological age.

d. Treatment: Reassure parents that deceleration is normal and expected, especially if both parents are short.

2. **Constitutional growth delay**

   a. General characteristics

   (1) The child is often called a "late bloomer" and may have a family history of delayed growth.

   (2) Family members may be of normal height.

   (3) Skeletal bone age will lag behind the chronological age.

   (4) Puberty may be delayed.

   b. Physical examination: Except for height, development is normal for age.

   c. Selected testing

   (1) Further testing is driven by the history and physical examination findings; testing is done to rule out other causes as mentioned in failure to thrive.

   (2) Radiography of the distal radius reveals chronological age greater than bone age.

   d. Treatment: Growth is delayed, but eventually the child will reach their expected height.

3. **GH deficiency**

   a. General characteristics

   (1) The anterior pituitary produces GH under stimulation from GH-releasing hormone and suppression of somatostatin. GH deficiency may be an isolated disorder or may occur as a result of other pituitary hormone deficiencies.

   (2) The most likely cause is idiopathic; other diagnoses to consider include congenital (empty sella syndrome) and acquired (craniopharyngioma).

   (3) Growth failure caused by GH deficiency may occur during infancy or appear later in childhood and is largely dependent on the underlying cause.

   (4) Laron syndrome is dwarfism that results from a mutation in the GH receptor.

   b. Physical examination

   (1) Decline in growth velocity or subnormal growth is characteristic.

   (2) Children with dwarfism have distinctive facial features.

   (3) Truncal obesity may be present because GH also promotes lipolysis.

   (4) Impaired peripheral vision with optic chiasm tumors is frequent.

   (5) Delayed puberty and webbed neck are seen in cases of Turner's syndrome.

   (6) Disproportionately short limbs compared with trunk suggest a skeletal dysplasia.

   c. Testing

   (1) Testing should be as suggested by the history and physical examination and to rule out other causes as mentioned in failure to thrive.

   (2) Radiography of the distal radius should be performed for bone age.

   (3) When other causes are ruled out and GH status is equivocal, more provocative studies are warranted.

   (4) In some cases, a trial of human GH may be warranted and may confirm the diagnosis.

   d. Treatment

   (1) Human GH has been approved for specific causes, such as Prader–Willi syndrome, Turner's syndrome, children born small for gestational age who fail to grow, and chronic renal failure.

> In growth delay, evaluate for failure to thrive and consider: familial short stature (matching short parents), constitutional growth delay (a "late bloomer"), and growth hormone (GH) deficiency (an endocrine deficiency warranting careful evaluation).

(2) Referral to a pediatric endocrinologist is recommended because tests for GH deficiency are often difficult to interpret and treatment with GH for other causes is controversial.

C. **Selected nutritional disorders**

1. General considerations

a. Nutritional deficiencies may result from internal causes (e.g., blood loss, malabsorption, chronic disease) or external causes (e.g., inappropriate feeding, psychosocial distress, inability to take in sufficient nutrition).

b. The ideal source of infant nutrition is breast milk because it contains the ideal mix of nutrients as well as protein, lipids, and carbohydrates; promotes bonding; and strengthens the infant's immune system. Infant formulas closely resemble breast milk in terms of providing energy and nutrition.

c. The typical infant diet should consist of breast milk or formula until 6 months of age. Solid foods should be introduced one at a time to avoid confusion and identify any sensitivities. There is no special order for introducing foods, but all food should be pureed to prevent choking.

d. Cow's milk with low fat (2%) content should be initiated not earlier than 1 year of age.

2. Calcium, fluoride, vitamin K, protein, and carbohydrate deficiencies (Table 17-10).

Table 17-10 | Selected Nutritional Disorders

Nutrient	Risk Factors for Development	Signs and Symptoms	Laboratory Examinations	Treatment
Protein	Body cannot store protein, so a daily supply is needed. Severe skin disease and burns Cystic fibrosis	Impaired growth velocity Severest form is kwashiorkor, resulting in lethargy, irritability, impaired growth velocity, edema, and hepatomegaly.	Chemistry panel (may suggest decreased albumin) CBC (may reveal other deficiencies)	Adjust diet; increase daily intake of protein
Carbohydrate	Daily supply is required because of the body's limited ability to store excess. Galactosemia (inborn error of metabolism) Diarrhea Malabsorption Improper diet Excess intake results in obesity and increased risk of type 2 diabetes mellitus	Impaired growth velocity Obesity Marasmus is a severe form of malnutrition resulting from multiple dietary deficiencies, including lack of carbohydrates.	Chemistry panel (electrolyte imbalances likely) CBC	Dietary adjustment
Vitamin K	Aids in the formulation of coagulation proteins Newborns Breastfed newborns who do not receive vitamin K prophylactically at birth	Hemorrhagic purpura involving skin, internal organs, and CNS, which may be fatal	Vitamin K levels Prolonged prothrombin time	IM vitamin K injection
Fluoride	Fluoride is incorporated into the tooth matrix, increasing resistance to dental caries. This element is contained in most public water sources.	Increased number of dental caries In case of fluorosis, look for undermineralization and discolored teeth.	Dental examinations	Consider supplementation after 6 months of age when the water source does not contain fluoride.
Iron	Breastfed infants Untreated maternal anemia Prematurity Blood loss during the neonatal period	Asymptomatic when mild Pallor Fatigue Impaired cognitive and motor development Pica	CBC with differential Serum ferritin Serum iron Total iron-binding capacity Reticulocyte count	Food with high iron content Supplementation For breastfed infants, introduce iron-fortified cereals at 4–6 months

CBC, complete blood count; CNS, central nervous system; IM, intramuscular.

Immunization of Infants and Children (Fig. 17-2)

A. General considerations

1. Combination products (one syringe containing multiple vaccines) are preferred and have not been found to diminish immune response or to increase the rate of adverse events.

2. Premature infants are immunized just as term newborns in regard to amount and timing. One exception is the hepatitis B vaccine, which is recommended for premature infants weighing ≥2 kg.

3. There are few contraindications to vaccines:

   a. Anaphylactic reaction to previous vaccine or component of a vaccine:

      (1) Neomycin and streptomycin are common preservatives in measles, mumps, and rubella (MMR) vaccine and inactivated polio vaccine (IPV) and have caused allergic reactions and anaphylaxis.

      (2) Baker's yeast allergy: Avoid hepatitis B vaccine.

      (3) Allergy to eggs: Avoid influenza vaccine if anaphylaxis has occurred with egg or egg-containing products. Children with relatively minor intolerance of eggs may be considered for vaccination.

Vaccine	Birth	1 mo	2 mos	4 mos	6 mos	9 mos	12 mos	15 mos	18 mos	19–23 mos	2–3 yrs	4–6 yrs	7–10 yrs	11–12 yrs	13–15 yrs	16–18 yrs
Hepatitis B[1] (HepB)	1st dose	◄---- 2nd dose ----►			◄---------------------- 3rd dose ----------------------►											
Rotavirus[2] (RV) RV1 (2-dose series); RV5 (3-dose series)			1st dose	2nd dose	See footnote 2											
Diphtheria, tetanus, & acellular pertussis[3] (DTaP: <7 yrs)			1st dose	2nd dose	3rd dose			◄----- 4th dose -----►				5th dose				
Haemophilus influenzae type b[4] (Hib)			1st dose	2nd dose	See footnote 4		◄--- 3rd or 4th dose, See footnote 4 ---►									
Pneumococcal conjugate[5] (PCV13)			1st dose	2nd dose	3rd dose		◄----- 4th dose -----►									
Inactivated poliovirus[6] (IPV: <18 yrs)			1st dose	2nd dose	◄---------------------- 3rd dose ----------------------►							4th dose				
Influenza[7] (IIV; LAIV)					Annual vaccination (IIV only) 1 or 2 doses						Annual vaccination (LAIV or IIV) 1 or 2 doses		Annual vaccination (LAIV or IIV) 1 dose only			
Measles, mumps, rubella[8] (MMR)					See footnote 8	◄----- 1st dose -----►						2nd dose				
Varicella[9] (VAR)						◄----- 1st dose -----►						2nd dose				
Hepatitis A[10] (HepA)						◄-------- 2-dose series, See footnote 10 --------►										
Meningococcal[11] (Hib-MenCY ≥6 weeks; MenACWY-D ≥9 mos; MenACWY-CRM ≥ 2 mos)					See footnote 11									1st dose		Booster
Tetanus, diphtheria, & acellular pertussis[12] (Tdap: ≥7 yrs)														(Tdap)		
Human papillomavirus[13] (2vHPV: females only; 4vHPV, 9vHPV: males and females)														(3-dose series)		
Meningococcal B[11]															See footnote 11	
Pneumococcal polysaccharide[5] (PPSV23)												See footnote 5				

| Range of recommended ages for all children | Range of recommended ages for catch-up immunization | Range of recommended ages for certain high-risk groups | Range of recommended ages for non-high-risk groups that may receive vaccine, subject to individual clinical decision making | No recommendation |

This schedule includes recommendations in effect as of January 1, 2016. Any dose not administered at the recommended age should be administered at a subsequent visit, when indicated and feasible. The use of a combination vaccine generally is preferred over separate injections of its equivalent component vaccines. Vaccination providers should consult the relevant Advisory Committee on Immunization Practices (ACIP) statement for detailed recommendations, available online at http://www.cdc.gov/vaccines/hcp/acip-recs/index.html. Clinically significant adverse events that follow vaccination should be reported to the Vaccine Adverse Event Reporting System (VAERS) online (http://www.vaers.hhs.gov) or by telephone (800-822-7967). Suspected cases of vaccine-preventable diseases should be reported to the state or local health department. Additional information, including precautions and contraindications for vaccination, is available from CDC online (http://www.cdc.gov/vaccines/recs/vac-admin/contraindications.htm) or by telephone (800-CDC-INFO [800-232-4636]).

This schedule is approved by the Advisory Committee on Immunization Practices (http://www.cdc.gov/vaccines/acip), the American Academy of Pediatrics (http://www.aap.org), the American Academy of Family Physicians (http://www.aafp.org), and the American College of Obstetricians and Gynecologists (http://www.acog.org).

NOTE: The above recommendations must be read along with the footnotes of this schedule.

Figure 17-2 ▶ Recommended immunization schedule for persons aged 0 to 18 years. Available along with schedules for ages 7 to 18 years and catchup at: http://www.cdc.gov/vaccines/schedules/hcp/child-adolescent.html.

(4) Gelatin allergy: Avoid varicella vaccine.

b. History of encephalopathy within 7 days of giving diphtheria, tetanus, and pertussis (DTaP) vaccine. The DTaP is the vaccine most likely to cause a febrile reaction, although this is rare and should not limit future vaccines.

c. Guillain–Barré syndrome following any vaccine.

d. Pregnancy: Avoid live vaccines, such as MMR and varicella, and live attenuated influenza vaccine.

e. Avoid MMR, varicella, and rotavirus vaccine if immunocompromised.

4. Precautions should be taken with the following vaccines under certain circumstances:

a. Consider rescheduling any vaccine in the presence of moderate to severe illness and/or fever ($\geq$102.5°F/39.0°C) or in the presence of rashes or exanthems.

b. Postpone MMR and varicella vaccine until 3 to 6 months after the administration of immunoglobulin.

c. Carefully consider readministration of DTaP or DTP when serious or severe side effects, such as high fever (40.5°C/104.5°F), shock-like state, seizure, prolonged and inconsolable crying, or Guillain–Barré syndrome, occur with any dose. Chronic seizure disorder is a contraindication to tetanus, diphtheria, and pertussis (Tdap)/DTaP.

d. Pregnant females should avoid human papillomavirus (HPV), live influenza, MMR, varicella, and polio vaccines. Generally, all other nonlive vaccines can be given during pregnancy.

e. Consider postponing MMR with a current or recent history of thrombocytopenic purpura.

f. The first dose of rotavirus vaccine is administered earlier than 15 weeks of age and the last by age 8 months.

g. MMR vaccine may decrease the response to a tuberculin (TB) skin testing, potentially causing a false-negative response in someone who actually has an infection with TB. MMR can be administered the same day as a TB skin test, but if MMR has been administered and 1 or more days have elapsed, in most situations, it is recommended to wait at least 4 weeks before conducting a routine TB skin test.

5. Personal or family history of seizures, mild illness with or without fever ($\leq$102.5°F/39.0°C), breastfeeding, recent positive TB skin testing, and use of antibiotics are not reasons to postpone vaccines.

B. Thimerosal

1. Since 2001, routine childhood vaccines in the United States are manufactured without the use of thimerosal.

2. Multidose vials of injectable influenza vaccine may contain thimerosal (depending on the manufacturer), whereas single-dose preparations are free of the preservative.

3. Numerous large studies have failed to link thimerosal or vaccines to autism as was initially reported in a refuted 1998 study. The MMR vaccine never contained thimerosal.

> If a patient is immuno-compromised or pregnant, avoid MMR, varicella, rotavirus, and live flu vaccine.

Common Pediatric Poisonings

A. General considerations

1. Every year, 85% of all poisonings occur in children <5 years of age; they generally are accidental and unwitnessed.

2. Mortality rates are low and likely to involve analgesics, household cleaning products, iron, hydrocarbons, and medications (over-the-counter, prescription, and illicit).

3. Adolescent ingestions are likely intentional and result from suicide attempts or use of illicit drugs and are 15-fold more fatal than accidental ingestions in small children.

4. Commonly ingested substances include cosmetic or hygiene products, cleaning products, analgesics, plants, cough or cold preparations, pesticides, vitamins, and hydrocarbons.

5. Children should be screened for lead poisoning.

   a. The primary source of lead exposure in the United States is lead-based paint, even though its use has been banned in residential buildings since the 1970s.

   b. Universal risk assessment screening is recommended for all children, with a focus on high prevalence areas. Targeted screening at older ages is recommended for communities with a greater prevalence of elevated lead levels or communities with a higher proportion of older homes.

   c. A venous sample is preferred over capillary blood. Levels <10 µg per dL require no further action; >14 µg per dL should prompt close developmental and cognitive monitoring, identification of possible sources, and removal of the child from exposure. Levels >45 µg per dL should be treated with chelation; >70 µg per dL results in severe health problems, seizure, and coma.

> Lead risk assessment screening is recommended as part of a well-child visit under age 6, with testing if the assessment is positive.

B. History and physical examination

   1. Obtain a history of what (and quantity), when, and how the ingestion or exposure occurred.

   a. If available, the offending substance should be brought to the emergency department.

   b. Inventories of household products as well as over-the-counter and prescription medicines should be conducted.

   c. History reveals the substance in about 90% of cases.

   2. Physical examination (see Table 17-11 for toxins and physical findings)

   a. Note any unusual breath odors (arsenic and organophosphates produce garlic breath).

   b. Check the skin for excessive dryness, sweating, discoloration, and fever (anticholinergics cause warm, dry skin, whereas organic phosphates produce salivation and urination).

   c. Pupillary size as well as lacrimation should be noted.

   d. Vomiting or excessive salivation should be noted.

   e. Neurologic changes, such as agitation, ataxia, tremors, convulsion, and coma, are often encountered.

   f. Tachycardia, tachypnea, and dysrhythmias (tricyclic antidepressants are notorious for causing prolonged QRS complexes) may occur in some settings.

C. Laboratory testing (see Table 17-11)

   1. Calculate the anion and osmolar gaps (alcohol causes an anion gap; methanol causes an osmolar gap).

   2. Perform initial and ongoing electrocardiography.

   3. When the substance is unknown, standard emergency department toxin panels may provide the diagnosis.

   4. Order specific toxicology screens, such as diuretics, ethylene glycol, lithium, aromatic hydrocarbons, and cyanide, as indicated.

   5. Abdominal radiographs, as a rule, are not helpful because very few agents are radio-opaque (e.g., heavy metals, iodine, enteric-coated tablets).

D. **Management** (see Table 17-11)

   1. Airway, breathing, and circulation should be the first concern.

   2. Additional management is predicated on the type of ingestion.

   3. General principles of management

   a. Induced vomiting and/or gastric lavage are not recommended.

Table 17-11 | **Common Toxidromes**

Toxin	Physical Findings	Special Tests	Antidotes/Management
Hydrocarbons (benzene, gasoline, petroleum distillates)	Mucosal irritation Vomiting, bloody diarrhea Cyanosis, respiratory distress Tachycardia Fever CNS depression	CXR Urinalysis ECG	Avoid emetics and lavage Oxygen with mist Antibiotics if pneumonia develops
Caustics (toilet bowl cleaners)	Skin, mucosal burns Hematemesis Abdominal pain Respiratory distress Convulsions, coma	EGD to determine the degree of esophageal injury ECG	Small amounts of water or milk Avoid vomiting Supportive care
Bases (Clorox, Drano)	Irritated mucous membranes Respiratory distress secondary to edematous epiglottis Perforation of stomach or esophagus	EGD to determine the degree of damage to the larynx, esophagus, and stomach	Small amounts of water as dilutant Avoid vomiting Supportive care
Acetaminophen	Hepatotoxic	Monitor APAP plasma concentration (use specific nomogram)	Acetylcysteine is the specific antidote
Aspirin (salicylates)	Vomiting Hyperpnea Fever Encephalopathy, convulsions, coma Renal failure Pulmonary edema	Check serum salicylate level Look for metabolic acidosis and decreased K^+ Elevated or reduced serum glucose	Induce emesis Charcoal to bind drug Correct dehydration Hemodialysis
Antihistamines	Agitation and hallucinations Miosis Red eye, dry skin Fever Respiratory failure CV collapse	EC6 ligase chains Pulse oximetry	Activated charcoal Whole-bowel irrigation Physostigmine
Organophosphates (chlorthion, diazinon)	Salivation, lacrimation Diaphoresis Urination, diarrhea Miosis Pulmonary congestion Twitching, convulsions, coma	Measure red cell cholinesterase levels Blood glucose levels	ABCs Decontamination of skin Atropine plus pralidoxime
Iron (vitamins, prenatal vitamins)	Intestinal bleeding Impaired coagulation Acidosis Shock Coma Red urine	Blood indices Metabolic panel Monitor urine output for renal damage Blood type and cross-match LFTs	Evoke emesis Gastric lavage Whole-bowel irrigation Desferoxamine Dialysis

CNS, central nervous system; CXR, chest radiography; ECG, electrocardiography; EGD, esophagogastroduodenoscopy; APAP, *N*-acetyl-*P*-aminophenol; CV, cardiovascular; ABCs, airway, breathing, circulation; LFTs, liver function tests.

    b. Activated charcoal is used to promote GI decontamination. It is the current first-line treatment for most ingested poisons.

    c. Use of sorbitol or other cathartics may accelerate elimination.

    d. Whole-bowel irrigation, dialysis, and hemoperfusion are rarely necessary.

    e. Antidotes exist for specific ingestions. Check with the local poison control center.

Common Pediatric Disorders

A. For further information and other disorders, see appropriate chapters.

B. Foreign bodies

1. Infants and children often place objects in orifices. Common objects include beads, buttons, nuts, foodstuff, and toy parts.

2. Ear, nose, and throat (ENT)

   a. Unilateral purulent rhinitis, persistent sinusitis, or a blocked nasal passage should prompt consideration of a foreign body in the nose.

   b. Ear pain, drainage, and acute hearing loss accompany foreign bodies in the ear.

   c. If the object is visible, remove it using a curette, forceps, or catheter. Be sure the child is restrained, and do not blindly probe.

3. Respiratory tract

   a. Upper airway: Obstruction causes abrupt onset of cough, stridor, choking, and cyanosis; complete obstruction leads to inability to cough or choke.

   b. Lower airway: Obstruction causes acute to subacute cough, unilateral persistent wheezing, and recurrent pneumonia; complete obstruction may cause a ball valve effect, resulting in distal hyperinflation and mediastinal shift, which is most apparent on expiratory films.

   c. Attempt the Heimlich maneuver if respiratory distress is apparent, and proceed with rigid bronchoscopy if the object is lodged in the lower airway.

4. GI tract

   a. Most objects pass through the GI tract. Large or irregularly shaped objects may become lodged; sharp objects, such as pins, may cause mucosal tearing.

   b. Prompt removal by EGD is recommended for caustic (e.g., batteries), sharp, or lodged objects. Small lithium button-type batteries can rapidly erode the esophagus or stomach lining, resulting in severe morbidity and death in as little as 3 hours.

> Most GI ingestions pass harmlessly, with the exception of batteries, which can erode mucosal lining and cause mortality. Ingested batteries require prompt removal with esophagogastroduodenoscopy (EGD).

C. **Functional (innocent) murmurs**

1. Approximately 40% to 45% of children have an innocent murmur at some point in their childhood.

2. Still's murmur is the most common innocent murmur of childhood.

   a. It is usually apparent from 2 years of age through preadolescence.

   b. It is the loudest in the apex and left sternal border. It is typically a grade I to III musical or vibratory, high-pitched, early systolic murmur that diminishes with sitting, standing, or Valsalva maneuvers, and it accentuates with fever.

3. Venous hum

   a. Grade I or II musical hum is heard best in the left and right infraclavicular areas and is usually louder on the right.

   b. It typically appears after 2 years of age.

   c. Best heard with the child sitting; diminishes with turning of the head, jugular compression, or supine position.

4. Innominate or carotid bruits

   a. This is typically found in older children and adolescents.

   b. A grade II or III, harsh, systolic ejection murmur is characteristic.

5. Pulmonary ejection murmur is a common innocent murmur in older children.

   a. It typically first appears around 3 years of age and continues through adolescence.

   b. Grade I or II, soft, systolic ejection murmur well localized to the upper left sternal border is heard.

   c. It typically becomes louder with the patient supine and diminishes with Valsalva maneuver.

6. Echocardiography is recommended to rule out pathologic murmurs; other testing should be selected based on patient history, physical exam, and echocardiography results.

7. The most important components of management are establishing the correct diagnosis and reassuring the parents.

   D. Infectious diseases

     1. Coxsackievirus

       a. Herpangina

         (1) There is acute onset of fever and posterior pharyngeal vesicles.

         (2) Vesicles are grayish white and quickly form ulcers with erythematous halos. Lesions may be linearly arranged on the palate, uvula, and tonsillar pillars.

         (3) Dysphagia, fever, vomiting, and anorexia occur. The child is irritable secondary to pain. Risk of dehydration is high.

         (4) Treatment is supportive (e.g., fluids, antipyretics, topical lidocaine).

       b. **Hand–foot–mouth disease caused by Coxsackievirus A16**

         (1) Red papules or vesicles occur on the tongue, oral mucosa, hands, feet, and buttocks.

         (2) Fever, sore throat, and malaise are usually mild.

         (3) Treatment is supportive.

     2. **Kawasaki disease** (mucocutaneous lymph node syndrome)

       a. Etiology is unknown, but a viral cause is suggested. A similar syndrome has been seen in pediatric patients post–COVID illness.

       b. Most patients are <5 years of age.

       c. Fever (>5 days) in addition to at least four of the following symptoms are needed to make a diagnosis: conjunctivitis; lip cracking and fissuring, strawberry tongue, or inflammation of the oral mucosa; cervical lymphadenopathy, usually unilateral; polymorphous exanthem; or redness and swelling of the hands and feet with subsequent desquamation.

       d. Cardiovascular manifestations are worrisome; myocarditis, pericarditis, valvular heart disease, and coronary arteritis and aneurysms are possible. Two-dimensional echocardiography or angiography is recommended in all the patients suspected of having Kawasaki disease.

       e. **Treatment** is with IV immunoglobulin and high-dose aspirin; early treatment reduces the chance of cardiac events. Patients with cardiac disease should receive long-term aspirin therapy and annual follow-up.

       f. Patients should be monitored through serial electrocardiography, chest radiography, and echocardiography until they recover.

     3. **Viral exanthems:** Table 17-12 depicts the characteristics of some common viral exanthems.

Table 17-12 | Common Viral Exanthems

Characteristics	Varicella (Chicken Pox)	Erythema Infectiosum (Fifth Disease, Slapped Cheek)	Roseola (Roseola Infantum, Exanthem Subitum)	Measles (Rubeola)	Rubella (German Measles)
Etiology	A human herpesvirus	Human parvovirus B19	Human herpesvirus 6 or 7	Measles virus	Rubella virus
Incubation period	10–21 days	4–14 days	10–14 days	8–14 days	14–21 days
Prodrome	Fever, respiratory symptoms (1–3 days)	None	Fever (4 days)	Fever, cough, anorexia, coryza (1–3 days)	None
Rash	Vesicular erythematous, torso and face to extremities (dewdrop on rose petal)	Red face ("slapped cheek"); lacy, pink, macular rash on torso	Pink, macular rash	Maculopapular, face to extremities; Koplik's spots in mouth	Maculopapular, from head to toe
Comments	Pruritic		Fever resolves before rash		Teratogenic

Caring for the Adolescent

1. Examination of the adolescents (13 to 19 years of age)

   a. Generally, it is an acceptable practice to screen adolescents every 3 years under normal conditions.

   b. Complete physical examinations are conducted looking for hearing and visual impairments, scoliosis, and heart defects that may prohibit sports participation along with Tanner Staging (see Table 17-8). Blood pressure, weight, height, body mass index, lipid measurements, and sexually transmitted infection testing may be performed.

   c. A complete social, behavioral, and educational history should be obtained at the well-child visit using what is commonly referred to as HEADSS assessment (see Table 17-13).

Table 17-13 │ HEADSS Assessment

Home	Where do you live? Details about home life.
Education	Tell me about your school.
Activities/employment	What do you do for fun/job/with friends?
Drugs	Smoking or drinking or drugs?
Suicidality	Have you ever thought of hurting yourself?
Sex	Dating? Boys/girls/both? Are you safe?

Practice Questions

Directions: *Each of the numbered items or incomplete statements in this section is followed by a list of answers or completions of the statement. Select the ONE lettered answer or completion that is BEST in each case.*

1. Examination of a newborn reveals flat facies, pale yellow spots at the periphery of the irises, upward-slanting palpebral fissures, and small abnormally shaped ears. What is the most likely diagnosis?
   A. Down syndrome
   B. Fetal alcohol syndrome
   C. Fragile X
   D. Klinefelter syndrome
   E. Turner's syndrome

2. A new mother is concerned about a rash that started on her 3-day-old son's arms and has spread to the neck and trunk. Examination reveals a sleeping baby with diffuse small pustules on erythematous halos. What is the recommended management?
   A. Apply low-dose topical corticosteroid cream daily
   B. Dress the child in loose clothing
   C. Reassure the mother that the rash is benign and will fade in 1 to 2 weeks
   D. Use moisturizing soaps without dyes or fragrance
   E. Wash clothes with hypoallergenic detergent and avoid fabric softener

3. A 4-year-old presents with a diffuse, pink, macular rash that developed today. The child's mother states that the child was cranky and feverish for 2 days but back to her usual activity today. Vitals in the office include T 98.4°F, P 80 and regular, R 16, BP 90/62. What is the most likely diagnosis?
   A. Erythema infectiosum
   B. Measles
   C. Roseola infantum
   D. Rubella
   E. Varicella

4. A baby undergoes well-child examination. She sits alone leaning forward on her arms, reaches for an object with a raking grasp, and responds to her name with babbling echoes. Given typical milestones, what is the likely age for this child?
   A. 3 to 4 months
   B. 6 to 8 months
   C. 10 to 12 months
   D. 12 to 14 months

5. A 4-week-old who is exclusively breastfed has loose maroon stools and scattered purpura. What is the next step in management of this child?
   A. Add over-the-counter multivitamin daily
   B. Avoid red meats in mother's diet
   C. Draw blood for thrombocyte workup
   D. Obtain stool for ova and parasites
   E. Vitamin K intramuscularly

6. A 3-year-old has a grade I/VI early systolic murmur. It is high-pitched, loudest at the apex, and diminishes with Valsalva. Echocardiography is unremarkable. Which of the following should be included in the education of this patient and parents?
   - **A.** Activity should be restricted.
   - **B.** Any fever should prompt nonsteroidal anti-inflammatory drug (NSAID) use.
   - **C.** The child is at an increased risk for cardiac complications.
   - **D.** It will disappear by adolescence.
   - **E.** Siblings should be evaluated as well.

7. A preadolescent boy presents for routine checkup. Examination reveals sparse pubic hairs that are coarse, dark, and curly. What Tanner stage does this represent?
   - **A.** Stage 1
   - **B.** Stage 2
   - **C.** Stage 3
   - **D.** Stage 4
   - **E.** Stage 5

8. A 3-year-old has experienced a significant decline in growth velocity. Radiographs of what area is best to evaluate this patient's bone age?
   - **A.** Cervical vertebrae
   - **B.** Distal femur
   - **C.** Distal radius
   - **D.** Ischial spine
   - **E.** Proximal humerus

9. During the newborn examination, a nasal catheter easily passes through the right nares but not the left. What is the next step?
   - **A.** CT scan of the area

   - **B.** Instill saline twice daily and reassess in 1 week
   - **C.** Instill topical steroid daily and reassess in 1 week
   - **D.** Place baby in a humidity tent
   - **E.** Waters view plain radiographs

10. A newborn is noted to have several small pearly nodules along the midline of the hard palate. What is the diagnosis?
    - **A.** Aphthous ulcers
    - **B.** Coxsackievirus
    - **C.** Epstein pearls
    - **D.** Natal teeth
    - **E.** Submucosal cleft

11. A newborn is exhibiting mild respiratory distress. Examination reveals a scaphoid abdomen. What is the most likely diagnosis?
    - **A.** Cystic hygroma
    - **B.** Diaphragmatic hernia
    - **C.** Hirschsprung's disease
    - **D.** Prune belly
    - **E.** Situs inversus

12. A 14-year-old has been diagnosed with congenital syndrome that causes defects in collagen and connective tissue. He is tall and lanky with lax joints, long digits, and myopia. What is the inheritance pattern of the most likely diagnosis?
    - **A.** Autosomal dominant
    - **B.** Autosomal recessive
    - **C.** X-linked dominant
    - **D.** X-linked recessive

Practice Answers

1. A. *Pediatrics; Diagnosis; Down Syndrome*

There are several characteristics that may indicate Down syndrome (trisomy 21) including flat facies, Brushfield spots, slanting palpebral fissures, abnormally shaped ears, hypermobile joints, excess skin on the posterior neck, a single transverse palmar crease (Simian crease), and digital dysplasia. Affected individuals have intellectual disability and are at risk of hearing loss and congenital cardiac disease. Fetal alcohol syndrome may be suspected in babies with microcephaly, long smooth philtrum, thin upper lip, small palpebral fissures, and small distal phalanges. Fragile X babies have pale blue irises, long narrow facies, large protruding ears and jaw, and flat feet. Turner's syndrome (single X) includes webbed neck, prominent ears, and a low posterior hairline. Klinefelter syndrome (XXY) is not associated with characteristic features at birth; later ataxia, mild developmental delay, and behavior problems develop.

2. C. *Pediatrics; Clinical Intervention; Erythema Toxicum*

Small scattered pustules with erythematous bases describe erythema toxicum, a benign rash of the newborn. No particular treatment or lifestyle change is needed; the rash fades away in 1 to 2 weeks. Milia consists of small white papules on the nose, cheeks, forehead, and chin; it is also benign and fades away

in 1 to 2 months. Miliaria ("heat rash") is caused by blockage of sweat glands and presents as a macular rash; light, loose clothes, and low humidity are recommended.

3. C. *Pediatrics; Diagnosis; Roseola*

Roseola (roseola infantum, exanthem subitum) is caused by human herpesvirus 6 or 7. The child typically has a fever for 2 to 5 days and breaks out in a fine macular rash when the fever breaks. It is benign and resolves with time. Erythema infectiosum (parvovirus) presents with fever and a red rash on the face ("slapped cheek"). Measles rash is preceded by 2 to 5 days of fever, cough, and coryza. Rubella (German measles) presents as a maculopapular rash that spreads from the head down to the toes. Varicella (chicken pox) presents with fever, mild respiratory symptoms, and a vesicular rash that crusts; lesions appear in crops.

4. B. *Pediatrics; History and PE; Developmental Milestones*

This child is exhibiting milestones typical of a 6- to 8-month-old. A 3- to 4-month-old can lift and hold their head up and look around for the source of sounds. A 10- to 12-month-old can stand alone, is able to bang two objects together, and use a rough grasp to pick up small objects. At 12 to 14 months, a fine pincer grasp is expected; the child can typically say one or two words with their meaning.

5. E. *Pediatrics; Clinical Intervention; Vitamin K Deficit*

Babies who are breastfed are at risk for vitamin K deficit, which manifests with bleeding. Infants who are breastfed should receive a multivitamin specifically designed to deliver needed minerals and vitamins. If the child does not respond to a vitamin K injection, consider further workup. Mother's diet does not need adjusting.

6. D. *Pediatrics; Health Maintenance; Still's Murmur*

Still's murmur is the most common innocent murmur of childhood. The murmur is early systolic, loudest at the base or left sternal border, and diminishes with Valsalva. No restrictions are needed, and the murmur typically resolves by adolescence. An echocardiography rules out other causes.

7. C. *Pediatrics; History and PE; Tanner Stage*

Fine vellus hair is present in stage 1. Straight hair at the base of the penis is stage 2. Stage 3 is characterized by sparse hairs that are coarse and curly. An almost full extent of hair is stage 4, and full adult appearance is stage 5.

8. C. *Pediatrics; Diagnostic Studies; Growth Delay*

The hand and wrist bones, including the distal radius, is the most sensitive area for assessing bone age because the pattern of ossification is predictable.

9. A. *Pediatrics; Diagnostic Studies; Choanal Atresia*

A CT scan is indicated in suspected choanal atresia to assess the full extent of the obstruction and guide corrective interventions.

10. B. *Pediatrics; Diagnosis; Epstein Pearls*

Epstein pearls are benign retention cysts; they resolve with time. Coxsackievirus causes hand–foot–mouth disease. Aphthous ulcers appear on the mucosa as superficial erosions with gray halos. Natal teeth appear in the gums. A submucosal cleft is evidenced by a bifid uvula.

11. B. *Pediatrics; Diagnosis; Diaphragmatic Hernia*

With a diaphragmatic hernia, the abdominal organs move into the chest cavity causing a scaphoid abdomen. A prune belly is caused by inadequate abdominal musculature and is often associated with renal anomalies. Hirschsprung's disease is exhibited by the lack of passage of meconium. A cystic hygroma appears as a mass posterior to the sternocleidomastoid muscle. Situs inversus is a complete reversal of the placement of thoracic and abdominal organs.

12. A. *Pediatrics; Scientific Concepts; Marfan Syndrome*

Marfan syndrome results in tall, lanky individuals who are likely to be very myopic. It is an autosomal dominant disorder.

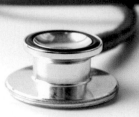

Index

Page numbers followed by *f* indicate figure; those followed by *t* indicate table.